# Dentofacial
# Orthopedics
# with Functional
# Appliances

# Dentofacial Orthopedics with Functional Appliances

Thomas M. Graber, D.M.D., M.S.D., PhD., Odont.Dr., D.Sc., Sc.D., FDSRCS (Eng)

**Clinical Professor, Orthodontics, University of Illinois, College of Dentistry**

Director, Kenilworth Dental Research Foundation; Editor-in-Chief, American Journal of Orthodontics and Dentofacial Orthopedics; Trustee, American Association of Orthodontics; Founder, former Professor and Chairman, Section of Orthodontics and Dentofacial Orthopedics, Pritzker School of Medicine, University of Chicago; formerly, Research Scientist, ADA Research Institute; Author, Researcher, Clinician

Thomas Rakosi, M.D., D.D.S., Ph.D.

**Professor and Head, Emeritus, Orthodontics and Jaw Orthopedics, University of Freiburg, Freiburg, Germany**

Author, Researcher, Lecturer, Clinician

Alexandre G. Petrovic, M.D., D.Sc.

**Professor, Director of Research, Emeritus, National Institute of Health and Medical Research, Louis Pasteur University Medical School, Strasbourg, France**

Director, Laboratory for Craniofacial Cartilage and Bone Growth Regulations (INSERM-U.213), Louis Pasteur University Medical School; formerly, Visiting Professor, Department of Orthodontics, Louisiana State University Medical Center; Researcher, Author, World Wide Lecturer

*with 1630 illustrations*

**Second Edition**

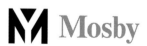

St. Louis  Baltimore  Boston  Carlsbad  Chicago  Naples  New York  Philadelphia  Portland
London  Madrid  Mexico City  Singapore  Sydney  Tokyo  Toronto  Wiesbaden

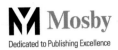

Dedicated to Publishing Excellence

A Times Mirror
Company

Vice President and Publisher: Don Ladig
Editor: Linda L. Duncan
Developmental Editor: Melba Steube
Project Manager: Linda McKinley
Production Editor: Jennifer Furey
Designer: Elizabeth Fett
Manufacturing Manager: Linda Ierardi

Second Edition

**Copyright © 1997 by Mosby–Year Book, Inc.**

Mosby–Year Book, Inc.
11830 Westline Industrial Drive
St. Louis, Missouri 63146

Printed in the United States of America
Composition by Graphic World, Inc.
Lithography by Top Graphics
Printing/binding by Maple-Vail Book Manufacturing Group

**Library of Congress Cataloging in Publication Data**

Graber, T. M. (Thomas M.), 1917-
    Dentofacial orthopedics with functional appliances / T.M. Graber,
Thomas Rakosi, Alexandre G. Petrovic. — 2nd ed.
        p.      cm.
    Includes bibliographical references and index.
    ISBN 0-8151-3558-0 (hardcover)
    1. Orthodontics.   2. Orthodontic appliances.
3. Malocclusion—Treatment.   I. Rakosi, Thomas.
II. Petrovic, Alexandre G.   III. Title.
[DNLM:   1. Orthodontic Appliances, Functional.
    2. Malocclusion—therapy.   3. Orthodontics, Corrective.   WU 426 G728d 1997]
    RK521.G688   1997
    617.6'43—dc21
    DNLM/DLC
for Library of Congress                                                96-49801
                                                                              CIP

97 98 99 00 01 / 9 8 7 6 5 4 3 2 1

# Contributors

Christoph Bourauel, Dr. Rer.nat,
Dipl.Physics
Department of Orthodontics
(Experimental Orthodontics),
University of Bonn,
Bonn, Germany

William J. Clark, B.D.S., D.D.O.,
RCPS (Glas)
Orthodontist and International
Lecturer,
Fife, Scotland

Dieter Drescher, D.M.D., Ph.D.
Head, Department of Orthodontics,
University of Bonn,
Bonn, Germany

Donald H. Enlow, Ph.D.
Professor Emeritus,
Case Western Reserve School of
Dentistry,
Cleveland, Ohio
Whispering Pines, North Carolina

David C. Hamilton, D.D.S., M.S.
President, American Association of
Orthodontics, 1996-1997,
New Castle, Pennsylvania

J. J. Jasper, D.D.S.
Clinical Orthodontist,
Santa Rosa, California

Sten Linder-Aronson, D.D.S.,
Ph.D., Ph.D. (h.c.)
University of Athens
Athens, Greece;
Sun Yat Sen University
Guangzhou, China; Professor Emeritus
Karolinska Institut,
Huddinge, Sweden

James A. McNamara, Jr.
D.D.S., Ph.D.
Professor of Orthodontics and Pediatric
Dentistry,
University of Michigan School of
Dentistry,
Ann Arbor, Michigan

Barry Mollenhauer, M.D.Sc.,
B.D.Sc., L.D.S., FRACDS
Clinical Editor,
Faculty, Emeritus Editor,
*Australian Orthodontic Journal,*
Private Practice
Ivanhoe, Victoria, Australia

Melvin L. Moss, D.D.S., Ph.D.
Professor Emeritus,
Department of Anatomy,
Columbia University School of
Dentistry,
New York, New York

Hans Pancherz, D.D.S.,
Odont. Dr.
Professor and Chair,
Department of Orthodontics,
University of Giessen,
Giessen, Germany

Gottfried P.F. Schmuth,
D.D.S., M.D.
Professor Emeritus,
Kieferorthopädie,
University of Bonn
Bonn, Germany

Jeanne J. Stutzmann,
A.B., M.S. D.Sc.
Research Scientist,
Louis Pasteur Medical School,
Strasbourg, France

Alexander D. Vardimon,
D.M.D., M.S.
Coordinator, International Graduate
Orthodontic Program,
Goldschlager School of Dentistry,
Tel Aviv University,
Tel Aviv, Israel

Donald G. Woodside, D.D.S.,
M.Sc., Ph.D. (h.c.) FRCDC,
FDSRCS (Eng)
Professor, Department of Orthodontics,
Faculty of Dentistry
University of Toronto,
Toronto, Ontario, Canada

To Robert Edison Moyers, *who has been an inspiration to us all. As a pioneer in electromyographic study of the neuromusculature of the stomatognathic system, Dr. Moyers provided scientific validation of functional orthopedic concepts and therapy. Throughout his productive life, he stimulated and inspired countless students and colleagues. Because of Bob Moyers, a champion of applied biology, orthodontics/dentofacial orthopedics stands at the forefront of dentistry today.*

# Preface

The welter of clinical reports in the orthodontic literature and the profusion of short courses being given on so-called functional appliances (often featuring "specialists" from other countries) have engendered great interest in this approach to orthodontic and orthopedic treatment of malocclusion. The popularity and large number of sales of the first edition of this book and of *Removable Orthodontic Appliances* by T.M. Graber are testimony to the enhanced desire to learn more about these appliances on the American side of the Atlantic. Functional jaw orthopedics has been used (and misused) for many years in Europe, ever since it was promulgated by Andresen of Norway. As in America, cultism, dogma, and the arbitrary follow-the-leader approaches have too often dominated the scene. The results have been spotty. There is an old aphorism "It is not the tool but how you use it that counts." This can be rephrased to cover one aspect of the topic at hand: although functional appliances may provide dramatic anecdotal examples of stable and balanced corrections of severe malocclusions, they also may show problems in which only partial correction was achieved or excessive lower incisor proclination was the result. Multiple factors may be responsible.

It is unfortunate that the glowing functional appliance "successes" have been emphasized and oversold by some American proponents. Weekend motel and "tailgate" courses also have been given too often by inadequately trained orthodontists, pediatric dentists, or would-be orthodontists who were interested more in the financial returns from these courses or the ego inflation that goes with standing behind a podium with a captive audience. Glitzy, glossy brochures promise as much as a $100,000 benefit to course attendees. Thus what has become a "hot number" for orthodontists and dentofacial orthopedists has effectively burned more than a few clinicians and patients who have been promised too much.

Despite the admonitions in the previous edition of this book and other books and articles on the subject by superbly qualified leaders such as Rakosi, Fränkel, Eirew, McNamara, Moss, Bimler, Vardimon, Clark, Hamilton, and others, hundreds of clinicians have succumbed to the blandishments of the domestic gurus and used these appliances indiscriminately and in shotgun style on their patients. The inexorable unfavorable patient response from excessive use by inadequately trained orthodontists and unqualified pediatric dentists and general practitioners has produced a wave of frustration and backlash to functional appliances in many quarters.

Yet if the clinician realizes that diagnosis is as demanding for functional orthopedics as it is for conventional fixed appliances, that case selection is critical, that construction bite details can make or break a treatment regimen (no matter how perfectly an appliance is constructed), that it takes time to learn how to manipulate these appliances, that mistakes will be made, that growth direction and growth amount as well as growth timing are major factors in the ultimate success or failure of a treatment regimen, and that patient compliance and motivation demand constant reinforcement after careful patient selection—if all of these are absorbed into the clinician's *modus cogitandi,* they cannot help engendering a warm glow of success and pride in the beautiful results attained on many patients, results not possible from fixed appliances alone. This is not a recommendation for a "one shot" approach, nor does it diminish the importance of fixed appliances as needed.

It is the purpose of this book to present those essential details on the Achilles' heel of functional appliances, or diagnosis, give detailed instructions on how to obtain a correct construction bite, describe fabrication and use of various types of functional appliances alone or in combination, and particularize specific treatment regimens for different malocclusion categories. We hope to be able to offset the antagonism engendered against functional appliances by the mixed experiences of the past 8 to 9 years.

It might appear unseemly that the qualifications of the authors should be extolled. However, this aspect is vitally important if the objectives elaborated in the previous paragraph are to be achieved.

Professor T. M. Graber, currently with the University of Illinois in Chicago, has spent a lifetime practicing, teaching, and writing about various aspects of orthodontics. He has published more books and articles than any other author in orthodontic history. He continues to teach, practice, write, direct research, and guide continuing education programs, as well as serve as editor or editorial advisor for a number of journals. An important facet of his routine is to serve as an educational consultant for institutions around the world. His lifetime of clinical practice has been a blend of fixed and removable appliance techniques that provide biologically oriented optimal service to his patients. His philosophy is simple: "Let the diagnosis dictate the appliances and their use, not vice versa." Working with Alexander Vardimon, now teaching at Tel Aviv University, their research team has explored gross and microscopic aspects of the use of rare earth magnets in orthodontic mechanotherapy.

Thomas Rakosi is Professor Emeritus of one of the finest orthodontic departments in the world at the University of Freiburg in Germany. With an eminent reputation, its orthodontic specialty training program has turned out some of the top clinicians and researchers in Europe, some who head other orthodontic departments. Professor Rakosi has had a rich experience, teaching and practicing early in Czechoslovakia before assuming the professorship at Freiburg. Two outstanding books, *Cephalometric Radiography* and a magnificently colored *Atlas on Orthodontic Diagnosis,* where he is joined by Professors Irmtrud Jonas and T.M. Graber, are translated into several languages and are used throughout the world. He continues to practice what he preaches. This book is a "must" for all dentists.

Professor Emeritus Alexandre Petrovic is former head of what many observers consider has been the top craniofacial growth and development research center in the world. The prolific, innovative, and meticulously clinically oriented basic research emanating from the Louis Pasteur Medical School in Strasbourg has profoundly affected all phases of orthodontics and orthopedics. Petrovic and Jeanne Stutzmann, joined by Claudine Oudet, Nicole Gasson, Jean Lavergne, and others, have produced a multitude of chapters in various books and a profusion of articles in the professional literature of Europe and the United States on the histochemical response of tissues to various appliances, as well as studies of various force values and their effect on craniofacial structures. This book brings together the unique, exciting, and provocative research of the past 20 years and allows the clinician to understand the raison d'être for all orthodontic and orthopedic therapy.

The list of contributing authors is a veritable "Who's Who" of the orthodontic world. Top scientists and clinicians in their own right, their contributions have literally shaped modern concepts of craniofacial growth, development and physiology, and clinical application of current biologically sound mechanotherapy. They are listed alphabetically so as not to do injustice to any of these world-class authorities: Christoph Bourauel, William C. Clark, Dieter Drescher, Donald H. Enlow, David Hamilton, J.J. Jasper, Sten Linder-Aronson, James A. McNamara, Barry Mollenhauer, Melvin L. Moss, Hans Pancherz, Gotfried P.F. Schmuth, Jeanne J. Stutzmann, Alexander D. Vardimon, and Donald G. Woodside.

A generation of orthodontists has been surfeited with two-dimensional cephalometrics. The majority of orthodontic graduate student research projects have been related to cephalometrics in one form or another. Although mensuration is commendable if it means more objectivity, making diagnostic decisions solely on the basis of linear and angular measurements gleaned from a two-dimensional profile radiograph has resulted in overly simplistic solutions to complex biologic problems. It is fair to say that the craniofacial complex, despite the thousands of graduate theses gathering dust on the library shelves, is an imperfectly observed variable.

Diagnosis requires manifold approaches to multisystem involvement. A broader approach to both research and diagnosis is imperative, if we are to advance beyond the "numbers racket" of traditional cephalometrics.

Chapter 1, by an internationally renowned team of T. M. Graber, Melvin L. Moss, Sten Linder-Aronson, and Donald H. Enlow, introduces the reader to the functional matrix hypothesis, the physiologic basis of functional appliances, and the biologic targets in the control of facial growth.

Chapter 2, by Alexandre G. Petrovic and Jeanne J. Stutzmann, is an updated insight into the potential of a cybernetically oriented approach to progress in orthodontics. Via this approach, that mythical "black box" is bound to become smaller. This chapter needs to be read and re-read so that it will input into the reader's own biologic computer the systematic analysis of oral physiology, growth and development, and the effects and counterreactions engendered by orthodontic treatment and the modus operandi of functional appliances.

Chapter 3, by Jeanne J. Stutzmann and Alexandre G. Petrovic, summarizes the most important research that has been done in their laboratory, specifically with regard to condylar growth and direction changes. This chapter alone justifies the existence of this book. Clinical implications and applications abound.

Chapter 4, by Donald G. Woodside, summarizes the many outstanding research projects on functional appliances at the University of Toronto. A number of them have won international recognition.

Chapter 5, by Thomas Rakosi, provides a thorough analysis of conventional functional appliances, so necessary for a full understanding of which appliances to use, when, and how. Not all functional appliances employ the same "functional orthopedic" approach, yet there are common denominators for most of them. Many a clinician would not have had the sad experiences of partial correction or iatrogenic consequences if Chapter 5 had been available and read before they followed the dictums of some of those ballyhooed weekend courses.

Cephalometrics properly used is a valuable diagnostic and treatment adjunct. Based on his recent widely used book on cephalometric analysis and the joint endeavor mentioned above, Professor Rakosi has synthesized the best combination of cephalometric criteria specifically for functional appliance use in Chapter 6. The functional appliance is not the proverbial procrustean bed into which all Class II malocclusions are crammed whether or not they fit. Certain cephalometric measurements, taken together, provide insight into both current morphology and future pattern expression, as well as the likely treatment response. Using the tool properly is the name of the game and Chapter 6 takes the clinician a long way toward that goal.

In Chapter 7, Professor Graber continues the diagnostic and analytical steps necessary before embarking on a therapeutic approach. A functional analysis makes eminently good sense for the use of a functional appliance, and yet, far too many clinicians have neglected this aspect of patient assessment before treatment. The various steps in this assessment are described in a manner permitting immediate clinical application. The role of the temporomandibular joint is explored and clarified. It's not the tool but how you use it!

Chapter 8, on the activator, is the first of a number of chapters on functional appliances per se. Professor Rakosi describes the philosophy, the physiologic justification, and the development of the basic appliance, which is the progenitor of all modern functional appliances. The minutiae of the all-important construction bite, along with the rationale and variances of vertical and horizontal jaw positioning, are detailed for specific cases. Treatment planning, the use of appliances, and problems encountered are all-important aspects to be found in this chapter, which serves as a prerequisite for subsequent activator appliance variations.

In Chapter 9, on the fabrication and management of the activator, Dr. Rakosi illustrates "how to do it." The information is valuable for both the neophyte and experienced clinician as details based on years of experience are elucidated.

Continuing the management aspects of activator use, Chapter 10 discusses the trimming of the acrylic portions of the activator to better guide the teeth into their proper positions after jaw posturing is achieved by the construction bite.

Chapter 11 describes the bionator, originally developed by Balters. It is the most widely used modification of the classical activator. The rationale for changes made in the construction is given in detail. The necessity of full-time wear due to the modifications made is an important part of bionator therapy. Drs. Clark and Hamilton stress this theme again in Chapters 13 and 15.

Chapter 12, by Dr. Graber, is a detailed discussion of the Fränkel appliance. Because of the tremendous exposure and use in the past 15 years, as well as the relatively more demanding aspects of fabrication and dependence on total patient compliance, specific step-by-step details are described and illustrated so that the clinician can avoid the pitfalls commonly encountered by the uninitiated and even the experienced clinician. Great care has been taken to weed out the propaganda, oversell, and overreliance on anecdotal claims. The approach presented is most likely to be successful for the various categories of malocclusion.

Chapter 13, by William J. Clark, on the twin block appliance is state of the art. The author particularizes the justification, construction, and use of this currently most popular "double plate" approach and its superiority in eliciting three-dimensional changes and enhancing patient compliance. Martin Schwarz, who developed the original double plate version, would be very happy indeed with the success of this appliance.

Chapter 14 is a team effort by Alexandre D. Vardimon, Dieter Drescher, Christoph Bourauel, Gottfried P.F. Schmuth, and T.M. Graber on the magnetic functional twin block appliance. The appliance has been developed after extensive National Institutes of Health (NIH) supported research on both laboratory animals and patients. The compilation of patient-tested and modified appliances from the United States, Germany, and Israel emphasizes the international effort. The use of rare earth magnets to enhance the functional aspect and mandibular posturing provides unique enhancement of neuromuscular accommodation.

Chapter 15, by David C. Hamilton, represents the culmination of years of clinical research and constant modification of appliances to achieve the best possible combination to achieve optimal elimination of skeletal problems. The appliance provides three-dimensional control, postural modification, and fixed appliance correction of the dental irregularities. Patient compliance is enhanced by bonding and full-time wear.

Chapter 16, by Professor Hans Pancherz, is the most complete discussion of this extremely efficient fixed functional mechanism for correction of skeletal dysplasias. Modern armamentaria make the fixed mandibular posturing feasible, while still allowing function and concomitant individual tooth movement. Long-term assessments are particularly of interest in assessing ultimate stability.

Chapter 17, by James A. McNamara, J.J. Jasper, and Barry Mollenhauer, is a logical continuation of the previous chapter by Pancherz. Based on the Jasper jumper, which is a modification of the Herbst appliance, dramatic results illustrate the potential for maxillomandibular basal control. The first part of the chapter is by McNamara and Jasper on routine use. The second part by Barry Mollenhauer discusses use in asymmetric situations.

Chapter 18, by Graber, shows the potential for melding European functional appliances with American extraoral force control for optimal sagittal and vertical control of the dentofacial structures. It is generally agreed that the primary effect of functional appliances is on the mandible. With the incorporation of extraoral force, maxillary retraction and depressive forces are possible with this combination. With bonded functional appliances, headgear use is even more effective.

Chapters 19 through 22, by Rakosi, describe and illustrate actual treatment of basal Class II, Class III, and open-bite malocclusions. These chapters are likely to be of greatest interest to the practicing orthodontist, because of the fine clinical orientation, based on a lifetime of experience with a variety of functional appliances by this eminent leader. They are unequaled in the literature. Together with Rakosi, Jonas, and Graber's colored *Atlas on Orthodontic Diagnosis,* these chapters could make a chairside manual and bible for modern day functional orthopedists and applied biologists.

Clearly, despite their misuse because of inadequate doctrination, oversell, inadequate attention to treatment details, and unwillingness to combine fixed and removable appliances for the highest degree of correction, the future is bright—provided that clinicians are willing to apply themselves assiduously to the principles and techniques expounded in this text. No book can be all things to all people. The sheer enormity of developing information makes it impossible for a single- or multiple-volume text to present all the research validation and clinical experience. It is our opinion that we can achieve results with less pain, less effort, less expense, more routinely, and with less iatrogenic potential. Proliferating managed care programs are likely to hasten more widespread use of these biologically oriented appliances.

For those who read this book, the dedication of all who had a hand in its production and the successful blending of efforts will be obvious.

T.M. Graber

# Contents

# Prologue

The emphasis of orthodontics has undergone a major shift in the past 25 years. We now recognize that a face-conscious society needs more than merely movement of the molars and the teeth in front of them to achieve optimal results. Part of this has been the realization that we are dealing with a multisystem environment in which the osseous and neuromuscular components are just as important in the overall picture as the dental structures. Lischer called attention to this obvious interrelationship as early as 1912, but the real impact did not sink in until functional appliances that could produce major three-dimensional changes were developed. Research on both primates and human patients substantiated the claims of the earlier users, and orthognathic surgery produced dramatic improvements that heretofore were not possible with conventional appliances. The public and the profession came to expect more than "straight teeth."

The speciality of orthodontics itself has made a fundamental change in direction and treatment emphasis with the greater stress on orthopedic goals and the changing of the specialty to *Dentofacial Orthopedics*. Nevertheless, the traditional, cultist, tooth-moving systems persist as dominant means of mechanotherapy. Realization that the teeth can literally be used as a handle to manipulate facial changes and changes in the neuromuscular and osseous supporting and motivating structures has been slow in some quarters and nonexistent in others. The lip service paid to growth and development has been replaced by convincing research validation that age-oriented therapy (i.e., early treatment) is vital. If we are to make the stable and dramatic three-dimensional alterations desired in the dentofacial complex, hard facts, clinical experience, and long-term records indicate that early growth guidance is essential. The importance of growth guidance is evident from a perusal of this book by the world's outstanding authorities.

Do dentistry and the orthodontic specialty realize that growth guidance and fundamental basal structural changes are essential for treatment of sagittal dysplasias? Is mixed dentition treatment really worthwhile to our patients? Even today, the literature is ambivalent.

We need a fuller appreciation of what the orthodontic specialty really thinks in this changing world of managed care–driven medical and dental services in which nonspecialists are demanding and taking over a larger share of orthodontic care that has heretofore been the province of the properly trained specialist. To this end, David Hamilton, President of the American Association of Orthodontists and long-time leader in functional appliance use, developed an extensive survey of some 54 questions that was completed by a sample of 90 randomly selected orthodontists out of residency at least 5 years, 100 personally selected orthodontists regarded as leaders by virtue of publications and clinical reputation, 59 department chairpersons, 59 senior residents selected by each chairperson, and 12 biologists familiar with facial growth.

The changing face of orthodontics is evident from a summary perusal of the results. Space limitations do not allow a full report of the study, which is available elsewhere.* However, salient points make a fitting prelude to this volume's multiauthored theme that functional appliances must be an integral part of the armamentaria of modern orthodontics.

The survey was constructed with five levels of response possible, ranging from strong disagreement to strong agreement. After a series of 14 general questions, maxillary, mandibular, vertical, transverse, and asymmetric growth modification statements were postulated. Statements on age of growth modification and etiologic and functional considerations completed the series.

As Hamilton says, "Orthodontists are an interesting, complex egocentric, 'almost' omniscient, quality oriented and stubborn group." Again, there is one caveat: "Opinion polls are just that. It should be noted that the fact that a significant number of orthodontists agree or disagree with any premise does not substantiate that their opinion is correct."

In answer to the first postulate that it is possible to determine with a fair degree of reliability that a 3- to 4-year-old child has a severe facial/skeletal dysplasia, 77% strongly or moderately agree, whereas only 13% disagree. Within the sample, believed that child's facial pattern could be predicted by viewing their parents, but 39% questioned the reliability of such a judgment. This latter group included one third of the department chairpersons.

The survey produced the following findings:

- Regarding the practitioner's ability to alter the skeletal pattern of a growing child, 85% agree and 7% disagree.
- Of the survey participants, 74% support the thesis that the earlier the correction of the skeletal problem, the greater the chances of success and stability; 11% disagree.
- Pliancy of sutures correlated positively with early age (95%). However, the high support does not necessarily translate into shortened treatment time for younger patients in the survey answers. The majority of respondents were ambiguous, with 76% replying in the middle three neutral responses.
- Only 25% of the respondents felt that our European colleagues were more advanced in growth guidance, whereas 46% disagreed and 28% were neutral; 64% of department chairpersons disagreed and 24% agreed.

*Hamilton D: *Keynote address,* Edward H. Angle Society, October 1995.

- A trend toward earlier orthodontics was predicted by 67%, with a similar number of department chairpersons agreeing, but there is little evidence of actually selecting cases for residents in this category. Of the respondents, 76% felt that patients between 3 and 6 years were good candidates for maxillary protraction appliances, but few actually treat patients in this age range. More education of referring dentists and the public is clearly needed in this area. Finally, the survey indicated that 86% felt facial growth guidance research should be prioritized.

In this era of managed care and nonspecialist treatment and inroads by pediatric dentists and general practitioners, 72% of the respondents still felt that growth guidance would help reduce this invasion because of the greater diagnostic and therapeutic demands on the practitioner. Of some significance is the fact that two thirds of the sample felt that research done on traditional permanent dentition cases should not be applied to growth guidance cases in the mixed dentition period. Equally significant, 71% agreed that problems of patient compliance constitute a chief deterrent to the successful use of removable orthopedic appliances. That this now can be handled by modern, bonded and cemented, 24-hour, truly functional appliances is evident from chapters in this book by McNamara, Mollenhauer, Pancherz, and Hamilton.

The survey sample showed wide disagreement on whether extraoral force could be substituted for functional appliances. Differential diagnosis is the key here and is discussed in a number of chapters in this book. Answers were equivocal on whether functional appliances had any inhibiting influence on the maxilla—but then, so is some of the research.

In the mandibular growth–modification series of statements the majority of respondents felt that differential diagnosis could determine the difference between true and pseudo Class III malocclusions. Little support was found for influencing true Class III problems.

Of the respondents, 78% supported the premise that a simple biteplate may act as an effective functional appliance in growing patients. Only 6% disagreed. Hamilton and McNamara both interpret this as support for the concept that maxillary constriction could produce mandibular entrapment and at the very least prevent optimal accomplishment of mandibular sagittal growth.

Hamilton felt that one of the most important concepts in the survey was the idea that alteration of the functional matrix could affect growth. Within the survey sample, 60% agreed, 34% took a neutral position, and only 6% disagreed. Only 21% felt that mandibular growth could be stimulated beyond its natural potential.

Despite all the morphologic, histologic, and radiographic evidence, only 59% of respondents felt that the condylar heads of the mandible could be remodeled. In addition, 28% were neutral and 12% disagreed. The biologists all concurred, however. Similar figures support remodeling of the glenoid fossa. In support of both, the chapters by Petrovic and Stutzmann, Woodside, Rakosi, and others provide convincing evidence.

For vertical dimension changes, use of high-pull headgear was accepted as a legitimate modality for intrusion of posterior teeth, but magnets had no support among the survey sample. The majority (69%) accepted forced eruption of posterior teeth to increase the vertical dimension.

Hamilton feels that the transverse dimension has been neglected too much because of orthodontic obsession with the lateral cephalogram. Do survey figures bear him out? Apparently not, as maxillary expansion was clearly the most widely accepted regimen (96%). Sutural expansion had support from 83% of the sample as a stable means of transverse modification; 81% also supported dental expansion. However, over half felt that beyond a certain age, sutural expansion is inappropriate. Only 74% supported dental expansion in the mandible, with 21% not agreeing that this is a viable modality. In addition, 90% supported the view that many transverse asymmetries are caused by maxillary constriction and convenience deviation of the mandible on closing. The longer we wait for correction, the less likelihood of success. Chapter 15 by Hamilton addresses this topic well.

The survey found that 98% of orthodontists felt severe dysplasias should be seen before 8 years of age; 61% lowered this to under 6 years, although few would institute treatment at this time. This is in contrast to the support for early treatment for mandibular prognathism.

In the final series of questions on etiology, 85% supported airway problems as one factor. However, 80% disagreed with the premise that functional treatment posed any risk in growing children. Approximately two thirds support the concept that airway control favorably affects the transverse dimension. Of the respondents, 91% supported prolonged thumb or finger sucking and dummy sucking, and 69% supported tongue thrust and posture as potential etiologic factors. Contrary to claims by contingency fee lawyers, 80% saw no causative relationship between functional appliances and temporomandibular dysfunction.

It should be emphasized again that this is only an opinion poll, not a scientific study. This type of survey is considered flawed because it uses vague or unequal quantifiers. Should a 10-point scale be used? Since this was not a truly random study, how much reliance can be placed on the opinions? In defense of the conclusions reported, it is the best assessment of specialty opinion of growth guidance and orthopedic appliances we have so far. Clearly, as this book attempts to show, the increasing body of research and clinical evidence has produced a serious consideration of growth guidance at an earlier age than time-honored tooth-moving mechanisms. Managed care trends only enhance the potential for this multisystem treatment regimen. Orthodontics no longer means only "straight teeth" (from the Greek words *ortho* and *dons*). Basal structural and neuromuscular considerations have made the term *Dentofacial Orthopedics* more appropriate for what the orthodontist does as we enter the new millennium.

# Part One

## Scientific Concepts and Validation of Functional Appliances

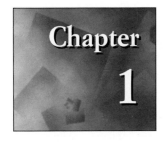

# Chapter 1 — Introduction

T.M. Graber

Melvin L. Moss

Sten Linder-Aronson

Donald H. Enlow

## EARLY TREATMENT

The past 20 years have seen an increasing awareness of the potential of functional appliances as valuable tools in the armamentaria of orthodontists. They are not the only tools any more than fixed edgewise brackets are able to answer all therapeutic demands in orthodontics, but they are important weapons in the arsenal and can accomplish results not possible without such appliances. An increasing recognition of the interrelationship of form and function, the realization that neuromuscular involvement is vital in treatment, the recognition of the importance of the airway in therapeutic considerations, and a growing understanding of head posture and the accomplishment of dentofacial pattern changes are all factors producing rapid growth in the use of functional appliances. Clinicians should seriously consider any mechanisms capable of influencing these factors favorably.

Certainly, abnormal and adaptive neuromuscular function can hinder the accomplishment of an optimal dentofacial pattern. However, the same forces created under control can be used to eliminate morphologic aberrations resulting from abnormal lip trap habits, tongue posture and function, and finger habits that have produced deviations from the normal growth and development of the stomatognathic system.

One early article in American orthodontic literature, "The 'Three Ms': Muscles, Malformation and Malocclusion," by Graber (1963) described the effects of function and malfunction to a mechanistically oriented profession that was at that time treating patients according to numbers gleaned from two-dimensional cephalograms. These numbers corresponded to predetermined norms based on ideal relationships established by lateral head films.

European orthodontists have long been aware of the role of perioral musculature in orthodontic problems. They also recognize the potential use of deforming forces to eliminate these problems. The Andresen activator, for instance, was designed to achieve the results its name implied—activate normal function while eliminating the spatial and morphologic malrelationships exacerbating the malocclusion. Although European orthodontists may have overemphasized the possibilities of functional appliances, this does not detract from their value any more than the American overreliance on fixed appliances placed in permanent dentition negates the corrective possibilities of these devices. Clearly, a perspective that transcends the relied-upon tools of the trade is needed. Arbitrary distinctions are unacceptable in a biologic continuum.

Half of all malocclusions treated in the United States are probably in the Class II category. This does not mean that the same percentage of these malocclusions occurs in society as a whole but only that the practice load is so constituted. The preponderance of Class II malocclusions seen in orthodontic practice is partly a result of public awareness of aberrant physiognomic characteristics associated with malocclusion, transient developmental attributes in mixed dentition (when large central incisors erupt and appear too big for the face), and education of the public by concerned dental practitioners.

Too often Class II malocclusions have been treated with extraoral force directed against the maxilla and with maxillary expansion (alone or with extreme force). However, abundant research shows that much of the problem lies in the mandible, which is underdeveloped, possibly retropositioned, or both. Although maxillary incisor procumbency is usually present locally, the sagittal basal malrelationship is the greater part of the problem. Unfortunately, many practitioners have largely ignored this condition and aimed their therapeutic resources at the relatively normal maxilla instead of the abnormal mandible. In using Class II elastics to augment extraoral force, orthodontists often slide the mandibular dentition forward on the deficient base or procline the lower incisors in a localized attempt to correct the anteroposterior malrelationship. Functional appliances, on the other hand, correct the localized maxillary incisor spacing and protrusion while directing their primary efforts toward the mandible, thus eliminating the deforming neuromuscular adaptive function. Functional appliances effect this change in the critical growth period, which is characterized by mixed and transitional dentition. Many articles in the literature show that dramatic results are possible. Careful research provides ample evidence of the potential of such treatment in properly chosen cases, with properly selected appliances, proper patient control, and maximal patient compliance.

3

Cephalometric and study cast measurements show clear evidence of significant expansion and sagittal correction that do not seem possible with conventional fixed appliances. Part of this is the result of treatment timing, occurring as the succedaneous teeth vie for space and optimal growth direction in the changing, expanding alveolar bony shell. Research evidence also indicates that functional appliances if used properly have less adverse iatrogenic potential and produce less root resorption, decalcification, gingival proliferation, temporomandibular dysfunctions (TMDs), and sheared alveolar crests than do fixed appliances. These advantages apply to removable appliances in general and functional appliances in particular. Although the efficacy of functional appliances does not obviate the need for fixed appliances, functional appliances may be used to reduce the time of wear of potentially compromising fixed devices in severe basal malrelationship Class II cases requiring protracted extraoral force and wear of Class II elastics. Functional appliances are not the answer to all the problems of orthodontic patients but perhaps are the best answer for problems resulting from a certain set of basal-neuromuscular attributes occurring in patients' developmental patterns. Fixed appliances to produce correct inclination, alignment, rotation, parallel roots, and torque are as important as ever, but only in their place and at the proper time. Limiting fixed appliances to the objectives they can best accomplish reduces the magnitude of correctional challenges as well as the time needed for treatment and the potential adverse iatrogenic response produced.

Another positive aspect of early treatment is that it can intercept a developing malocclusion at a time when the maxillary incisors are more vulnerable to fracture and loss. Protecting these teeth with functional appliances eliminates functional aberrations, trains the perioral musculature to assist in optimal dentofacial development, and helps the mandible, through spatial posturing achieved with a properly taken construction bite, to attain the most favorable growth increments and direction. It also helps eliminate increasing arch-length deficiencies by establishing a normal, functional matrix and functional spaces. Proffit (1995) has shown that many abnormal muscle patterns (particularly those involving the tongue) disappear in later life; functional appliance therapy accelerates this trend to normality at a critical time.

The apparent simplicity of functional appliances does not mean any less diagnostic acuity is required for their use. If anything, they demand more attention to the patient and the cephalogram, as well as to functional analysis, growth projection, and assessment of behavioral patterns, motivational potential, long-range treatment goals, future mechanotherapeutic considerations, and study cast measurements. Enlow's book *The Human Face* is essential preparatory material for anyone using functional appliances. It emphasizes biologic factors in controlling the process of facial growth.

Because of the claims and counterclaims made about functional appliances and the proliferation of their use by poorly trained or nontrained practitioners, a discussion of the basic physiologic aspects of these appliances is urgently needed. Even in Europe, considerable controversy exists concerning the effects of these appliances. Their effects on condylar growth, the role of different magnitudes of sagittal and vertical posturing, the efficacy of daytime versus nighttime or all-the-time wear, the results of working with the conventional activator from within the dental arch instead of from the vestibular area, and the determination of different times for beginning treatment all evoke differing answers from clinicians.

Practitioners must therefore direct their efforts to finding common denominators of functional appliance treatment and determining rules that apply to all appliances and the biologic, biomechanic, and physiologic aspects of their use. Then, with a proper perspective, proper diagnosis, and reasonable expectations, American orthodontists can make the best use of the functional jaw orthopedics approach. Using this treatment in conjunction with fixed appliances and extraoral force, they can produce the best possible results for patients, with less possibility of problems and greater long-term stability, a stability depending on the balance of teeth, bone, and muscle attained during treatment and not on an artificial retaining splint that must be worn indefinitely (or until the third molars start erupting and provide the orthodontist with a convenient alibi for the inevitable relapse).

## THE FUNCTIONAL MATRIX HYPOTHESIS AND EPIGENETICS

A discussion of the regulation of craniofacial growth seems an appropriate place to outline the conceptual milieu within which the functional matrix hypothesis originated and exists. The hypothesis derives from the century-old work of His and Roux and is compatible with recent epigenetic concepts associated with Waddington, Blechschmidt, and Lovtrup. The functional matrix hypothesis serves as a conceptual bridge between the concepts of function and epigenesis.

The functional matrix hypothesis claims that the origin, growth, and maintenance of skeletal tissues and organs are always secondary, compensatory, and mechanically obligatory responses to temporally and operationally prior events and processes occurring in related nonskeletal tissues, organs, and functioning spaces (e.g., in functional matrices, either periosteal or capsular). Unless explicitly stated otherwise, the assumption of the theory is that endocrinologic, nutritional, and all other internal and external (environmental) parameters are within normal ranges.

This hypothesis may be considered a modern restatement of the central position of His, who in 1874 enunciated the doctrine of the "physiology of the plastic," indicating that biologic structure was alterable and could be intentionally changed. Roux and Driesch discussed the hypothesis at the turn of the century using the term *Entwicklungsmechanik* (developmental mechanism); their principal theme was that both normal and abnormal development is capable of experimental study and subsequent analysis and description as a series of temporally and operationally sequential events. Each event or process can be shown to be productive of or followed by specific morphologic and functional results. In this view, *development* can be described as the result of a hierarchic series of proximate, efficient, extrinsic, and necessary causes. The extremely active field of experimental embryology is derived from this concept.

Such efficiently causal events and processes are similar to those currently termed *epigenetic*. This term may be used generally to describe the sum of all biomechanic, bioelectrical, biochemical, and biophysical parameters, (intracellularly, intercellularly, and extracellularly) produced by the functioning of cells, tissues, organs and organisms. These epigenetic factors serve as an internal environment and must be considered in addition to the classical external environment of genetics. Epigenetic factors are thought to act on the products of the genome to regulate all developmental processes leading to the production, increase, and maintenance of biologic structural complexity. These epigenetic factors provide feedback regulation of the genome.

The implications of this hypothesis are considerable. The functional matrix hypothesis denies that the genome of skeletogenic cells itself contains sufficient information to regulate the type, site, rate, direction, and duration of skeletal tissue growth. Hypotheses that assert the primacy of the genome are perceived as subscribing to a modern form of preformationism. Attributing all structural information to combinations of the genetic code is a type of reductionism that contains its own falsification. A rigorous reduction would not stop at the complex structures of the codons but seek the basis for developmental information at the subatomic level of charms and quarks. The rejection of this type of extreme neodarwinism is based on data drawn from many fields and reviewed extensively elsewhere.

To be sure, the modern epigeneticist accepts both the data and fundamental concepts of modern molecular biology, derived chiefly from studies of *Escherichia coli*. What is denied, however, is the view that the diploid genome at the moment of fertilization contains all the information necessary to regulate skeletal size, shape, and location—a blueprint merely requiring a permissive environment in which to express itself. Instead, epigenetics views the genome as providing a set of formal, prior, intrinsic, and necessary causal factors that, when combined with the efficient, proximate, extrinsic, and necessary epigenetic causal factors, together are sufficient to account for the regulation of development. No essential conflict exists between the genomic and epigenetic hypotheses except in the minds of those unwilling to engage in semantic clarification to draw distinctions among the types of causation.

A further explication of the epigenetic hypothesis and a conclusion with some possible clinical implications may be helpful. Within the hypothesis, development is considered a continuum of efficiently causally related events from the fertilization of the ovum onward. For example, in the two-celled stage the epigenetic parameters differ significantly between mutually opposed cell surfaces and those lying freely exposed; these differences significantly regulate the next developmental event and so on in an ever more specific series of interactions, a cascade of ontogenesis. As biologic structure and order (negentropy) is accumulating in a vital system, this structural order regulates successive developmental processes and also may regulate the genome. For example, Hall has shown that

when motion is produced between two normally nonmobile membrane bones, secondary cartilage is produced and maintained as long as motion (the epigenetic stimulus) is continued; the cartilage disappears and is replaced by bone when the motion ceases. Indeed, much orthopedic therapy on the postcranial skeleton is based on an analogous epigenetic interpretation of the regulatory role of what may be termed *functional matrices,* a therapeutic concept that received classical expression as Wolff's law. To the extent that any therapeutic modality can alter (within appropriate homeostatic limits) the epigenetic milieu of the craniofacial skeleton, practitioners may expect an appropriate response by the skeleton. However, such factors as the type of stimulus and its strength, duration, rate, period of application, and direction are presently unknown for any proposed prosthetic functional matrix and are at best only empirically estimated. Such ignorance, however, should not preclude a search for these factors and a determination of the quantitative and qualitative aspects of their parameters. A substantial body of clinical and experimental data suggests strongly that the understanding and application of such epigenetic stimuli are potentially useful.

## THE PHYSIOLOGIC BASIS OF FUNCTIONAL APPLIANCES: THE ROLE OF RESPIRATION

In discussing the physiologic basis of functional appliances, a consideration of respiratory function is important. The size and shape of the nasopharyngeal space must be adequate for functional demands. Opinions regarding the mode of respiration and its effect on dentition and facial morphology have usually been based on an association found between the mode of breathing and anteroposterior jaw relations. However, much interest has recently been directed to the relationship between breathing patterns and the vertical development of the face. This section of the chapter concentrates on Linder-Aronson's findings concerning the relationship between respiratory function and vertical development of the face and dentition.

In his first study on this subject in 1960, Linder-Aronson found that mouth breathing was associated with crowding of narrow upper jaws in patients with long, narrow faces. At that time these findings were explained as being secondary to facial morphology. In a second study on adenoidectomies performed in 1970 on 81 children with nasal obstruction problems, a comparison of mouth breathers was made with an equal number of nose breathers of similar gender and age (Figure 1-1). Children with obstructed nasal breathing were characterized by increases in both lower and total facial heights. The greatest difference between the two groups was in the vertical development of the face and not in anteroposterior jaw relations. However, the differences between the two groups could be the result of differences in morphogenetic type.

An intraindividual follow-up study was then carried out. The facial heights of the children in both groups were compared initially and then 1 and 5 years postoperatively. Because adenoidectomies had been performed on the children in the

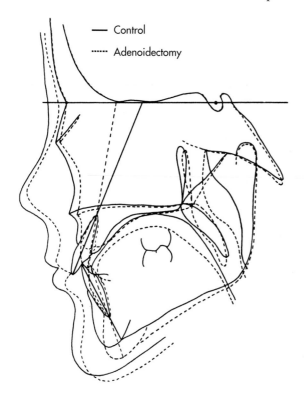

**Figure 1-1.** Tracings of lateral cephalometric radiographs showing significant differences between children who are mouth breathers (*dotted lines*) and nose breathers (*solid lines*).

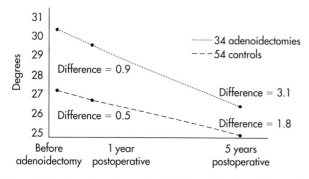

**Figure 1-2.** Angular changes in children with adenoidectomies and in controls between mandibular lines (ML) and nasal lines (NL) preoperative and 1 year and 5 years postoperative.

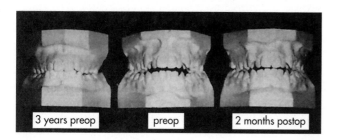

**Figure 1-3.** Casts at 10 years of age (before nasal obstruction problems), at 13 years of age (with nasal obstruction problems occurring during the 3 intervening years), and at 13 years of age (2 months after adenoidectomy with no subsequent nasal obstruction).

**TABLE 1-1. • STEPWISE REGRESSION ANALYSIS—REGRESS AND ANGLE BETWEEN MANDIBULAR AND NASAL LINES**

| Regressor | t Value | Partial Correlation |
|---|---|---|
| Constant | 5.24 | — |
| Preoperative airflow | −2.57* | −0.20 |
| Nasal line | −3.51† | −0.27 |
| Height of upper lip | 3.69† | 0.28 |
| Height of lower lip | 4.10† | 0.31 |
| ^SS-N-SM‡ | 4.99† | 0.37 |
| ^SS-N-BA§ | −4.20† | −0.31 |

$r_2$ (coefficient determinant) = 0.45.

\* = < 0.05.

† = < 0.001.

‡ ANB angle, Bjørk measurement.

§ ANBA angle, Bjørk measurement.

nasal obstruction group, the mode of breathing changed from mouth breathing to nose breathing. This change was recorded 1 month after adenoidectomy and remained unchanged during the 5-year observation period.

Figure 1-2 illustrates the way the angle between the mandibular line (ML) and nasal line (NL) changed after a change in mode of breathing. The actual difference during the first year was 0.4 degrees, which was not significant. However, during the 5-year postoperative observation period a greater change in the ML/NL angle (significant at the 0.01 level) occurred in the adenoidectomy group compared with the control group. A process of normalization appears to have taken place throughout the observation period. Therefore the size of the ML/NL angle, if influenced by the mode of breathing, can probably decrease after a change from mouth to nose breathing and come closer to normal values.

The size of the ML/NL angle also is related to changes in lower facial height. A correlation analysis between reductions in the ML/NL angle and changes in lower facial height was found to be significant at the 0.01 level.

Figure 1-3 shows the dentition of a girl who had nasal obstruction problems between 10 and 13 years of age. During this period an open-bite malocclusion developed. In the 2 months after adenoidectomy and a change in the mode of breathing from mouth to nose, the open bite decreased by 1.5 mm. After adenoidectomy a normalization of the posture of the mandible seems to have occurred.

Stepwise regression analysis reveals that reduced nasal airflow to some extent explains the size of the ML/NL angle (Table 1-1). In this form of regression analysis the ML/NL angle is the dependent variable and the airflow through the nose is one of the explanatory variables. The negative sign indicates that nasal airflow is reduced in patients with large ML/NL angles. These findings have been supported by Vig et al (1980), who found higher nasal resistance in a group of children with increased vertical facial heights.

Reduced nasal airflow that encourages mouth breathing is caused by frequent respiratory infections, nasal septum deviations, or narrow maxillary arches. All these factors can con-

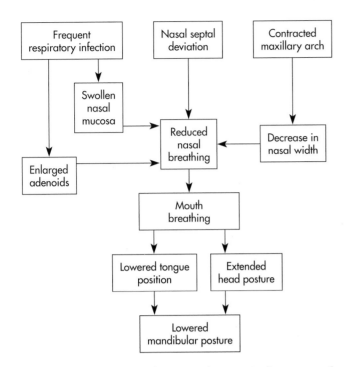

Figure 1-4. Factors contributing to alteration in the posture of the mandible.

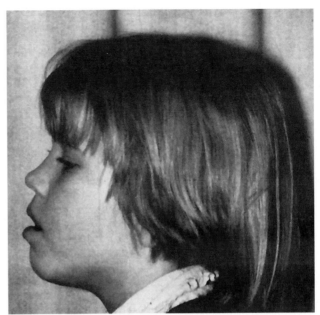

Figure 1-5. Extended head posture to maintain patent airway.

tribute to alterations in the postural position of the mandible (Figure 1-4). However, to what extent mouth breathers unconsciously maintain an extended or upwardly rotated head position to improve the oropharyngeal airway has become a question of great interest (Figure 1-5).

The head postures of 16 patients who had undergone adenoidectomy to improve nasal airflow were studied to examine this question. They were compared with the same number of control subjects of similar age and gender. The inclination of the sella-nasion (S-N) line was measured relative to a vertical reference line included in the lateral skull radiographs (Figure 1-6). The S-N/vertical angle decreased in patients with extended head postures. Measurements were made before and 1 month after surgery.

In spite of the small number of cases examined, a significant difference in the size of the S-N/vertical angle was found when the two groups were compared before surgery (Figure 1-7). This difference could not be found 1 month after adenoidectomy (Figure 1-8). Solow and Greve (1979) carried out a similar study independently in 1979 and got the same results concerning head posture before and after adenoidectomy.

Figures 1-9 and 1-10 illustrate the S-N/vertical angle for mouth breathers and controls relative to lower and upper facial heights, respectively. Norms for facial height were taken from Canadian population standards. Most of the mouth breathers have small S-N/vertical angles and large lower facial heights in comparison with the controls.

Thus a significant increase in the lower facial height but no significant change in the upper facial height occurs among mouth breathers. The head postures of patients with obstructed nose breathing seem to be somewhat more extended; this can influence the position of the mandible.

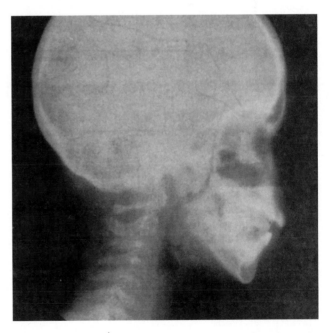

Figure 1-6. Vertical reference line included in lateral skull radiograph.

Linder-Aronson's hypothesis is that extended head posture stretches the soft tissues, leading to a retrusive and downward force generated against the facial complex (Figure 1-11). Nasal airway maintenance therefore dictates the postural performance of the muscular barrier formed by the soft palate and tongue. As suggested by Bosma, the necessity of airway maintenance also is reflected in all mechanisms affecting head and neck posture.

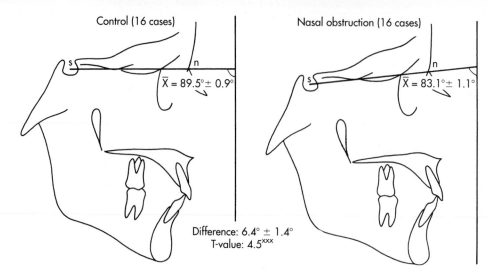

**Figure 1-7.** Values for the S-N/vertical angle before adenoidectomy.

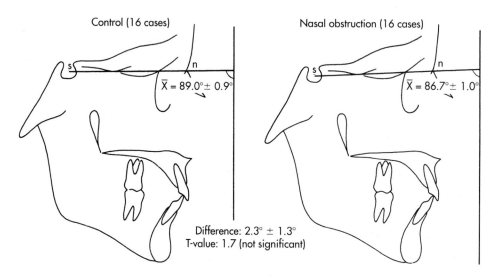

**Figure 1-8.** Values for the S-N/vertical angle 1 month after adenoidectomy.

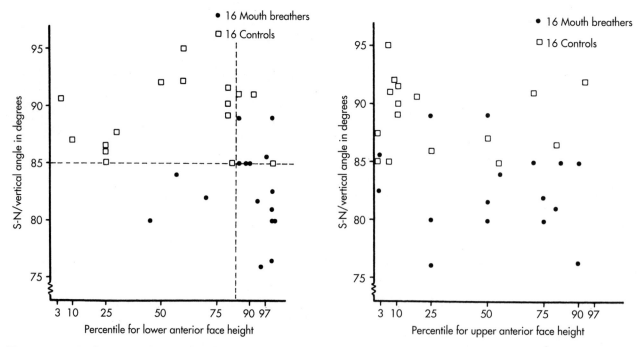

**Figure 1-9.** Head postures of mouth breathers and controls relative to lower facial heights. The subjects were Swedish children.

**Figure 1-10.** Head postures of mouth breathers and controls relative to upper facial heights. The subjects were Swedish children.

In 1974, Bushey studied a pair of monozygotic twins who were 8 years and 11 months old with different anterior facial heights and tongue postures (Figure 1-12). One of the twins had difficulty with nose breathing for several years. His anterior facial height was higher than that of the child without nose breathing problems.

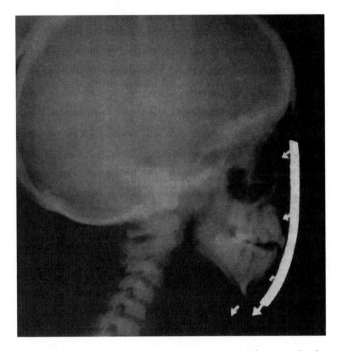

**Figure 1-11.** Soft tissue stretching and retrusive force on the facial complex resulting from extended head posture.

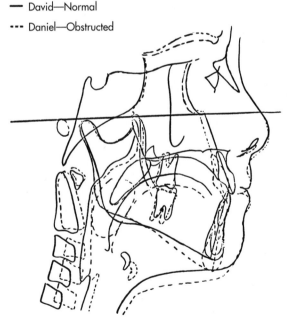

**Figure 1-12.** Superimposed cephalometric tracings showing differences in the facial morphologies of monozygotic twins, one of whom had obstructed nose-breathing capacity.

(Bushey R: personal communication, July 1996.)

As early as the turn of the century, Case (1894) asserted that in cases of open-bite malocclusion caused by continued mouth breathing during the years of childhood development, the mandible is pulled down and held open by the hyoid muscles attached beneath the chin. This force is principally opposed by the lifting actions of the masseter and internal pterygoid muscles near the angle between the mandibular ramus and corpus. This explanation for increased anterior facial height among mouth breathers may still be valid. Obstructed nose breathing with a subsequent switch to mouth breathing has been shown in several investigations to lead to a lowered posture of the tongue and hyoid bone.

Statements regarding a lowered position of the tongue and mandible usually imply the lowering is in relation to the cranial base/maxillary complex. The same findings also may be described as a raised cranial base/maxillary position relative to the tongue and mandible.

The distinction between the descriptions of this postural relationship is important. The neuromuscular patterns of activity are not the same when the head is tilted up relative to a stable linguomandibulocervical complex as they are when the tongue and mandible are lowered relative to a stable craniocervical complex. Davies (1979) has studied this phenomenon electromyographically.

The change from open to closed lip function after normalization from mouth to nose breathing establishes proper physiologic conditions in the orofacial area. If the anterior oral seal is incompetent, the pressure conditions are beyond the physiologic range in both the oral and nasopharyngeal spaces. The changed function in the orbicularis oris and its surrounding muscles when the lip posture is switched from open to closed also may affect the vertical development of the face and dentition, as has been shown by Fränkel (1980b). The postural performance of those muscles in their provision of the anterior oral seal is of great importance in functional analysis and therapy.

In a study by Woodside and Linder-Aronson (1979), normal percentile population standards were calculated for upper and lower anterior face heights in males from a previous study sample. A subgroup of 22 males showed distance curves for lower anterior face height that followed the 90th or 97th population standard curve or ascended from a lower percentile to a higher percentile between the ages of 6 and 20 years. They were analyzed separately and their airways through the nasopharynx and nose were assessed from lateral and anteroposterior cephalograms.

In cases with high or increasing percentiles for lower anterior face height (Figure 1-13), the following questions were asked:

1. Is airway obstruction in either the nasopharynx or nasal cavity associated with a large lower anterior facial height relative to upper facial height?
2. Is airway obstruction in either the nasopharynx or nasal cavity associated with an increasing lower anterior face height?
3. Is airway obstruction in either the nasopharynx or nasal cavity associated with an open-bite tendency?

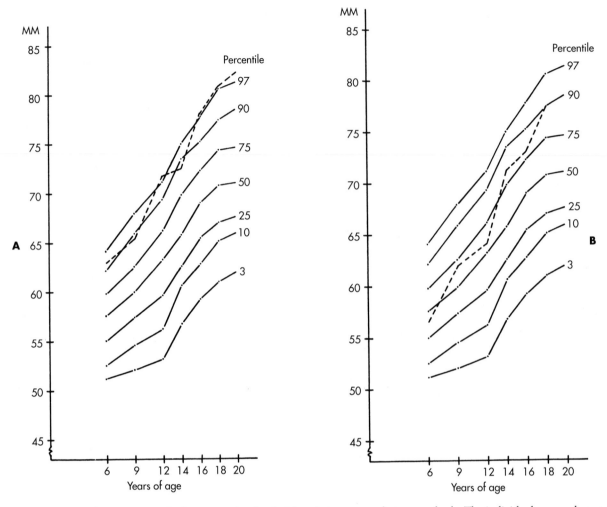

**Figure 1-13.** Serial distance curves for lower anterior face height relative to population standards. The individual curves do not channelize. **A,** Curve ascends from the 90th percentile to above the 97th percentile. **B,** Curve ascends from the 25th percentile to the 90th percentile.

**TABLE 1-2. • NUMBER AND PERCENTAGE OF ANSWERS TO THREE QUESTIONS ON AIR OBSTRUCTION FOR 22 MALES WITH HIGH OR INCREASING PERCENTILES FOR LOWER ANTERIOR FACE HEIGHT**

| | Answer: Yes | | Answer: No | | Differential Answer |
| Question | Number | Percentage | Number | Percentage | Yes-No t Value |
|---|---|---|---|---|---|
| 1 | 13 | 59.1 ± 10.5 | 9 | 40.9 ± 10.5 | 1.22 NS |
| 2 | 16 | 72.7 ± 9.5 | 6 | 27.3 ± 9.5 | 3.38* |
| 3 | 14 | 63.6 ± 10.3 | 8 | 36.4 ± 10.3 | 1.86 NS |

*NS,* Not significant.
* < 0.01.

The answers to these questions for the 22 males in the study with high or increasing percentiles for lower anterior face height are shown in Table 1-2. The response to question 1 reveals that this study was unable to establish a relationship between a consistently large lower anterior face height relative

to upper anterior facial height and airway obstruction between the ages of 6 and 20 years.

Neither could airway obstruction be related to an openbite tendency (question 3). A significant difference at the 1% level for question 2 shows, however, that airway obstruction can to a certain extent explain the reason the distance curve for the lower anterior face height progressively ascended from a lower to a higher percentile between the ages of 6 and 20 years in 16 of the 22 males.

Therefore, diagnostically, much emphasis should be placed on respiratory function. The results presented here clearly support the theory that disturbed nasal respiration may affect facial morphology.

These study findings seem to lend support to the concept that some facial characteristics previously thought to be strictly governed by genetic factors may also be products of environmental influences. This statement, however, does not imply that certain environmental conditions are necessary prerequisites for excessive lower anterior face heights. The mode of breathing and its effect on facial morphology and dentition is only one factor of a multifactorial complex. Respiratory function influences the posture of the mandible; therefore the tongue, hyoid bone, head and neck posture, and nasal airway maintenance provide important physiologic bases for functional appliance therapy.

## BIOLOGIC TARGETS IN THE CONTROL PROCESS OF FACIAL GROWTH

Every scientific field has its share of aphorisms for theoretic concepts. These aphorisms were once working keystones but are now obsolete; nevertheless, they linger in each discipline's everyday vocabulary and thinking. In the field of facial growth, "foward and downward" and "condylar growth" are frequently encountered examples of outdated aphorisms. Such clichés are not actually incorrect but instead connote viewpoints now known to be inaccurate, incomplete, oversimplified, or misleading. They have led to nonproductive and false directions in the ongoing attempt to better understand the basis for complex biologic systems.

Two other proverbs also are pertinent to the present discussion: "pressure and tension on bone produce resorption and deposition" and "a tooth moves toward the pressure side of a socket and away from the tension side." The actual biomechanic circumstances are of course multifactorial and far more complex than those implied by these proverbs. In fact, if the collagenous fibers of the periodontal membrane are under tension, the key cells and other tissue components among them are being compressed. Also, a cell membrane under surface pressure can be in a state of tension. A bone surface undergoing flexure by a force is in a state of tension on convex surfaces but under compression on concave surfaces. A concave surface undergoing a decrease in the curvature of concavity is in a state of compression, but the magnitude is decreasing and the surface can behave as if in a tension state. Questions naturally arise: Is the primary target of a mechanical force the bone matrix or the bone's membrane? If both are involved, what is the primary response in the sequence? How can a force acting on the periosteum become translocated to trigger activity of the endosteum?

One cannot simply suggest that pressure or tension on bone explains the biomechanic processes of growth and change. The primary components involved must be stated and multifactorial biomechanic circumstances taken into account. A number of targets affect the chain of events relating to physical forces. The effects often appear different and even contradictory among these different targets; that is, tension acting on the fibrous matrix of a bone's periosteal membrane appears in some circumstances to relate to bone resorption but in others to tension. Also, pressure on the membrane and tension within the bone's calcified surface relate to resorption, whereas pressure alone relates to deposition. The piezo factor is believed to relate to the latter changes, but the primary trigger for action on bone membranes is not presently known. The way a "first messenger" triggers an osetoblast's or osteoclast's surface receptors also is not understood. Moreover, the way seemingly contradictory responses elicited by the composite of different localized mechanical forces on tissue components (fibers, cells, bone matrices, blood vessels, nerve receptors) become expressed as coordinated growth processes is not clearly understood. The way equilibrium is established has not been explained, and the parameters comprising biomechanic, bioelectrical, physiologic, morphogenic, cytogenic, neurotropic, and vascular equilibrium have not been described. However, that different expressions of forces can act on different targets in different ways to produce different responses is well established. A vague statement such as "pressures or tensions acting on a bone" does not encourage new ideas now needed if control processes in facial growth and clinical procedures related to them are ever to be explained.

### Growth Movements

"Working with growth" is another phrase heard repeatedly in the field of facial growth. One significant aspect of this phrase, however, is not usually taken into account. Growth and development involve growth movements of cells, tissues, and organs. Two basic kinds of movement take place with respect to bones and teeth. The first is a remodeling movement in which combinations of inside and outside bone deposition and resorption move all surfaces and parts to new locations. For example, the hard palate moves and rotates by progressive resorptive and depository remodeling in conjunction with the growth of the overlying nasal chambers. The second type of movement is a displacement process in which a whole bone is moved collaterally (i.e., passively in concert) with the growth expansion of its functional matrix. Thus as the soft tissue mass associated with a bone continues to grow and enlarge, the bone is moved with it. "Separation" of bones then occurs at articular junctions, and the membranes and cartilages of the bones are presumably triggered to simultaneously enlarge and remodel themselves to match the distances moved and the extents of soft tissue enlargement involved. This remodeling process is now widely believed to be secondary to a generalized, widespread displacement process taking place throughout the face and cranium and not merely related to a primary growth control provided by the bones' immediate membranes or other contiguous, closely associated soft tissues.

Therefore the practitioner must consider toward which target a given clinical or experimental procedure is directed:

(1) a remodeling process involving bone or tooth membranes (periodontal membrane, periosteum-endosteum) or (2) a bone or tooth displacement process? For example, as the palate and maxillary arch progressively remodel in an inferior direction, the whole maxilla simultaneously becomes displaced in an anteroinferior direction. An orthodontic procedure can involve manipulation of the bone remodeling process to place an individual tooth, in which case the periodontal membrane and contiguous periosteum-endosteum are among the primary targets. On the other hand, a procedure can inhibit or accelerate the displacement process, in which case the translatory movement of the entire bone is affected and the sutures and cartilages are among the primary targets. The positioning of the dental arch as a whole is manipulated, not an individual tooth and its socket. The practitioner must consider the following questions in planning therapy: In using a functional intraoral appliance, which of the two types of movement is affected? Are both involved? What is the nature of the balance between them?

## Primary and Secondary Principles

The preceding discussion and most of the literature assume the primacy of the old concepts of primary and secondary actions, cause-and-effect relationships, and pacemaker control. However, this conceptual direction may be biologically inappropriate. Practitioners and researchers are always implying that in any biologic system some factor must necessarily be a dominant, regulating pacesetter, with all other components passive, subordinate, or secondary to it. To what extent this is true has not been determined and clinging to this idea closes more doors to understanding. A concept of progressive interrelationships among all components may more accurately reflect the biology involved. The primary/secondary concept may be conceptually constraining.

## The Myofibroblast

The manner in which histologists teach the structure and function of connective tissue to students does not always emphasize the full significance of this tissue. Connective tissue does much more than merely connect parts while providing a sort of fill or packing among these parts. Histologists teach that this tissue is composed of three basic components: fibers, ground substance, and cells. What is usually not taught is that many varieties and functional types of fibroblasts exist and that extensive changes often occur in fibers and the ground substance, changes associated with complex circumstances relating to the multiple activities of connective tissues and the dynamic role they play in growth and development. Connective tissue is ubiquitous throughout the body and provides almost uninterrupted continuity. As other tissues and organs grow and remodel, the growth and extensive remodeling of the connective tissue sustain this continuity and allow the operation of functional interrelations among the different gross and microanatomic parts.

Connective tissue is responsible for the placement and mobility of the different anatomic parts undergoing the growth movements previously mentioned. Connective tissue has its own intrinsic, complex remodeling process that not only accompanies growth but also allows uninterrupted function during the growth movements and enlargement of bones, muscles, cartilage, glands, vessels, nerves, and epithelia.

A more recently recognized and important function also is associated with connective tissue. In addition to accommodating mobility for growth movements, this tissue appears to provide motility as well. Bones, teeth, muscles, tendons, and glands are placed and continuously re-placed as they continue to grow, enlarge, and change their positions. One hypothesis for the source of this motion is that cells called *myofibroblasts* may be directly involved. These cells are a type of fibroblast that contain contractile actin-myosin filaments. They have been observed in many locations in the connective tissue stroma throughout the body, including the periosteal and periodontal membranes. Research shows that myofibroblasts participate in tooth movements, displacement movements of bones, shifts of muscles and tendons along growing bone surfaces, relocation movements of bones relative to the functional matrix, and movement and placement of the connective tissue stroma relative to the movements of these parts. A new and promising research and clinical direction has been opened to practitioners. In the years ahead, the clinician's arena of operation will be expanded to include biochemical control of growth-stimulating and mediating agents because of increased knowledge of the tissue elements involved.

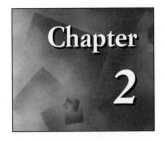

# Chapter 2

# Research Methodology and Findings in Applied Craniofacial Growth Studies

Alexandre G. Petrovic

Jeanne J. Stutzmann

This chapter discusses findings concerning facial growth as relates to the method of operation of functional appliances. As a new millenium approaches, an extraordinary evolution of the art and science of orthodontic and dentofacial orthopedics has occurred, resulting mainly from the willingness of researchers to ask questions concerning the relationships among craniofacial growth mechanisms and the methods of operation of orthodontic and dentofacial orthopedic appliances. The use of modern conceptual and instrumental tools in such investigations makes the search for answers conceivable and feasible.

The explanation for this progress lies less in technology than in the questions investigators are asking. Investigators are no longer restricted by arbitrary limits within the specialty. Instead, orthodontists are confronted with a challenging, interdisciplinary environment that encompasses anatomy, physiology, and molecular biology. The wide spectrum of current research is bringing orthodontists closer to understanding the pathogenetic and therapeutic aspects of orthodontics and dentofacial orthopedics.

Findings concerning the biologic peculiarities of mammalian condylar cartilage have helped fuel this understanding. In the late 1960s, Petrovic and co-workers (Charlier, Petrovic, 1967b; Charlier et al, 1968, 1969ab) produced the first rigorous demonstrations that the condylar cartilage's growth rate and amount can be modified using appropriate functional and orthopedic appliances. Since then, many other clinicians, researchers, and experimenters have inquired about the possibility of modifying the condylar cartilage's growth rate and direction.

Research also has shown that the lateral pterygoid muscle (LPM) apparently plays a regulating role in the control of the condylar cartilage's growth rate (Petrovic, Stutzmann, 1972; Stutzmann, Petrovic, 1974ab, 1975c). This finding was further investigated and confirmed by McNamara et al in the early 1980s. Earlier, Stutzmann et al (1976) discovered that the retrodiscal pad apparently has a mediator role in the efforts of the LPM to control condylar growth.

To represent as broadly and precisely as possible the many interdisciplinary findings that have become accepted in modern orthodontics and dentofacial orthopedics, Petrovic has employed the terminology of cybernetics and control theory to describe craniofacial growth mechanisms and the method of operation of functional and orthopedic appliances. Cybernetic theory refines orthodontic concepts by demonstrating the qualitative and quantitative relationships between observationally and experimentally collected findings. It also provides a conceptual tool for a broader understanding of clinical orthodontic problems, particularly because the rigorous language of cybernetics is compatible with the rapidly expanding use of computers among clinicians. Most recently the molecular biology approach to the method of operation of functional appliances has provided new insights for experimental investigations.

The emergence of dentofacial orthopedics as a major field of the biomedical sciences also has led to great progress. In the mid-1970s, using cellular, tissue culture, and organ culture methods of studying human alveolar bone taken from the distal and mesial sides of the premolars and molars both before and during treatment with orthodontic or functional appliances, the authors introduced precise quantitative evaluations of different parameters of the bone turnover rate (1979, 1980). No systematic inquiry into the quantitative aspects of these parameters had been performed before these investigations.

The chronobiologic aspects of cartilage and bone growth and the effectiveness of functional and orthodontic appliances also are areas of serious inquiry. Oudet and co-workers (Oudet, Petrovic, 1978a, 1982; Petrovic et al, 1981ce, 1984) demonstrated the significant variations produced by these appliances on condylar cartilage growth and alveolar bone turnover in both rats and humans during the day-night cycle and seasonal sequence. The reduced growth rate in a rat's LPM produced during treatment with functional appliances is significantly greater in the resting phase than it is in the activity phase. This diminished rate of increase (with analogous variations in other masticatory muscles) plays an important role in the mechanism of action of some functional appliances by maintaining the mandible in a more forward position, even during the daily period when the appliance is not worn (Petrovic et al, 1982ab).

The rapid increase in research efforts has produced a new understanding of the mechanism of action of functional appliances. Nevertheless, much about the etiology and pathology of major dentofacial malrelations is still unknown. Answers to these inquiries are not likely to come solely from observations of the patient; biomedical research is required as well. Undoubtedly the biologic analysis of craniofacial growth mechanisms and the method of dentofacial orthopedic operation of appliances is assuming a more important role in treatment decision making.

The data in this chapter are based primarily on experimental research investigations pursued in the Laboratory for Craniofacial Growth Mechanisms in Strasbourg, France, with the assistance of several leading clinically oriented researchers and research-oriented clinicians from around the world. This chapter provides readers with information to help them master the structure and meaning of developments in orthodontics and dentofacial orthopedics.

## COGNITIVE STATUS OF BIOMEDICAL AND MEDICAL CONCEPTS, PROPOSITIONS, AND THEORIES

The goal of research is the increase of knowledge. Moreover, knowledge and its growth also is an area for research.

### Epistemologic Features

The branch of philosophy that deals with the possibility, nature, origin, structure, and validity of knowledge is called *epistemology.* In biomedical sciences, epistemology concerns mainly the relations between the "subject" and the "object," between the expected and the normal or pathologic reality.

Biomedical research distinguishes among several disciplines. Logic is a formal discipline of inquiry into the principles guiding reasoning. Epistemology is a philosophic branch inquiring into the nature and validity of knowledge. Psychology investigates the conscious aspects of cognitive processes exclusively as they relate to mental life, whereas epistemology deals with the relation of cognitive processes to reality.

Epistemology may be divided into areas of inquiry: the possibility and limits of knowledge, origin of knowledge (empiricism versus rationalism), methodologic* problems of acquiring knowledge, varieties of knowledge, structure of knowledge, and problem of truth. Orthodontists and other practitioners may be tempted to consider epistemologic problems as having no connection to their specialties and activities. Nevertheless, at every step of biomedical and clinical research

*Methodology should not be mistaken for technology or technique. Methodology refers to the analysis of conceptual, observational, and experimental principles and processes that guide a scientific, biomedical, or clinical inquiry. Each branch of science, medicine, and dentistry has specific methodologic problems that require investigation.

and activity, practitioners are confronted with epistemologic and methodologic problems; often such practitioners are not even aware they are dealing with an epistemologic or methodologic obstacle or difficulty.

Epistemologic inquiry within the biomedical sciences corresponds for the most part to the philosophic vision of Popper (1963), who held that science is not a static acceptance of truth but rather the permanent search for truth. No theory or statement may be irrefutably verified; however, if efforts to refute a working hypothesis fail, the hypothesis is corroborated. Corroboration indicates the strengthening of a theory or concept but not its definite, unmistakable truth. In other words, the criterion of a hypothesis's validity is its resistance to refutation. Orthodontists must therefore not only seek support for working hypotheses but also be alert to biomedical concepts and clinical cases that may refute them.

In *Conjectures and Refutations, the Growth of Scientific Knowledge* (1963), Popper states the following:

Clinical observations, like all other observations, are interpretations in the light of theories; and for this reason alone they are apt to seem to support those theories in the light of which they are interpreted. But real support can be obtained only from observations undertaken as tests (by attempted refutations); and for this purpose, criteria of refutation have to be laid down beforehand: it must be agreed which observable situations, if actually observed, mean that the theory is refuted.

This statement may be considered a guiding rule in medical and orthodontic research. It implies that any theory or concept in orthodontics is conjectural and—to use Kuhn's language (1962)—based on a paradigm (a model used as a thinking pattern). A paradigm-free fact does not exist.

In compliance with Popper's thinking, Petrovic (1982) affirms that any refutation-corroboration process in medicine and orthodontics is not a cognitive act but a decision-making procedure; the distinction between the normal and the pathologic results from an operational definition rather than from an appreciation of biomedical reality.

According to Popper (1963) the degree of refutability is the measure of the heuristic fruitfulness of a working hypothesis. As a corollary the irrefutability of a theory or concept is an expression of its informational emptiness or meagerness. Decisional analysis in medicine and orthodontics implies in both diagnosis and therapeutics the progressive refutation of erroneous hypotheses.

### Methodologic Features

Orthodontic methodology and research design is built on the following assertions (Figure 2-1):

1. Biomedical theories and concepts illuminate only part of the clinical reality. Therefore decision-making procedures in dentofacial orthopedics are based both on scientific biomedical knowledge and empirical clinical evidence. The authors (1980a) make the following epistemologic distinction between the two:
   a. Biomedical knowledge is established according to rigorous rules of scientific inquiry; reasoning validates the basis of orthodontic decision making.

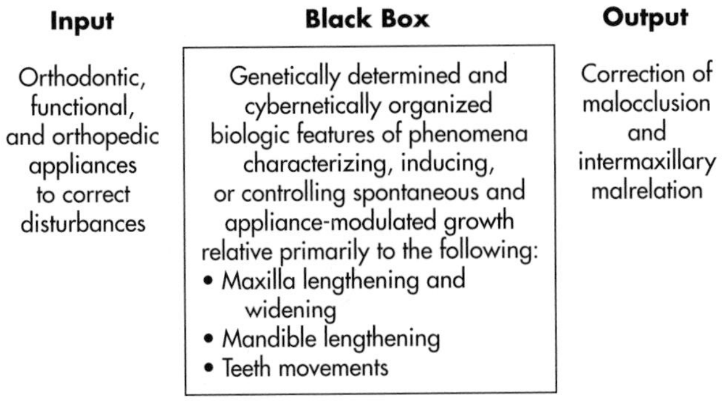

| Input | Black Box | Output |
|---|---|---|
| Orthodontic, functional, and orthopedic appliances to correct disturbances | Genetically determined and cybernetically organized biologic features of phenomena characterizing, inducing, or controlling spontaneous and appliance-modulated growth relative primarily to the following:<br>• Maxilla lengthening and widening<br>• Mandible lengthening<br>• Teeth movements | Correction of malocclusion and intermaxillary malrelation |

**Figure 2-1.** Research design: clinical versus biologic approach.

b. Clinical evidence flows from a collection of clinical procedures, guidelines, and experience established and evaluated according to their effectiveness. Reasoning is only an intellectual attempt to account for clinical effectiveness—it cannot validate or invalidate orthodontic decision making.

2. The etiology of dentofacial malrelations and the method of operation of functional appliances is more likely to be found in the morphophysiologic peculiarities of different growth sites than in the agents and events that play triggering roles (Petrovic, 1972).

3. The distinction between the normal and abnormal is an operation of decision rather than a cognitive act. Indeed, for an isolated morphologic or physiologic parameter the limit between the normal and abnormal is rarely apprehensible or ascertainable. A discontinuity may be detectable at the system level (e.g., during the transition phase from an optimal, stable occlusal relationship to a suboptimal one). However, such a discontinuity is not necessarily the threshold of the abnormal.

4. In dentofacial orthopedics, which is founded mainly on empirical and anecdotal procedures, explanation often has the strength of doctrine. In biomedical orthodontics, explanation has taken the forms encountered in biologic sciences:
   a. Deductive
   b. Deductivoprobabilistic
   c. Functional
   d. Phylogenetic

5. Biomedical explanation is the process of fitting a factual statement into the framework of systematically organized knowledge. Clinical explanation consists mostly of accounting for a singular phenomenon by making reference to corresponding general statements (theories, concepts) and specific conditions under which the involved biomedical statements operate. Orthodontists are necessarily interested in forecasting (i.e., attributing an explanatory scheme for future occurrences) and theorizing that if the conjecture and the appropriate set of initial requirements are fulfilled, the anticipated event will occur.

6. Research investigators and clinicians must account for the individual variability of the sample, uncontrolled or unknown disturbing factors, and unexpected secondary effects. Hence a carefully prepared research design, including whenever possible a quantitative variation of input variables (e.g., a functional appliance) and a quantitative evaluation of output parameters (e.g., growth rate, amount, direction and the lengths and angles of specific cephalometric criteria), is a necessity. Methodologically, causal research is a search leading to identification and analysis of disturbing factors.

7. The word *theory* has two meanings:
   a. It refers to systematically organized knowledge (e.g., the cybernetic theory of craniofacial growth).
   b. It refers to a set of logically formulated assumptions that have yet to be tested (e.g., the functional matrix theory).

   In epistemology the distinction is made between laws (valid, corroborated, empirical generalizations) and principles (axioms, postulates [i.e., sets of unproven or undemonstrable propositions], theories).

8. Any working hypothesis is methodologically useful as long as it is unambiguously testable and can be either corroborated or refuted. If it cannot meet these criteria, it is inoperative—informationally meaningless and practically worthless.

In medical and orthodontic research, including dentofacial orthopedics, objectivity does not imply a hesitancy to formulate imaginative, fanciful, and even extravagant working hypotheses but rather an eagerness to abandon a concept of preference if tested evidence does not confirm fundamental anticipations. Passion and controversy may have a place in discussion and interpretation but certainly not in the study of rigorously collected biomedical and clinical data.

As teachers, most orthodontists are storytelling lecturers and case reporters rather than scientifically minded investigators. Indeed, their style for organizing presentations of clinical experiences and thoughts is too often narrative (vivid, glib, anecdotal) rather than argumentative (logically legitimate).

Four types of explanation are current in literature concerning craniofacial growth and orthodontic questions (Petrovic, 1982, 1984ab):

1. Deductive—The item to be explained appears as a necessary consequence of certain premises. Such an explanation may be used for description and classification of observations and for the forecast of future events, including degree of probability. A deductive explanation requires a logically organized framework of knowledge (e.g., a cybernetic diagram containing precise quantitative data).

2. Deductivoprobabilistic—In this type of explanation, at least one of the premises consists of probabilistic statements concerning specific categories of individual occurrences. The deductivoprobabilistic type does not assess the degree of validity of the premises but instead notes the relationship between the premises and the items to be explained. This type of explanation is the most common in medicine and orthodontics. It forms the basis of differential diagnosis and prognosis. The computer-based orthodontic diagnosis is an illustration of such reasoning.

3. Functional—In this case the explanation specifies the function an element performs in maintaining major elements of the system to which it belongs and in protecting the system against random variations and intrinsic or extrinsic disturbances. This type of explanation corresponds to the goal-seeking description of technologic systems. Various components of the system that control craniofacial growth and development interact and provide feedback in precise, causal interdependence and responsiveness. Thus the functional explanation again presupposes a cybernetically organized knowledge.

Because morphophysiologic systems are almost always nonlinear, quantitative descriptions may only occasionally be restricted to differential equations; discontinuities must be taken into account. The mathematic theory of catastrophe is an excellent topologic tool to account for discontinuities (i.e., bifurcation situations during growth and development).

4. Phylogenetic—This type of explanation holds that the morphophysiologic entity, such as the temporomandibular joint, that characterizes mammals may be accounted for by describing the way it evolved from earlier phylogenetic forms. In this evolutionary type of explanation the first step is the setting out of a sequence of major events through which a system has evolved. The second step is the discovery of events that are causally pertinent to the transformation of the system. The third step is the presentation of reasons for the transformation by detecting the morphophysiologic appropriateness of the newly evolved system. The fourth step is elucidating the evolutionary successfulness of the transformation. An evolutionary explanation is at best presumptive; because an evolutionary transformation is generally a nonrecurring event, its hypothetic explanation is hard to test.

Nevertheless, the evolutionary explanation for the peculiarities of the condylar cartilage is intellectually tempting. In reptiles the joint between the skull and lower jaw is formed by two bones originating from the primary cartilages, the quadratus and the articular. In mammals this joint is formed by two dermal bones, the squamosal and the dentary (i.e., mandible), the latter developing from three posterior secondary cartilages (coronoid, condylar, angular—the last one differentiating only in small mammals).

According to Symons (1951), in the mammalian embryo, the condylar cartilage also develops independently of the chondrocranium. Thus phylogenetic data illuminate ontogenetic data. However, phylogenetically and ontogenetically the prechondroblastic zone of the condylar cartilage (and of any secondary cartilage) appears to be closer to the craniofacial sutures and subperiosteal zone than to the epiphyseal cartilage.

The response of condylar cartilage growth to local factors may explain the extraordinary success of the phylogenetically new mammalian joint between the skull and the lower jaw. Condylar cartilage growth is integrated into an organized, functional whole that has the form of a servosystem and is able to modulate the lengthening of the condyle so that the lower jaw adapts to the upper jaw during growth. Indeed, the confrontation between the positions of the upper and lower dental arches is the comparator of the servosystem. The comparator is the origin of correction signals intended to modulate the postural activity of the LPM to place the mandible in an optimal or a suboptimal occlusal adjustment. Variations in the postural activity of the LPM and the iterative activity of the retrodiscal pad modify the condylar cartilage's growth rate and the condylar growth direction, producing a more anterior or posterior growth rotation of the mandible.

The ability of the lower jaw to adjust in length to the upper jaw during growth certainly favored the genetic variations that led to anteroposterior facial shortening, molarization of the postcanine teeth, and subsequent mastication. In the absence of adjustment of mandibular teeth to maxillary teeth, the occlusal forces expose the periodontal structures to repeated traumas that can result in the loss of the teeth. The responsiveness of condylar cartilage growth to local factors (and fossa and eminence adaptation as shown in Chapter 4) increases the possibility of mastication and this facilitates a high metabolism and the maintenance of a constant body temperature.

Research investigations have led to the following theorizations regarding growth mechanisms of the mandible:

- A relatively stable periosteal contribution exists that is subordinated to both orders affecting the organism and local control factors represented primarily by muscular contractions. Thus by the nature of bone growth and remodeling the periosteal growth of the mandible is commanded rather than regulated.

- A cartilaginous contribution (condylar, coronoid, and angular) exists that is more easily modifiable and subject to local control systems through feedback loops. Integrated within the local regulative loop, the cartilaginous contribution to mandibular growth is more rapidly established; it is intended for fine growth adjustment to ensure an efficient occlusion. The growth of the condylar cartilage may therefore be seen as a mechanism that at each moment depends partly on messages of local origin. Thus the expression of a regional structural homeostasis is the enabling factor in the coordinated growth of the masticatory apparatus. This does not mean that periosteal deposition of bone is only an accessory mechanism; the consequences of condylectomy and acromegaly indicate the opposite (see Chapter 1). However, because in both these situations the increase in size of the mandible is more subject to an overall command than to local regulation, mandibular overgrowth from an intense and prolonged subperiosteal ossification may lead to occlusal disharmony.

Stutzmann (1976) emphasizes the following: primary cartilages exist in the axial skeleton, skull base, and limbs; the dividing cells, differentiated chondroblasts, are surrounded by a cartilaginous matrix that isolates them from local factors able to restrain or stimulate cartilaginous growth. Secondary cartilages (Figures 2-2 and 2-3) exist in condylar and coronoid (and, in small mammals, in angular) processes and sometimes in sutures; the dividing cells, prechondroblasts, are not surrounded by a cartilaginous matrix and thus are not isolated

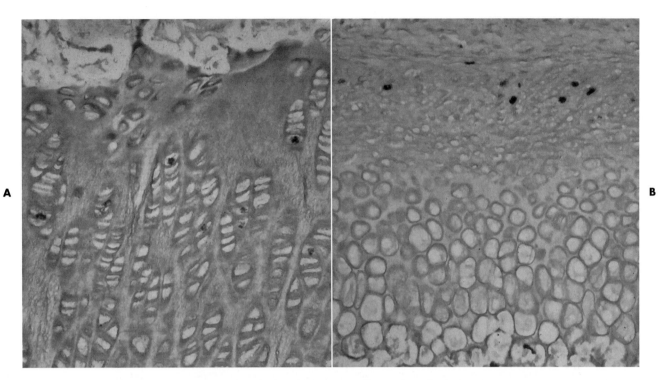

**Figure 2-2.** Radioautographs of a histologic section. **A,** Epiphyseal cartilage. In primary cartilages the chondroblasts divide and synthesize the intercellular matrix. **B,** Condylar cartilage of the mandible. In secondary cartilages the cells that divide the prechondroblasts are not yet surrounded by the cartilaginous matrix.

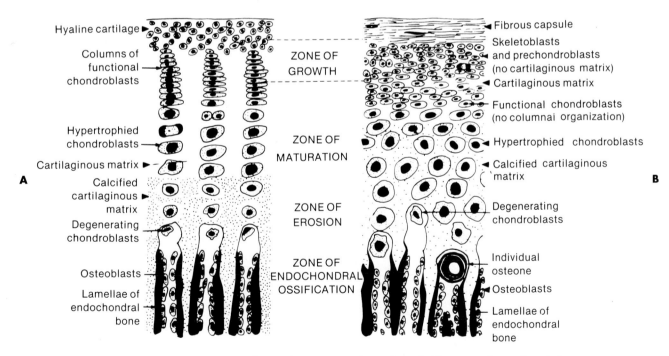

**Figure 2-3.** Primary (**A**) and secondary (**B**) growth cartilage. **A,** The zone of growth includes functional chondroblasts, cells that divide and synthesize a cartilaginous matrix. Functional chondroblasts are surrounded by collagen II but no collagen I. Hypertrophied chondroblasts are surrounded by collagen II and collagen X. **B,** The zone of growth includes skeletoblasts and prechondroblasts, cells that divide but do not synthesize a cartilaginous matrix. They are surrounded by collagen I. Functional chondroblasts synthesize a cartilaginous matrix but usually do not divide. They are surrounded by collagen II and collagen I. Hypertrophied chondroblasts are surrounded by collagen I, II, and X.

from local factor influences. In conclusion, the findings regarding the singular biologic behavior of the condylar cartilage help explain the evolutionary supremacy of the new joint between the skull and the lower jaw: it characterizes mammals and allows their phylogenetic success.

Another osteologic character of mammals should be noted: the so-called secondary bony palate separating the nasal cavity from the oral cavity. This structure facilitates mastication. A phylogenetic origin of the human bony palate helps explain biologic and pathologic peculiarities of the midpalatal suture.

## Cybernetic Features

Craniofacial growth is an extremely complex process. In the accounting for scientific findings its mechanisms and the method of operation of orthopedic and orthodontic appliances, the following set of approaches is useful:

1. Discoveries may be related by placing the observations next to each other. This approach is still quite common but is becoming outdated if not obsolete in modern practice.
2. Diagrams (Figures 2-4 and 2-5) displaying the qualitative relations between observations can be constructed. This approach, the first step toward modeling, is not only more helpful but also more heuristic, with greater fact-finding potential.

3. Diagrams may be improved by making the relationships illustrated by the model either continuous or discontinuous. This approach is time consuming and therefore unpopular (especially for busy clinicians).
4. Diagrams may be further improved by using matrices in mathematic language to describe interactions among parts of the morphophysiologic system. In these matrices the output is usually proportional to the input. Such an image implies a proper research approach that is often difficult to practice but is indisputably rewarding for both biologists and clinicians.
5. Cybernetics based on communication and information theory—particularly on feedback control systems—provides another useful research approach. Cybernetics has brought new and beneficial concepts (e.g., negative and positive feedback, self-regulation, reference input, open and closed loop, regulation versus servosystem, gain [amplification of attenuation], systems and circuit analysis) to the biologic and biomedical sciences. This approach also relies on linear differential equations. A relevant and well-chosen investigatory strategy is therefore important. Once disregarded as a pointless sophistication in accounting for biologic and biomedical findings, the cybernetic approach is in fact a major breakthrough in the decision-making process and problem solving in scientific and clinical orthodontics and dentofacial orthopedics.

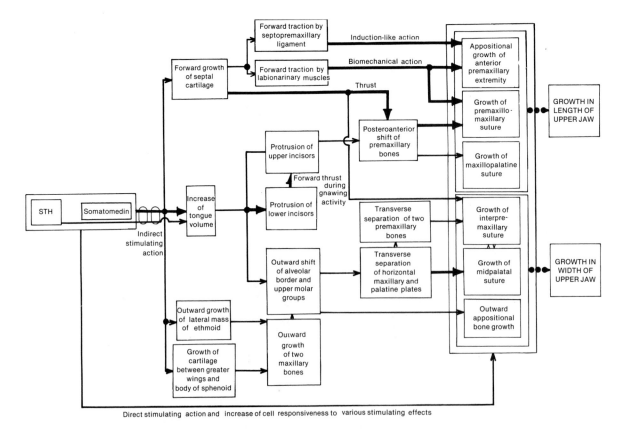

**Figure 2-4.**   Functional diagram for the sequential analysis of upper jaw growth control by STH-somatomedin.

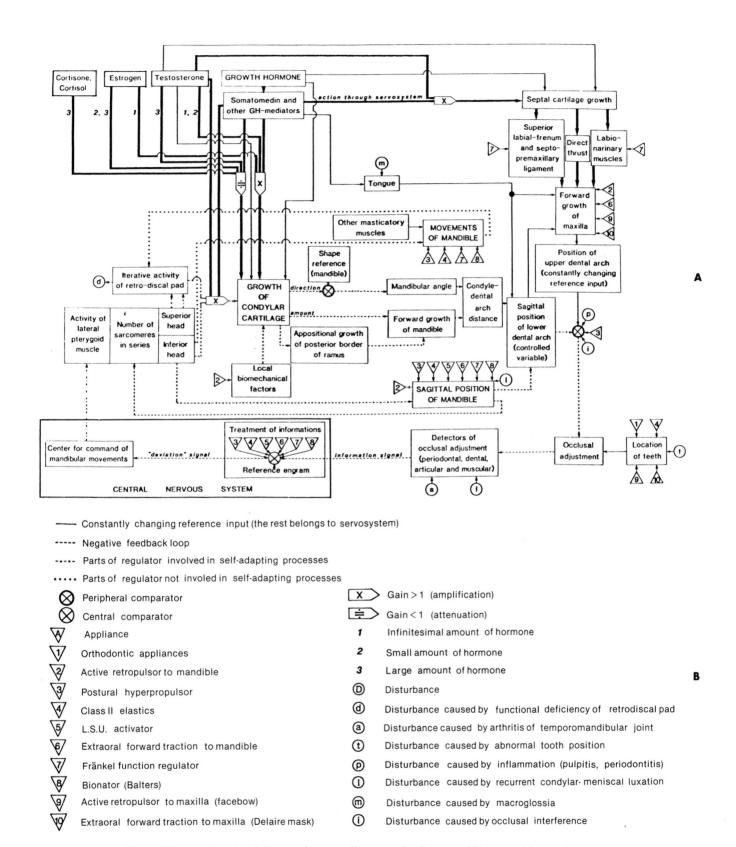

**Figure 2-5.** **A,** Functional diagram for controlling growth of the mandibular condylar cartilage. **B,** Key.

*Continued*

| Category | Rotation Group | Occlusion | Comparator | Extraction | 1 | 2 | 3 | 4 | 5 | 6 | 7 | 8 | 9 | 10 |
|---|---|---|---|---|---|---|---|---|---|---|---|---|---|---|
| 1 | P2 DOB | I | M | + | | | | | | | | | | |
| 1 | P2 DN | c/c | M | + | | | | | | | | | * | |
| | | II | M | ++ | | | | | | | | | * | |
| 2 | P1 NOB | I | M | | | | | | | | | | | |
| 2 | P1 NN | c/c | M | | | * | | | | | | | | |
| | | III | M | | | * | | | | | | | | |
| 2 | A2 DN | II | I | ++ | | | | | | | | | * | |
| 2 | A2 DDB | II | I or P | ++ | | | | | | | | | * | |
| 3 | R2 DN | I | M ▲ | | | | | | | | | | | |
| 3 | R2 DOB | c/c | M ▲ | + | * + 9 | | | | | | | | | |
| | | II | M ▲ | ++ | | | | | | | | | | |
| 3 | R2 DDB | II | M ▲ | ++ | | | | | | | | | | |
| 4 | R1 NN | I | M ▲ | | | | | | | | | | * | |
| 4 | R1 NOB | c/c | M ▲ | ++ | * + 9 | | | | | | | | | |
| 4 | R1 NDB | II | M ▲ | ++ | * + 9 | | | | | | | | | |
| 5 | R3 MDB | I | M | | | | | | | | | | | |
| 5 | R3 MN | III | M | | * + 10 | | | | | | | | | |
| 5 | R3 MOB | III | M | | * + 10 | | | | | | | | | |
| | | I | I | | | | | | | | | | | |
| 5 | A1 NN | c/c | I | | * | | | | | | | | | |
| | | II | I | + | | | (*) | * | (*) | * | * | | | |
| | | I | I or P | 0 | | | | | | | | | | |
| 5 | A1 NDB | c/c | I or P | 0 | | | (*) | * | (*) | * | * | | | |
| | | II | I or P | 0 | | | (*) | * | (*) | * | * | | | |
| | | II | I | + | | | (*) | * | (*) | * | * | | | |
| 5 | A1 DN | c/c | I | + | | | (*) | * | (*) | * | * | | | |
| | | I | I | | | | | | | | | | | |
| 5 | A1 DDB | II | I or P | + | | | (*) | * | (*) | * | * | | | |
| 5 | P1 MOB | III | M | | | * | | | | | | | | |
| 5 | P1 MN | III | M | | | * | | | | | | | | |
| 6 | A3 MN | I | I | | | | | | | | | | | |
| 6 | A3 MDB | III | I | | | | | | | | | | | * |
| 6 | P3 MN | III | M | | * + 10 | | | | | | | | | |
| 6 | P3 MOB | III | M | | * + 10 | | | | | | | | | |

Note: Treatment and extractions are considered only with regards to a basal discrepancy correction.
Groups P3 MN and P3 MOB require orthognathic surgery.
Category—Expression of the tissue level growth potential.
Comparator—I,P,M, incisors; I,P,M, premolars; I,P,M, molars; I + P + M when occlusion is completed.
Extraction—++, unavoidable; + often indicated; 0, contraindicated.
Suggested appliance—1, orthodontic appliance; 2, active retropulsor of the mandible; 3, postural hyperpropulsor of the mandible; 4, class II elastics; 5, LSU activator; 6, extraoral forward traction of the mandible; 7, Fränkel function regulator; 8, bionator; 9, active maxillary retropulsor; 10, extraoral forward maxillary traction.
* = First choice; (*) = alternative choice.

**Figure 2-5, cont'd.**    **C,** Treatment decision relating to facial growth rotation group.

6. Catastrophe theory, a topologic concept designed to describe discontinuities (Figure 2-6), is another powerful research approach. In cybernetic models, discontinuities correspond to sudden changes in references of the control system. Catastrophe theory allows the researcher to relate either qualitatively or quantitatively nonlinear relationships that would be difficult to describe by manipulating classical differential equations (see Chapter 1). Dentofacial orthopedics' representation of craniofacial growth mechanisms and the method of operation of orthodontic and orthopedic appliances has made significant progress through the use of cybernetics and catastrophe theory. Modern decision making in orthodontics and dentofacial orthopedics is grounded in a highly sophisticated portrayal of biologic and biomedical realities.

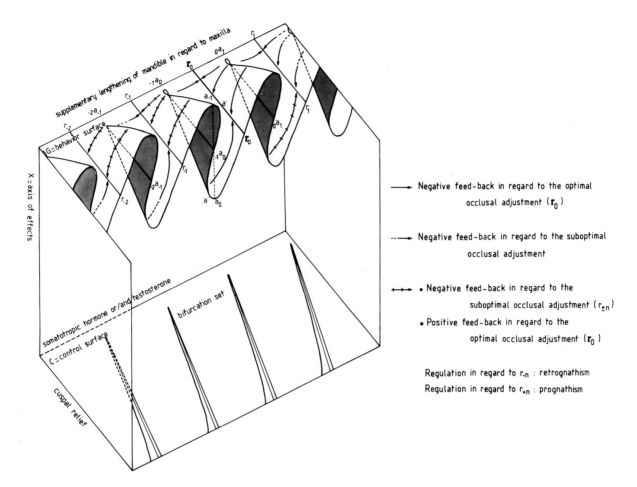

**Figure 2-6.** Topologic representation of increasing hormone levels (testosterone or STH-somatomedin) resulting in supplementary growth of the mandible combined with lengthening of the maxilla as modulated by the comparator of the servosystem (cuspal relief). Experimental results are expressed in terms of catastrophe theory. $\gamma\alpha$ Position of the optimal occlusal adjustment; $\gamma \pm \gamma v$ position of suboptimal occlusal adjustment; **a,** position of cuspal opposition.

A rational, intellectually consistent, and cohesive understanding of dentofacial malrelations is still far from supplanting the unshaken, anecdotal, self-confidence–based doctrinal statements of some clinicians. Indeed, many controversies in the contemporary history of orthodontics and dentofacial orthopedics are more a matter of conflicts between individuals than confrontations between theories and concepts.

One cause of this situation is the frequently encountered, ambiguous, and inarticulate accounts of the orthodontist's assumed position and reasoning. Nevertheless, the epistemologic consistency of any newly formulated theory cannot be legitimately established and evaluated without the unequivocal expression of the principles of reasoning applied throughout the research investigation. No sound research achievement can leave out a circumspect and well-advised epistemologic and methodologic inquiry into the theoretical basis and structure of a discipline such as dentofacial orthopedics. Otherwise, professional communication remains difficult. The rationalization of all orthodontic diagnostic and treatment procedures is a difficult task with ordinary language, especially

when problems of immediate clinical effectiveness outweigh conceptual coherence. However, no efficient clinical activity in orthodontics and dentofacial orthopedics can occur without the realization that dentofacial malrelations occur as part of an indivisible whole, even though clinicians often deal with different diagnostic and treatment approaches.

Cybernetics and control theory are in this respect new and powerful tools. They help clinicians rigorously address the study of communications, control mechanisms, and organizations in both living and technologic systems. In other words they provide a language of combined analysis and a systemic approach to biology and the biomedical sciences. They make it possible to account for the properties of normal or abnormal systems as an emergence from the organization of connectivity relations. Modern orthodontists must become acquainted with the cybernetic language, because cybernetic thinking is the primary route to data processing and computerizing for the twenty-first century.

A cybernetically organized system operates through signals that transmit information. A physiologic signal may be of a physical, chemical, or electromagnetic nature. Usually it possesses very little energy. Craniofacial growth and development are information-processing phenomena that include production, perception, transmission, and storage of information. Petrovic (1977, 1982) was the first to promulgate a cybernetic model to account for the physiologic phenomena involved in facial growth and the method of operation of orthodontic and functional appliances (see Figure 2-5); however, this model is only one of several possible rational descriptions. According to Popperian epistemologic precepts, no cybernetic model or set of equations can describe craniofacial growth and the method of operation of orthodontic and functional appliances exclusively and definitively. Petrovic has noted that cybernetics is a part of orthodontics but his own cybernetic model is not.

The formation and renewal of the craniofacial skeleton are many-faceted phenomena. The connections between constituents are complex, although the constituents themselves are not. The complexity results from the organization, the structured whole that is infinitely more complex than the sum of its constituents. The physiologic properties of the craniofacial skeleton are not simply related to the cells and intercellular substances or to elementary intercellular actions but originate from the tissue and organ system with all its interactions and feedbacks. The identification and analysis of feedback loops (i.e., regulation processes) are among the main tasks in the field of craniofacial growth. So far, cybernetic language has been the best tool to render accurately the intricacy and complexity of craniofacial morphogenesis and the means to influence it clinically.

The study of a morphophysiologic system involves describing its properties. Usually the researcher measures simultaneously the spontaneous or experimentally and therapeutically induced variations of a stimulus (input) and the varia-

tions of one or several responses (output). The output is related to the input by a transfer function that characterizes the system under investigation. The system is thus described as a function of changes affecting the various parameters.

The following details may be useful in understanding the cybernetic approach to research:

- Inputs and outputs are generally represented by arrows. In the study of time-dependent phenomena, each arrow represents a signal; at some point the signal may become a message. The percentage of data that are not indispensable to the message but contribute to the reliability of its transmission is called the *redundancy*. The translation of a message from one language into another is called *transcodage*.
- The physiologic system under investigation is represented by a black box. The content of the black box is usually unknown (see Figure 2-1).
- If a physiologic system is designed to maintain a specific correspondence between outputs and inputs in spite of disturbances, it is a closed-loop control system. The closed-loop system is characterized by the presence of a feedback loop and comparator. An open-loop system has no feedback loop or comparator.

The closed-loop control system has two variations:

1. The regulator—In this system the main input is a constant. The comparator detects disturbances and their effects. The regulator is a negative feedback system; disturbances cause changes that tend to restore the state of the disturbed system to initial conditions.
2. The servosystem or follow-up system (Figure 2-7)—In this system the main input is not a constant but varies across time.

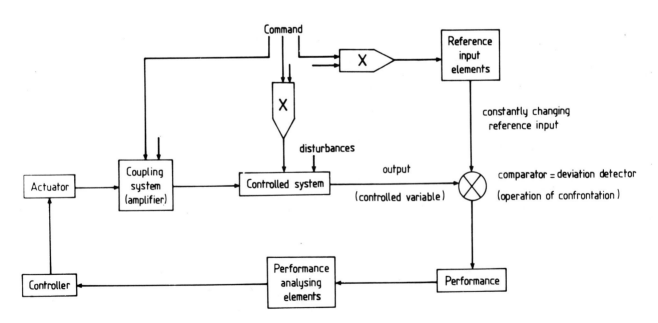

**Figure 2-7.** Elements and organization of a servosystem.

Control theory is becoming the common language of science and technology. The definitions vary across disciplines and authors. The definitions of concepts and terms formulated by the authors (1977, 1982) for the field of craniofacial growth and the method of operation of orthodontic and functional appliances are used here:

- The command—The command is a signal established independent of the feedback system under scrutiny. It affects the behavior of the control system without being affected by the consequences of this behavior. For instance, the secretion rates of growth hormone–somatomedin, testosterone, and estrogen do not seem to be modulated by variations of craniofacial growth.
- Reference input elements—Reference input elements establish the relationship between the command (e.g., growth hormone–somatomedin) and the reference input (the sagittal position of the upper dental arch). They include the septal cartilage, septopremaxillary frenum, labionarinary muscles, and premaxillary and maxillary bones.
- Reference input—The reference input is a signal established as a standard of comparison. Ideally it should be independent of the feedback.
- The controller—The controller is located between the deviation signal and the actuating signal.
- Actuating signal—The actuating signal corresponds to the output signal of the controller (i.e., to the input signal of the controlled system). The activity of the LPM and retrodiscal pad corresponds to the actuating signal.
- Controlled system—The controlled system is part of the control system between the actuating signal and the directly controlled variable. An example is the growth of condylar cartilage via metabolic blood interchange in the retrodiscal pad.
- Controlled variable—This is the output signal of the system. The best example is the sagittal position of the mandible.
- The gain—The gain of a system is the output divided by the input. If the gain is greater than one, amplification is present; if it is less than one, attenuation is the result. The pterygocondylar coupling is an example of gain. According to Petrovic's investigation, the basal value of the gain is determined genetically but may be amplified by growth hormone-somatomedin and testosterone or attenuated by estrogen. This is of great clinical significance.
- Feedback signal—The feedback signal is the function of the controlled variable that is compared to the reference input. In a regulator or servosystem, it is negative.
- The disturbance—Any input other than the reference chosen by the researcher is considered a disturbance. The disturbance is responsible for deviation of the output signal. It may act on any element of the regulating system. The concept of disturbance is sometimes difficult to grasp. For instance, the supplementary lengthening caused by growth hormone–somatomedin is greater for the mandible than it is for the maxilla. This implies that an increase in hormone level may have a disturbing effect on occlusal adjustment.
- The attractor—This is the final structurally stable steady state in a dynamic system. An example is the full interdigitation type of occlusal relationship (full Class I and also to a degree full Class II or III).
- The repeller—This is the set of all unstable equilibrium states, including their limit points. An example is the cusp-to-cusp type of occlusal relationship.
- The fractal—The mathematician Mandelbrot coined the term *fractal* from the Latin adjective *fractus* corresponding to the verb *frangere,* which means to break creating irregular fragments. *Fractal* thus means both *fragmented* and *irregular.* The fractal approach to form goes beyond the topologic approach, although fractal and topologic features are complementary.

The interdental relationship produces a natural shape that may be represented by fractal geometry. The semiquantitative evaluation of electromyographic records also is based on an analysis using fractal geometry. The following terms are common in fractal geometry:

- Fractal curve—This is the curve for which the fractal dimension exceeds the topologic dimension.
- Noise—This is a chance fluctuation of a signal and its subsequent manifestation. The weaker the signal, the greater the relative weight of the noise.
- Scaling fractals—The word *fractals* indicates disorder and is used for cases of intractable irregularity, whereas the term *scaling* indicates some degree of order. Indeed, according to Mandelbrot, most fractals are invariable under certain transformations of scale.

## Final Methodologic Comments

The cybernetic theory of craniofacial growth mechanisms is based on analytic and synthetic approaches. The proposed functional diagrams (see Figures 2-4 and 2-5) are not static conceptual viewpoints but dynamic representations of experimental findings concerning the detected and investigated phenomena of growth and growth determinism in the postnatal period. Such cybernetic models have much heuristic value; they open new perspectives and provide new working hypotheses to be tested. Within the methodology of scientific investigation the construction of a general model must precede any lengthy experimental work designed to refute or corroborate the working hypothesis resulting from the model. New cybernetic models that are continuously being revised to conform to new findings offer a general overview while enabling close critical scrutiny to leave no opportunity for confusion.

In methodology, animal experimentation is designed to detect causal relationships. In clinical research, conditions do not always allow the establishments that a phenomenon is actually produced orthodontically or orthopedically. For instance, selecting a given parameter of facial growth and comparing an individual to a population is not an ideal procedure for describing therapeutically produced variations. Nevertheless, much modern orthodontic research does just that. Also, the clinician's failure to detect the effect of a functional appliance does not necessarily indicate that the given parameter is genetically determined. The temporal organization of tissue growth is another important research parameter.

The condylar cartilages and alveolar bones of growing children exhibit a higher percentage of cells in the DNA-synthesis phase during the night than they do during the day. In other words the first sleeping hours (deep plane of sleep) are the most favorable for therapeutically triggering an increased number of cell divisions in condylar cartilage and alveolar bone. Logically, the mitosis rate is highest during breakfast time. Also, the lengthening of the masticatory muscles, especially the LPMs, appears more active during the night than during the day. In fact, the L.S.U. activator and similar appliances appear more efficient when worn during the night. Such general methodologic considerations enable the clinician to take a valid approach to problems concerning the biologic mechanisms of facial growth and the method of operation of functional appliances.

## METHOD OF OPERATION OF FUNCTIONAL APPLIANCES

No universal agreement exists concerning the mechanisms of craniofacial skeletal growth. Nevertheless, various theoretic explanations can be tentatively categorized.

### Genetic Control Theory

Genetic control theory stipulates that the genotype supplies all information required for phenotypic expression. However, although the role of genes is widely acknowledged, disagreement exists concerning whether general, regional, and local factors modify the gene expression and the way in which such modification occurs. Genomic control of *size* is not as important as epigenetic factors (Burdi, 1995).

### Cartilage-Directed Growth Theory

According to Scott (1953, 1954, 1967), cartilage is the primary factor in craniofacial growth control (i.e., the synchondrosis, nasal septum, and mandibular condyle are the centers of growth). Sutural growth is considered compensatory in cartilage-directed growth theory.

### Functional Matrix Theory

According to the functional matrix theory (M.L. Moss, 1960, 1962, 1997), regional and local factors play a role in craniofacial morphogenesis (see Chapter 1). The growth of cartilage and bone seems to be a compensatory response to functional matrix growth; the functional matrix includes muscles, nerves, glands, and teeth. Two types of functional matrix are recognized: periosteal and capsular. The growth of the functional matrix is primary, whereas that of a skeletal unit is secondary. The functional matrix theory has produced many experimental and clinical investigations but also has led to fruitful controversy (Johnston, 1972).

### Servosystem Theory

A further step in understanding the mechanisms of craniofacial growth was made when Charlier, Petrovic, and Stutzmann detected in organ culture (in both transplantation and in situ investigations) the following dissimilarities concerning different growth cartilages:

- If growth results from cell division of differentiated chondroblasts (epiphyseal cartilages of the long bones and cartilages of the synchondroses of the cranial base and nasal septum, all stemming from the primary cartilaginous skeleton of the organism), it appears to be subject to general extrinsic factors and more specifically to somatotropic hormone (STH)-somatomedin, sexual hormones, and thyroxinel. In this case the effect of local biomechanic factors is reduced to modulation of the direction of growth (with no effect on the amount of growth).

- If growth results from cell divisions of prechondroblasts (condylar, coronoid, and angular cartilages of the mandible; the midpalatal suture cartilage; and all secondary formation during phylogenesis and ontogenesis), it is somewhat subject to local extrinsic factors. In this case the amount of growth can be modulated by appropriate orthopedic devices.

Further research based on factorial quantitative analysis has led to a servosystem theory of the processes controlling postnatal craniofacial growth. According to this theory the influence of the STH-somatomedian complex on the growth of the primary cartilages (epiphyseal cartilages of the long bones, cartilages of the nasal septum and sphenoccipital synchondrosis, lateral cartilaginous masses of the ethmoid, cartilage between the body and greater wings of the sphenoid) has the cybernetic form of a command. The influence of the STH-somatomedin complex on the growth of the secondary cartilages (condylar, coronoid, and angular cartilages of the mandible; cartilages of the midpalatal suture; some other craniofacial sutures; the provisional callus during bone fracture repair; and to some extent rib growth cartilages) comprises direct and indirect effects on cell multiplication. In condylar, coronoid, and angular cartilages the indirect effects correspond to regional and local factors involving primarily neuromuscular mechanisms affecting postural occlusal adjustment (i.e., epigenetic influence) (see Figure 2-5).

Defects in mandibular growth resulting from condylectomy and resection of the pterygoid and masseter muscles and excision of the retrodiscal pad have been extensively investigated. A summary of the investigations may be found in Petrovic et al (1982b).

The sagittal growth rates of the maxilla and mandible are represented as a function of STH-somatomedin and testosterone levels within the servosystem theory (Figure 2-8). For each level of activity of the LPM the slope of the straight line for condylar cartilage growth and mandible lengthening is

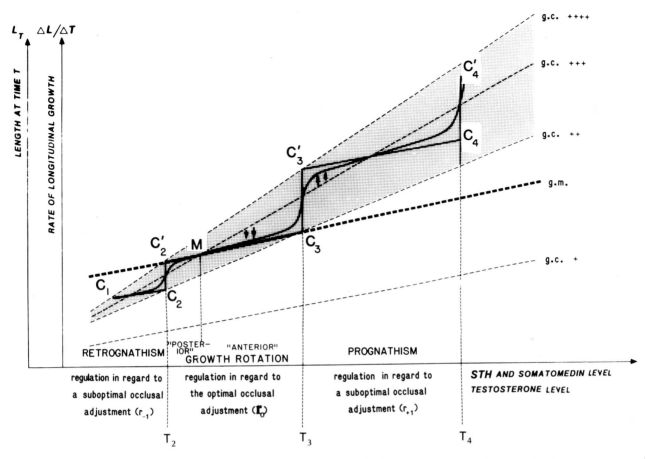

**Figure 2-8.** Semihypothetical diagram of the multiplicative interaction between STH-somatomedin or testosterone secretion rates and lateral pterygoid muscle activity on the condylar cartilage growth rate. A comparison with the action of the same hormones on septal cartilage and maxillary growth rates (bidimensional presentation of a phenomenon with three variables). *g.m.,* Lengthening of the maxilla (correlates directly with lengthening of the septal cartilage); *g.c.*+, growth of the condylar cartilage after the lateral pterygoid muscle is removed; *g.c.*++, growth of the condylar cartilage for minimal contractile activity of the lateral pterygoid muscle; *g.c.*+++, growth of the condylar cartilage for mean contractile activity of the lateral pterygoid; *g.c.*++++, growth of the condylar cartilage for maximal contractile activity of the lateral pterygoid:, position of cuspal opposition:, growth of the condylar cartilage.

greater than that required for maxillary growth (except after resection of the lateral pterygoid). In the case of the normal STH-somatomedin level and the usual contractile activity of the LPM the straight lines for maxillary and condylar cartilage growth cross at $M$. As the testosterone level varies from $T_2$ to $T_3$, the growth rate of the condylar cartilage varies from $C_2$ to $C_3$, partly as a result of the regulatory functioning of the servosystem. If the STH-somatomedin or testosterone level is greater than $T_3$, prognathism is no longer corrected because the activity of the LPM is already at a minimum. However, if the STH-somatomedin or testosterone level is lower than $T_2$, retrognathism is no longer corrected because the activity of the LPM cannot exceed its maximum.

In discussing condylar cartilage growth, two components in the servosystem are essential: the peripheral comparator, which is represented by the confrontation between the respective positions of the upper and lower dental arches, and the output (i.e., the rate and the direction of condylar carti-

lage growth). The upper dental arch is the constantly changing reference input, and the lower arch provides the controlled variable. The gain of the servosystem corresponds roughly to the coupling between the LPM activity and the iterative activity of the retrodiscal pad on one side and the rate and orientation of cell multiplication in the condylar cartilage on the other. Fossa and eminence modification must be considered.

## BIOLOGIC FEATURES OF PRIMARY AND SECONDARY CARTILAGES

In primary cartilages (e.g., epiphyseal, sphenoccipital synchondrosis, nasal septal) the chondroblasts divide and synthesize intercellular matrix (see Figures 2-2 and 2-3). In secondary cartilages (e.g., condylar, coronoid, angular, those in some craniofacial sutures) the prechondroblasts are not yet surrounded by cartilaginous matrix (see Figures 2-2 and 2-3). When the secondary prechondroblasts begin synthesizing the cartilaginous matrix, they usually stop dividing. In primary cartilages the cartilaginous matrix seems to isolate the dividing chondroblasts from local factors able to restrain or stimulate the cartilage growth rate, whereas in secondary cartilages the dividing cells are not surrounded by the cartilaginous matrix and thus not isolated from the influence of local factors. Local extrinsic factors may modify the growth rate of secondary cartilage. Experiments carried out since 1968 have demonstrated that some masticatory muscles and appropriate orthopedic appliances can modify the rate and amount of condylar cartilage growth. Experiments performed on juvenile rats were later confirmed by Demner and Nassibulin (1977), L. Graber (1975), Komposch (1978, 1991), Komposch and Hockenjos (1979), McNamara et al (1975), Stöckli and Willert (1971), and Vardimon et al (1997) on monkeys.

Because of its particular biologic features, the secondary prechondroblast is similar to the preosteoblast. Both the type II prechondroblast and the preosteoblast are able to divide. Neither the type II prechondroblast nor the preosteoblast is surrounded by intercellular matrix (cartilage or bone). When either starts to synthesize intercellular matrix, it stops dividing and becomes type II chondroblast or an osteoblast. The multiplication rate of both the type II prechondroblast and preosteoblast can be modified by intrinsic and local extrinsic factors.

## Nature of Cells Belonging to the Mitotic Compartment of Secondary Cartilage

Experiments carried out by the authors (1976, 1982) show that in vivo, cell culture, and transplantation, the mitotic compartment of secondary cartilage contains two cell varieties. The first is the skeletoblast, a fibroblast-like pluripotential stem cell originating from the embryonic mesenchymal cell. In cell culture, migrating skeletoblasts form a loose arrangement. Their intermitotic interval is relatively long (Figure 2-9). The maximum number of cell divisions may reach 60. The skeletoblast usually spontaneously differentiates into a preosteoblast, but under specific conditions, it may differentiate into a secondary prechondroblast or an osteoclast (by fusion). The second variety is the prechondroblast, a round cell originating from the skeletoblast. In cell culture, migrating prechondroblasts form a compact arrangement. Their intermitotic interval is relatively short (see Figure 2-9). The prechondroblast is a differentiated cell; it matures into only a secondary chondroblast. The maximum number of cell divisions is less than 10. Prechondroblast multiplication is controlled by general and local extrinsic or intrinsic factors. The cytoplasmic factor IV calcium ($Ca^{++}$) concentration is lower and the sodium ion ($Na^+$) concentration is higher in prechondroblasts and preosteoblasts than they are in skeletoblasts.

Investigations have shown a continuing need for the prechondroblast to perceive its environment and monitor the requirements of mass tissue in relation to those of whole condylar cartilage. If part of the chondroblast mass is lost by resection or hypertrophy and death, an increased multiplication of prechondroblasts occurs. Clearly, in such a case, signals occur that respond to a sensing of the volume of the chondroblastic zone. Short-range interactions have been detected biologically, but no regulator action has been identified.

## Condylar Cartilage Before and After Resection of the Lateral Pterygoid Muscle and Retrodiscal Pad

In the normal condylar cartilage of growing individuals, skeletoblasts multiply; some differentiate into prechondroblasts. The resection of the LPM produces a significant slowing of the condylar cartilage growth rate (Stutzmann, Petrovic, 1974ab). The skeletoblasts no longer differentiate into pre-

| | cell cycle time (Tc) | observed maximal number of cell generations (nG) |
|---|---|---|
| flattened stem cell — SKELETOBLAST | 5 to 10 days | > 30 |
| globular cell — PREOSTEOBLAST or PRECHONDROBLAST TYPE II | 1 to 2 days | < 10 |

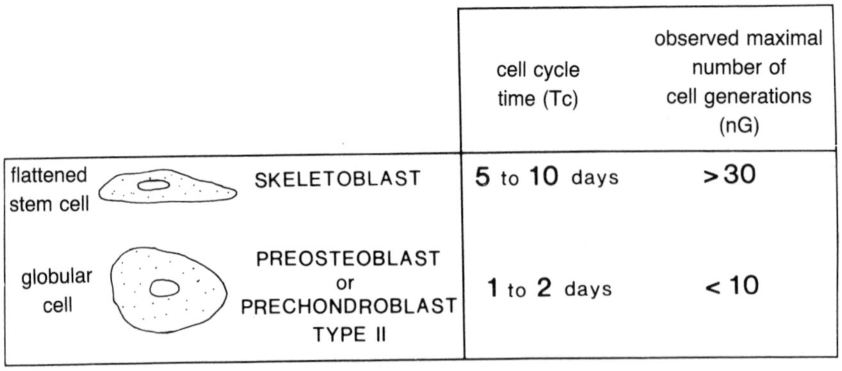

**Figure 2-9.**   The mitotic compartment of secondary cartilage contains two cell varieties. The first is a fibroblast-like pluripotential stem cell, the skeletoblast. In cell culture the cell cycle time (*Tc*) of this type is relatively long (5 to 10 days). The maximal number of cell generations (*nG*) seen is more than 30. The second variety also is a globular cell, the preosteoblast or type II prechondroblast. In cell culture the cell cycle time of this type is relatively short (1 to 2 days), and the maximum number of cell generations is less than 10.

chondroblasts. Consequently the percentage of skeletoblasts increases to the detriment of the prechondroblasts. When the maximum number of prechondroblast cell divisions reaches about 8 to 10, the stock of prechondroblasts progressively decreases. When the stock is completely exhausted, skeletoblasts begin differentiating into preosteoblasts and osteoblasts. The condyle then increases further in size through periosteal-type growth. The prechondroblasts may have an inhibiting effect on the differentiation of skeletoblasts into preosteoblasts (Figure 2-10) (Stutzmann and Petrovic, 1982, 1990).

Because these findings have elicited controversy and some misunderstanding, their proper interpretation is essential. The interruption of the circulatory dependence on the blood supply originating directly from the LPM and indirectly through the retrodiscal pad may contribute to the inhibited differentiation of skeletoblasts. Surgical excision of the retrodiscal pad and anteriorly displaced articular disks, destroying intracapsular metabolism and the metabolic pump function of the retrodiscal pad, dramatically demonstrates the mechanistic iatrogenic potential of nonphysiologic surgery. Further experimental investigations involving destruction of metabolic and catabolic functions within the TMJ have led to new findings concerning this problem (Stutzmann, Petrovic, 1990). Experimental studies have been performed on juvenile rats in an attempt to elucidate the roles of the LPM, retrodiscal pad, and postural hyperpropulsor in the control the condylar cartilage's growth rate, direction, and amount. After surgical resection of the LPM the growth of the condylar cartilage and lengthening of the mandible continue but are significantly decreased. Also, the potential stimulating effect of postural hyperpropulsion on condylar cartilage and mandibular growth is much less intense after the resection of the LPM.

The retrodiscal pad is at least partly a physiologic mediator of the LPM because the blood supply is through the LPM. After surgical resection of the retrodiscal tissue, the growth of the condylar cartilage and lengthening of the mandible con-

tinue at a significantly diminished rate. The effect of the functioning retrodistal attachment on mandibular growth seems to have both a blood-circulating and biomechanic component (Stutzmann, Petrovic, 1990).

The blood-circulating effect of the retrodiscal pad is relatively easy to understand: an intensification of activity is associated with an increase in blood flow and lymph flow (i.e., an increase in the open-loop nutritive and growth-stimulating factor supply (STH-somatomedin, testosterone and estrogen in low doses, insulin, prostaglandin $F_2$, mitogenic peptides) and a decrease in locally produced cell catabolites and other negative feedback factors (the prechondroblast's multiplication-restraining signal, cyclic adenosine monophosphate [cAMP], and prostaglandin $E_2$, a somatostatin-like substance). These iterative changes account at least partly for the supplementary growth of the condylar cartilage produced by functional appliances. In ultrasoft nipple–fed newborn rats the retrodiscal pad is found to be morphologically less developed than that observed in breastfed rats. Positron emission tomography (PET) scans of these rats revealed notably decreased blood flow. Reduction of nutrient supply to the retrodiscal pad and condylar head has obviously deleterious consequences.

The biomechanic effect of the retrodiscal pad is more difficult to understand. It is probably partly responsible for posterior growth rotation and supplementary lengthening of the mandible (Paulsen, 1996) because of increased bone apposition at the posterior border of the ramus (Stutzmann, Petrovic, 1990). Research investigations strongly suggest the following explanation for the biomechanic effect (Figure 2-11). The increase of the condylar cartilage growth rate and more posterior growth direction of the condyle therapeutically induced with functional appliances correspond to the accentuation of the concavity of the ramus' posterior border. As a result of piezoelectric and other effects, an increase of negative electric charges occurs along the posterior border of the ra-

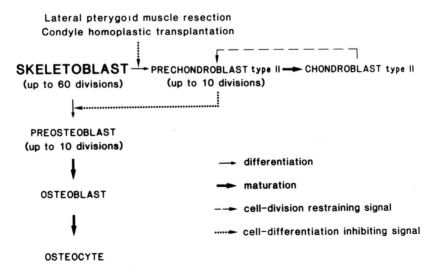

**Figure 2-10.** Double differentiating potential of skeletoblasts. According to local biologic conditions, skeletoblasts may differentiate into type II prechondroblasts or preosteoblasts.

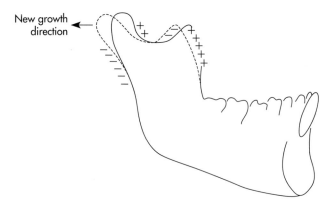

New growth
direction

**Figure 2-11.** The retrodiscal pad controls mandibular growth in two ways. Its vascular component controls the condylar cartilage growth rate and endochondral ossification rate; an increase in iterative activity of the retrodiscal pad produces an increase in condylar cartilage growth and endochondral ossification. Its biomechanic component governs bone apposition and condylar growth direction at the posterior border of the ramus. An increase in iterative activity of the retrodiscal pad produces an accentuation of the ramus' posterior concavity and a local increase in bone apposition and the number of negative charges at the ramus' posterior concave surface. It also produces an accentuation of the ramus' anterior convexity and a local increase in bone resorption and the number of positive charges at the ramus' posterior convex surface.

mus, producing increased periosteal bone formation, and, reciprocally, the anterior border becomes more electropositive (with increased bone resorption). This causal chain may account for the supplementary lengthening of the mandible produced by functional appliances. It gives some support to the interpretation that the functional appliance–induced increased contractile activity of the LPM causes local bone resorption and not bone formation. Nevertheless, the mechanisms of piezoelectric and other effects have still to be properly investigated.

## Condylar Cartilage After Homoplastic Transplantation into the Rat's Testis or Anterior Chamber of the Eye

After intratesticular or intraocular transplantation the condyle undergoes histologic modifications similar to those observed after resection of the LPM (see Figure 2-10). The mitotic compartment contains mostly skeletoblasts 3 weeks after transplantation. A few prechondroblasts continue to divide before becoming chondroblasts, and a few skeletoblasts start differentiating into osteoblasts. The mitotic compartment consists of only skeletoblasts 5 weeks after transplantation; these later differentiate exclusively into preosteoblasts and osteoblasts. Reduced metabolic activity is an important factor.

## Development of the Rat's Midpalatal Suture

The double differentiating potentiality of the skeletoblast also has been indicated clearly in the rat midpalatal suture.

The intermaxillary portion of the fast-growing midpalatal suture includes secondary cartilage. During this growth period the skeletoblasts differentiate exclusively into prechondroblasts, however, from the age of 37 to 40 days, as the growth rate slows, the skeletoblasts begin to differentiate into preosteoblasts. Accordingly the cartilaginous suture becomes a boneline suture, similar to the other craniofacial sutures. If growth at the midpalatal suture is restrained experimentally before the age of 37 to 40 days by either local mechanical constraint or resection of the primary cartilages between the body and greater wings of the sphenoid and lateral cartilaginous masses of the ethmoid, skeletoblasts differentiate into preosteoblasts instead of prechondroblasts.

## Homology Between the Preosteoblastic Layer of the Mandibular Periosteum and the Prechondroblastic Layer of the Condylar Cartilage

At the boundary between the condylar cartilage and the condylar periosteum, skeletoblasts stop differentiating into prechondroblasts belonging to the mitotic compartment of the condylar cartilage and begin differentiating into preosteoblasts belonging to the subperiosteal layer of the condyle. Researchers have studied the response of the growing rat after resection of the condylar cartilage, superior head of the LPM, disc, and retrodiscal pad with the condylar bone remaining intact. Initially, skeletoblasts originating from the subperiosteal layer multiply, migrate, and eventually completely cover the resected surface. Then, if no inflammation has occurred and mandibular mobility is maintained, the newly formed skeletoblasts differentiate locally into secondary cartilage. To some extent this newly formed condylar cartilage corresponds to cartilage formed temporarily during fracture repair. However, growth intensity is reduced because of the limited metabolic nutrients supplied by the compromised blood supply.

## Growth Hormone and its Mediators—Mode of Action on Different Varieties of Cartilage

Investigations carried out in the Strasbourg laboratory since 1967 have demonstrated the following:

1. The growth of the epiphyseal cartilage of the long bones, cartilage of the sphenoccipital synchondroses, lateral cartilaginous masses of the ethmoid, and cartilage between the body and greater wings of the sphenoid (all of which stem from the primary cartilaginous skeleton of the organism) is subject to general extrinsic factors and the effects of STH-somatomedin. In this case, orthopedic devices can modify the direction but not the amount of growth.
2. The growth of condylar, coronoid, and angular cartilages of the mandible; cartilage in some cranial sutures; and cartilage in the postfracture callus (all secondarily formed during phylogenesis and ontogenesis) is subject to local extrinsic (epigenetic) factors and the effects of

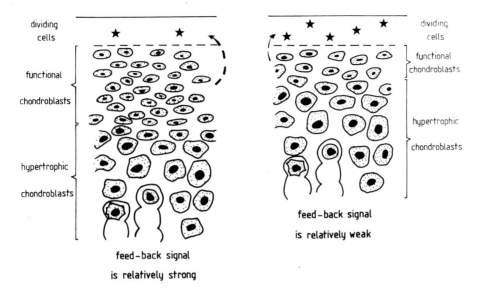

**Figure 2-12.** Intrinsic regulation of the condylar cartilage growth rate. Variations in the rate of chondroblastic hypertrophy and subsequent variations in prechondroblastic multiplication result from a restraining feedback signal.

STH-somatomedin. In this latter case, appropriate orthopedic devices may modify both the direction and amount of growth (Burdi, 1995).

## Intrinsic Regulation of the Condylar Cartilage Growth Rate

Experimental studies have shown the existence of an intrinsic regulatory mechanism for the condylar cartilage growth rate. Variations of cell density cannot completely account for this finding. In other words a negative feedback signal originates from the proximal part of the chondroblastic zone and exerts a restraining effect on the prechondroblastic multiplication rate (Figure 2-12). The concept of an intrinsic regulation of the condylar cartilage growth rate can help explain the effects of some orthopedic or orthodontic appliances and of a hormone such as thyroxine: the earlier commencement of chondroblastic hypertrophy and the subsequent decrease in the prechondroblast division–restraining signal appear to be important intermediary steps in the growth-stimulating effect of Class II elastics, the mandibular postural hyperpropulsor, and similar appliances. The acceleration of the chondroblastic maturation rate is similarly an intermediary step for the growth rate–stimulating effect of thyroxine (Stutzmann, Petrovic, 1975b, 1979).

## Osteochondral Rib Transplant

Whether an osteochondral rib transplant is an appropriate biologic substitute for condylar cartilage in the surgical treatment of temporomandibular ankylosis is an important research question. Human rib cartilage near the sternum is composed of cells designated *precursor chondroblasts* (Petrovic, 1984a) (Figures 2-13 and 2-14). In the postnatal period these cells become quiescent; mitoses are infrequent. Nevertheless,

in cell culture, each precursor chondroblast may divide 35 to 50 times. During the growth period, a few millimeters from the osteochondral junction, the precursor chondroblast differentiates into a cell Petrovic calls a *progenitor chondroblast*. After it is fully differentiated, each progenitor chondroblast divides no more than 8 to 11 times, but cell division occurs at short intervals. The chondroblasts issuing from a progenitor chondroblast produce a pyramid-like structure that is a component of the primary growth cartilage of the rib. The cartilage matrix surrounding the cells issuing from the progenitor chondroblast is biochemically different from the matrix surrounding the precursor chondroblasts.

Using rib cartilage fragments removed from growing children (2 to 14 years old) during surgery, the authors performed several organ culture experiments that produced provocative observations (Figure 2-15). When an osteochondral junction fragment was exposed to light pressure, the cells belonging to the area in which precursor chondroblasts differentiate into progenitor chondroblasts displayed the following variations compared with identical rib fragments cultivated as controls:

1. Intracellular concentrations of $Na^+$ tended to decrease.
2. Intracellular concentrations of $Ca^{++}$ and hydrogen ions ($H^+$) tended to increase.
3. Intracellular pH was lowered.
4. $Na^+$ and potassium ion ($K^+$)-adenosine triphosphatase activity was intensified.
5. $Ca^{++}$, $Mg^{++}$-ATPase, and $H^+$-adenosine triphosphatase activities were diminished.
6. The numbers of cell divisions declined slightly and demonstrated a significant slowing of the growth rate.

When the juvenile human or rat condylar cartilage was exposed in organ culture to an identical pressure, similar but much more pronounced variations were observed. However, such variations were never detected in the growth cartilage of

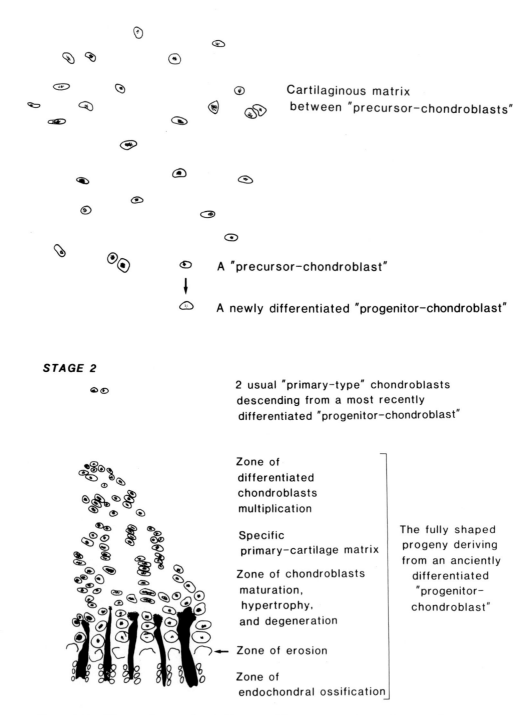

**STAGE 1**

Cartilaginous matrix
between "precursor-chondroblasts"

A "precursor-chondroblast"

A newly differentiated "progenitor-chondroblast"

**STAGE 2**

2 usual "primary-type" chondroblasts
descending from a most recently
differentiated "progenitor-chondroblast"

Zone of
differentiated
chondroblasts
multiplication

Specific
primary-cartilage matrix

Zone of chondroblasts
maturation,
hypertrophy,
and degeneration

Zone of erosion

Zone of
endochondral ossification

The fully shaped
progeny deriving
from an anciently
differentiated
"progenitor-
chondroblast"

**Figure 2-13.** Human rib osteochondral junction. The two stages observed in the differentiation of precursor chondroblasts into progenitor chondroblasts.

**STAGE 3**

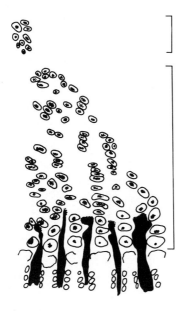

A new-formed progeny originating
from a recently differentiated
"progenitor-chondroblast"

The completed progeny of
an anciently differentiated
"progenitor-chondroblast"

**STAGE 4**

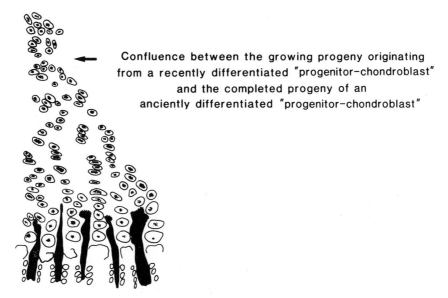

Confluence between the growing progeny originating
from a recently differentiated "progenitor-chondroblast"
and the completed progeny of an
anciently differentiated "progenitor-chondroblast"

**Figure 2-14.**   Final two stages in the differentiation in the progeny of progenitor chondroblasts.

| | Mandibular Condylar Cartilage | Callus Cartilage | Osteochondral Junction of the Rib | | | Growth Cartilages of Long Bones, Metatarsals, Metacarpals, Sphenooccipital Synchondrosis |
| --- | --- | --- | --- | --- | --- | --- |
| | | | Area of precursor chondroblasts | Area of differentiation of precursor chondroblasts into progenitor chondroblasts | Area of primary chondroblast differentiation from progenitor chondroblasts | |
| Membrane-linked activity $Na^+$ and $K^+$ adenosine triphosphatase $Ca^{++}$ and $Mg^{++}$ adenosine triphosphatase $H^+$ adenosine triphosphatase | ↗ ↘ ↘ | ↗ ↘ ↘ | --→ --→ --→ | ↗ ↘ ↘ | --→ --→ --→ | --→ --→ --→ |
| Cytosolic concentration $Na^+$ $Ca^{++}$ $H^+$ | ↘ ↗ ↗ | ↘ ↗ ↗ | --→ --→ --→ | ↘ ↗ ↗ | --→ --→ --→ | --→ --→ --→ |
| Intracellular pH | ↘ | ↘ | --→ | ↘ | --→ | --→ |
| Cell volume | ↘ | ↘ | --→ | ↘ | --→ | --→ |
| Intracellular water content | ↘ | ↘ | --→ | ↘ | --→ | --→ |
| Intracellular cAMP | ↗ | ↗ | --→ | ↗ | --→ | --→ |
| Number of cell divisions | ↘ | ↘ | --→ | ↘ | --→ | --→ |

→ Strong variation          → Moderate variation          --→ No significant variation

**Figure 2-15.** Schematic representation of the effects of appropriate continuous pressure on cells belonging to the mitotic compartment of human and animal (rat, mouse, guinea pig, rabbits, squirrel monkey) cartilage placed in organ culture. Only callus cartilage and the area of differentiation of precursor chondroblasts into progenitor chondroblasts exhibit biologic behavior similar to the behavior of the mitotic compartment of the condylar cartilage.

the metatarsal, tibia, fibula, radius, and cubitus (endochondral bone) (Petrovic, 1982, 1984a). In other words the differentiation rate of the precursor chondroblast into a progenitor chondroblast is submitted not only to the command represented by genetic, hormonal, and humoral factors but also to local regulation that includes regional epigenetic biomechanic factors. This finding implies that an autologous osteochondral rib transplant is preferable to a metatarsal cartilage transplant in the treatment of temporomandibular ankylosis and similar conditions in which a substitute for the condylar cartilage is required. This finding also implies that the rib transplant must include a sufficient portion of precursor chondroblasts, which are able to divide 35 to 50 times and whose growth rate is modifiable by local biomechanic factors as the cell reaches the transient stage of differentiation into the progenitor chondroblast. However, this is not always the case, as Rabie (1996) shows.

## CONTROL OF MAXILLARY GROWTH

The increase in length of the maxilla in mammals is caused by growth at the premaxillomaxillary and maxillopalatine sutures and by subperiosteal deposition of bone in the anterior region. The premaxillomaxillary suture persists much longer in young rats and monkeys than it does in humans. Therefore its participation in the forward growth of the upper jaw ceases much later in rats and monkeys than it does in human children. In all cases the stem cell skeletoblast differentiates into a preosteoblast, and the preosteoblast multiplies and becomes an osteoblast which surrounds itself with bone matrix and becomes an osteocyte. The increase in width of the maxilla is attributed to growth at the midpalatal suture and bone deposition along the lateral areas of the alveolar ridge. In the young, rapidly growing rat the midpalatal suture is unusual; it is composed of secondary cartilage on each side of the median line.

In this case the skeletoblast differentiates into a prechondroblast, and the prechondroblast divides and matures into a secondary chondroblast; the cartilage formed is later replaced by bone.

The mechanisms controlling the growth of the upper jaw are presently under investigation. Divergence of opinion exists on several points:

1. According to Prahl (1968) and Weinmann and Sicher (1955) sutural tissue has an autonomous growth potential. However, according to M.L. Moss (1962, 1995), Persson (1973), Petrovic et al (1969, 1991), and Scott (1956), sutural growth is subject to extrinsic factors.
2. According to Baume (1961), Kvinnsland (1974), Petrovic et al (1969), Ronning (1971), Scott (1953), and Wexler and Sarnat (1961), the growth of the nasal septal cartilage constitutes an important factor in the control mechanisms of vertical and horizontal facial growth, including that of the maxilla. This opinion is not shared by Melsen et al (1981) and Moss (1976, 1995).
3. According to Scott (1967) the cartilage of the midpalatal suture is capable of separating adjacent bones. However, according to Stutzmann and Petrovic the separation of the horizontal processes of the two maxillae stimulates the growth of this suture.

As represented by the functional diagram in Figure 2-4, STH-somatomedin, testosterone, and estrogen play primary roles in the extrinsic control of postnatal growth of the upper jaw. Their effects are both direct and indirect.

## Direct Effect

The direct effect represents almost the entire influence of STH-somatomedin on the growth of the sphenoccipital synchondrosis and nasal septal cartilage, the lateral masses of the ethmoid bone, and between the body and greater wings of the sphenoid. A small part of the effect of STH-somatomedin on the growth of the cranial and facial sutures is a direct effect; in these areas, STH-somatomedin has a direct effect primarily on the responsiveness of the preosteoblasts to regional and local factors, stimulating the skeletal cell multiplication rate. In areas composed of secondary cartilage the direct effect of STH-somatomedin is seen in both the multiplication and responsiveness of the prechondroblasts.

## Indirect Effect

The indirect effects of STH-somatomedin occur through a number of intermediaries. They are discussed in the following paragraphs.

**Forward growth of the septal cartilage.** The forward growth of the septal cartilage in the rat produces a forward shift of the premaxillary bone that leads to an increase in the growth of the premaxillomaxillary suture and to a lesser extent that of the maxillopalatal suture. It also results in a forward traction by means of the septopremaxillary ligament and the labionarinary muscles on the anterior end of the premaxilla, resulting in local stimulation of bone growth. This phenomenon has functional implications.

*Thrust effect.* The anterior extremity of the nasal septal cartilage spreads laterally on both sides of the median line in an anteroinferior direction to penetrate directly into the premaxillary bone. Such a configuration supports the hypothesis that forward growth of the nasal septal cartilage produces a sufficient thrust on the premaxillary bone to stimulate the growth of the premaxillomaxillary suture and to a lesser extent that of the maxillopalatal suture. The thrust effect on the premaxillary bone consists of a histologic traction component represented by collagen fibers connecting the cartilage and bone trabeculae located immediately behind it.

*Septopremaxillary ligament traction effect.* The study of human fetuses led Latham (1970) to formulate the hypothesis that forward growth of the nasal septal cartilage has a traction effect on the premaxillary bone through the septopremaxillary ligament. According to studies of the septopremaxillary ligaments of young rats (Stutzmann, Petrovic, 1976, 1978a) the number of dividing preosteoblasts and the level of osteoblastic activity are significantly greater where this ligament contacts the premaxillary bone. In any case the histologic characteristics of the septopremaxillary ligament imply that this ligament is hardly able to provide necessary traction on the premaxillary bone to produce increased growth at the premaxillomaxillary suture. In other words, histologically it is misnamed a ligament.

Findings after resection of the septopremaxillary ligament in young rats clearly show that a stimulating action on growth at the premaxillomaxillary suture must be excluded. However, the ligament does seem to have a local, induction-like, stimulating effect on subperiosteal growth.

*Labionarinary muscle traction effect.* The forward growth of the septal cartilage produces a forward traction on the premaxillary bone through the labionarinary muscles, resulting in a biomechanic promotion of the forward growth of the upper jaw. In humans the absence of labial muscle attachment on the nasal septum in cleft lip could be responsible for bone malformations. Surgical reattachment of the orbicularis oris and alar muscles is an essential part of the repair of cleft lip and palate (Delaire, 1961, 1978; Delaire, Chateau, 1977).

Unilateral resection of the labionarinary muscles in the young rat produces a unilaterally decreased forward growth on the operated side. On the opposite side the outward growth of the premaxilla is slightly increased.

Experimental investigations in young rats on the mechanisms of action of the Fränkel appliance (Table 2-1) show that the superior labial frenum and labionarinary muscles are the mediators of the superior retrolabial lip pads (Fränkel retrolabial vestibular shields) in their stimulating effects on sagittal growth of the maxilla.

**TABLE 2-1. • EFFECTS OF THE FRVS ON SAGITTAL GROWTH OF THE UPPER JAW***

| Experimental Group | Surgical Interventions | | | Standard Error |
| --- | --- | --- | --- | --- |
| | No Operation | Resection of Labial Frenum | Resection of Labial Frenum and Labionarinary Muscle | |
| **Mean dividing cell index at the anterior extremity of premaxillary bone (%)†** | | | | |
| FRVS | 29.65 | 22.40 | 14.40 | |
| No appliance | 17.04 | 15.37 | 13.68 | 1.3976 |
| **Mean length of the premaxillomaxillary suture (as measured by the distance between two visible tetracycline-labeled surfaces on each side of the suture) (mm)‡** | | | | |
| FRVS | 1.80 | 1.74 | 0.95 | |
| No appliance | 1.30 | 1.28 | 0.90 | 0.0487 |
| **Mean length of the maxillopalatal suture (as measured by the distance between two visible tetracycline-labeled surfaces on each side of the suture) (mm)§** | | | | |
| FRVS | 0.79 | 0.76 | 0.35 | |
| No appliance | 0.60 | 0.60 | 0.32 | 0.011 |
| **Mean length of the jaw (mm)‖** | | | | |
| FRVS | 18.14 | 17.49 | 14.90 | |
| No appliance | 16.66 | 16.27 | 14.74 | 0.0996 |

*A total of 12 48-day-old male rats were in each group.

†Smallest significant difference between two means: 5% level, 2.79; 1% level, 3.71; 0.1% level, 4.81.

‡Smallest significant difference between two means: 5% level, 0.10; 1% level, 0.13; 0.1% level, 0.17.

§Smallest significant difference between two means: 5% level, 0.02; 1% level, 0.03; 0.1% level, 0.04.

‖Smallest significant difference between two means: 5% level, 0.19; 1% level, 0.26; 0.1% level, 0.34.

**Outward growth—effects of Fränkel lateral vestibular shields on widening of the upper jaw.** The outward growth of the lateral cartilaginous masses of the ethmoid and the cartilage between the body and greater wings of the sphenoid produces a lateralization of the alveolar ridges on both the left and right sides; this in turn stimulates the growth of the midpalatal suture (i.e., the outward growth of the maxilla) (see Figure 2-4).

Experimental findings reported by Stutzmann et al (1983) demonstrate that the Fränkel lateral vestibular shields (FLVS) produce an enhanced and supplementary widening of the upper jaw. This was corroborated by Graber et al in 1991. The appliance acts by stimulating midpalatal suture growth and to a lesser extent by increasing bone apposition on the external subperiosteal layer of the maxilla. Another effect of the buccal shields stressed by Fränkel is their influence on the eruptive path of the succedaneous teeth at a critical time in their development. The relief of pressure from the cheeks in the dentoalveolar area seems to allow a more downward and outward eruptive path at a time of maximal viability, permitting horizontal and vertical adjustment of the osseous tissues involved.

The stimulating effect on sutural growth can be observed even after the cartilaginous midpalatal suture has become a bony suture (i.e., when it is in a phase of less rapid growth). The results are similar in nature but not in extent. Indeed, the effect is proportionally more intense during the period from day 20 to 48 of the rat's life span, a prepubertal period when suture growth is naturally more rapid, than during the

period from day 40 to 180, when sutural growth progressively slows. In extrapolating this result to human beings, researchers have noted that the period coincides with the transitional period before puberty, when Fränkel feels the greatest potential exists for width increase. In other words the greatest change occurs during the period encompassing the tooth exchange time.

At the end of the experimental period (180 days) when all growth is finished, the width of the upper jaw remains greater in animals treated with lateral vestibular shields than it does in nontreated ones. The supplementary widening of the upper jaw persists and seems stable after growth is completed. The results clearly demonstrate that the three investigated factors are differentially involved in the spontaneous lateral growth of the upper jaw.

The lateral vestibular sulcus seems to play only a minor role; after bilateral sectioning, lateral growth is only slightly affected. This same observation has been made in the study of *Saimiri scirius* monkeys by Graber (1983c), who found that vestibular shields initially enhanced proliferation in the sulcus after appliance placement (a possible adaptation) but that their effects disappeared quickly, with less activity subperiosteally than in the alveolar process covering the buccal surfaces of the posterior teeth. Significantly greater proliferation occurred in the experimental animals in this area than in the controls; this proliferation remained stable, as shown in the rat study.

Although studies indicate that the sulcus area is not a major growth area regardless of the resection of sulcular tissue, little doubt exists that the cheeks and tongue influence jaw growth. Under normal conditions a dynamic balance exists between the restraining buccinator mechanism on the outside (the cheeks) and the tongue on the inside; the tongue exerts a positive outward pressure both during rest and active function. Research has shown that any perturbation of this balance, produced by either resection of the cheek muscles or a reduced tongue mass, modifies the lateral growth of the upper jaw. Thus the resection of the cheeks favors bone deposition on the external subperiosteal layer of the maxilla and the outward thrust effect of the functioning tongue on the contiguous buccal segments, resulting in significant supplemental upper jaw widening. A narrowed or reduced tongue produced by surgical stenoglossia no longer exerts a sufficient outward thrust on the adjacent molar segments to maintain the usual growth of the midpalatal suture. The wearing of lingual shields also reduces the outward thrust effect of the tongue, which may affect the eruption of the succedaneous teeth, because the tendency is to erupt in a more vertical inclination and lingual direction if tongue pressure is reduced or absent.

Nevertheless, the effect produced by surgical narrowing of the tongue on the widening of the upper jaw is less pronounced than that elicited by the wearing of lateral lingual shields. Indeed, when the volume of the tongue was experimentally reduced in growing rats (i.e., when either the longitudinal dimension [partial glossectomy] [Stutzmann, Petrovic, 1976] or the transverse dimension [experimental stenoglossal] was changed), with time the tongue presented the tendency to recover its usual position. The partial glossectomy that had been done in previous experiments was repeated 2 weeks after the initial operation. For technical reasons the experimental stenoglossia was not redone. After several weeks the increased transverse dimension of the tongue was great enough to exert again an outward thrust on the two molar groups and stimulate midpalatal suture growth. This happened even after this suture had become a bony type. Consequently, 4 weeks after the operation, no difference could be found in midpalatal suture growth rates between the control group and the stenoglossia group. This finding implies that for therapeutic purposes, the surgical reduction of tongue volume is justified only in the presence of genuine macroglossia.

Quantitative analysis revealed an amplification type of interaction between the morphologic factors investigated and vestibular shield treatment. Quantitative experimentation such as this is useful as a statistical tool for establishing the existence of possible interactions between different physiologic factors and between these factors and specific functional or fixed types of orthodontic appliances.

These experiments demonstrated beyond any doubt that the effect of lateral vestibular shields on the transverse growth of the maxilla is relayed, partly through passive resistance against the pressure of the buccinators and the anterior portion of the masseters and partly through the tension created in the vestibular sulcus. Clearly if the pressure of the tongue on the two molar groups is usual (i.e., if no stenoglossia has been surgically created and no lingual shields are in place), the re-

sult is significantly increased transverse growth of the maxilla without the potentially iatrogenic "suture splitting" too often employed.

Quantitative analysis shows that if one of the three factors investigated in this study (tongue, vestibular sulcus, cheek muscles) was modified, the appliance-produced effect on the widening of the maxilla was of similar magnitude. However, depending on the factor that was experimentally modified, the appliance-produced supplementary widening of the upper jaw resulted either from supplementary growth of the midpalatal suture only or from both a supplementary growth of the midpalatal suture and supplementary bone apposition on the lateral vestibular side of the maxilla.

Only if the two opposing factors (pressure of the tongue on one side and pressure of the buccinators and anterior portion of the masseters on the other) were modified simultaneously did the appliance become ineffective. In this case the tension of the sulcus from the wearing of vestibular shields was insufficient to stimulate the growth rate of the midpalatal suture and produce a supplementary widening of the upper jaw.

In animals in which the buccinators and the anterior portion of the masseters were bilaterally resected, the wearing of lateral vestibular shields produced a supplementary widening of the upper jaw; however, the sutural contribution appears to have been meager and new bone apposition on the vestibular side of the maxilla was hardly different from that observed in the reference animals. This apparent contradiction may be tentatively explained in the following two ways:

1. Because the ³H-methyl-thymidine–labeled preosteoblast index is a "snapshot" only of occurrences during the hour before sacrifice, researchers can assume that in this experimental variety the sum of the snapshots during the 4 weeks after the onset of the experiment is sufficient to account for the appliance-produced additional widening of the maxilla.
2. Researchers also can assume that the tension effect of the sulcus is more operative immediately after the muscle resection than it is at the end of the experiment. Indeed, postoperative edema probably made the sulcus less elastic, and thus its pulling effect was increased during this transient period.

These two tentative explanations are not mutually exclusive.

Finally, this study was certainly not an exhaustive one with regard to factors involved in the aberrant morphology and correction of the transverse dimension. For instance, previous investigations in growing rats had shown that the number of dividing cells in the midpalatal suture is much higher in the oral region than it is in the nasal region but that this difference tends to decrease after removal of the nasal septal cartilage. After the cartilage is removed, the transverse growth of the upper jaw is slightly (but still significantly) reduced, and even the appositional bone on the oral surface of the palate (as revealed by tetracycline labeling) is slowed. In other words, further investigations on the potential lateral expansion and mechanical action of the Fränkel appliance should take into account the role of the septal cartilage.

Reported findings help illustrate the mechanism of maxillary widening produced by the Fränkel appliance. They display the complexity of the appliance's action at the tissue level. Above all, they provide a conceptual tool for the clinician facing the common problem of the narrow maxillary arch.

## CONTROL OF MANDIBULAR GROWTH

Growth control involves a multitude of factors. These factors do not form independent causal chains. Rather, the interaction that occurs among them is often highly important. For this reason, these factors are usually studied together whenever possible so that their possible interactions can be detected.

Any research investigation on the control mechanisms of craniofacial growth should take into account not only local and regional extrinsic factors (tissue contacts, muscles, blood supply, and nerve signals) but also general factors (STH-somatomedin, thyroxine, and sex hormones). Moreover, previous researchers have found the simultaneous study of both the effects of these hormones and effects caused by regional and local extrinsic factors to be indispensable. For instance, the roles of STH-somatomedin and nasal septal cartilage in the lengthening of the upper jaw cannot be studied separately; indeed, the effect of STH-somatomedin is relayed and expressed through the forward growth of the nasal septal cartilage (Stutzmann, Petrovic, 1976). In addition, growth hormone–somatomedin and testosterone or estrogen have not only direct effects on condylar cartilage growth but also indirect ones. Both the magnitude and direction of condylar growth present quantitative variations in response to physiologic stimuli or experimentally or therapeutically implanted lip pads that produce changes in the sagittal growth of the maxilla. As long as growth variations do not exceed a certain limit, no significant alterations in the sagittal relationship of the dental arches occur. Effective operation of the servosystem can take place only through slow, gradual changes.

### Servosystem Theory of Facial Growth

The variation in direction and magnitude of condylar growth is partly a quantitative response to experimentally effected changes in the lengthening of the maxilla. Variations in maxillary growth may be induced through resection of the nasal septal cartilage or administration of growth hormone or testosterone or by orthopedic appliances. As long as growth alteration does not exceed a certain limit, no significant changes in the sagittal relationship of the dental arches occur (see Figure 2-5). This action can be considered part of a servosystem in which the upper dental arch is the constantly changing reference input and the lower arch is the controlled variable. Effective operation of the servosystem can take place only through gradual changes between the dental arches.

The operation of confrontation between the dental arches elicits in certain cases a deviation signal that modifies the activity of the LPM and other muscles of mastication, allowing the mandible to adjust to the optimal occlusal position. This change in LPM activity probably influences the growth rate of the condylar cartilage. To some extent, experimental devices (e.g., mandibular protraction, Class II elastics) can elicit similar condylar responses. The hyperpropulsor positions the reference input in a more anterior direction. After an experimentally induced latent period the growth rate increases relative to the degree of appliance activation. The receptors associated with the deviation signal are therefore involved with the regulation of condylar growth. Although little research has been conducted on this aspect of receptor function, clearly the elicited signal not only causes an improvement in masticatory function but also synchronizes the growth between the maxilla and mandible during the entire developmental period of the facial skeleton.

The physiologic adaptation of mandibular length to maxillary length occurs through a variation in both growth rate and direction of the condylar cartilage. Growth hormone–somatomedin affects the lengthening of the mandible (through condylar growth) to a greater extent than it affects the lengthening of the maxilla (see Figure 2-5). If this hormonal effect remains within physiologic limits, the occlusion is not significantly altered, because a concomitant reduction in the angle between the ramus and corpus decreases the length of the mandible. The explanation for the adjustment mechanism may be found in the servosystem.

Another clinically important observation seen in growing children should be reported: in anterior growth rotation, both the subperiosteal ossification rate and alveolar bone turnover are generally increased; in posterior growth rotation, they are decreased. Because the subperiosteal ossification rate usually parallels the condylar cartilage growth rate, this finding may account for a greater responsiveness to orthopedic and orthodontic appliances in cases of anterior growth rotation.

The elastic retrodiscal pad and its condylar attachment (Figure 2-16) are predominant intermediaries between the variations of LPM activity and the growth of the condylar cartilage (see Figure 2-5) in rats and humans. If the LPM is missing or nonfunctional, direct, repetitive stimulation of the retrodiscal pad elicits the same condylar response as if the muscle were intact. However, physiologically the LPM appears essential for fine occlusal adjustment. This newly discovered role of the retrodiscal pad helps explain the way Class II elastics increase the condylar cartilage growth rate, provided the mandible is not immobilized in the protruded position. Adequate blood supply and function are essential.

The peripheral comparator (see Figure 2-5) adjusts the sagittal anterior growth of the facial skeleton so that an optimal (or suboptimal) occlusal relationship is maintained between the upper and lower incisors, canines, and molar cusps. Such relationships correspond to a stable situation for masticatory function. The transposition from one stable situation to another is accompanied by a physiologic discontinuity (i.e., a topologic, bifurcation-type instability [see Figure 2-6] whose critical point lies in the edge-to-edge or cusp-to-cusp relationship; this instability corresponds to the repeller). Lack of interdental contacts corresponds to the absence of stable and unstable bifurcation-type situations.

The existence of bifurcation-type situations at the periph-

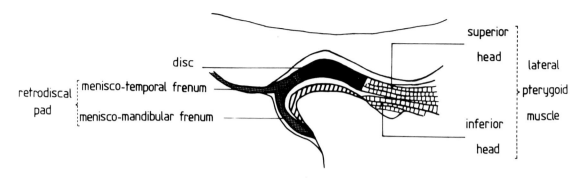

**Figure 2-16.**   Sagittal section of the temporomandibular joint of the rat.

eral comparator of the servosystem implies that facial growth should be accounted for by using unpredetermined and discontinuous models rather than deterministic, continuous ones. This precept also applies to models designed for growth forecasting in orthodontic practice but is ignored too often.

The existence of bifurcation-type situations at the peripheral comparator also makes intelligible the evidence that the genome only partially determines the phenome. Indeed, a given genome codes not for a single phenotype but for a regulatory pattern. In other words, at critical moments of facial development, small fluctuations around the bifurcation can produce different types of occlusal relationships. This situation is observed in orthodontic practice most often in patients between 8 and 10 years old. Mixed dentition therapy is thus strongly supported biologically. Obviously the cybernetic theory of facial growth and the crucial topologic concept of structural and functional stability and instability are highly useful in a systematic and increasingly computerized approach to clinical situations.

In addition to the peripheral comparator, a central comparator of the servosystem also has been described (see Figure 2-5). The reference for this is a sensory engram for the postural activity of the masticatory muscles corresponding to a habitual anteroposterior mandibular position. This engram develops from repeated mandibular posturing for which the minimal deviation signal of the peripheral receptors results. This posturing has occasionally been called the *postural rest position.* Such an engram allows the detection and correction of deviations from optimal or suboptimal occlusal position.

## Postural Hyperpropulsor

Appropriate functional appliances that place the rat mandible in a forward postural position increase the condylar cartilage growth rate and amount. During the growth period the sagittal deviation produced by the postural hyperpropulsor decreases through the supplementary forward growth of the mandible. This implies that the deviation signal simultaneously decreases; in other words the supplementary growth rate of the conylar cartilage and supplementary lengthening of the mandible also decrease. Periodic increases in the thickness of the postural hyperpropulsor produce increases in LPM activity and in the activity of the retrodiscal pad as recorded electromyographically; these, consequently, bring

about increases in the rate and amount of condylar cartilage growth. If the appliance is removed after the growth of the animal is completed, little or no relapse is observed. If the appliance is removed before growth is completed, no significant relapse is detected if a good intercuspation is achieved during the experimental phase. However, if a good intercuspation is not achieved, the comparator of the servosystem imposes an increased or decreased condylar growth rate until a state of intercuspal stability is established. Functional maxipropulsion involving periodic forward repositioning appears to be the best procedure for eliciting a supplementary lengthening of the mandible. No genetically predetermined final length of the mandible has been detected in these experiments (see Chapter 1).

If a young rat is fitted with a postural hyperpropulsor and similar functional appliances for 10 to 12 hours daily, changes occur as if the upper dental arch (the constantly changing reference input) were in a more anterior position than is actually the case (see Figure 2-5). The confrontation between the dental arches then produces a deviation signal that is reduced by an appropriate forward positioning of the lower dental arch through the propulsion of the mandible. The increased contractile activity of the LPM produces supplementary growth in the condylar cartilage and a subsequent supplementary lengthening of the mandible. With time this supplementary lengthening reduces the anatomic retropositioning of the mandible and the intensity of the deviation signal. Consequently the increased activity of the LPM and the supplementary growth of the condylar cartilage also tend to diminish. If the mandible reaches a length corresponding to the new occlusal relationship imposed by the postural hyperpropulsor, the intensity of the deviation signal in treated animals no longer differs significantly from that observed in untreated animals; henceforth the condylar cartilage growth rate in the treated animals becomes virtually the same as that observed in the untreated animals. Nevertheless, as long as the rat wears the postural hyperpropulsor, its mandible remains longer than that of the untreated animal.

When young rats were treated for 4 weeks with a mandibular postural hyperpropulsor, an appliance designed to increase the condylar cartilage growth rate, the proportion of indefatigable fibers in the LPM increased significantly (Oudet et al, 1988). Concomitantly the amount of slow myosin–light chains increased in the fiber extract. This slow myosin originated

## TABLE 2-2. • FORWARD REPOSITIONING OF THE MANDIBLE

The following data are from a study of periodic forward repositioning of the mandible (12 male rats in each experimental group, sacrificed at day 48 or 180).

In experimental group $O_s$ the following therapy was applied*:
- No treatment was applied from birth to day 20 (0.0).
- A 2-mm thick postural hyperpropulsor was worn from day 20 to 48 (2.0).
- A 3-mm thick postural hyperpropulsor was worn from day 48 to 76 (3.0).
- A 4-mm thick postural hyperpropulsor was worn from day 76 to 120 (4.0).
- The postural hyperpropulsor was removed at day 120; from day 120 to 180, no treatment was applied (0.0).
- The rats were sacrificed at day 180.

| | Thickness of Postural Hyperpropulsor (mm) | | | | | | |
| --- | --- | --- | --- | --- | --- | --- | --- |
| Group | 20 Days | 48 Days | 76 Days | 120 Days | 180 Days | Mean | Standard Error |
| **Number of $^3$H-methyl-thymidine–labeled cells in condylar cartilage—sacrifice at 48 days†** | | | | | | | |
| $A_1$ | 0.0 | 0.0 | | | | 878 cells | |
| $B_1$ | 0.0 | 0.5 | | | | 1049 cells | |
| $C_1$ | 0.0 | 1.0 | | | | 1316 cells | |
| $D_1$ | 0.0 | 2.0 | | | | 1499 cells | 40.63 |
| $E_1$ | 0.0 | 3.0 | | | | 818 cells | |
| **Angle between growth direction of condyle and mandibular plane (Stuzmann's angle)—sacrifice at 48 days‡** | | | | | | | |
| $A_1$ | 0.0 | 0.0 | | | | 128.9 degrees | |
| $B_1$ | 0.0 | 0.5 | | | | 136.0 degrees | |
| $C_1$ | 0.0 | 1.0 | | | | 136.9 degrees | |
| $D_1$ | 0.0 | 2.0 | | | | 140.5 degrees | 0.6880 |
| $E_1$ | 0.0 | 3.0 | | | | 129.2 degrees | |
| **Angle between growth direction of condyle and mandibular plane (Stuzmann's angle)—sacrifice at 180 days§** | | | | | | | |
| $A_4$ | 0.0 | 0.0 | 0.0 | 0.0 | 0.0 | 131.9 degrees | |
| $B_4$ | 0.0 | 0.5 | 0.5 | 0.5 | 0.5 | 131.8 degrees | |
| $C_4$ | 0.0 | 0.5 | 0.5 | 0.5 | 0.0 | 132.0 degrees | |
| $D_4$ | 0.0 | 0.5 | 0.5 | 0.0 | 0.0 | 132.0 degrees | |
| $E_4$ | 0.0 | 0.5 | 0.0 | 0.0 | 0.0 | 132.2 degrees | |
| $F_4$ | 0.0 | 1.0 | 1.0 | 1.0 | 1.0 | 133.1 degrees | |
| $G_4$ | 0.0 | 1.0 | 2.0 | 3.0 | 3.0 | 134.9 degrees | |
| $H_4$ | 0.0 | 1.0 | 2.0 | 3.0 | 0.0 | 133.0 degrees | |
| $I_4$ | 0.0 | 1.0 | 1.0 | 1.0 | 0.0 | 132.3 degrees | 0.4378 |
| $J_4$ | 0.0 | 1.0 | 1.0 | 0.0 | 0.0 | 131.8 degrees | |
| $K_4$ | 0.0 | 1.0 | 0.0 | 0.0 | 0.0 | 132.0 degrees | |
| $L_4$ | 0.0 | 2.0 | 2.0 | 2.0 | 2.0 | 133.9 degrees | |
| $M_4$ | 0.0 | 2.0 | 3.0 | 3.0 | 3.0 | 134.7 degrees | |
| $N_4$ | 0.0 | 2.0 | 3.0 | 4.0 | 4.0 | 135.9 degrees | |
| $O_4$ | 0.0 | 2.0 | 3.0 | 4.0 | 0.0 | 135.0 degrees | |
| $P_4$ | 0.0 | 2.0 | 2.0 | 2.0 | 0.0 | 133.3 degrees | |
| $Q_4$ | 0.0 | 2.0 | 2.0 | 0.0 | 0.0 | 131.9 degrees | |
| $R_4$ | 0.0 | 2.0 | 0.0 | 0.0 | 0.0 | 132.0 degrees | |

*Based on the analysis of variance, a standard error was calculated for the 48-day-old popoulation and the 180-day-old population. The difference (experimental group $0_s$, control group $A_s$, under the first table subheading) was equal to 3.30 mm (23.35 mm − 20.05 mm). This difference, which is greater than 0.24 mm, is significant at the 1% level.

†Smallest significance difference between two means (cells): 5% level, 81; 1% level, 108; 0.1% level, 141.

‡Smallest significant difference between two means (degrees): 5% level, 1.4; 1% level, 1.8; 0.1% level, 2.4.

§Smallest significant difference between two means (degrees): 5% level, 0.9; 1% level, 1.1; 0.1% level, 1.5.

from IIA fibers. Through functional orthopedic treatment the LPM was enriched with less fatigueable fibers; the changes observed in the LPM were similar to those observed in other muscles after training. Carlson et al (1990) corroborated these results. This is a fertile area for future research.

If the postural hyperpropulsor is then removed, the confrontation between the two dental arches detects the appliance-produced excessive anterior position of the lower dental arch and produces another deviation signal, which is reduced by a diminution in the contractile activity of the LPM and

## TABLE 2-2. • FORWARD REPOSITIONING OF THE MANDIBLE—cont'd

The following data are from a study of periodic forward repositioning of the mandible (12 male rats in each experimental group, sacrificed at day 48 or 180).

In experimental group O$_s$ the following therapy was applied*:
- No treatment was applied from birth to day 20 (0.0).
- A 2-mm thick postural hyperpropulsor was worn from day 20 to 48 (2.0).
- A 3-mm thick postural hyperpropulsor was worn from day 48 to 76 (3.0).
- A 4-mm thick postural hyperpropulsor was worn from day 76 to 120 (4.0).
- The postural hyperpropulsor was removed at day 120; from day 120 to 180, no treatment was applied (0.0).
- The rats were sacrificed at day 180.

| | Thickness of Postural Hyperpropulsor (mm) | | | | | | |
| --- | --- | --- | --- | --- | --- | --- | --- |
| Group | 20 Days | 48 Days | 76 Days | 120 Days | 180 Days | Mean | Standard Error |
| **Length of mandible (as measured by the distance between the mental foramen and the posterior border of the condylar cartilage)—sacrifice at 48 days‖** | | | | | | | |
| A$_1$ | 0.0 | 0.0 | | | | 13.95 mm | |
| B$_1$ | 0.0 | 0.5 | | | | 14.95 mm | |
| C$_1$ | 0.0 | 1.0 | | | | 15.25 mm | 0.0754 |
| D$_1$ | 0.0 | 2.0 | | | | 15.44 mm | |
| E$_1$ | 0.0 | 3.0 | | | | 13.58 mm | |
| **Length of mandible (as measured by the distance between the mental foramen and the posterior border of the condylar cartilage)—sacrifice 180 days¶** | | | | | | | |
| A$_4$ | 0.0 | 0.0 | 0.0 | 0.0 | 0.0 | 20.05 mm | |
| B$_4$ | 0.0 | 0.5 | 0.5 | 0.5 | 0.5 | 21.12 mm | |
| C$_4$ | 0.0 | 0.5 | 0.5 | 0.5 | 0.0 | 21.06 mm | |
| D$_4$ | 0.0 | 0.5 | 0.5 | 0.0 | 0.0 | 20.50 mm | |
| E$_4$ | 0.0 | 0.5 | 0.0 | 0.0 | 0.0 | 20.15 mm | |
| F$_4$ | 0.0 | 1.0 | 1.0 | 1.0 | 1.0 | 21.62 mm | |
| G$_4$ | 0.0 | 1.0 | 2.0 | 3.0 | 3.0 | 21.93 mm | |
| H$_4$ | 0.0 | 1.0 | 2.0 | 3.0 | 0.0 | 21.91 mm | |
| I$_4$ | 0.0 | 1.0 | 1.0 | 1.0 | 0.0 | 21.48 mm | 0.0734 |
| J$_4$ | 0.0 | 1.0 | 1.0 | 0.0 | 0.0 | 20.65 mm | |
| K$_4$ | 0.0 | 1.0 | 0.0 | 0.0 | 0.0 | 20.28 mm | |
| L$_4$ | 0.0 | 2.0 | 2.0 | 2.0 | 2.0 | 22.57 mm | |
| M$_4$ | 0.0 | 2.0 | 3.0 | 3.0 | 3.0 | 23.68 mm | |
| N$_4$ | 0.0 | 2.0 | 3.0 | 4.0 | 4.0 | 23.67 mm | |
| O$_4$ | 0.0 | 2.0 | 3.0 | 4.0 | 0.0 | 23.35 mm | |
| P$_4$ | 0.0 | 2.0 | 2.0 | 2.0 | 0.0 | 22.29 mm | |
| Q$_4$ | 0.0 | 2.0 | 2.0 | 0.0 | 0.0 | 22.02 mm | |
| R$_4$ | 0.0 | 2.0 | 0.0 | 0.0 | 0.0 | 21.44 mm | |

‖Smallest significant difference between two means (mm): 5% level, 0.15; 1% level, 0.20; 0.1% level, 0.26.

¶Smallest significant difference between two means (mm): 5% level, 0.14; 1% level, 0.19; 0.1% level, 0.24.

thereby through a reduction in the condylar cartilage growth rate. The mandible then tends to reach the length it would have attained in the absence of treatment with the functional appliance (Table 2-2). Under these conditions, relapse after removal of a functional appliance from a growing animal appears, in the light of cybernetic theory, to be the expression of regulatory mechanism that rends to minimize the deviation from the optimal occlusal adjustment. Obviously, however, not all change occurs in the condyle; the fossa and eminence are other areas of significant change (see Chapter 4).

The angle between the mandibular plane and the main orientation of newly formed endochondral bone trabeculae under the condylar cartilage (Stutzmann's angle) increases at the beginning of treatment (see Table 2-2). With time, however, the difference between treated and control animals becomes undetectable (see Tables 2-2 and 2-3). In other words the

TABLE 2-3. • EFFECTS OF VARIOUS FUNCTIONAL APPLIANCES ON GROWTH OF THE RAT MANDIBLE (12 ANIMALS IN EACH GROUP)

| Treatment | Mean | Standard Error |
|---|---|---|
| **Treatment number of $^3$H-methyl-thymidine–labeled cells in condylar cartilage** | | |
| *Bionator and Fränkel appliance\** | | |
| No appliance | 859 cells | |
| Bionator (end to end) | 988 cells | 25.47 |
| Bionator (1 mm forward) | 1199 cells | |
| Fränkel superior retrolabial vestibular shields (lip pads) | 1236 cells | |
| *Postural hyperpropulsor and intraoral elastics†* | | |
| No appliance | 878 cells | |
| Postural hyperpropulsor (0.5 mm) | 1049 cells | 41.73 |
| Postural hyperpropulsor (1 mm) | 1316 cells | |
| Intraoral elastic forces | 1336 cells | |
| **Angle between growth direction of rat condyle and mandibular plane (Stuzmann's angle) at 48 days** | | |
| *Bionator and Fränkel appliance‡* | | |
| No appliance | 126.3 degrees | |
| Bionator (end to end) | 130.5 degrees | 0.437 |
| Bionator (1 mm forward) | 132.9 degrees | |
| Fränkel superior retrolabial vestibular shields (lip pads) | 131.2 degrees | |
| *Postural hyperpropulsor and intraoralelastics§* | | |
| No appliance | 128.9 degrees | |
| Postural hyperpropulsor (0.5 mm) | 136.0 degrees | 0.569 |
| Postural hyperpropulsor (1 mm) | 136.9 degrees | |
| Intraoral elastic forces | 137.6 degrees | |
| **Length of rat mandible (distance between mental foramen and posterior border of condylar cartilage) at 48 days** | | |
| *Bionator and Fränkel appliance‖* | | |
| No appliance | 14.24 mm | |
| Bionator (end to end) | 14.67 mm | 0.1596 |
| Bionator (1 mm forward) | 15.29 mm | |
| Fränkel superior retrolabial vestibular shields (lip pads) | 15.22 mm | |
| *Postural hyperpropulsor and intraoral elastics¶* | | |
| No appliance | 13.95 mm | |
| Postural hyperpropulsor (0.5 mm) | 14.87 mm | 0.0730 |
| Postural hyperpropulsor (1 mm) | 15.25 mm | |
| Intraoral elastic forces | 15.26 mm | |

*Smallest significant difference between two means (cells): 5% level, 51; 1% level, 69; 0.1% level, 90.

†Smallest significant difference between two means (cells): 5% level, 84; 1% level, 112; 0.1% level, 147.

‡Smallest significant difference between two means (degrees): 5% level, 0.9; 1% level, 1.2; 1% level without appliance; 1.5.

§Smallest significant difference between two means (degrees): 5% level, 1.1; 1% level, 1.5; 0.1% level, 2.0.

‖Smallest significant difference between two means (mm): 5% level, 0.32; 1% level, 0.43; 0.1% level, 0.56.

¶Smallest significant difference between two means (mm): 5% level, 0.15; 1% level, 0.20; 0.1% level, 0.26.

opening of the trabecular orientation angle is only a transient remedial event. Change occurs as if the shape (in cybernetic language the *reference input*), rate, and amount of growth in the regulatory system controlling mandibular morphogenesis were controlled variables. Indeed, a deviation from the normal shape (e.g., the opening of Stutzmann's angle) that occurs as a transient phenomenon in response to the placing of a functional appliance tends to be reduced and is observed only over a long period through the increase in growth rate and amount, translated primarily into directional changes.

These findings imply that variations in the growth direction of the condylar cartilage and condyle produced by a functional appliance account for only a small part of the differences observed at the end of growth between treated and untreated individuals. No significant effect of the postural hyperpropulsor can be detected histologically in the condyle after growth is completed.

The mechanisms of action of the Fränkel appliance and other appliances such as the Herbst or Clark twin block on the sagittal growth of the mandible are physiologically similar to the mechanism of action of the postural hyperpropulsor. The total time of appliance wear also has been postulated as a factor in growth variation, with increased iterative activity in the retrodiscal pad and greater potential for adaptive changes in the fossa and articular eminence.

A young patient with a retropositioned lower dental arch presents different conditions because the fitting of a postural hyperpropulsor is intended to reduce the sagittal malrelation. From these observations, clinicians can infer that rational orthodontic treatment must lead to the minimization of deviation from the optimal occlusal adjustment so that the risk of relapse is decreased.

The future of orthodontics is not only therapy and interception but also prevention. Certainly, genetic engineering is not a treatment option for the immediate future, but other methods of prevention are feasible. An animal experiment designed by Stutzmann and Petrovic may provide functional implications for the feeding of infants (breastfeeding or stiff- or soft-nipple bottle feeding).

Experimental rats were sacrificed at 20 days, and the following observations were made:

1. The growth rate of the condylar cartilage was greatest in breast-fed and lowest in gavage-fed rats.
2. Stutzmann's angle (the direction of the trabecular orientation, indicating condylar growth) was more vertical in gavage-fed rats and more horizontal in breast-fed rats.
3. The length of the mandible was comparable in the stiff-nipple–fed and ultrasoft nipple–fed rats and in gavage-fed rats, but all three mandibles were significantly shorter than those of the breast-fed rats. This is a classical epigenetic functional effect with significant preventive implications for treatment of malocclusions.

The breastfed, stiff nipple–fed, ultrasoft nipple–fed, and gavage-fed rats were then exposed to usual feeding after reaching the age of 20 days. In addition, half of the animals in each category were treated with the postural hyperpropulsor (construction bite, 2-mm forward positioning of the mandible for 12 hours daily); the other half served as controls. Some treated animals were killed at 48 days (pubertal period) and some at 180 days (adult animal).

Observational results concerning the mandible are summarized as follows:

1. Regardless of the age of sacrifice (48 or 180 days), little difference is evident between breastfeeding and stiff nipple feeding (highest level of functional activity). However, mandibular growth is obviously impaired by ultrasoft nipple feeding and in a more pronounced manner by gavage feeding (lowest functional activity level). Nipple design and use also are important.
2. Regardless of the age of sacrifice (48 or 180 days) the responsiveness of the mandible to the stimulating effect of the functional appliance was of the same order of magnitude in breast-fed and stiff nipple–fed rats; however, it was greatly reduced in ultrasoft nipple–fed and

gavage-fed rats. Reduced functional stimulus produced reduced growth. This is substantiated by Burdi (1995).

## Class II Elastics

Intermaxillary intraoral elastics, placed bilaterally for 14 hours daily, in rats between the upper first molar and the lower third molar, are not only orthodontic devices capable of moving teeth but also functional appliances capable of stimulating the growth rate and amount of the condylar cartilage (see Table 2-3). The clinician is thus dealing with the influence on growth of the mandible because no such effect can be detected after growth is completed.

The postural hyperpropulsor and similar mandibular protraction appliances produce a significant and electromyographically detectable increase in the contractile activity of the LPM; the Class II elastics do not. The stimulating action of the Class II elastics on the lengthening of the condyle is mediated primarily through the retrodiscal pad, a structure that according to previous investigations also partly mediates the stimulating effect of the increased contractile activity of the LPM on condylar cartilage growth. Indeed, only in the presence of the retrodiscal pad (the metabolic pump) are the Class II elastics able to elicit an earlier start of the chondroblasts' hypertrophy and an increased growth rate of the condylar cartilage. The concept of an intrinsic regulation of the prechondroblasts' multiplication accounts partly for the phenomenon. Only functional (i.e., not yet hypertrophied) chondroblasts produce a prechondroblast multiplication restraining signal so that when the number of functional chondroblasts decreases, the negative feedback signal also decreases and consequently the prechondroblast multiplication rate increases.

The intraoral Class II elastics significantly stimulate the growth rate of the condylar cartilage and the lengthening of the mandible (see Table 2-3), whereas the extraoral elastics designed to produce active hyperpropulsion of the mandible have little effect. In the first case, however, the mandible remains mobile; in the second case, it is immobilized. Function is the essential element.

The LPM is a major intermediary in maintaining the optimal occlusal adjustment during growth and in facilitating the action of functional appliances (e.g., the postural hyperpropulsor, Herbst appliance). However, the biologic activator for the stimulating effect of the Class II elastics seems to be the retrodiscal pad and its role as a metabolic pump.

## Herren (L.S.U.) Activator

The word *activator* is misleading because it refers to various appliances operating in different biologic ways. The Herren activator, or the Louisiana State University modification of it, is different from a postural hyperpropulsor; it opens the construction bite well beyond the postural rest position, similar to that achieved by the Harvold-Woodside activator (see Chapter 4). Indeed, according to Auf der Maur (1978) and Herren (1953) the wearing of this appliance does not bring about any increased activity of the LPM.

In one research experiment, male rats wore either a Herren or L.S.U. activator for 12, 18, or 22½ hours daily. The appliance was fixed to the maxilla. A 2.0-mm forward positioning of the mandible was obtained through the construction bite, and the vertical increase in the molar bite was 0.4 mm, or 1.8 mm. The mobility of the lower jaw was lessened by extending the sides of the appliance lingually as deep as possible toward the bottom of the oral cavity. No free movement of the mandible was possible without a minimal opening of several millimeters. In fact, no increase in the electromyographically recorded activity of the LPM was detected during the wearing of the Herren activator (Figure 2-17), corroborating the observations of Herren and Auf der Maur.

Nevertheless, both the Herren and L.S.U. activator produced an increased growth rate and amount of condylar cartilage and a supplementary lengthening of the mandible at the posterior border if the appliance was worn for 12 or 18 hours daily and the molar bite height was 0.4 mm or 0.8 mm (Figure 2-18). If the vertical dimension of the appliance was increased to 1.8 mm the condylar cartilage growth and lengthening of the mandible were no longer promoted. The clinical implications are clear.

The analysis of these experimental findings strongly suggests that the Herren and L.S.U. activators' actions have two-step effects. Indeed, during the time the appliance is worn, the forward positioning of the mandible is the cause of the reduced increase in length of the LPM (Figure 2-19). At the same time a sensory engram is formed for the new positioning of the mandible. The corollary to this is that during the period in which the activator is not worn, the mandible is functioning in a more forward position so that the retrodiscal pad is much more stimulated than it is in controls (i.e., increased metabolic activity occurs). The increased repetitive activity of the pad produces an earlier onset of hypertrophy of the condylar chondroblasts. This earlier commencement and the simultaneous decrease in the number of functional chondroblasts implies that the decrease of the negative feedback signal has a restraining effect on the prechondroblast multiplication rate. Consequently the growth rate of the condylar cartilage is accelerated. In other words the LPM partly mediates the action of the appliance. However, in the case of the Herren or L.S.U. activator the stimulating effect on condylar growth appears to be produced mostly during the time the appliance is not worn. Indeed, if either the Herren or L.S.U. activator is worn for 22½ hours daily, or almost full time, the length of the LPM is decreased, but no stimulating effect on the condylar cartilage growth rate is detected. Furthermore, if the vertical dimension of the activator used in juvenile rat experiments is opened to 1.8 mm or beyond, mandibular lengthening is not promoted. In this case the growth of the LPM as estimated by the number of serial sarcomeres is not significantly reduced.

Research investigations (some still in progress) have shown that the Planas approach to the management of distoclusions as applied by Simoes may be validated using the cybernetic understanding of facial growth (Simoes et al, 1992):

1. The Planas appliance—regardless of its association with the grinding of canines and premolar and molar cusps—produces a phenomen observed in animal experiments. The mandible presents a physiologic tendency to a more forward position, implying a supplementary contractile activity of the LPM.
2. The resulting incisor contact inhibits the contraction of the LPM. The backward movement of the mandible, which cancels the incisor contact, allows a new contraction of the LPM.
3. The repetitive forward-backward movements of the mandible cause, by solicitation of the iterative activity of the retrodiscal pad, a supplementary growth of the posterior border of the ramus (i.e., supplementary lengthening of the mandible).
4. The Planas appliance, by allowing lateral movements of the mandible, magnifies alternately the repetitive contractile activity of the LPM on the left and right side and consequently the stimulation of the retrodiscal pad's iterative activity and the condylar cartilage's growth. The lateral functional movement of the

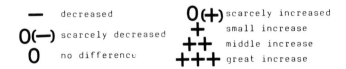

| | During the daily wear of the appliance | Without appliance |
|---|---|---|
| POSTURAL HYPERPROPULSOR | +++ | ++ |
| FRAENKEL APPLIANCE (small shields labial to lower incisors) | +++ | ++ |
| ELASTICS CLASS II | + | ++ |
| ACTIVATORS characterized by 0.4mm and 0.8mm high molar bite plate | 0 or O(+) | + |
| ACTIVATORS characterized by 1.6mm high molar bite plate | O(−) or − | 0 |

− decreased

O(−) scarcely decreased

0 no difference

O(+) scarcely increased

+ small increase

++ middle increase

+++ great increase

**Figure 2-17.** Semiquantitative evaluation of electromyographic activity in the lateral pterygoid muscle of the juvenile rat during the weeks after the commencement of treatment.

**Figure 2-18.** Effects of the L.S.U. activator and extraoral forward traction on mandibular growth. The activator had a sagittal deviation of 2 mm and a vertical deviation of 0.8 mm; forward traction had a sagittal deviation of 2 mm. Each group consists of 12 48-day-old male rats. The degree of significance at the top of the columns corresponds to the comparison of treated animals with controls. *NS,* Not significant.

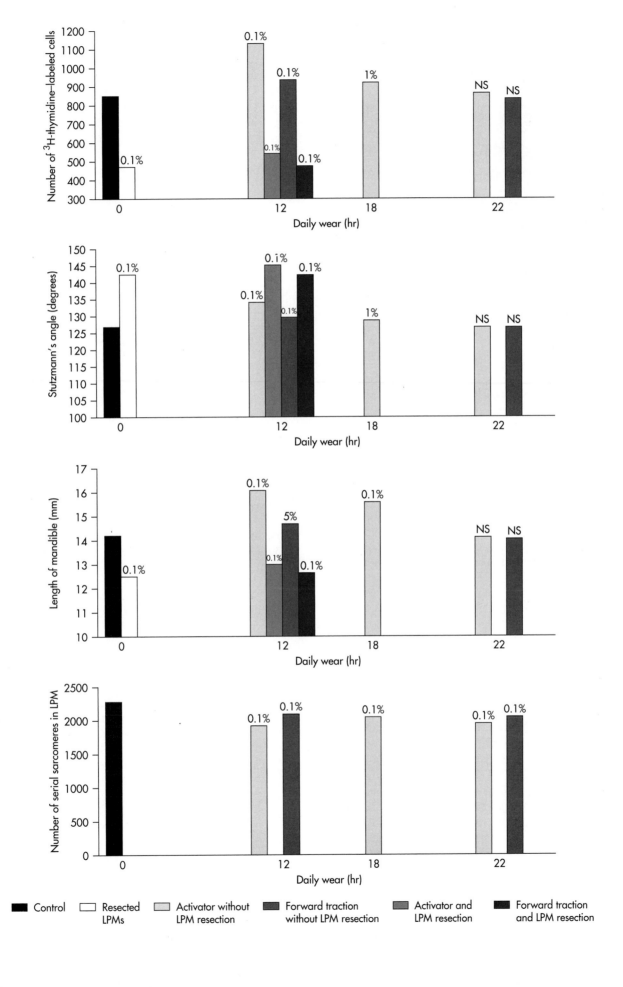

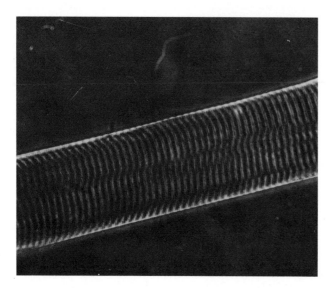

**Figure 2-19.** Segment of isolated muscle fiber from the LPM. Phase-contrast microscopy clearly illuminates the sarcomeres.

mandible apparently amplifies growth in the midpalatal suture of the maxilla. In some cases this supplementary widening of the maxilla in turn facilitates a more forward positioning of the mandible. At the very least, mandibular entrapment is eliminated.

5. Planas appliance treatment may start at different ages. Physiologically and cybernetically, if treatment starts several years before puberty, the main result consists of a supplementary increase in mandibular lengthening leading to an improvement in the functioning of the comparator of the servosystem that controls the growth of the condylar cartilage and lengthening of the mandible. If treatment starts or continues during the pubertal growth acceleration, the supplementary lengthening of the mandible is great enough to reduce the distoclusion in biologic growth category 2 and correct it completely in growth category 5. The treatment of a distoclusion intermaxillary malrelation with conventional fixed appliances and Class II elastics also stimulates the growth of the condylar cartilage and lengthening of the mandible. (For clinical details, see Petrovic, Stutzmann, 1994.)

## TENTATIVE CAUSAL INTERPRETATION OF THE METHOD OF OPERATION OF FUNCTIONAL APPLIANCES

The servosystem concept accounts not only for biologic organization but also for the mechanisms of action of appliances used in dentofacial orthopedics. According to experimental investigations, functional appliances may be tentatively divided into two categories (Figure 2-20):

1. The postural hyperpropulsor, activator, Class II elastics, Fränkel appliance, Clark twin block, and Balters biona-

tor all exert their effects mainly through the movements of the mandible. Indeed, their stimulating effects on condylar cartilage growth are produced mainly during the wearing of the appliance.

2. The Herren and L.S.U. activators and by inference the Harvold and Hamilton activators and extraoral forward traction on the mandible seem to exert their effects mostly through sagittal repositioning of the mandible.

Regardless of the differences in mode of action of the various functional appliances, the following causal chain is involved:

Functional appliance
↓
Increased contractile activity of the LPM
↓
Intensification of the repetitive activity of the retrodiscal pad (bilaminar zone)
↓
Increase in growth-stimulating factors
- Enhancement of local mediators
- Reduction of local regulators (factors having negative feedback effects on cell multiplication rate)
↓
- Change in condylar trabecular orientation
- Additional growth of condylar cartilage
- Additional subperiosteal ossification of the posterior border of the mandible
↓
Supplementary lengthening of the mandible

Investigations underway concerning the signals locally affecting the condylar cartilage-stimulating action of the postural hyperpropulsor, Fränkel appliance, L.S.U. activator, bionator, Clark twin block, and Class II elastics have led to several findings:

1. Electron micrographs of the condylar cartilage show that cytoplasmic junctions between skeletoblasts become quantitatively reduced. Consequently, possibilities of inhibitory intercellular communications are reduced; the cell division rate increases. Simultaneously the rate of differentiation of skeletoblasts into prechondroblasts also increases.

2. Characteristic and consistent transmembrane ion flux variations are detected: the intracellular $Na^+$ concentration is raised; the intracellular $K^+$ concentration is lowered; and the discharge of $H^+$ from both skeletoblasts and prechondroblasts is increased, leading to an increase in intracytoplasmic pH. Intracytoplasmic $Ca^{++}$, however, is maintained at a lower level.

3. Calmodulin and $Ca^{++}$, $Mg^{++}$-ATPase, and $H^+$-adenosine triphosophatase activities are promoted, whereas cAMP, fibronectin, $Na^+$ and $K^+$-adenosine-triphosphatase activity, cell transglutaminase, heparan sulfate, and other glucosaminoglycan levels are reduced. Nevertheless, the antimultiplicative effect of cAMP is not direct but results from the amplification of specific growth-

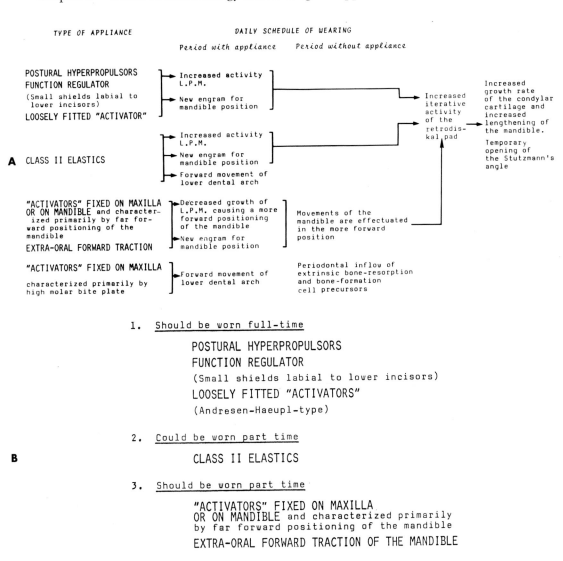

TYPE OF APPLIANCE                    DAILY SCHEDULE OF WEARING

Period with appliance    Period without appliance

**Figure 2-20.    A,** Tentative classification of orthopedic appliances according to their effects on condylar growth and mandibular lengthening. **B,** Daily duration of wear of the orthopedic appliances.

regulating signals (detected biologically but not yet identified), and the cell division process is initiated through a momentary surge of cytoplasmic $Ca^{++}$ and endogenous cAMP.

4. Local coupling mechanisms include the following:

a. The first is an open-loop part of the control system, which has a stimulating effect on cell multiplication and consists of growth hormone, testosterone, estrogen (in low doses), insulin, insulin-like substances (including liver-synthesized and locally produced somatomedins), glucagon, parathormone, calcitonin, calmodulin, and prostaglandin $F_{2\alpha}$. Mitogenic peptides also can correspond operationally to the fibroblast, endothelial cell-derived, platelet-derived, and monocyte-derived growth factors. Unexpectedly, these growth-promoting factors operate primarily by counteracting or even canceling the effects of agents that amplify the intercellular signal restraining skeletoblast and preosteoblast multiplication. In other words, these mitogenic peptides are not initiators of cell division but are instead required for $G_1$ (or rather $G_0$) skeletoblasts and preosteoblasts either to become responsive again to the specific gene-produced messenger initiating a new cell cycle or to directly repress the gene that controls the production of the agent amplifying the cell division–restraining signal. Whatever the mechanism involved, the cell is converted from a quiescent to a new cycle stage.

b. The second is a feedback part of the control system that has an inhibitory effect on cell multiplication and consists of regulators of local origin: skeletoblast or prechondroblast multiplication–restraining signals of unknown nature, contact inhibition–type signals, cAMP, prostaglandin $F_2$, and somatostatin-like substances.

5. The intensification of retrodiscal pad activity is associated with an increase in blood and lymph flow (i.e., in the supply of open-loop factors) and a decrease in cell catabolite concentration and negative feedback factors. These changes enhance the supplementary growth of the condylar cartilage caused by functional appliances. LPM activity is essential.

**Active retropulsion of the mandible.** The active retropulsion of the mandible (with chincaps) is more orthopedic than functional. However, the position of the condyle in the glenoid fossa is affected in a manner similar to that seen with the Class III activator and the Fränkel FR III.

If growing rats are subjected to active retropulsion with chincap therapy, the number of dividing cells in the mandibular condylar cartilage decreases dramatically. The direction of growth becomes more vertical, as evidenced by the closing of the Stutzmann's angle, which measures trabecular alignment with the mandibular plane. The length of the mandible decreases markedly (Table 2-4). In comparing chincap-treated and control animals for both 48-day and 180-day periods of wear, researchers noted that at 48 days the number of labeled cells, the length of the mandible, and the number of serial sarcomeres is greater in the treated group. By 180 days the angle between the trabeculae of the growing condyle and the mandibular plane still shows a difference that is significant at the 0.1% level. Mandibular length is decreased in the chincap-treated animals. The serial sarcomere count is greater for the treated animals but is not statistically significant.

Chincap therapy performs an orthopedic function, restraining the condylar cartilage growth rate as the condyle grows in an upward and forward direction. This research substantiates the experimental and clinical studies by Graber (1983c) and Graber et al (1967) on squirrel monkeys and large numbers of young patients with Class III malocclusions. A final adjustment factor is the effect on the fossa and articular eminence, where adaptive changes produce a more posteriorly placed condyle (see Chapter 4).

Investigations in juvenile rats (see Table 2-5) have shown that compared with controls, partial immobilization of the mandible and retractive chincap therapy produced a highly significant decrease in the growth rate and number of ³H-thymidine–labeled cells in the condylar cartilage and also a significant decrease in the lengthening of the mandible (amount of growth).

Complete immobilization of the mandible without the use of a chincap produces a reduction in the number of dividing cells in the condylar cartilage and the lengthening of the mandible compared with controls. However, this reduction is not statistically significantly different from that obtained using partial immobilization and a chincap.

Complete immobilization and the use of a chincap induces the greatest decrease in the growth rate of the condylar cartilage and the lengthening of the mandible. All effects are much

| TABLE 2-4. • EFFECTS OF A CHINCAP APPLIANCE AND PARTIAL AND COMPLETE IMMOBILIZATION ON THE GROWTH OF THE MANDIBLE* | | |
|---|---|---|
| **Experimental Group** | **Mean** | **Standard Error** |
| **Number of ³H-thymidine–labeled cells in the condylar-cartilage†** | | |
| Control | 935 cells | |
| Chincap and partial mandibular immobilization | 711 cells | |
| Complete mandibular immobilization | 667 cells | 24.78 |
| Chincap and complete mandibular immobilization | 620 cells | |
| **Angle between the growth direction of the condyle and the mandibular plane (Stuzmann's angle)‡** | | |
| Control | 125.7 degrees | |
| Chincap and partial mandibular immobilization | 124.9 degrees | |
| Complete mandibular immobilization | 124.5 degrees | 0.52 |
| Chincap and complete mandibular immobilization | 122.1 degrees | |
| **Length of the mandible (as measured by the distance from the mental foramen to the posterior border of the condylar cartilage)§** | | |
| Control | 14.33 mm | |
| Chincap and partial mandibular immobilization | 13.27 mm | |
| Complete mandibular immobilization | 12.97 mm | 0.1687 |
| Chincap and complete mandibular immobilization | 12.49 mm | |

*A total of 15 48-day-old male rats were in each group.

†Smallest significant difference between two means; 5% level, 70; 1% level, 93; 0.1% level, 122.

‡Smallest significant difference between two means: 5% level, 1.5; 1% level, 2.0; 0.1% level, 2.6.

§Smallest significant difference between two means: 5% level, 0.48; 1% level, 0.64; 0.1% level, 0.83.

more marked if the chincap is associated with complete rather than partial immobilization of the mandible. Functional appliances that modulate the growth rate of the condylar cartilage also influence bone formation and mineralization in the mandible of the growing rat.

# SPONTANEOUS AND THERAPEUTICALLY INDUCED VARIATIONS IN HUMAN ALVEOLAR BONE TURNOVER— A QUANTITATIVE STUDY

Variations in human alveolar bone turnover resulting from many physiologic functions can easily be investigated. Understandably, biopsies are performed on human bone only for medical reasons such as if a probability of pathology exists.

However, one common exception exists to this guideline. During tooth extraction the examination of alveolar bone fragments is easy. Furthermore, if the tooth is extracted for orthodontic purposes, the alveolar bone is generally normal and the turnover rate is superior to that found in other parts in the skeleton. Finally, because alveolar bone fragments are a by-product of tooth extraction, the researcher may use them in any appropriate way.

The investigation of alveolar bone turnover using organ culture and measuring appropriate physiologic parameters is a common research choice. In the following discussion, only data relative to the mandibular first premolar are reported.

The literature contains a large number of studies regarding the response of alveolar bone to both physiologic and orthodontically induced tooth movement (Baron, 1973; Baumrind, 1969, 1970; Gianelly, 1969; Graber et al, 1967; Kvam, 1970; Macapanpan et al, 1954; Markostamou, 1974, Reitan, 1947, 1960, 1964, 1974; Roberts, 1994; Rygh, 1973; Stein, Weinmann, 1925; Storey, 1955). These investigations are based on histologic descriptions; only a few were designed to quantify alveolar bone formation and resorption (Baron, 1973; Kingler, 1971; Markostamou, Baron, 1973, Roberts, 1994).

Orthodontically induced tooth movement depends on bone density, the number of cells involved in bone formation and resorption, and the magnitude and timing of the applied force. It also depends on the rate of physiologic bone remodeling activity and the possibility of increasing this remodeling orthodontically.

In addition, according to various experiments, mononuclear cells of extrinsic origin also appear to be involved in alveolar bone remodeling activity.

The purpose of the investigation under discussion is as follows:

1. To analyze quantitatively the physiologic alveolar bone turnover rate in 11- to 13-year-old boys as a function of the timing of extraction (morning or evening), season (spring or fall), growth rotation* of the mandible, and location of the bone (mesial or distal) with regard to the extracted premolar
2. To analyze quantitatively the variations of alveolar bone turnover as a function of orthodontic treatment variety (light or heavy and intermittent or continuous forces)

## Choice of Parameters in the Quantitative Evaluation of Human Alveolar Bone Turnover

The mitotic index is not useful in evaluating alveolar bone turnover. Indeed, determining whether the dividing cell is a preosteoblast or preosteoclast is often impossible, and many of the bone-forming or bone-resorbing cells in alveolar

bone are of extrinsic origin (Stutzmann et al, 1979, 1980b; Stutzmann, Petrovic, 1981).

Alkaline phosphatase activity was used as a parameter of osteoblast activity; calcium-45 uptake was used as a parameter of bone mineralization. β-Glucuronidase and acid phenylphosphatase activities were used as parameters of bone resorption intensity.

These choices do not imply that these two enzymes are involved directly in the resorption of bone; previous experiments (Stutzmann et al, 1979, 1980b) have shown that their activities vary directly with the intensity of bone resorption regardless of the relationship between enzyme activities and bone resorption.* The osteoclast count is therefore a poor parameter of bone resorption because some mononuclear cells, mainly of extrinsic origin, also participate in this phenomenon.

## Research Design

Human alveolar bone fragments and adjacent periodontal tissue were obtained from 11- to 13-year-old boys during the extraction for orthodontic purposes of mandibular first premolars. Specimens were taken from both mesial and distal sides of the extracted tooth and immediately placed into organ culture for 72 hours using a modified version of the Petrovic-Heusner apparatus (Heusner, Petrovic, 1964; Petrovic, Heusner, 1961). TC 199 medium was supplemented with 0.15 mg/ml ascorbic acid and 15% calf serum. In addition, 0.05 μCi calcium-45 was added to the culture medium. After a 3-day organ culture, the following procedures were performed:

- Calcium-45 uptake (in counts per minute) was measured.
- Alkaline and acid phenylphosphatase activities (in enzyme units per g of fresh bone) were estimated.
- β-Glucuronidase activity (in Fishmann units per mg of protein) was estimated.

In this way, the quantitative estimation of the spontaneous turnover rate of the alveolar bone was accurately performed.

Therapeutically induced variations in the human alveolar bone turnover rate were evaluated as follows (Figure 2-21):

1. The first mandibular premolar was extracted and contiguous mesially and distally located alveolar bone was collected on one side of the tooth before orthodontic treatment began. The specimens were immediately organ-cultured for 72 hours and assessed for the three parameters mentioned previously.
2. After the premolar extraction, only the subjects from Group I (spring group with anteriorly or posteriorly inclined mandibles) were fitted with Class II elastics on the contralateral side of the mandible.

---

*In the strictest sense, *growth rotation* refers only to the time-related variations observed during the growth of an individual. When dealing with the features of a given individual, the clinician or researcher should use the term *inclination* as more appropriate.

*According to experimental observations (Stutzmann et al, 1979, 1980) the turnover of bone-resorbing cells (osteoclasts and mononuclear cells) is significantly accelerated if bone resorption is stimulated. In other words the increase in lysosomal enzyme activities can be related to the shortened life-span of bone-resorbing cells.

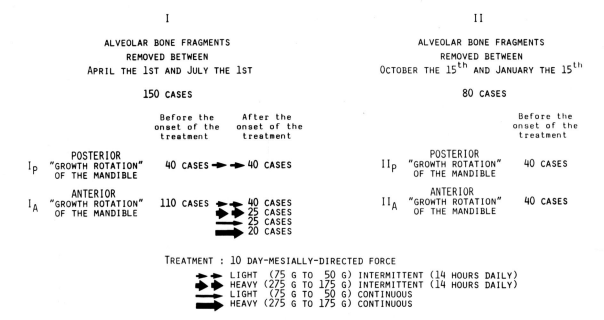

**Figure 2-21.** Experimental design.

3. Different forces were applied:
   - Light (75 g to 50 g), intermittent (14 hours daily) force
   - Heavy (275 g to 175 g), intermittent force
   - Light (75 g to 50 g), continuous force
   - Heavy (275 g to 175 g), continuous force

After 10 days of orthodontic treatment, the remaining mandibular first premolar and contiguous alveolar bone fragments were removed and studied in organ culture.

## Experimental Findings

The results of investigations using the organ culture method show that human alveolar bone turnover displays diverse but consistent variations. Some of the factors responsible have been identified; others have not. For this reason, experimental data are not distributed normally. Earlier research (Stutzmann et al, 1979, 1980a) suggests the selected parameters of the alveolar bone turnover rate appear preferable to histomorphometric analysis; however, such a quantitative evaluation certainly needs further improvement.

Significant nyctohemeral variations in bone turnover have been discovered during spontaneous sagittal tooth movement (Table 2-5); these variations are important in the biologic understanding of rhythmic fluctuations in human bone turnover and in medical decisions concerning the best time to apply a given therapeutic agent. For instance, if orthodontic forces must be applied only during part of the day, the practitioner must be able to choose the time of greatest effect.

Significant seasonal variations in the alveolar bone turnover rate also have been discovered (Table 2-6); these variations have obvious clinical interest. For example, when investigating the alveolar bone turnover rate in 20- to 25-year-old male patients before and after a 21-day orthodontic treatment

with Class II elastics, researchers discovered that the orthodontically induced increase in cell activity is significantly greater in the spring than in the fall.

A puzzling observation was made during the investigation (Table 2-7): in the anteriorly rotating mandible the alveolar bone formation rate is usually notably greater on the mesial side than on the distal, and the resorption rate is markedly greater on the distal side. This implies that in most anteriorly rotating mandibles the first premolar undergoes a physiologic distalization rather than a mesialization during growth. Only in the posteriorly rotating mandible do the parameters of alveolar bone turnover support the classic concept of mesialization during growth.

A strong correlation between the alveolar bone turnover rate and the direction of mandibular growth rotation was detected (see Table 2-7). High bone formation and resorption rates are associated mostly with anteriorly rotating mandibles; conversely, low bone formation and resorption rates are generally associated with posterior rotation.

Previous experiments on juvenile rats may help explain the correlation; they show that the direction of mandibular growth rotation is related to the magnitude of the mandibular growth rate. In anterior growth rotation the response of cells (prechondroblasts of secondary cartilage and subperiosteal and trabecular preosteoblasts of the mandible) to stimulating factors such as growth hormone–somatomedin, testosterone, and muscle activity is higher than if the mandible is undergoing posterior rotation. This concept is consistent with the clinical observation of a thick, massive mandible seen in extreme anterior rotation and a slender, gracile ramus and corpus seen in extreme posterior rotation.

The rate of alveolar bone turnover and the direction of mandibular growth rotation are important to the clinician. Indeed, if orthodontic forces are applied (Table 2-8), the magnitude of an orthodontically induced increase in alveolar bone

**TABLE 2-5. • VARIATIONS IN ALVEOLAR BONE TURNOVER DURING SPONTANEOUS SAGITTAL TOOTH MOVEMENT AS A FUNCTION OF TIME OF EXTRACTION\***

| Time of Extraction | Number of Subjects | Median | Median Difference (Evening to Morning) | Wilcoxon Value of Z† |
|---|---|---|---|---|
| **Alkaline phenylphosphatase activity (enzyme units)** | | | | |
| Morning‡ | 30 | 157.5 (117 to 183) | 24 (−7 to 87) | −4.47 |
| Evening§ | 30 | 183.5 (146 to 227) | | ($p < 0.001$) |
| **Calcum-45 uptake (counts per minute)** | | | | |
| Morning | 30 | 12,433 (6871 to 16,550) | 646 (−2166 to 3716) | −1.24 |
| Evening | 30 | 12,631 (9147 to 15,625) | | ($p = 0.11$) NS |
| **β-Glucuronidase activity (Fishman units)** | | | | |
| Morning | 30 | 35.17 (22.46 to 42.48) | 2.87 (−2.43 to 8.93) | −4.44 |
| Evening | 30 | 38.25 (22.79 to 46.46) | | ($p < 0.001$) |
| **Acid phenylphosphatase activity (enzyme units)** | | | | |
| Morning | 30 | 14.98 (10.45 to 17.84) | 0.51 (−0.89 to 2.16) | −3.89 |
| Evening | 30 | 16.16 (10.87 to 19.50) | | ($p < 0.001$) |

*NS*, Not significant.

*Subjects were 11- to 13-year-old boys.

†Wilcoxon matched-pairs signed rank test.

‡Alveolar bone removed between 10:00 AM and 12:30 PM.

§Alveolar bone removed between 10:00 PM and 12:30 AM.

**TABLE 2-6. • VARIATIONS IN ALVEOLAR BONE TURNOVER DURING SPONTANEOUS SAGITTAL TOOTH MOVEMENT AS A FUNCTION OF THE SEASON\***

| Season of Extraction | Number of Subjects | Median | Range | Mann-Whitney U Test Value of Z |
|---|---|---|---|---|
| **Alkaline phenylphosphatase activity (enzyme units)** | | | | |
| Spring† | 80 | 160 | 128 to 212 | 9.86 |
| Fall‡ | 80 | 132 | 120 to 158 | ($p < 0.001$) |
| **Calcium-45 uptake (counts per minute)** | | | | |
| Spring | 80 | 12,461 | 4156 to 23,196 | 4.12 |
| Fall | 80 | 9585 | 3172 to 18,238 | ($p < 0.001$) |
| **β-Glucuronidase activity (Fishman units)** | | | | |
| Spring | 80 | 38.15 | 20.32 to 54.15 | 9.10 |
| Fall | 80 | 24.14 | 12.83 to 37.49 | ($p < 0.001$) |
| **Acid phenylphosphatase activity (enzyme units)** | | | | |
| Spring | 80 | 15.66 | 7.09 to 25.93 | 4.69 |
| Fall | 80 | 12.38 | 6.42 to 21.72 | ($p < 0.001$) |

*Subjects were 11- to 13-year-old boys.

†Alveolar bone removed between April 1 and July 1.

‡Alveolar bone removed between October 15 and January 15.

turnover is statistically greater in the anteriorly rotating mandible than in the jaw with posterior rotation. Furthermore, the magnitude of the increase is greater if the applied forces are light than if they are heavy (Table 2-9). In addition, the effectiveness of light forces is enhanced if the forces are applied intermittently. Clinical implications are obvious.

These findings can be interpreted as follows:

1. Light and intermittent forces have a less adverse effect on local periodontal tissue and local circulatory conditions. Consequently, local cell multiplication and differentiation are less impaired.

TABLE 2-7. • VARIATIONS IN ALVEOLAR BONE TURNOVER DURING SPONTANEOUS SAGITTAL TOOTH MOVEMENTS AS A FUNCTION OF THE GROWTH ROTATION OF THE MANDIBLE*

| Growth Rotation of Mandible | Number of Subjects | Median | Range | Mann-Whitney U Test Value of Z |
|---|---|---|---|---|
| **Alkaline phenylphosphatase activity (enzyme units)** | | | | |
| Anterior | 80 | 152 | 123 to 212 | 5.04 |
| Posterior | 80 | 134 | 120 to 173 | ($p < 0.001$) |
| **Calcium-45 uptake (counts per minute)** | | | | |
| Anterior | 80 | 12,795 | 4738 to 23,196 | 6.65 |
| Posterior | 80 | 8233 | 3172 to 19,293 | ($p < 0.001$) |
| **$\beta$-Glucuronidase activity (Fishman units)** | | | | |
| Anterior | 80 | 32.34 | 17.82 to 54.15 | 4.72 |
| Posterior | 80 | 25.74 | 12.83 to 42.65 | ($p < 0.001$) |
| **Acid phenylphosphatase activity (enzyme units)** | | | | |
| Anterior | 80 | 14.27 | 6.42 to 25.93 | 1.83 |
| Posterior | 80 | 13.09 | 6.83 to 22.28 | ($p = 0.034$) |

NOTE: The Wilcoxon test is used for matched pairs (e.g., morning and evening), whereas the Mann-Whitney test is used for independent samples (e.g., spring and fall).

*Subjects were 11- to 13-year-old boys.

TABLE 2-8. • VARIATIONS IN ALVEOLAR BONE TURNOVER DURING ORTHODONTIC TREATMENT USING LIGHT, INTERMITTENT, MESIALLY DIRECTED FORCES*

| Growth Rotation | Number of Subjects | Difference Before and After Treatment | | Mann-Whitney U Test Value of Z |
|---|---|---|---|---|
| | | Median | Range | |
| **Alkaline phenylphosphatase activity (enzyme units)** | | | | |
| Anterior | 40 | 1062 | 334 to 1410 | 5.96 |
| Posterior | 40 | 387 | 93 to 1151 | ($p < 0.001$) |
| **Calcium-45 uptake (counts per minute)** | | | | |
| Anterior | 40 | 51,377 | 14,709 to 85,480 | 6.77 |
| Posterior | 40 | 15,121 | 2297 to 44,004 | ($p < 0.001$) |
| **$\beta$-Glucuronidase activity (Fishman units)** | | | | |
| Anterior | 40 | 306.27 | 100.55 to 418.64 | 5.01 |
| Posterior | 40 | 147.45 | 47.50 to 304.72 | ($p < 0.001$) |
| **Acid phenylphosphatase activity (enzyme units)** | | | | |
| Anterior | 40 | 131.85 | 45.87 to 170.46 | 7.27 |
| Posterior | 40 | 39.95 | 19.71 to 88.50 | ($p < 0.001$) |

NOTE: The distal side is the locus of bone formation, whereas the mesial side is the locus of bone resorption.

*Subjects were 11- to 13-year-old boys.

2. Previous research, however, indicates another important factor: the increased alveolar bone resorption rate on the mesial side and increased alveolar bone formation on the distal side (produced orthodontically by mesially directed forces) involve cells of extrinsic origin (circulating monocyte-type cells). This extrinsic contribution of bone-resorption and bone-formation cell precursors may account for the effectiveness of light and intermittent orthodontic forces in tooth movement, because light and intermittent forces have less adverse effect on local circulatory conditions.

3. By using antisera against the four types of collagen, researchers found type I collagen (as detected by immunofluorescence in the periodontal ligament) predominant on the mesial and distal sides of the extracted first premolar both before orthodontic treatment and during Class II elastics treatment with light forces (75 g to 50 g) applied intermittently (Figure 2-22). However,

**TABLE 2-9.** • VARIATIONS IN ALVEOLAR BONE TURNOVER DURING ORTHODONTIC TREATMENT AS A FUNCTION OF INTENSITY AND DURATION OF APPLIED FORCES*

| Intensity and Direction of Mesially Directed Forces | Number of Subjects | Difference Before and After Treatment | | Mann-Whitney U Test Value of Z | | |
|---|---|---|---|---|---|---|
| | | Median | Range | HI | LC | HC |
| **Alkaline phenylphosphatase activity (enzyme units)** | | | | | | |
| LI | 40 | 1062 | 334 to 1410 | 1.80 ($p = 0.04$) | 5.65 ($p < 0.001$) | 5.88 ($p < 0.001$) |
| HI | 25 | 885 | 285 to 1360 | | 3.95 ($p < 0.001$) | 4.82 ($p < 0.001$) |
| LC | 25 | 436 | 231 to 962 | | | 2.54 ($p = 0.005$) |
| HC | 20 | 322 | 127 to 743 | | | |
| **Calcium-45 uptake (counts per minute)** | | | | | | |
| LI | 40 | 51,377 | 14,709 to 85,480 | 1.79 ($p = 0.04$) | 5.92 ($p < 0.001$) | 5.96 ($p < 0.001$) |
| HI | 25 | 42,703 | 12,412 to 74,386 | | 4.82 ($p < 0.001$) | 5.57 ($p < 0.001$) |
| LC | 25 | 22,781 | 4349 to 40,307 | | | 3.68 ($p < 0.001$) |
| HC | 20 | 8065 | 1684 to 27,544 | | | |
| **β-Glucuronidase activity (Fishman units)** | | | | | | |
| LI | 40 | 306.27 | 100.55 to 418.64 | 2.56 ($p = 0.005$) | 5.25 ($p < 0.001$) | 5.23 ($p < 0.001$) |
| HI | 25 | 19100 | 103.10 to 398.33 | | 2.86 ($p = 0.002$) | 5.28 ($p < 0.001$) |
| LC | 25 | 158.26 | 71.66 to 205.28 | | | 4.59 ($p < 0.001$) |
| HC | 20 | 68.80 | 16.17 to 173.90 | | | |
| **Acid phenylphosphatase activity (enzyme units)** | | | | | | |
| LI | 40 | 131.85 | 45.87 to 170.46 | 4.30 ($p < 0.001$) | 6.45 ($p < 0.001$) | 6.26 ($p < 0.001$) |
| HI | 25 | 83.29 | 40.10 to 120.88 | | 5.25 ($p < 0.001$) | 5.60 ($p < 0.001$) |
| LC | 25 | 37.68 | 22.47 to 72.15 | | | 3.79 ($p = 0.001$) |
| HC | 20 | 24.86 | 5.55 to 47.48 | | | |

NOTE: The distal side is the locus of bone formation, whereas the mesial side is the locus of bone resorption.

*LI,* Light intermittent; *HI,* heavy intermittent; *LC,* light continuous; *HC,* heavy continuous.

*Subjects were 11- to 13-year-old boys.

**TYPE OF COLLAGEN**

★ Before any orthodontic treatment — Collagen I

★ During an orthodontic treatment

- Class II elastics *light* forces (50 to 75 g) applied intermittently
- LSU–Activator
- Fränkel appliance

⎤ Collagen I

- Class II elastics *heavy* forces (250 to 275 g) applied continuously
- Edgewise or straight–wire variety of fixed appliances (*heavy* forces)

⎤ Collagen III and Collagen I

**Figure 2-22.** Type of collagen in the periodontal ligament as a function of orthodontic treatment.

when 11- to 13-year-old boys are treated with heavy forces applied continuously, either with Class II elastics (275 g to 250 g) or fixed appliances (edgewise, straight wire), the type III collagen tends to become predominant in the mesially located periodontal ligament. This finding strongly suggests that light, intermittent orthodontic forces amplify the usual collagen turnover in the periodontal ligament, whereas heavy orthodontic forces induce the synthesis of a collagen type different from the normal one. To be more precise, type III collagen may be detected during connective tissue repair after local injury.

Further investigation now underway should elucidate the relationship between the intensity of orthodontic forces and the type of collagen synthesized in the human periodontium. But the question of whether a specific, deleterious effect occurs if the force used is too strong cannot be ignored in future investigations relative to various orthodontic appliances. Studies into this question afford insights into the biologic mechanisms involved in the acute-phase response of local tissues to orthodontic treatment. The molecular biologic approach to orthodontic problems is becoming an operative conceptual tool for the research-oriented clinician.

Do the findings reported by Stutzmann and Petrovic relative to alveolar bone turnover correspond to clinical observations? Orthodontists who treated patients in whom the alveolar bone had been investigated were asked to evaluate semiquantitatively for each individual the clinical effectiveness (0 to +4) of the treatment 1 year later. In this way the clinical effectiveness of treatment could be compared with findings relative to alveolar bone turnover. Researchers were in strong agreement that the higher the alveolar bone turnover rate, the faster the movement of teeth and the shorter the duration of treatment.

Duration of treatment is of paramount importance because it means that, independent of the variety and modality of orthodontic treatment, the rapidity and duration of treatment depend on the alveolar bone turnover rate which is unique to each individual. Clinical orthodontic researchers must now further test the validity and applicability of these conclusions based on physiologic findings relative to human alveolar bone turnover before and during orthodontic treatment.

A high turnover rate of mandibular alveolar bone is generally associated with anterior growth rotation, standard turnover rate with neutral growth rotation, and a low turnover rate with posterior growth rotation. These findings are confirmed in 11- to 13-year-old boys who have undergone surgical treatment of mandibular fractures near the ramus: in anterior growth rotation the subperiosteal ossification is significantly higher than it is in posterior growth rotation (Table 2-10).

Investigations of alveolar bone turnover before and 10 days after the onset of orthodontic treatment indicate greater treatment effectiveness for patients whose mandibles follow anterior rather than posterior growth rotations. However, clinical situations are always more complex than the general

| Growth Rotation of the Mandible | Number of Subjects | Median (%) | Range (%) | Median Test (×2) |
|---|---|---|---|---|
| Anterior | 65 | 7.5 | 0.4 to 14.5 | |
| | | | | 24.81 (p < 0.001) |
| Posterior | 64 | 4.1 | 0.2 to 14.9 | |

**TABLE 2-10. • QUANTITATIVE ESTIMATION OF $^3$H-THYMIDINE–LABELED CELLS IN THE MANDIBULAR SUPERIOSTEAL LAYER***

*Subjects were 11- to 13-year-old boys.

biomedical and orthodontic rules suggest. Indeed, about 20% of 11- to 13-year-old boys with a high turnover rate of mandibular alveolar bone display posterior growth rotation. Interestingly, in about two thirds of such cases the children suffer from respiratory or allergic problems.

A better knowledge of underlying physiologic and pathophysiologic mechanisms should lead to a better use of therapeutic armamentaria. Orthodontic control of biologic laws implies an accurate and detailed understanding of the normal order of living matter.

An organ culture study of human alveolar bone turnover rate has been performed to test whether the Fränkel appliance and similar functional appliances effect results in forward movement of the mandibular premolars. According to its findings the therapeutic effect of the Fränkel function regulator is certainly not solely the result of dentoalveolar changes in the mandible. An orthopedically elicited supplement of mandibular growth is postulated and has been demonstrated in growing rats and recently in children.

## BIFURCATION DURING FACIAL GROWTH—ITS MEANING IN THE PATHOGENESIS OF MALOCCLUSION AND IN TREATMENT PLANNING

Most orthodontic treatment plans involve growth prediction. Amazingly, most growth prediction methods implicitly take as a precondition the continuity of facial development. Experimental investigations have long indicated the existence of nonlinear and unanticipated variations in the growth rate and direction of the mandible resulting from bifurcation-type alterations of the intercuspal relationship. The experimental and cybernetic approach to this finding has revealed, furthermore, that among all the conceivable occlusion-forming patterns, only a limited number are within the realm of biologic possibility and commonly seen during the process of postnatal facial growth and development. In addition, clinical findings have led to a morphogenetic classification of human facial development that presupposes biologic discontinuities.

Moss and Salentijn (1970) have described a logarithm for the growth of the human mandible, and no major cause exists to refute (in the Popperian sense) such a logarithm. However, this logarithm and the growth predictions of Ricketts, which are based on just three reference points, are still poorly substantiated.

Todd and Mark (1981ab) have published a topologic method to describe facial development using a transformation equation (cardioidal strain) between two stages of facial development. This method, although conceptually productive, has raised controversy (Bookstein, 1981; Todd, Mark, 1981ab) and reconsideration (Moiroud, 1981).

### Cardioidal strain

$$\theta' = \theta$$

$$R' = R[1 + k(1 - \cos \theta)]$$

According to Todd and Mark (1981ab) this method reflects the "global regularity of the biologic mechanisms that control growth." The same cardioidal strain transformation equation has been used by Lavergne and Petrovic (1983) to test the existence of a global regularity during postnatal craniofacial skeleton growth in children.

Experimental investigations have conclusively demonstrated that the occlusal relationship plays a significant role in the processes controlling facial growth. According to the servosystem theory (Petrovic, Stutzmann, 1975, 1977) the growth of the mandible is subject to the modulating effects of regional and local factors, including mechanisms regulating the occlusal relationship. The peripheral comparator of the servosystem is represented by the operation of confrontation between the upper and lower dental arches (see Figure 2-5). The peripheral comparator has several stable positions, each corresponding to some type of Class I, II, or III intercuspation. Any given occlusal relationship is stable with respect to limited fluctuations and disturbances. The stable positions are separated by unbalanced states corresponding generally to cuspal occlusion. Each cusp-to-cusp unstable position corresponds to a functional discontinuity (i.e., to a topologic bifurcation-type instability as described by Thom [1972] and Zeemann [1976]). Lack of interdental contacts corresponds to the absence of both stable and bifurcation situations. The topologic concept of discontinuity connotes that at critical points the servosystem behavior goes through some basic switch, implying the existence of continuous quantitative variations that appear qualitative.

The values of the coefficient K have been calculated from cephalometric measurements. Careful analysis of the transformation coefficient K reveals that if no change occurs in the molar relationship, the value of the coefficient K does not vary significantly from one reference point to another on the bony profile; however, as soon as a shift occurs in the molar relationship, the coefficient value is not the same for points on the mandible, midface, and skull. This finding highlights the existence of discontinuities during postnatal facial growth in children. It also strongly suggests the existence of a correlation and perhaps a causal dependence between the occlusal rela-

tionship and the growth of the facial skeleton, especially the mandible.

Occlusal development appears to involve two phases:

1. The first phase consists of all morphogenetic processes leading to a stable occlusion. During this phase, different parts of the servosystem are already existent and functional, but a stable occlusal development capable of serving as a peripheral comparator has not yet been achieved. Without an operational peripheral comparator having a stable position between the lower and upper dental arches for a reference point, the creation of an engram* for the adequate postural activity of the masticatory muscles is not possible. The engram serves as a reference for the central comparator. In other words, during the first phase, mandibular morphogenesis cannot be regulated through information originating from the occlusal relationships.

2. The beginning of the second phase coincides with the establishment of a stable occlusion to serve as a peripheral comparator; this comparator is required for the formation of the central comparator reference (engram) (see Figure 2-5). The subsequent morphogenesis of the face is regulated to minimize possible deviations from the achieved stable occlusal adjustment, regardless of whether this occlusal relationship corresponds to a Class I, II, or III intercuspation.

The duration of the first phase may vary; it is short in some children but long in others and may even be permanent in those in whom a peripheral comparator is never established.

Depending on the relationship between the maxilla and mandible the dentition as a whole or in part may be operating as a peripheral comparator of the servosystem. In the latter case, findings show the existence of a clinically interesting consistency: the peripheral comparator may be located near the molars or incisors or sometimes near the canines.

In the posteriorly rotating mandible, special therapeutic attention should be given to the molar group, whereas in anterior rotation, major consideration should be assigned to the incisor and canine group. Indeed, the action of the peripheral comparator is important in both orthodontic and orthopedic treatment. Whenever a curative measure alters the position of the group of teeth operating as a part of the peripheral comparator in a growing child (incisor-canine group in anteriorly rotating mandibles, molar group in posteriorly rotating mandibles, or dentition as a whole in many cases), the clinician is dealing not only with an orthodontic treatment (moving the teeth) but also with a functional or orthopedic one (modifying the rate, amount, and direction of growth in the facial skeleton).

---

*This engram is developed through repeated sagittal positioning of the mandible coincident with the minimizing of deviation signals originating from the occlusal adjustment. Deviation is detected by appropriate periodontal, dental, muscular, and temporomandibular joint capsule receptors. Such minimization is achieved in a stable optimal (Class I) or suboptimal (full Class II or III) occlusal relationship.

The pathogenesis of many interjaw malrelations may be found in the malfunctioning of the servosystem. Although several malfunctions may occur, two situations are more common:

1. The malfunctioning of the servosystem appears to involve mainly the peripheral comparator, which may be morphologically defective (e.g., multiple caries, extreme bruxism) or morphologically acceptable but have an inadequate reference basis (e.g., an anteriorly rotating mandible associated with a distal basal interjaw relationship, a posteriorly rotating mandible associated with a mesial basal interjaw relationship).

2. The malfunctioning of the growth process control appears to result mainly from the shortcomings of the servosystem. Basically, the control system operates faultlessly but is unable fully to correct the discrepancy between the growth rates of the upper and lower jaws. This may be observed in an anteriorly rotating mandible associated with a mesial basal interjaw relationship (Class III). It also may be seen in a posteriorly rotating mandible associated with a distal basal interjaw relationship (Class II).

Needless to say, the second situation may be coupled with either peripheral comparator condition in the first situation.

The orthodontist should keep the following conclusions in mind: the cybernetic theory of facial growth and the crucial topologic concept of structural and functional stability and instability are useful tools in a systematic and computerized approach to clinical situations with regard to diagnosis, prognosis, and therapeutics.

Discontinuities on the functioning of the peripheral comparator of the servosystem controlling the growth of the facial skeleton are unquestionably salient points in growth prediction, treatment planning, and decision making. A factor that may appear during the growth period as an invariant may in fact result from a physiologic regulation; for a given occlusal relationship, random (purposeless but not causeless) growth fluctuations are detected and counterbalanced. The final pattern of occlusal relationships emerges in a series of bifurcations having to some extent a random character. A given occlusal pattern (Class I, II, or III) may have been initiated by nonessential or fortuitous influences, however, once formed, it remains relatively unaltered because random growth fluctuations are neutralized by regulatory mechanisms and local optimization processes. In other words, a full Class II relationship with a stable occlusal relationship will rarely grow into a Class I relationship. Only appropriate orthodontic or orthopedic treatment may successfully achieve such a conversion.

The existence of discontinuities implies that facial growth can be accounted for using stochastic, discrete models rather than deterministic, continuous ones (i.e., the Ricketts approach). This implication also bears on models designed for growth projection in orthodontic treatment programs and follow-up.

The existence of discontinuities at the peripheral comparator also makes intelligible the genotype's partial determinating of the phenotype. Indeed, a specific genome is encoded

for an overall regulatory pattern, not for a singular phenotype (i.e., for an inventory of possible stable situations). Under such conditions, very small fluctuations taking place around the bifurcation at crucial moments of facial development can lead to two very different types of occlusal relationships. One example is the ultimate status of the occlusion resulting from a flush terminal plane occlusal relationship. Depending on a number of local factors, this bifurcation-type condition can lead to a Class I, II, or III malocclusion.

## CLINICAL MEANING OF EXPERIMENTAL FINDINGS RELATIVE TO CRANIOFACIAL GROWTH MECHANISMS AND THE METHOD OF OPERATION OF FUNCTIONAL APPLIANCES

The question often arises of the interest for clinicians of concepts based on experimental research findings. Animal experimentation seeks to formulate biologic and biomedical laws and explain biologic mechanisms underlying specific pathologic states. These goals do not imply endorsement of extrapolation-type statements applying to humans in specific situations, either normal or pathologic. However, if no significant morphologic difference can be detected between specific mammalian species for a given element of the tissue cell or molecular level, rejection of biologic similarity is unscientific and methodologically unsound. Some clinicians make an even more serious methodologic error. They seem to disregard the biologic differences between the behavior of the condylar cartilage and the behavior of primary cartilages.

A number of remarkable observations based on animal and human experimentation have been made regarding molecular biology:

1. In growing rats and children the cytosolic level of $Na^+$ is higher in secondary cartilage prechondroblasts and primary chondroblasts than it is in secondary chondroblasts. Lower cytosolic levels of $Na^+$ account to a large extent for the repression of mitogenesis-specific genes in secondary chondroblasts.

2. In growing rats and children the cytosolic $Ca^{++}$ concentration is lower in preosteoblasts and secondary prechondroblasts than it is in skeletoblasts.

3. In growing rats and children the cytosolic level of $Ca^{++}$ is lower in actively dividing secondary prechondroblasts than it is in prechondroblasts about to mature into secondary chondroblasts.

4. In growing rats and children an appropriate force applied to the condylar cartilage in organ culture experiments produces a significant decrease in cytosolic $Na^+$ concentration in condylar cartilage prechondroblasts. Compressive forces of similar or higher magnitude do not produce detectable changes of cytosolic $Na^+$ concentration in metatarsal growth cartilage or the epiphyseal plate chondroblasts of the tibia, fibula, and radius.

5. In growing rats and children the osteochondral zone of the rib displays a biologic peculiarity. The area where

the precursor chondroblast differentiates into the progenitor chondroblast is responsive to local biomechanic factors. Indeed, in organ culture experiments, if appropriate pressure is applied to the rib fragment, a decrease in both the number of mitoses and corresponding variations in ionic fluxes is observed in the area of differentiation. The biomechanically caused modifiability of the rat and infant osteochondral rib zone is smaller than that detected in the condylar cartilage. Nevertheless, such a biomechanically induced modifiability appears to be totally lacking in the metatarsal growth cartilage and other so-called primary cartilages.

Therefore in organ culture experiments each variety of rat and human cartilage can be said to display a similar responsiveness to biomechanic factors; this responsiveness is especially evident at the molecular biologic level. Accordingly, the postural hyperpropulsor, functional appliances, and Class II elastics all produce a significant decrease of cytosolic $Ca^{++}$ concentration in the skeletoblasts and prechondroblasts of growing rats and a significant increase in cytosolic $Na^+$ concentration in condylar cartilage prechondroblasts. Tensile forces of similar or higher magnitude do not produce detectable changes of cytosolic $Na^+$ concentration in metatarsal growth cartilage and in the tibia's, fibula's, and radius' epiphyseal plate chondroblasts. This also holds true if no valid reason exists to discount the ability of functional appliances to modulate the subperiosteal ossification rate at the posterior border of the mandible and the growth rate of the human condylar cartilage (Figure 2-23).

A provocative challenge to the biologic similarity of animals and humans at the tissue and cell level is represented by the mode of lengthening of the maxilla. In rats, monkeys, and almost all other mammals the premaxillomaxillary suture contributes substantially to the sagittal growth of the maxilla during the major part of the postnatal period; however, in the human the premaxillomaxillary suture cannot be considered as contributing to the lengthening of the maxilla.

In other words the interspecies validity of experimental findings depends not so much on the zoologic and evolutionary relationship between two mammals as it does on the morphophysiologic similarity between the tissues and cells under scrutiny. However, even in the case of biologic similarity, experimental findings are merely powerful conceptual tools in clinical investigations; the methodologically valid corroboration of a working hypothesis formulated from animal experimentation can be gathered only in the human species itself, and then only in specific and appropriate observational conditions. Even in the human species, significant differences may exist between individuals. For instance, between individuals with anteriorly rotating mandibles (highly responsive to functional appliances) and those with posteriorly rotating mandibles (much less responsive to functional appliances) a marked variability in response can be seen.

The quantitative aspects of comparing the effects of a factor in two different mammals should be elaborated. In their experimental and clinical investigations of the relationship between the sodium fluoride (NaF) dose administered and the

| Affected parameter | Area of effects | |
|---|---|---|
| | Condylar cartilage | Subperiosteal layer, ramus, posterior border |
| Cytosolic concentration $Na^+$ $Ca^{++}$ $H^+$ | ↗ ↘ ↘ | ↗ ↘ ↘ |
| Intracellular pH | ↗ | ↗ |
| Intracellular water content (significant increases may be detected by using magnetic resonance imaging) | ↗ | ↗ |
| Cell volume | ↗ | ↗ |
| Number of cell divisions | ↗ | ↗ |

**Figure 2-23.** Effects of a functional appliance on cells in the mitotic compartment.

bone turnover rate, Petrovic and Shambaugh (1966, 1968) made an interesting observation. They were able to determine which daily dose of NaF optimally and safely stimulated bone formation and mineralization in rats and humans. Taking into account the difference in body size between rats and humans, Petrovic and Shambaugh then considered which parameter should be selected as the reference for the quantitative comparison of the optimal doses as empirically detected:

- Body weight—In this case the optimal daily dose of NaF is relatively much lower in the human than it is in the rat. With body weight as reference, the optimal dose in rats is toxic in humans.
- Body surface—In this case the optimal daily dose of NaF appears similar in rats and humans. This finding is perfectly logical: mathematically, the metabolic rate is a function of the body surface; it is physiologically and pharmacologically legitimate and plausible that the action of NaF depends on the metabolic rate.

It follows from this example that the effect of a factor in two animal species (rat and human) may be compared not only qualitatively but also quantitatively, provided the mechanism of action is known and the proper reference of quantitative comparison is selected.

## BIOLOGIC PECULIARITIES OF THE MANDIBLE—OCCLUSAL PATTERN AND CEPHALOMETRIC FINDINGS

The description of functional relationships between tissue and cell determinants of the growing mandible on the one side and between general and local extrinsic factors (biomechanic agents) on the other is a crucial problem in clinical orthodontics. The orthodontist may be able to alter the local biomechanic situation, but so far the modification of specific tissue and cell characteristics has not been possible because they seem to be determined genetically. Nevertheless, the inability to modify specific features of the mandibular tissues does not bestow the right to ignore them. On the contrary, the orthodontist must make a special effort to recognize and understand the distinctive features of the facial skeleton and consider their involvement in the treatment's effect. A better knowledge and understanding of mandibular tissue behavior and responsiveness to intrinsic and extrinsic factors make the diagnosis of skeletal malrelations and malocclusions more accurate; moreover, the choice of the most appropriate therapeutic procedure depends primarily on the biologic responsiveness of the involved tissues. The difficult problem is deciding the way the orthodontist can acquire information about the biologic peculiarities of an individual patient's facial skeleton tissues.

Several approaches to this problem have been described and widely discussed in the orthodontic community. In the following paragraphs an approach founded on cephalometric analysis is presented and compared with animal experiments and cell and molecular biology findings in different mammals, including humans.

Previous investigations have provided a new way of categorizing children that takes into consideration both the mandible and maxilla and directs attention to individuals who are morphogenetically and morphologically alike and grow and respond similarly to orthopedic or functional treatment. This systematization has been further elaborated and presently takes the form of a three-level arborization (Figure 2-24):

1. The first level, based on the quantitative determination of the difference between maxillary and mandibular sagittal growth, likewise has three main branches:

    a. In about 70% of the children in the sample, sagittal growth of the mandible and maxilla remained quantitatively in the same range. Any tendency toward sagittal deviation from the normal occlusal relationship during growth was either physiologically corrected through the peripheral comparator of the servosystem or orthopedically curable by appropriate functional appliances.

    b. In about 3% of the children, sagittal growth of the mandible was far greater than that of the maxilla.

    c. In about 25% of the children, sagittal growth of the mandible was far less than that of the maxilla.

        In the latter two situations the spontaneous servosystem correction of the discrepancy is moderate (clinically insufficient). Even orthopedic treatment using a functional appliance is usually not fully efficient; the ultimate solution is orthognathic surgery.

        Cell and organ culture investigations strongly suggest that the first-level trifurcation results from quantitative differences at the cell and molecular biology level. For example (Petrovic, 1982), changes in ionic ($Na^+$, $Ca^{++}$, $H^+$) flux rates and in the percentage of mitoses in human condylar cartilage under the

influence of hormones (STH-somatomedin, insulin) and local biomechanic factors are much smaller in the $c$ branch than those in the $A$ branch. The mitotic index in the mandibular subperiosteal layer and the turnover rate of the alveolar bone also are smaller in the $c$ branch.

2. The second level, based on variations in the direction of mandibular and maxillary growth, affects each of the three main branches. It relates to growth inclination and growth rotation of both the mandible and maxilla. The variations observed at this level depend at least partly on respiration, phonation, and deglutition factors. The occlusal relationship that functions as the peripheral comparator of the physiologic servosystem regulating the growth rate of the mandible plays a subordinate role; however, in some clinical situations, it can markedly modify the direction of growth of the condyle and ramus.

3. The third level, based on the occlusal relationship that functions as the peripheral comparator of the servosystem, has subdivisions representing either an aggravation or a melioration of malocclusions resulting from the first two arborizational levels. Both full Class I and II intercuspations correspond to a stable occlusal situation; they are separated by unstable occlusions (cusp-to-cusp) representing functional discontinuities. A stable occlusion coincides with a well-established comparator reference that functions cybernetically as an attractor; that is, any tendency toward sagittal deviation from stable occlusion is detected by the peripheral comparator and, reduced or canceled through the servosystem. From this point of view the sagittal deviation appears to be the first cause initiating regulatory physiologic processes, and a stable occlusion (either Class I or II) is the ultimate outcome. Logically a full Class II intercuspation with a stable occlusal relationship will seldom if ever be allowed to grow spontaneously into a Class I intercuspation.

An unstable occlusal relationship corresponds topologically to a bifurcation type of situation and acts as a repeller. For example, in the second-level arborization a group exists in which 50% of the children have an unstable (i.e., bifurcation-type) situation at the time of permanent first molar eruption. In half these children the occlusal relationship later develops into a Class I in the other half, it develops into a Class II intercuspation. In the unstable occlusal situation (the repeller) a minimal fluctuation in molar position can lead to a stable situation; in other words, it can be the source of two types of occlusal relationships. This minimal fluctuation can be either spontaneous (resulting from dental disharmonies such as variations in tooth size and form, caries, early loss of teeth) or therapeutically induced (i.e., by the face-bow, the appliance indicated in this example).

This way of reasoning in dentofacial orthopedics leads to two conclusions:

1. The occlusal situation, including skeletal and dental malrelations, is determined by morphophysiologic

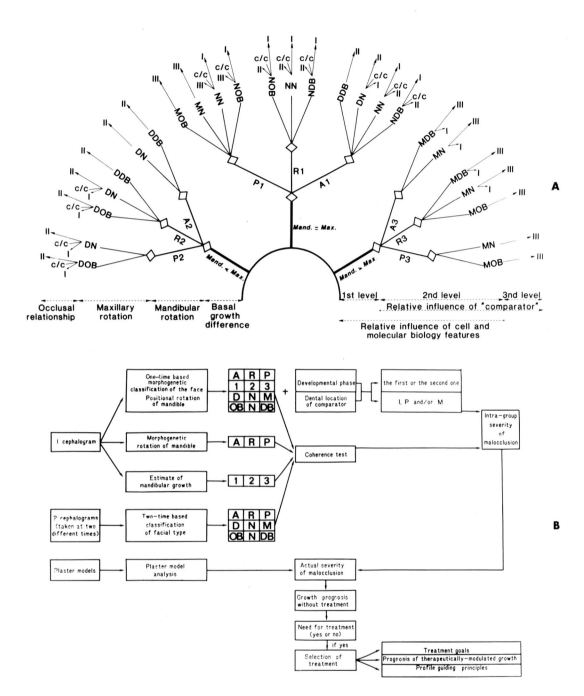

**Figure 2-24.** Morphogenetic classification of human facial development according to Lavergne and Petrovic (1983). **A,** Three-level arborization. *I, II,* and *III,* First molar occlusal relationships (stable); *c/c,* cusp-to-cusp molar relationships (unstable); *long straight arrow,* main outcome; *short arrow,* less frequent outcome; *straight line,* unachieved outcome. **B,** Flow diagram of orthodontic planning. Only 25 of the 33 outcomes at the second level are represented; 8 outcomes (constituting 3% of the population studied) are omitted. *A, R,* and *P,* Anterior, neutral, and posterior mandibular rotation; *1, 2,* and *3,* mandible equal to, less than, or greater than maxilla; *D, N,* and *M,* posteroanterior state distal, normal, or mesial; *OB, N,* and *DB,* open-bite, normal, and deep bite.; *R1NN,* neutral mandibular growth rotation, small basal growth difference, normal basal posteroanterior relationship, and normal basal vertical relationship.

*Continued*

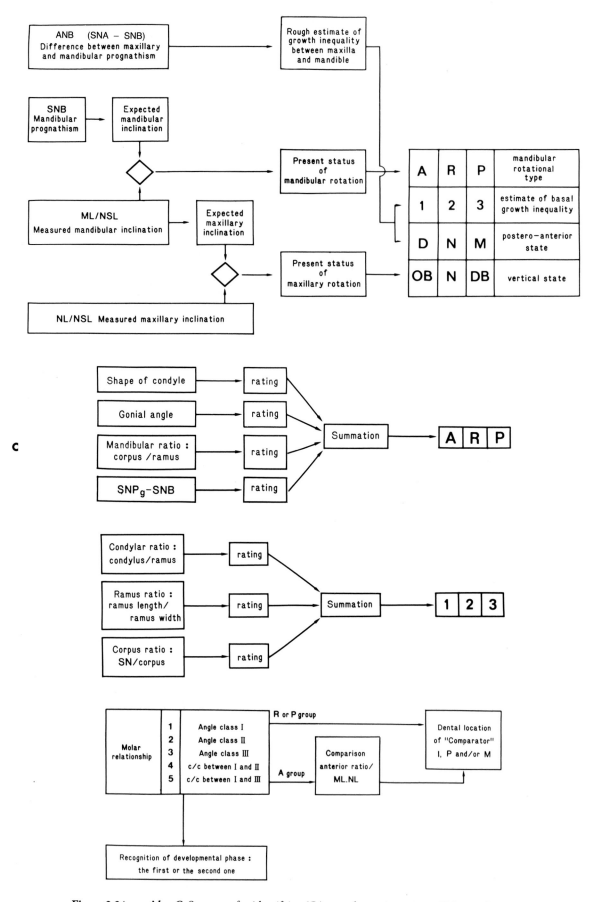

**Figure 2-24, cont'd.**   **C,** Sequence for identifying ($C_1$) growth rotation group, ($C_2$) morphogenetic rotation of the mandible, ($C_3$) growth of the mandible, and ($C_4$) location of the comparator. Each group consists of patients who are morphogenetically and morphologically similar.

characteristics (represented formally by the three-level arborization). In the shift from the first to the third level the proportion of tissue and cell peculiarities decreases, whereas the proportion of the interdental relation pattern increases. Because of vertical feedback connections among the three levels of arborization, any appropriate physiologic or orthopedic operation that uses the comparator and servosystem and aims at modifying the occlusal adjustment exerts a mild regulating effect on the morphogenetic rotation of the mandible (Lavergne, Gasson, 1977). Accordingly, treatment of skeletal malrelations could be greatly facilitated if therapeutic agents were able to amplify mandibular tissue and cell responsiveness to functional appliances. Needless to say, such amplifying agents remain to be discovered and carefully investigated.

2. A Class I or II occlusal situation may have been initiated by casual fluctuations at the peripheral comparator of the servosystem; however, once established, a given occlusal pattern remains basically unaltered. Indeed, random growth fluctuations are constantly regulated by regional and local feedback mechanisms and local optimization processes.

## RECENT PHYSIOLOGIC AND CLINICAL FINDINGS RELATIVE TO THE METHOD OF OPERATION OF FUNCTIONAL APPLIANCES

Clinical research indicates well-established correlations between orthopedic, functional, and orthodontic appliances and their macroscopically observable effects. The experimental research approach allows researchers to discover hidden biologic processes that facilitate spontaneous and appliance-induced effects (see Figure 2-1). In this way, biologic research investigation contributes conceptually to a better understanding of clinical situations and thus to more rational clinical decision making. Nevertheless, some still affirm that few applications of scientific method exist in clinical orthodontic research (Bookstein, 1991).

The research approach, outcomes, and cognitive status of medical and orthodontic concepts and theories can be formulated as follows:

- Description and classification—Classically, characterization and recognition of pathologic states require the classification of morbid conditions by observable symptoms and signs. The natural history of a disease is the description of its specific character, origin, onset, progression, termination, and mode of treatment. Methodologically, this approach contributes to expertise in diagnosis and therapeutics for trial-and-error medicine and orthodontics.
- Experimental approach—This approach allows the detection of causal relationships, usually through investigations of animals and organ culture (animal and human tissues).
- Molecular biology approach—This approach allows the

explanation of causal relationships. Methodologically, it contributes to reduction-type medical and orthodontic knowledge.
- Systemic approach—This approach allows the construction and testing of comprehensive but explicit and unequivocally articulated systems of knowledge with logically integrated relations of dependence, including interactions and negative and positive feedbacks. Methodologically, it contributes to modern, physiopathology-oriented, biomedical thinking and conceptualization as well as cybernetically conditioned decision making in medicine and orthodontics.

The effectiveness and safety of functional and orthopedic appliances are tested using both classical clinical procedures and the findings of research based on animals and human tissue cultures. The continuing development of dentofacial orthopedic appliances requires a better understanding of the biologic features of craniofacial growth mechanisms.

Research investigations at the tissue, cell, and molecular level in organ culture have established that the responsiveness of various growing human cartilages to appropriate biomechanic factors does not differ significantly from that seen in the corresponding growing animal cartilages (Petrovic, Stutzmann, 1982, 1984, 1985, 1986, 1988a, 1990, 1994). The application of functional appliances in growing rats and humans causes an increase in cytosolic $Na^+$ and intracytoplasmic water in the cells of the mitotic compartment of the condylar cartilage and in the cells of the subperiosteal zone of the posterior border of the ramus (Petrovic, Stutzmann, 1988ab). The phenomenon may be detected using magnetic resonance imaging (MRI). Research studies clearly demonstrate that biologically no reason exists to claim that human condylar cartilage reacts differently from animal condylar cartilage.

Results of long-term experimental investigations with appropriate functional appliances show that an increase in overall mandibular length may be achieved in growing rats and monkeys. Whether this applies to children is a difficult question to answer. No research approach is flawless, and various investigators express opposing views. Quantitative investigations (Baumrind et al, 1978, 1981; De Vincenzo et al, 1987; McNamara, 1986; Petrovic, Stutzmann, 1988, 1990, 1991, 1992) have found that the growth of the mandible in children can be altered; this alteration can be detected through well-designed clinical procedures. However, several researchers (Janson, 1983; Mills, 1983; Teuscher, 1986; Wieslander, Lagerström, 1979) do not consider the therapeutic effects of functional appliances on the lengthening of the mandible significant. According to Pancherz the alteration of growth direction may be the most significant long-term effect.

Without discussing the reported negative findings in detail, accounting for discrepancies in the literature concerning the effects of functional appliances on the lengthening of the human mandible is difficult. Individual differences in the responsiveness of the growing mandible to biomechanic factors are much greater in children than they are in pure strains of rats (for example, the Sprague-Dawley strain). Accordingly, the responsiveness of different children to functional appliances also is variable. The biologic concept of auxologic (i.e., of mandibular tissue–level growth potential* and responsiveness† to orthopedic and functional appliances) change, based on investigations on human mandibular tissues (Table 2-11), is an attempt to account for the differences among individuals the clinician faces in daily practice.

Comparative studies on the human ramus' subperiosteal ossification rate; the alveolar bone turnover rate and its orthodontically induced variations; and the clinical effectiveness of various techniques show that biologic features of mandibular tissues and the level of tissue growth potential and responsiveness are essential for treatment effectiveness. Björk (1955, 1969) described two varieties of mandibular growth rotation: anterior and posterior. Lavergne and Gasson (1977) introduced the concept of morphogenetic and positional‡ rotations. They also classified growth rotations as posterior, neutral, and anterior (1982). After investigating the mandibular tissue-level growth potential and responsiveness to orthodontic, orthopedic, and functional appliances, they described six auxologic (tissue-level growth potential) categories (Figure 2-25). They also identified the 11 rotation types described cephalometrically (see Table 2-11 and Figure 2-25). This categorization helps define the biologic, interindividual variations of the growing mandible. The result of this research is that the identification of a given rotation type is in fact an indirect identification of the auxologic category. In other words, when dealing with the mandible, clinicians must place greater emphasis on recognizing the tissue-level growth responsiveness to an appliance than on determining the growth direction (see Table 2-11 and Figure 2-25).

As previously noted, the supplement of anteroposterior growth in rats as induced by growth hormone (small amounts of testosterone or estrogen) is always greater in the mandible than it is in the maxilla. In children, interindividual variability of growth potential and responsiveness also is much greater in the mandible than it is in the maxilla. Interindividual tissue-level variations (as subdivided into six auxologic categories) are pronounced in the mandible but are less discernible in the maxilla.

The difficult problem in determining the effectiveness of an orthopedic or functional appliance is choosing the appropriate controls. For instance, in evaluating the effects of the activator on mandibular growth, Teuscher (1986) used a corresponding general population of children as controls. Such a methodologic choice may partly account for Teuscher's conclusion that the activator has no clinically significant effect on the lengthening of the mandible. Petrovic and Stutzmann pre-

---

*Tissue-level growth potential corresponds to the level of the subperiosteal ossification rate and the level of the alveolar bone turnover rate (Petrovic, Stutzmann, 1986).

†Tissue-level growth responsiveness corresponds to the degree of augmentation of alveolar bone turnover resulting from orthodontic treatment (Class II or III elastics) (Petrovic, Stutzmann, 1986).

‡Morphogenetic rotation describes the change in shape of the mandible. Positional rotation describes the change in position of the mandible relative to adjacent facial structures. (For details, see Lavergne, Gasson, 1977.)

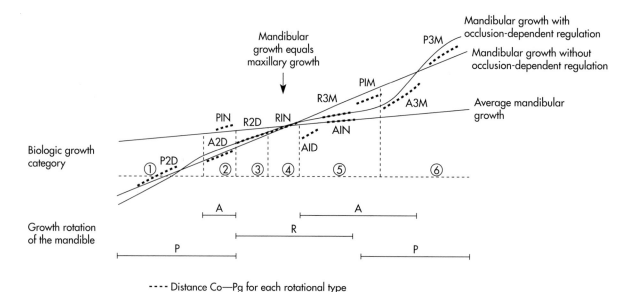

---- Distance Co—Pg for each rotational type

**Figure 2-25.**   The six auxologic categories of the human mandible, with rotational types and corresponding condylion-pogonion (co-Pg) distances. On the left side the auxologic potential of the mandible is inferior to that of the maxilla auxologic tendency to Class II. On the right side the auxologic potential of the mandible is superior to that of the maxilla auxologic tendency to Class III. With respect to the neutral growth rotation of the mandible (R) a posterior growth rotation (P) increases the condylion-pogonion distance by opening the angle between the corpus and ramus, whereas an anterior growth rotation (A) decreases this distance by closing the angle. The vertical relation is normal.

TABLE 2-11. • CELL DIVISION INDEX IN THE SUBPERIOSTEAL LAYER LOCATED BELOW THE CONDYLAR CARTILAGE ON THE VESTIBULAR SIDE OF THE RAMUS IN BOYS, AS RELATED TO AUXOLOGIC GROWTH CATEGORIES, ROTATIONAL TYPE, AND PREPUBERTAL GROWTH CURVE*

Time of Bone Biopsy

| Auxologic Category | Growth Rotation Type | Around Point M | | | Between Points 2 and 3 | | | Between Points 4 and 6 | | | Between Points 7 and 8 | | |
|---|---|---|---|---|---|---|---|---|---|---|---|---|---|
| | | Number of Observations | Median | Range | Number of Observations | Median | Range | Number of Observations | Median | Range | Number of Observations | Median | Range |
| 1 | P2D | 9 | 1.1 | (0.8-1.3) | 9 | 2.3 | (1.7-2.5) | 17 | 2.9 | (1.7-3.5) | 10 | 1.3 | (0.7-2.1) |
| 2 | A2D | 6 | 1.4 | (1.2-1.8) | 9 | 2.8 | (2.6-3.8) | 11 | 4.3 | (3.8-5.1) | 7 | 1.8 | (1.1-3.2) |
| 2 | P1N | 6 | 1.6 | (1.4-1.9) | 9 | 3.2 | (2.9-3.8) | 9 | 4.6 | (4.1-4.9) | 3 | 1.9 | (1.2-2.9) |
| 3 | R2D | 9 | 1.5 | (1.3-1.8) | 10 | 4.1 | (3.7-4.8) | 13 | 5.2 | (4.6-5.9) | 14 | 2.0 | (1.2-4.5) |
| 4 | R1N | 7 | 1.6 | (1.4-2.1) | 11 | 4.6 | (4.2-5.6) | 11 | 6.3 | (5.8-7.0) | 11 | 2.2 | (1.3-5.0) |
| 5 | A1D | 9 | 1.6 | (1.3-2.0) | 11 | 6.0 | (4.2-6.8) | 19 | 7.6 | (5.8-8.3) | 15 | 2.3 | (1.2-5.1) |
| 5 | A1N | 8 | 1.7 | (1.5-2.2) | 9 | 6.3 | (5.8-7.2) | 11 | 7.7 | (7.3-8.6) | 12 | 2.9 | (1.4-5.8) |
| 5 | R3M | 5 | 1.9 | (1.7-2.5) | 6 | 6.8 | (5.9-7.4) | 7 | 8.3 | (7.5-8.9) | 5 | 4.4 | (3.8-7.2) |
| 5 | P1M | 5 | 1.7 | (1.6-2.4) | 6 | 6.6 | (5.6-7.7) | 7 | 7.9 | (7.1-8.2) | 6 | 5.1 | (4.0-7.4) |
| 6 | A3M | 3 | 2.0 | (1.8-2.8) | 3 | 7.7 | (6.9-8.4) | 3 | 8.9 | (9.4-10.9) | 1 | 6.2 | |
| 6 | P3M | 1 | 2.2 | | 3 | 8.1 | (7.2-8.9) | 3 | 10.7 | (9.2-12.3) | 1 | 5.7 | |

*Bone biopsies were taken 6 to 12 months after functional therapy began. Points are located on the puberty-linked growth spurt. Each bone fragment was organ-cultured for 1 hour in a culture medium containing $^{3}$H-methyl-thymidine. The index is assessed on radioautographed histologic sections.

fer another approach in choosing controls. The treatment of skeletal Class II malocclusions with functional appliances usually starts much earlier than fixed mechanotherapy does. Therefore children who will be treated later with fixed appliances can in the meantime be used for 18 months as controls for children treated with functional appliances. For research purposes, Petrovic and Stutzmann took four cephalographs at approximately 6-month intervals on the ascending portion of the statural growth curve of 9- to 10-year-old boys with normal vertical dimensions and skeletal Class II malocclusions. The rotation group was determined using the flow diagram designed by Lavergne and Petrovic. In this way the auxologic category can be indirectly determined.

The following points should be emphasized:

- The choice of expected values and limits separating either biologically determined auxologic categories or cephalometrically determined rotation groups is inevitably somewhat arbitrary.
- Hasund's "floating norms" (1973) have to be reevaluated for each anthropologic population. Well-chosen esthetic criteria also have to be considered.

These reported observations lead to the conclusion that in standardized clinical conditions the supplementary lengthening of the mandible induced by functional or fixed appliances depends primarily on the tissue-level growth category. However, the effects of various functional appliances on mandibular lengthening appear much more marked. However, in addition to their effects on the condylion-pogonion (Co-Pg) distance, the bionator and Begg appliance by construction also provokes a mesially directed bodily movement or tipping movement of the teeth, especially in the posterior rotating mandible. The same is true for the Herbst appliance. Thus a methodologically rigorous evaluation of the effectiveness of a functional appliance has to take into account the interindividual biologic variability of human mandibular tissues and the effects of the appliance of choice. These results correlate with Petrovic and Stutzmann's previous investigations that noted the remarkable parallelism between variations in the subperiosteal ossification rate, alveolar bone turnover rate, and clinical effectiveness of functional appliances and corresponding variations in the condylar cartilage growth rate and responsiveness in growing children.

Fixed appliance Class II elastics also have a clinically relevant stimulating effect on the growth of the condylar cartilage and condylion-pogonion lengthening if treatment is initiated at the appropriate time (i.e., during the ascending portion of the puberty-linked growth spurt and in auxologic category 5) (Petrovic, 1994; Petrovic, Stutzmann, 1993).

Another interesting finding should be reported: of the 84 control boys belonging to different auxologic growth categories, 12 were never treated (for reasons not related to the study). In reexamining these individuals when they were between 18 and 22 years of age, in no case did the researchers find spontaneous "catch-up" growth to be equal to or even to approach the supplementary appliance-induced lengthening of the mandible, which led to the correction of the initial skeletal Class II malrelation. The importance of functional appliances in biologically pertinent situations is further corroborated by this observation.

After determining the rotation group (i.e., the trinomial label) the researcher must complete the study by considering the developmental phase and dental location of the servosystem comparator (Lavergne, Petrovic, 1983). After identifying the rotation group, the clinician can use a treatment decision chart. The suggested treatment on such a chart is related to the tissue-level growth potential and responsiveness identified indirectly by the cephalometrically detected rotation group.

## CONCLUSION

The treatment of dentofacial malrelations requires considerable insight into the modalities of craniofacial growth. This growth cannot be adequately understood without a knowledge of the mechanisms controlling it, the essential role played by hormones (e.g., STH-somatomedin, sexual hormones, thyroxine), the roles of the LPM and retrodiscal pad, and the contributions of local mediator-type and regulator-type chemical factors.

Research has therefore concentrated on the simultaneous study of the effects of hormones and orthopedic and functional appliances on craniofacial growth. Results have demonstrated that the interaction between functional and orthodontic appliances and certain hormones governing craniofacial skeletal growth is so vital that no rational planning of therapy is possible without taking it into account.

According to experimental investigations in rats and other laboratory animals, appropriate functional appliances that place the mandible in a forward postural position increase the condylar cartilage growth rate and subperiosteal ossification rate at the posterior border of the mandible. Consequently the mandibles of treated animals become longer than those of control animals. Some fossa–articular eminence adaptation is likely to occur.

With time the sagittal deviation produced by the postural hyperpropulsor during the growth period decreases through the supplementary forward growth of the mandible. This implies that simultaneously the deviation signal also will decrease.

Recurrent reactivation (increasing the thickness) of the postural hyperpropulsor involves a new increase in LPM activity as recorded electromyographically and consequently brings about a new increase in the rate and amount of condylar cartilage and mandibular growth. In other words, functional maxipropulsion involving periodic forward repositioning appears to be the best procedure for eliciting orthopedic mandibular lengthening.

If the appliance is removed after the growth of the animal is completed, no relapse is observed. If the appliance is removed before growth is completed, no significant relapse is detected if a good intercuspation has been achieved during the experimental phase; if a good intercuspation has not been achieved, the comparator of the servosystem imposes either an increased or decreased condylar growth rate until a given state of intercuspal stability is established.

No genetically predetermined final length of the mandible was detected in these experiments. Functional and orthopedic appliances may cause an increased or decreased final length of the mandible. However, a genetically determined responsiveness of various growth sites to growth-stimulating or growth-inhibiting factors has been noted (see Figure 2-17).

Experimental research investigations lead to the following tentative clinical implications regarding functional appliances:

- The postural hyperpropulsor, Andresen-Häupl activator, Fränkel appliance, bionator, Clark twin block, and Class II elastics all exert their actions mainly through the movements of the mandible. Their stimulating effects on condylar cartilage growth are produced chiefly during the wearing of the appliance.
- The Herren and L.S.U. activator and extraoral forward traction exert their actions mainly through sagittal repositioning of the mandible. These kinds of functional appliances seem to have two-step effects: during wear the more forward positioning of the mandible is the cause of reduced growth of the LPM; simultaneously a new sensory engram is formed for the new positioning of the lower jaw. During the time the activator is not worn, the mandible functions in the more forward position in such a way that the retrodiscal pad is much more stimulated than it is in the controls. The increased, repetitive activity of the retrodiscal pad produces an earlier beginning of condylar chondroblast hypertrophy and consequently an increased growth rate of the condylar cartilage. In other words, the LPM seems to mediate the action of the activator, but the stimulating effect on condylar growth appears to be produced almost exclusively during the time the appliance is not worn.

Research clearly indicates that the difference between normal occlusion and malocclusion is not qualitative but quantitative in nature. Nevertheless, at crucial moments of facial development, very small fluctuations around a bifurcation point in the intercuspal relationship can result in two very different occlusal patterns.

The potential pathogenesis of interjaw malrelations should therefore be sought at all levels of biologic organization. Recent cell and molecular biology advances are supplemental research tools that elaborate helpful concepts, theories, and treatment rationales in dentofacial orthopedics. No sector of dentistry has been as totally revised conceptually as dentofacial orthopedics. Several scientific and biomedical disciplines have been brought together in this revision. New research approaches have been added. The progress of knowledge about functional appliances will in the near future largely depend on further advances in highly sophisticated image-processing, microscopic, physiologic, biophysical, biochemical, and genetic engineering research procedures.

However, these scientific and biomedical achievements, marvelous as they are, will not take the place of clinical observation. They will merely promote understanding of the reasons and the ways malocclusions and interjaw malrelations appear and are treated. They will help develop the field of craniofacial growth mechanisms beyond the imagination of present-day orthodontists. Forward-looking clinicians will be obliged to upgrade their knowledge in this increasingly complex field and cease their reliance on outdated empirical information.

## FUTURE DIRECTIONS

A new technique is available for obtaining three-dimensional cross-sectional pictures of thin slices of the human head: MRI spectroscopy. In this procedure, only the resonance of hydrogen nuclei is employed, which yields images of internal structure without the use of x-rays. In the future the administration of MRI tracers (short-lived, radioactive phosphorus, carbon, sodium, manganese) will provide information on dynamic biochemical phenomena. The orthodontist will then be able to analyze the functioning of human tissue in situ, without biopsy. Many problems currently studied in animals will be investigated directly in human patients, without exposing them to danger.

Computerized axial tomography (CAT) is a new approach in craniofacial growth investigation. Automatic compilation of information provided by CAT and other technologies different from those currently used in clinical orthodontics is becoming useful in daily practice as new computer programs for pattern recognition are developed.

Unfortunately, decision making is not always a completely rational process. The modern psychology of individual preferences has shown that deviations from pure discursive reasoning often follow regular patterns; these patterns should be investigated so that discrepancies between subjective and objective elements in clinical decisions can be discerned. "Risk quest" or "risk reluctance" (sometimes based on the threat of legal action) may influence a surgical decision. Nevertheless, the orthodontist must be aware of the cognitive operations by which alternative realities are fabricated to be able to recognize biases that may misrepresent a set of clinical data and cloud judgment and therapeutic choice.

# Chapter 3

# A New Parameter for Estimating Condylar Growth Direction

Jeanne J. Stutzmann

Alexandre G. Petrovic

Using metallic implants to permit accurate longitudinal cephalometric analysis, Bjørk (1955), Isaacson et al (1977), Lavergne and Gasson (1976), and others have studied sagittal cephalometric radiographs to assess facial growth rotation during maxillary and mandibular growth. This chapter analyzes experimental investigations concerning the biologic mechanisms contributing to growth rotation of the mandible.

Work on this chapter was done with the technical assistance of M. Lecerf, biochemist-biologist, Institut National de la Santé et de la Recherche Médicale (INSERM), and D. George, biologist, Centre National de la Recherche Scientifique (CNRS), and was supported by grants INSERM. CRL : 80 40 09 and ATP : 42 76 74 13.

Anatomic, microscopic, and histologic studies of growing rat mandibles have shown that the growth direction of the condyle coincides in general with the axes of the individual trabeculae, located just inferior to the central part of the condylar cartilage (Stutzmann, 1976). Consequently, to determine the variations of condylar growth direction the researcher or clinician can measure the main axis of the endo-

**TABLE 3-1. • MITOSIS DISTRIBUTION IN A SAGITTAL SECTION OF CONDYLAR CARTILAGE***

| Treatment Group | Mean | Standard Error |
|---|---|---|
| Control | | |
| $S_1$ | 70 | 3.76 |
| $S_2$ | 300 | 13.89 |
| $S_3$ | 335 | 15.36 |
| $S_4$ | 173 | 8.34 |
| TOTAL | 878 | 39.91 |
| Postural hyperpropulsion | | |
| $S_1$ | 68 | 4.03 |
| $S_2$ | 400 | 15.65 |
| $S_3$ | 514 | 19.12 |
| $S_4$ | 363 | 21.72 |
| TOTAL | 1345 | 56.76 |
| Growth hormone (STH) | | |
| $S_1$ | 175 | 3.52 |
| $S_2$ | 610 | 16.46 |
| $S_3$ | 597 | 22.07 |
| $S_4$ | 190 | 6.09 |
| TOTAL | 1592 | 43.71 |

*The cartilage surface was divided into four sections; the first section was the most anterior. Each group was observed 10 times.

**Figure 3-1.** Radiograph of the mandible of a 48-day-old rat. **A,** Control. **B,** After resection of the LPM. Condylar bone trabeculae become oriented posteriorly.

chondral bone trabeculae in the condyle and the angle it forms with the mandibular plane as viewed on lateral radiographic cephalograms (Figure 3-1). The mandibular plane is not the most reliable cephalometric criterion, but such an angle can easily be constructed and measured on cephalometric films of experimental subjects. The pictures are quite clear if the soft tissue is removed and nonscreen film is used.

## CORRELATION BETWEEN THE GROWTH DIRECTION OF THE CONDYLE AND THE SAGITTAL DISTRIBUTION OF DIVIDING CELLS IN CONDYLAR CARTILAGE

A histologic and radioautographic study was made of the distribution of dividing cells in a sagittal section of the condylar cartilage of juvenile rats. The condylar cartilage surface was divided into four equal sections from an anterior to a posterior direction. The cells were then counted in each section in the control and experimental animals; each experimental group was subjected to specific orthopedic treatment (Figure 3-2).

A statistical analysis of the results showed that both treatment with the postural hyperpropulsor and with growth hormone produced a significant increase in the growth rate of the condylar cartilage as compared with that seen in the control animals (Charlier et al, 1968, 1969a; Petrovic et al, 1975b). However, the location of the increase in dividing cells was not the same after treatment with the postural hyperpropulsor (a forward-posturing appliance) as after treatment with growth hormone (Tables 3-1 and 3-2). Indeed, animals wearing the postural hyperpropulsor experienced the most supplementation of dividing cells in sections 2, 3, and 4 (mostly in sections 3 and 4) (see Figure 3-2 and Table 3-1).

The supplement of dividing cells mainly occurred in the posterior part of the condylar cartilage. The growth direction of the condyle was simultaneously modified: the newly formed endochondral bone trabeculae became oriented in a more horizontal direction, corresponding to an opening of the angle between them and the mandibular plane. In Bjørk's terminology (1955) this modification is called a *posterior growth rotation of the condyle* (Figure 3-3). If the experimental animal was treated with growth hormone (25 μg of somatotropic hormone [STH] daily), the supplement of dividing cells occurred in sections 1, 2, and 3, the superior part of the condylar cartilage.

This histologic study produced another important observation: condylar growth is not exclusively a result of the lengthening of preexisting endochondral bone trabeculae under the condylar cartilage but also a result of the growth of bone trabeculae that are formed in parallel and posteriorly oriented to the condylar cartilage (Figure 3-4). However, according to research findings this addition of new bone trabeculae does not seem to be a constant phenomenon; it is observed almost exclusively if the condyle is undergoing posterior growth rotation.

**TABLE 3-2. • VALUES OF EXPERIMENTAL ANIMALS COMPARED WITH THOSE OF CONTROLS**

| | Treatment | | | | | | | |
|---|---|---|---|---|---|---|---|---|
| | Postural Hyperpropulsion | | | | Growth Hormone (STH) | | | |
| Control | $S_1$ | $S_2$ | $S_3$ | $S_4$ | $S_1$ | $S_2$ | $S_3$ | $S_4$ |
| $S_1$ | 0.54 (NS) | | | | 20.37 | | | |
| $S_2$ | | 4.77 | | | | 14.39 | | |
| $S_3$ | | | 7.33 | | | | 9.74 | |
| $S_4$ | | | | 8.19 | | | | 1.66 (NS) |

*NS,* Not significant.

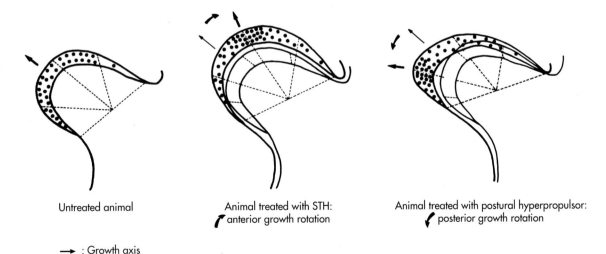

Untreated animal

Animal treated with STH: ↗ anterior growth rotation

Animal treated with postural hyperpropulsor: ↖ posterior growth rotation

→ : Growth axis

**Figure 3-2.** Mitosis distribution and area of concentration in a sagittal section of condylar cartilage. The cartilage surface is divided into four sections.

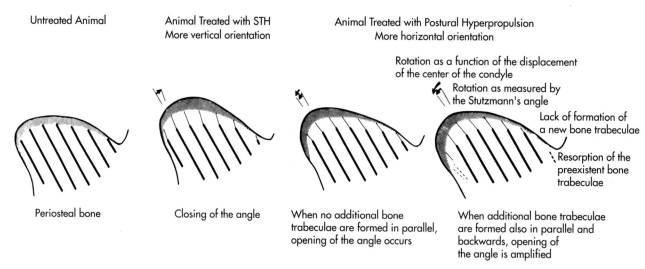

**Figure 3-3.** Variations in the direction of serially oriented, newly formed endochondral bone trabeculae in the mandibular condyle.

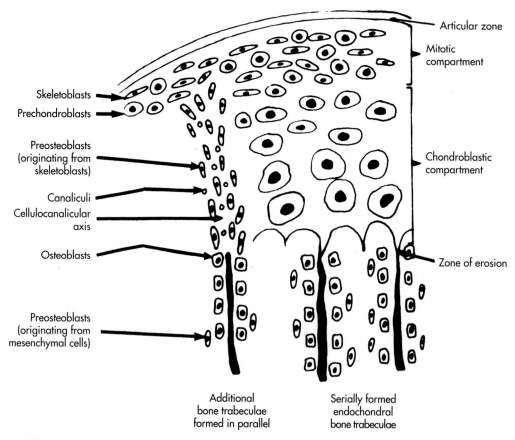

**Figure 3-4.** Genesis of additional endochondral bone trabeculae that are formed in parallel behind preexisting, serially formed endochondral bone trabeculae. In a given area of the mitotic compartment of condylar cartilage, skeletoblasts differentiate locally into preosteoblasts and subsequently mature into functional osteoblasts. This phenomenon occurs periodically and produces a cellulocanalicular axis in continuity with the newly formed additional bone trabeculae. It occurs more often if the condyle is undergoing posterior growth rotation and less often if it is undergoing anterior growth rotation.

## The Formation of Additional Trabeculae

The skeletoblasts of condylar cartilage generally differentiate into prechondroblasts that then become chondroblasts (see Figure 3-4). However, in a narrow zone of the posterior part of the condylar cartilage, skeletoblasts occasionally differentiate into preosteoblasts and arrange themselves into a cellulocanalicular duct or axis. After crossing the cartilage layer, the preosteoblasts become osteoblasts and synthesize bone matrix. The preosteoblasts that produce this parallel formation of additional bone trabeculae do not necessarily have the same origin as the preosteoblasts that produce endochondral bone trabeculae in the more common way. The first group originates from the skeletoblasts, the second from mesenchymal cells in the bone marrow spaces.

If these additional bone trabeculae are formed in a backward direction, the growth direction of the condyle is more posterior than that estimated by measuring the angle between the trabeculae and the mandibular plane. Nevertheless, the use of angle estimation enables the early detection of any variation in the growth direction of the condyle.

## VARIATION IN CONDYLAR CARTILAGE DIVIDING CELL NUMBER, MANDIBULAR LENGTH, AND TRABECULAR-MANDIBULAR PLANE ANGLE

### Results after Experimental Treatments

In all their experiments, Petrovic and Stutzmann (1992) first estimated mandibular growth by measuring the condylar cartilage growth rate and counting the number of dividing cells in the mitotic compartment of the condylar cartilage. They then measured the distance between the posterior edge of the condylar cartilage and the mental foramen. These two parameters are correlated, but the degree of correlation obviously depends on variations in the angle between the direction of the newly formed endochondral bone trabeculae and the mandibular plane.

**Administration of growth hormone and treatment by postural hyperpropulsor.** In one investigation, Petrovic and Stutzmann (1977) sacrificed 10 male experimental rats that had worn the postural hyperpropulsor for 2 weeks and 10 male control rats every 5 days; the age of sacrifice varied from 33 to 58 days. They sacrificed 10 48-day-old rats that had been treated daily for 2 weeks with 25 μg of STH.

Statistical analysis of the results (Figure 3-5 and Tables 3-3 and 3-4) reveals the following:

1. During the normal growth of the juvenile rat, both the condylar cartilage growth rate and the mandibular angle vary between the age of 23 and 58 days. These variations are not analogous; if the growth rate quickens, the angle has a tendency to close (and vice versa).

2. Both growth hormone and the postural hyperpropulsor quicken the condylar cartilage growth rate. However, if growth hormone is given, the angle has a tendency to close, whereas if the postural hyperpropulsor is applied, the angle has a tendency to open.

All other factors being equal, the lengthening of the mandible as measured by the distance between the posterior edge of the condylar cartilage and the mental foramen is greater if the angle has a tendency to open than if it has a tendency to close (Figure 3-6).

**Administration of testosterone.** Testosterone administered for 3 weeks to male rats (1.5 μg of testosterone per gram of body weight daily) starting on day 28 stimulated both the growth rate of the condylar cartilage and the lengthening of the mandible (Petrovic, Stutzmann, 1977; Stutzmann, 1976; Stutzmann, Petrovic, 1977, 1978a). Simultaneously, the angle between the main axis of the newly formed endochondral bone trabeculae and the mandibular plane decreased (Table 3-5).

**Resection of the lateral pterygoid muscle.** Resection of the lateral pterygoid muscle (LPM) was followed by a significant

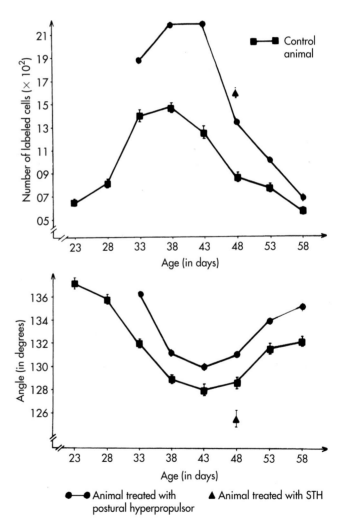

**Figure 3-5.** Growth rate of condylar cartilage in rats (as measured by the number of ³H-thymidine–labeled cells) and variations in the angle between the condyle-lengthening axis and the mandibular plane as functions of age and treatment by STH or postural hyperpropulsor.

**TABLE 3-3. • GROWTH RATE OF THE CONDYLAR CARTILAGE AND VARIATION OF THE ANGLE BETWEEN THE CONDYLE-LENGTHENING AXIS AND THE MANDIBULAR PLANE AS A FUNCTION OF AGE AND TREATMENT BY STH OR POSTURAL HYPERPROPULSION**

| Group* | Treatment | Agent Sacrifice (Days) | Mean (Degrees) | Standard Error | t Test |
|---|---|---|---|---|---|
| | | | | | Comparison for means of groups 1, 2, 3 |
| 1 | Control | 23 | 137.2 | 0.5121 | 1.99†    8.27‡    7.13‡ |
| 2 | Control | 28 | 135.9 | 0.4069 | |
| 3 | Control | 33 | 132.0 | 0.3651 | |
| 4 | Hyperpropulsion | 33 | 136.3 | 0.5783 | |
| 38 | Control | 38 | 128.9 | 0.3786 | |
| 38 | Hyperpropulsion | 38 | 131.2 | 0.2494 | |
| 43 | Control | 43 | 128.0 | 0.4714 | |
| 43 | Hyperpropulsion | 43 | 130.0 | 0.2981 | |
| | | | | | Comparison for means of groups 9, 10, 11 |
| 48 | Control | 48 | 128.6 | 0.5207 | 3.15§    3.80§    3.44§ |
| 48 | Hyperpropulsion | 48 | 131.0 | 0.5578 | |
| 48 | STH | 48 | 125.7 | 0.5588 | |
| 53 | Control | 53 | 131.6 | 0.3712 | |
| 53 | Hyperpropulsion | 53 | 134.0 | 0.5164 | |
| 58 | Control | 58 | 132.2 | 0.3590 | |
| 58 | Hyperpropulsion | 58 | 135.3 | 0.3667 | |

*Subjects each group.
†Hardly significant.
‡Most significant.
§Very significant.

**TABLE 3-4. • COMPARISON OF THE MEANS FOR DIFFERENT TREATMENTS BY ANALYSIS OF VARIANCE**

| Source of Variation | Sum of Squares | Degrees of Freedom | Mean Square | F Test |
|---|---|---|---|---|
| Age (33 to 58 days) | 499 | 5 | 100.00 | 53.63 |
| Hyperpropulsion | 227 | 1 | 226.00 | 121.83* |
| Interaction | 18 | 5 | 3.53 | 1.90 (NS) |
| Error | 201 | 108 | 1.86 | |
| TOTAL | 945 | 119 | | |

NOTE: Only groups 1, 2, and 11 are not included in this analysis. Smallest significant difference between two means at the level of 5% = 0.78 degree, of 1% = 1.03 degrees, and of 0.01% = 1.33 degrees.
*Highly significant
NS, Not significant.

**TABLE 3-5. • EFFECT OF ADMINISTRATION OF TESTOSTERONE ON CONDYLAR GROWTH***

| Experimental Group | Mean | Standard Error | t Test |
|---|---|---|---|
| **Number of $^3$H-thymidine–labeled condylar cartilage cells** | | | |
| Controls | 548 cells | 17.38 | 2.60† |
| Treated | 618 cells | 20.49 | |
| **Angle between condyle-lengthening axis and mandibular plane** | | | |
| Controls | 131 degrees | 0.75 | 4.60‡ |
| Treated | 127 degrees | 0.48 | |

*A total of 12 observations were made of each experimental group.
†Significant increase.
‡Highly significant decrease.

decrease in the condylar cartilage growth rate and a reduction in the lengthening of the mandible (Petrovic, Stutzmann, 1972; Stutzmann, Petrovic, 1974a). Simultaneously, the angle between the endochondral bone trabeculae and the mandibular plane opened (Table 3-6).

## Seasonal Variations

According to experiments carried out by Petrovic and co-workers (Oudet, Petrovic, 1976, 1977a, 1978a; Petrovic et al, 1981d), growth rate and direction of the condylar cartilage exhibited seasonal variations. The number of dividing cells was

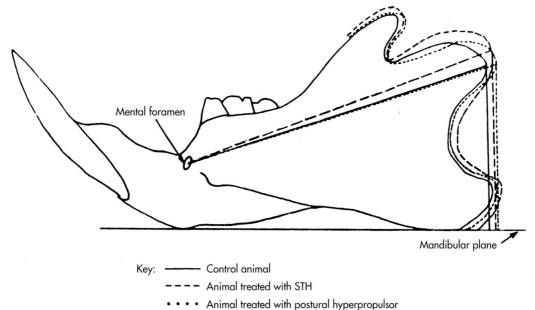

Key: ———— Control animal

‑ ‑ ‑ ‑ Animal treated with STH

• • • • Animal treated with postural hyperpropulsor

**Figure 3-6.** Types of mandibular lengthening observed in rats treated with STH or the postural hyperpropulsor.

**TABLE 3-6. • STUDY OF 58-DAY-OLD RATS WHOSE LPMs WERE RESECTED BILATERALLY AT 23 DAYS***

| Experimental Group | Mean | Standard Error | t Test |
|---|---|---|---|
| **Number of ³H-thymidine–labeled condylar cartilage cells** | | | |
| Controls | 917 cells | 25.31 | 26.94† |
| Treated | 220 cells | 5.11 | |
| **Distance between posterior edge of condyle and mental foramen** | | | |
| Controls | 16.71 mm | 0.021 | 60.89† |
| Treated | 15.11 mm | 0.017 | |
| **Angle between condyle-lengthening axis and mandibular plane** | | | |
| Controls | 133 degrees | 0.16 | 79.80‡ |
| Treated | 153 degrees | 0.20 | |

*A total of 16 observations were made of each experimental group.

†Highly significant increase.

‡Highly significant decrease.

**TABLE 3-7. • SEASONAL VARIATIONS IN CONDYLAR GROWTH***

| Month of Observation | Mean | Standard Error | t Test |
|---|---|---|---|
| **Number of 3H-thymidine–labeled condylar cartilage cells** | | | |
| May | 644 cells | 11.00 | 7.61 |
| November | 539 cells | 8.29 | |
| **Angle between condyle-lengthening axis and mandibular plane** | | | |
| May | 131.9 degrees | 0.295 | 8.23 |
| November | 136.4 degrees | 0.460 | |

*A total of 8 observations were made in each month under study.

## CYBERNETIC MODEL OF THE CONTROL MECHANISMS OF THE CONDYLAR CARTILAGE GROWTH RATE

### Effects of STH and Testosterone

greater in May than in November, whereas the angle between the endochondral bone trabeculae and the mandibular plane was smaller in May than in November (Table 3-7).

Thus during the normal growth of the animal, condylar growth direction varies after treatment with STH, testosterone, or the postural hyperpropulsor or after resection of the LPM. These treatments alter the condylar growth direction as measured by Stutzmann's angle. If treatment using the postural hyperpropulsor of the mandible is excluded from consideration, in the remaining categories, if the growth rate increases, the angle has the tendency to close, and if the growth rate decreases, the angle has the tendency to open.

Generally, if the blood level of STH or testosterone increases, the supplementary lengthening of the mandible is relatively greater than the supplementary lengthening of the maxilla (Figure 3-7) (Gasson et al, 1975; Petrovic, 1974; Petrovic et al, 1975b; Stutzmann, Petrovic, 1978a). However, at the beginning of the experiments, researchers did not observe a greater lengthening of the mandible; the optimal occlusal adjustment was maintained. Indeed, the operation of confrontation between the two dental arches showed a tendency to an anterior positioning of the mandible, which then produced a deviation signal that decreased the contractile ac-

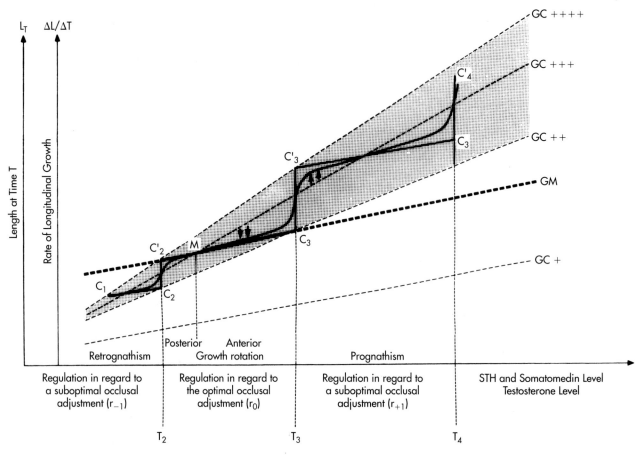

**Figure 3-7.** Semihypothetical diagram of the multiplicative interaction between STH and somatomedin level or testosterone level and LPM activity and the way the interaction affects the condylar cartilage growth rate.

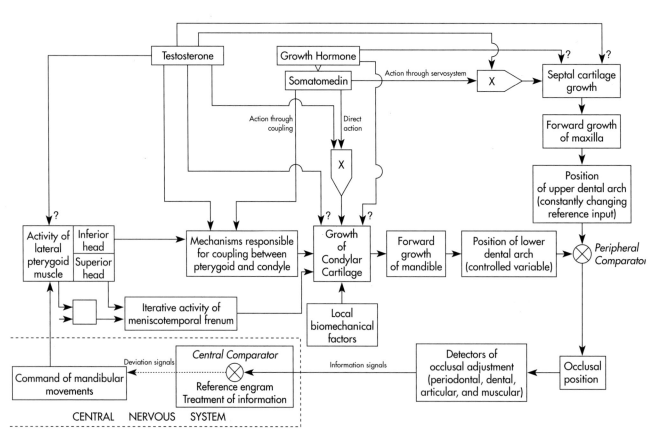

**Figure 3-8.** Cybernetic functional diagram of the effects of testosterone and STH on the condylar cartilage growth rate.

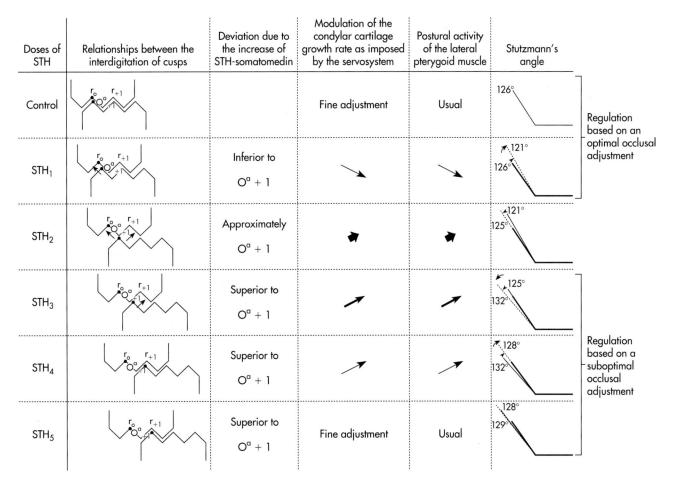

**Figure 3-9.** Variations in condylar growth direction and cuspal interdigitation as a function of STH blood level.

tivity of the LPM and the movements of the retrodiscal pad (Figure 3-8), resulting in a decreased condylar cartilage growth rate.

Experimental findings strongly suggest that the increased stimulation and participation of the retrodiscal pad through the meniscal part of the LPM is responsible for the more posterior location of mitoses in the condylar cartilage. Consequently, if the stimulation of the retrodiscal pad is reduced, the dividing cells are relocated in a less posterior direction and the newly formed endochondral bone trabeculae become vertically oriented, producing a closing of the angle, or an anterior growth rotation.

Such a closing of the angle corresponds to a smaller increase in mandibular length. In this manner the excess of mandibular growth that would be produced by STH or testosterone administration if the comparator of the servosystem were inoperative does not disturb the optimal occlusal adjustment between the dental arches. As an adaptive phenomenon the dental occlusion "locks" the mandible in its functional position. A similar adaptation occurs if the STH or testosterone level decreases: the optimal occlusal adjustment is maintained by the opening of the angle despite the decreased growth of the condylar cartilage.

However, if the STH or testosterone level rises beyond a certain hormonal level (Figure 3-9, *doses STH₃ and STH₄*), the regulatory or adaptive power of the servosystem is overwhelmed and "jumping of the bite" occurs. The reference point of the servosystem is then represented by a new, suboptimal occlusal adjustment. During the transition phase the experimental animal is constantly moving the mandible; the increased contractile activity of the LPM produces an increase in the number of dividing cells in the condylar cartilage. Simultaneously, the stimulation of the retrodiscal pad also is increased; dividing cells are relocated in a more posterior direction and the growth direction of the condyle becomes more posterior, producing an opening of the angle between the main axis of the newly formed endochondral bone trabeculae and the mandibular plane, or a posterior growth rotation. If the suboptimal occlusal adjustment is completely achieved after jumping the bite, or changing intercuspation forwardly, the angle closes again (Figure 3-9, *dose STH₅*).

## Effect of the Postural Hyperpropulsor

If the experimental animal wears the postural hyperpropulsor, growth occurs as if the upper dental arch (the constantly changing reference input of the servosystem) were in a more anterior position than normal. The operation of con-

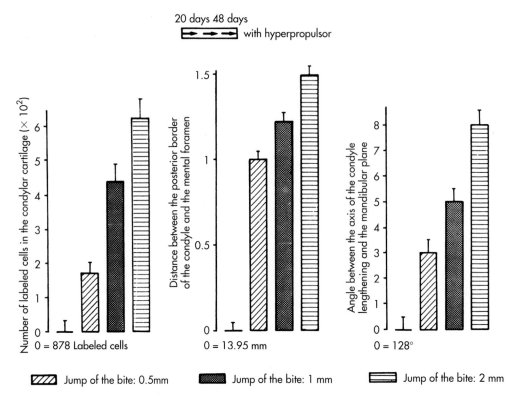

**Figure 3-10.** Variations in the condylar growth direction and condylar cartilage growth rate as a function of postural hyperpropulsor thickness.

frontation of the two dental arches then produces the deviation signal. During this time, the deviation signal is reduced through increased postural activity of the LPM and an increase in the condylar cartilage growth rate. The retrodiscal pad is thus overstimulated, producing a more posterior relocation of the supplementary dividing cells. The result is that the angle between the newly formed endochondral bone trabeculae and the mandibular plane opens (posterior rotation) (Tables 3-1 through 3-4).

If the sagittal thickness of the postural hyperpropulsor is altered, the following may be observed (Petrovic, Stutzmann, 1977; Stutzmann, 1976; Stutzmann, Petrovic, 1978a): the greater the alteration created orthodontically, the greater the supplementation of the condylar cartilage growth rate and mandibular lengthening. It thus follows that a greater opening of the angle occurs between the newly formed endochondral bone trabeculae and mandibular plane (Figure 3-10). However, with time the difference in the angle between treated and control animals tends to decrease and may even become undetectable. This implies that the sagittal deviation produced by the postural hyperpropulsor and detected by the comparator of the servosystem is reduced at the start of the experiment through the opening of the angle but in the end through the supplementary growth of the mandible. In other words the opening of the angle appears only as a transient, remedial occurrence (Petrovic et al, 1981d). Ultimately the mandibular lengthening elicited by the postural hyperpropul-

sor results substantially if not exclusively from growth phenomena (Figure 3-11).

Clinicians must understand that posterior growth rotation is usually the expression of a decreased growth level that already involves increased activity of the LPM. Therefore if retrognathism is associated with posterior growth rotation, little chance exists that the postural hyperpropulsor will be effective. However, if retrognathism is associated with anterior growth rotation, the postural hyperpropulsor will be quite effective.

## GROWTH ROTATION AND ALVEOLAR BONE TURNOVER OF THE MANDIBLE

A study of mandibular alveolar bone that was organ cultured for 3 days to assess its turnover rate showed that the formation rate of alveolar bone adjacent to the mandibular first premolar is greater in anterior mandibular growth rotation than in posterior growth rotation (Stutzmann et al, 1979, 1980b). This difference is statistically significant. Of the mandibles exhibiting posterior growth rotation studied, 80% had a relatively low bone formation rate. The remaining 20% displayed bone formation activity similar or even superior to the mean value of the anterior-rotating type; nearly half of the individuals of this latter group were either mouth breathers or individuals suffering from allergies. The resorption rate ap-

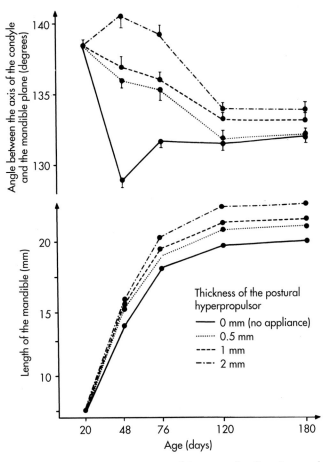

**Figure 3-11.** Variations in condylar growth direction and mandibular lengthening as a function of postural hyperpropulsor thickness and duration of treatment.

**TABLE 3-8. • VARIATIONS IN HUMAN ALVEOLAR BONE TURNOVER AS A FUNCTION OF THE GROWTH ROTATION OF THE MANDIBLE***

| Growth Rotation Group | Median | Range | Mann-Whitney U Test Value of Z |
|---|---|---|---|
| **Alkaline phenylphosphatase activity in enzyme units (eu)** | | | |
| Anterior | 152 | 123–212 | 5.04 |
| Posterior | 134 | 120–173 | $p < 0.001$ |
| **Calcium-45 uptake in counts per minute (cpm)** | | | |
| Anterior | 12,795 | 4738–23,196 | 6.65 |
| Posterior | 8233 | 3172–19,293 | $p < 0.001$ |
| **$\beta$-Glucuronidase activity in Fishmann units (Fu)** | | | |
| Anterior | 32.34 | 17.82–54.15 | 4.72 |
| Posterior | 25.74 | 12.83–42.65 | $p < 0.001$ |
| **Acid phenylphosphatase activity (eu)** | | | |
| Anterior | 14.27 | 6.42–25.93 | 1.83 |
| Posterior | 13.09 | 6.83–22.28 | $p = 0.034$ |

*Mandibular first premolar alveolar bone was removed from 11- to 13-year-old boys and organ cultured for 3 days for this study. Each growth rotation group was observed 80 times.

**TABLE 3-9. • QUANTITATIVE ESTIMATE OF ³H-THYMIDINE–LABELED CELLS IN THE MANDIBULAR SUBPERIOSTEAL LAYER***

| Growth Rotation of the Mandible | Number of Subjects | Median (%) | Range | Median Test ($\chi^2$) |
|---|---|---|---|---|
| Anterior | 65 | 7.5 | 0.4–14.5 | 24.81 |
| Posterior | 64 | 4.1 | 0.2–14.9 | $p < 0.001$ |

*Subjects were 11- to 13-year-old boys.

peared only slightly greater in the anterior rotation cases than in the posterior rotation cases, and although the difference did not achieve statistical significance, it was in the indicative range (Table 3-8).

In other words a high alveolar bone formation rate seems to coincide with anterior growth rotation, and a low alveolar bone formation rate seems to coincide with posterior growth rotation. These observations concerning human alveolar bone correlate with research findings in juvenile rats (i.e., that anterior growth rotation results from an increased mandibular growth rate). In fact, in anterior rotation the responsiveness of the cells (preosteoblasts of the alveolar bone and prechondroblasts of the condylar cartilage) to growth-stimulating factors is rather high.

To the degree that anterior growth rotation coincides with an increased bone formation rate in alveolar bone (without an increased bone resorption rate), the supplementation of alveolar bone formation over resorption contributes to the constitution of a massive mandible. Another factor contributes to the massive appearance of such a mandible: surgical biopsies of the periosteal zone in cases of mandibular fracture have shown that the mitotic index in the ramus is higher in anterior growth rotation than in posterior growth rotation (Table 3-9).

## CONCLUSION

Condylar growth direction presents spontaneous variations as a function of the age of the animal and the time of year (seasonal variation); it can be modified by different experimental conditions: administration of STH or testosterone, treatment with the postural hyperpropulsor, and resection of the LPMs. The cybernetic model of the mechanisms controlling mandibular growth based on research findings enables a better understanding of the biologic phenomena involved in mandibular growth rotation.

The measurement of this parameter (main axis of the newly formed condylar bone trabeculae) in estimating condylar cartilage growth direction may become a valuable element in diagnosis and projection of treatment effectiveness in dentofacial orthopedics. Such measurement includes the use of xerography and magnetic resonance imaging (MRI) alone or with appropriate bone-seeking radioactive elements.

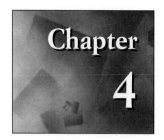
# Studies of Functional Appliance Therapy

Donald G. Woodside

A total of 13 studies carried out in recent years have provided some of the concepts influencing the functional appliance therapy practiced at the University of Toronto. This chapter summarizes these findings.

The first study assessed the effect of activator treatment applied during the evening and night on mandibular length (Woodside et al, 1975). Measurements of mandibular length were taken from 45-degree-rotated cephalometric radiographs using serial samples from the Burlington Growth Centre; the ages of the subjects varied from 3 to 18 years. Distance curves of mandibular length were established for large samples of male and female subjects to provide population standards. Mandibular growth curves established for each individual were smoothed by computer and plotted for each tenth of a year based on these population standards (Figure 4-1). The population standards for acceleration in mandibular length were then derived by computer from the mandibular length data, and each individual's acceleration curve was plotted based on these standards. Figure 4-2 shows a typical male subject with two marked accelerations in mandibular growth superimposed on the 50th percentile population standard for velocity. This velocity curve clearly illustrates that an individual may have accessory accelerations in mandibular growth in addition to the prepubertal growth acceleration. In fact, all but 5 male subjects in total sample of 140 showed these juvenile accelerations at age 9 years; many also showed a third, or childhood, acceleration occurring between ages 5 and 6 years. Of the total female subject sample, two-thirds also showed accessory accelerations in mandibular growth.

The sample in this study produced 30 instances of activator treatment in which annual 45-degree-rotated cephalometric radiographs were available for individuals from the ages of 3 to 18 years. Figure 4-3 illustrates a period of activator treatment coincident with a sharp acceleration in mandibular length. However, this was the only instance in which this correspondence occurred. Figure 4-4 shows the more typical situation in which two periods of activator treatment were not coincident with mandibular growth accelerations. Such naturally occurring multiple accelerations in mandibular length make proving the responsibility of an individual functional appliance treatment for a specific acceleration in mandibular length difficult. Thus in describing treatment concurrent with

one of the accessory accelerations, clinicians often assume the therapy is responsible for the accelerated growth.

Table 4-1 shows that no significant difference is discernible in the ultimate mandibular length achieved at early maturity in experimental and control samples. This first study showed that activator treatment applied during the evening and night

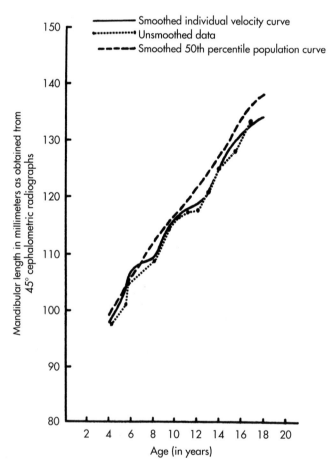

**Figure 4-1.** Distance curve of mandibular length for one individual from age 3 to 18 years plotted against the 50th percentile population standard. Mandibular length increases during periods of acceleration, which alternate with plateaus of growth.

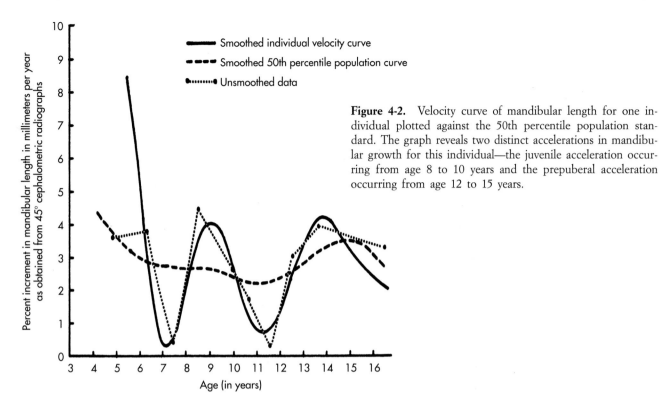

**Figure 4-2.** Velocity curve of mandibular length for one individual plotted against the 50th percentile population standard. The graph reveals two distinct accelerations in mandibular growth for this individual—the juvenile acceleration occurring from age 8 to 10 years and the prepuberal acceleration occurring from age 12 to 15 years.

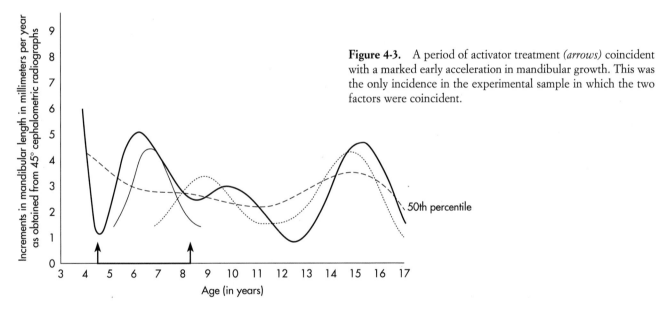

**Figure 4-3.** A period of activator treatment *(arrows)* coincident with a marked early acceleration in mandibular growth. This was the only incidence in the experimental sample in which the two factors were coincident.

TABLE 4-1. • COMPARISON OF FINAL MANDIBULAR LENGTH (IN MILLIMETERS) ACHIEVED AT EARLY MATURITY BETWEEN A SAMPLE OF ACTIVATOR-TREATED PATIENTS AND MATCHED CONTROLS

| | Age (years) | | | | Increment | |
| | 3 | | 17 | | | |
| **Experimental Group** | **Mean** | **Standard Deviation** | **Mean** | **Standard Deviation** | **Mean** | **Standard Deviation** |
|---|---|---|---|---|---|---|
| Treated males (*n* = 18) | 92.9* | 3.9 | 132.8 | 5.8 | 39.9 | 4.6 |
| Control males (*n* = 18) | 95.4 | 2.6 | 135.7 | 5.5 | 40.2 | 5.3 |
| Treated females (*n* = 9) | 93.5 | 3.3 | 124.7 | 3.9 | 31.2* | 3.8 |
| Control females (*n* = 9) | 92.6 | 1.9 | 127.3 | 2.2 | 34.7 | 2.3 |

*Significant difference at 0.05 level.

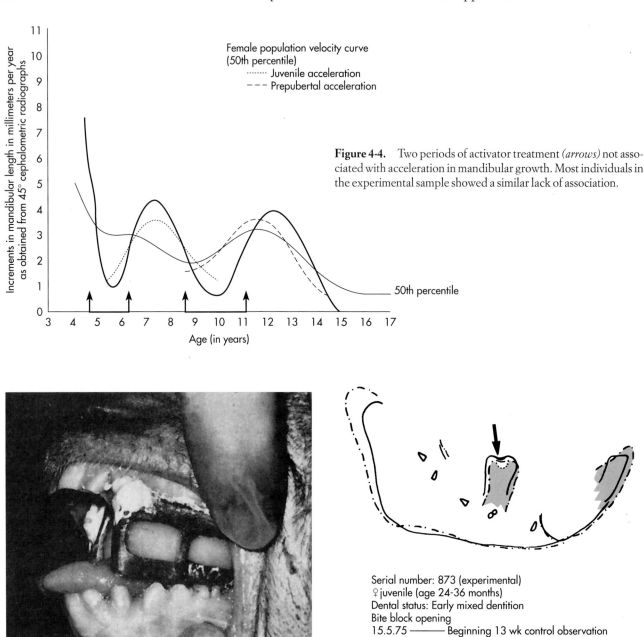

Female population velocity curve
(50th percentile)
.......... Juvenile acceleration
– – – Prepubertal acceleration

**Figure 4-4.** Two periods of activator treatment *(arrows)* not associated with acceleration in mandibular growth. Most individuals in the experimental sample showed a similar lack of association.

50th percentile

Increments in mandibular length in millimeters per year as obtained from 45° cephalometric radiographs

Age (in years)

A

B

Serial number: 873 (experimental)
♀juvenile (age 24-36 months)
Dental status: Early mixed dentition
Bite block opening
15.5.75 ———— Beginning 13 wk control observation
15.1.76 –·–·–·– End 13 wk experimental

**Figure 4-5.** **A,** *Macaca cynomulgus* monkey wearing an 8-mm posterior occlusal bite block attached to the maxillary arch. The mandible is rotated down and back so that closing movements of the mandible are limited to the dimension shown. Minimal condylar extension occurred during a 13-week control period (superimposition on metallic implants). **B,** Extensive condylar remodeling produced increased mandibular length after 13 weeks of posterior occlusal bite block wear.

did not result in clinically useful increases in mandibular length. Thus clinicians should not depend on therapeutically induced increases in mandibular length to achieve results in functional appliance treatment applied during the evening and night. Rather, they should attempt treatment coincident with naturally occurring accessory accelerations in mandibular length.

The second and third studies (Altuna, Woodside, 1977; 1985) attempted to clarify the experimental conditions neces-

sary to achieve increased mandibular length. These studies were primate experiments using juvenile and adult animals in which the mandible was opened 2.0, 4.0, 8.0, and 12.0 mm through the use of posterior occlusal bite blocks without any attempt to advance the mandible. Because the animals were unable to close the mandible, the postural relation of condyle to the glenoid fossa was continuously altered. The altered stress in the condylar area was generated by holding the mandible open and chewing in this position. Openings larger

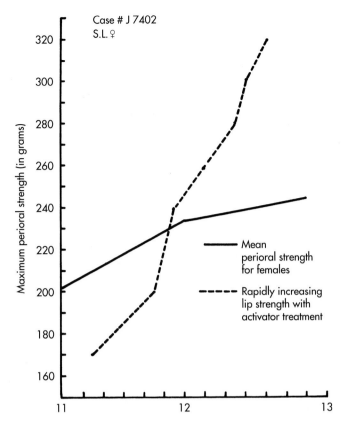

**Figure 4-6.** Rapidly increasing perioral strength in a patient receiving treatment with an activator with a large vertical opening (8 mm beyond rest) in the construction bite. Lip strength reached normal values in 6 months. The bite was then closed to a conventional vertical opening (2 to 4 mm beyond rest), and lip strength continued to increase with further treatment.

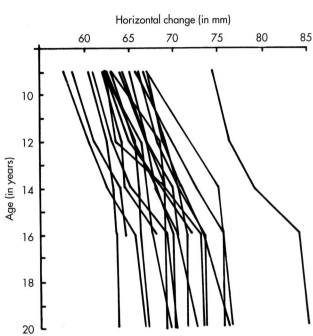

**Figure 4-7.** Horizontal changes at subnasale for each control individual.

than 2.0 mm produced increases in mandibular length of as much as 5.0 mm after 15 weeks in both young and young adult animals (Figure 4-5). These two studies support the hypothesis that a **continuous** change in condylar stress **without any active attempt to advance the mandible** consistently results in a large increase in mandibular length. However, few removable functional appliances currently in popular use meet the criterion of truly continuous change in condylar stress; fixed functional appliances are probably required to achieve this goal. At the University of Toronto, modified functional appliances are sometimes bonded to the maxillary dentition to achieve this goal.

The fourth study (Woodside et al, 1975) tested the effect of activators with wide vertical openings in the construction bite (8.0 mm beyond the rest) by comparing them with appliances with small vertical openings (3.0 to 4.0 mm). Activators were used for short periods in patients with flaccid and hypotonic lips to induce a rapid increase in lip strength (Posen, 1972; 1976). Figure 4-6 shows the progress of one individual whose maximum lip strength increased to a very high level after an activator was used. Large vertical opening bite registrations were used only until normal lip strength was

achieved; the construction bite was then changed to a small vertical opening. The position of the midface was recorded on a grid system, and population standards for the direction of midface growth were established from the Burlington Growth Centre samples (Figure 4-7). The growth directions of the midface for small samples of patients treated with activators with both large and small vertical openings were then plotted on the population standards. Figure 4-8 shows that in some instances both small and large vertical openings were capable of restricting forward development of the midface. (More restriction may have been produced by wide vertical openings.) Because this apparent restriction seems to result from an undesirable down and back tipping of the anterior part of the palate and maxilla, wide vertical openings in construction bites are not currently used.

A fifth study (Shapera, 1974) demonstrated a recovery from midface restriction within 5 years of treatment in a sample of patients who had all experienced this restriction during their treatment. Figure 4-9 shows that if midface growth is redirected, a rebound occurs during the posttreatment period so that the midface tends to return to a normal growth direction. However, full horizontal recovery does not occur, and a net restriction in midface position results. No reliable method is currently available to help the practitioner predict either the amount of redirection of maxillary growth or the amount of rebound that occurs during the posttreatment period.

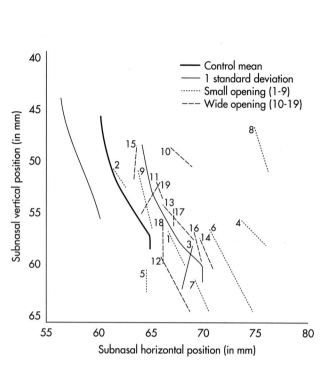

**Figure 4-8.** Vertical and horizontal changes in midface growth direction in two groups of patients treated with appliances with small (2 to 4 mm beyond rest) vertical and wide (8 mm beyond rest) vertical openings in the construction bite. Midface restriction was seen with both types of bite registrations, although predicting when such restrictions would occur was impossible.

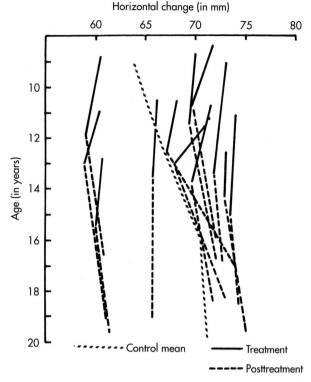

**Figure 4-9.** Posttreatment horizontal changes for the midface (subnasale) in a sample of individuals who showed alteration in growth direction in this area during orthodontic treatment. Each individual showed posterior positioning of the midface during treatment and moderate amounts of recovery during the posttreatment period. Such changes were not seen in the control individuals represented in Figure 4-7.

The types of functional appliances used in the author's practice have changed over the years as the redesigning of appliances and their concurrent use with fixed appliances have become possible. Thus tooth alignment and arch form can now be established concurrent with dysplasia correction. In 1978, 20% of patients in the author's practice received primarily functional appliance therapy with emphasis on the use of the Fränkel function regulator. By 1982 this percentage had reached 28% as a result of the introduction of the Herbst appliance and elastic open activator. By 1996 the percentage had increased to approximately 35%. Appliances currently in use include the elastic open activator and its derivatives, the bite director and speed repositioner (Figures 4-10 through 4-12). Elimination of extraneous labial bow wires without loss of the bite registration permits great flexibility in the control of tooth alignment, arch form, and incisor torque concurrent with functional appliance therapy.

A sixth investigation (Woodside, 1985) was conducted to compare differences in electromyographic (EMG) activity generated in the lateral pterygoid muscles (LPMs) by the Fränkel function regulator and the activator. These differences were compared to test the hypothesis that activity in these muscles was associated with proliferation of condylar tissue. Some researchers also had suggested that the function

regulator could produce this proliferation but that the activator could not. Needle electrodes were placed in the LPMs of a small sample of human subjects. After confirming the proper placement of the electrodes (Figure 4-13), researchers sequentially placed a Fränkel appliance and an activator made to the same construction bite and then made EMG records of muscle activity. Figure 4-14 clearly shows that both appliances generated similar amounts of LPM activity after initial appliance insertion. Whether this similarity continued after several weeks' wear was not known.

In a seventh study (Sessle et al, 1990) a sample of six juvenile female monkeys (*Macaca fascicularis*) was studied to test the longitudinal effect of functional appliances on jaw muscle activity. The EMG activity of masticatory muscles was monitored longitudinally with permanently implanted EMG electrodes to determine whether functional appliances produce a change in postural EMG muscle activity (Figure 4-15). Preappliance and postappliance EMG levels in four experimental animals fitted with functional appliances were compared with EMG levels in control animals. The insertion of Herbst and functional protrusive appliances to induce mandibular protrusion was associated with a statistically significant decrease in postural EMG activity in the superior and inferior heads of the LPM, superficial masseter, and anterior digastric

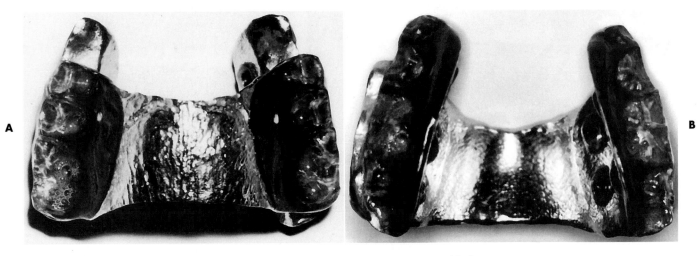

**Figure 4-10.** Speed repositioner. **A,** Palatal view. **B,** Mandibular aspect.

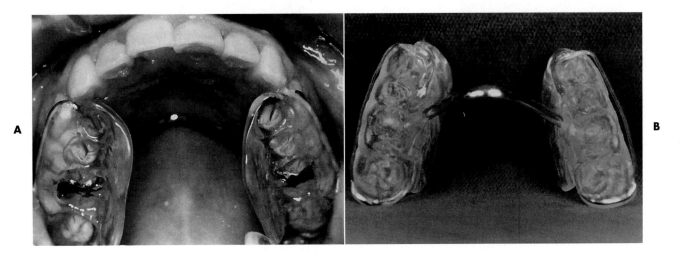

**Figure 4-11.** Bite director. **A,** View from below. **B,** Palatal aspect.

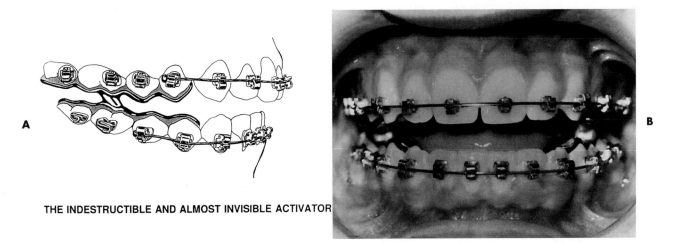

THE INDESTRUCTIBLE AND ALMOST INVISIBLE ACTIVATOR

**Figure 4-12.** **A,** Almost invisible activator. **B,** Activator in place.

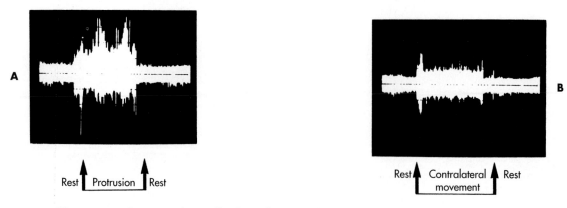

Rest ↑ Protrusion ↑ Rest

Rest ↑ Contralateral ↑ Rest
movement

**Figure 4-13.** In one study, needle electrodes were placed in the human LPM. EMG tracings taken during (**A**) protrusion and (**B**) contralateral movement confirm the proper placement of the electrodes.

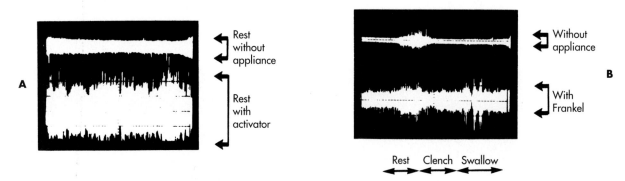

Rest
without
appliance

Rest
with
activator

Without
appliance

With
Fränkel

Rest  Clench  Swallow

**Figure 4-14.** EMG tracings illustrate clearly that both (**A**) the activator and (**B**) Fränkel appliance are able to stimulate increased LPM activity. However, the activity shown may simply be an initial response not maintained over long periods.

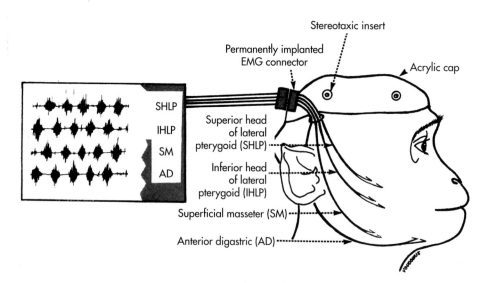

**Figure 4-15.** Permanently implanted EMG electrode technique used in one study. Bipolar fine-wire electrodes were surgically placed into the superior and inferior heads of the LPM, superficial masseter muscle, and anterior digastric muscle. They were then passed under the dermis to a connector secured in an acrylic cap attached to the calvaria. The male connector from the EMG recording instrumentation was inserted into the female connector permanently implanted in the acrylic cap during each EMG recording session.

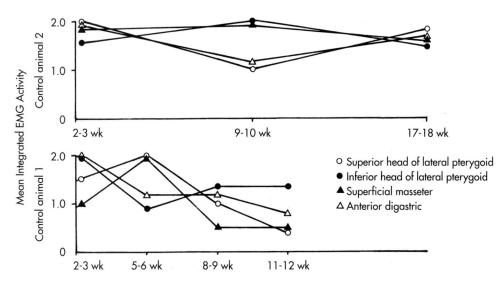

**Figure 4-16.** Masticatory muscle postural EMG activity in control animals. In control animal 1, EMG recordings were made at 2 to 3, 9 to 10, and 17 to 18 weeks after the permanent implantation of EMG electrodes in the superior and inferior heads of the LPM, superficial masseter, and anterior digastric muscles. In control animal 2, EMG recordings were made at 2 to 3, 5 to 6, 8 to 9, and 11 to 12 weeks after electrode insertion. At each recording, EMG signals for each muscle were similarly rectified, integrated, expressed as a mean level of activity (in arbitrary units), and normalized for each animal. The EMG electrodes in control animal 2 were removed and surgically reinserted at some of the recording sessions. The variability in EMG activity over time in this animal is evident compared with that in control animal 1, whose EMG electrodes were left in place.

muscles. This decreased postural EMG activity persisted for approximately 6 weeks, gradually returning to preappliance levels during a subsequent 6-week observation period. Progressive mandibular advancement of 1.5 to 2 mm every 10 to 15 days did not prevent a decrease in postural EMG activity (Figures 4-16 and 4-17). Similar results were obtained in similar experiments (the eighth and ninth studies) that tested functional activity in the muscles of mastication after the insertion of a functional appliance (Sectakof, 1992; Yamin, 1991). Because increased muscle activity was absent in the studies, this activity could not have promoted condylar growth. The promotion of chronic condylar unloading as an alternative strategy thus became advisable. All these studies led to the redesigning of working functional appliances to permit 24-hour wear during the initial months of therapy.

A tenth study (Organ, 1979) tested the hypothesis that extension of the buccal shield into the soft tissues of the oral vestibule results in increased arch width and bone formation at the apical base. A stainless steel functional regulator was placed in the experimental animal's mouth with the buccal shields extended. This experiment was unable to demonstrate bone formation at the apical base, although small amounts of bone formation were evident at the alveolar crest. These results were not conclusive because the monkey species chosen for the study has large buccal food pouches that make effectively stretching tissues difficult. However, the theory remains that large increases in arch width after functional regulator therapy may occur primarily within the alveoli.

Because their previous work was unable to show clinically useful increases in mandibular length with functional appliance therapy, the author and co-workers theorized that the dramatic changes seen dentally, skeletally, and facially in some patients treated with these appliances might result from a downward and forward remodeling of the glenoid fossa. In the eleventh study (Woodside et al, 1987) a sample of juvenile monkeys was studied to assess the remodeling changes in the condyle and glenoid fossa after a period of progressively activated and continuously maintained mandibular advancement using the Herbst appliance. Progressive mandibular advancement was achieved through the addition of stops to the telescopic arms of the appliance; total activation reached 7.0 to 10.0 mm depending on the length of the treatment phase. This mandibular advancement produced extensive remodeling and anterior relocation of the glenoid fossa, which contributed to anterior mandibular positioning and altered jaw relationships (Figure 4-18).

A twelfth study (Voudouris, 1988) found similar changes in mixed dentition animals, and a thirteenth study (Angelopoulos, 1991) showed that these changes are stable. Thus glenoid fossa relocation has been shown to be a powerful tool in the correction of Class II dysplasia. Continuous, 24-hour wear of functional appliances during the first 3 to 4 months of therapy produces rapid correction of Class II malocclusion. A longer period of continuous wear is not indicated because of changes observed in condylar form.

The studies summarized in this chapter have led to the fol-

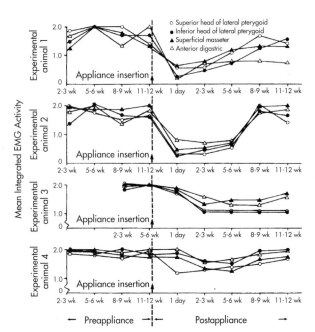

**Figure 4-17.** Masticatory muscle postural EMG activity in experimental animals. EMG activity was recorded in the four muscle groups indicated. Animals 1 and 2 received a Herbst appliance after a 12-week control period and were studied over the subsequent 12-week period. Animals 3 and 4 received protrusive appliances after control periods of 6 and 12 weeks, respectively, and were studied for a further 12 weeks. A decrease in EMG activity is evident in all four animals within 2 to 3 weeks of appliance insertion, as is a gradual return to control levels in most muscles. Many of these decreases in EMG activity reached statistical significance.

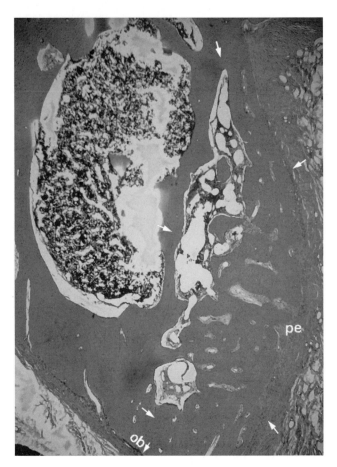

**Figure 4-18.** Section of the temporomandibular joint of a 12-week-old experimental adolescent animal. Extensive bone formation occurred along the anterior border of the postglenoid spine. Arrows indicate the location of newly formed bone. Increased cellular activity occurred in the inner (osteogenic) layer of periosteum *(pe)* and in rows of osteoblasts *(ob)* along the lower border of the spine. (Hematoxylin-eosin stain; × 42.)

lowing conclusions, which may influence the clinician's approach to functional appliance treatment:

1. Removable functional appliances used part time do not routinely create clinically useful increases in mandibular length.
2. Redirection of maxillary growth direction may occur with either a large or moderate vertical opening of the construction bite.
3. Successful redirection of maxillary growth direction is always followed by recovery toward the normal path of growth direction. However, a net restriction in midface position occurs.

4. The function regulator does not increase bone formation in the apical base but rather at the alveolar crest in primate experimentation.
5. Both the function regulator and bionator activator create similarly increased amounts of LPM activity at appliance insertion.
6. The insertion and progressive activation of a functional appliance produce a decrease in the resting and functional activity of the muscles of mastication.
7. Chronic condylar unloading produces a rapid downward and forward relocation of the glenoid fossa; this relocation contributes to large changes in jaw relationships and occlusions. Such changes remain stable.

# Part Two

# Functional Appliance Diagnosis and Treatment

# Chapter 5

# Principles of Functional Appliances

Thomas Rakosi

Functional appliances are considered by most authorities to be primarily orthopedic tools to influence the facial skeleton of the growing child in the condylar and sutural areas. However, these appliances also exert orthodontic effects on the dentoalveolar area. The uniqueness of functional appliances lies in their mode of force application. They do not act on the teeth in a similar manner to conventional appliances, which use mechanical elements such as springs, elastics, or ligatures, but rather transmit, eliminate, and guide natural forces (e.g., muscle activity, growth, tooth eruption).

The influences of natural forces and functional stimulation on form were first reported by Roux in 1883 as results of studies he performed on the tail fins of dolphins. He described the characteristics of functional stimuli as they build, mold, remold, and preserve tissue. His working hypothesis became the background of both general orthopedic and functional dental orthopedic procedures.

Häupl (1938) saw the potential of the Roux hypothesis and applied his concepts to the correction of jaw and dental arch deformities using functional stimuli. The clinical aspects of the Roux hypothesis had already been applied by Robin (1902) and Andresen (1936, 1939), and the capabilities of the appliances were already apparent; Häupl's contribution was to explain the way functional appliances worked through the activity of the orofacial muscles. Function is inherent in all cells, tissues, and organs and influences these media as a functional stimulus. The goal of functional dental orthopedics is to use this functional stimulus, channeling it to the greatest extent the tissues, jaws, condyles, and teeth allow. The mode of channeling is passive in the sense that mechanical, force-producing elements are unnecessary. The forces that arise are purely functional and intermittent in most cases. According to Häupl (1938), this is the only mode of force application that can build up tissue because bone remodeling cannot take place in the presence of continuous active forces. Because of their abilities to transfer muscle forces from one area to another, functional orthopedic appliances are considered transformators. Force deprivation also plays a role in functional appliance therapy, particularly with the Fränkel and Balters appliances.

Despite this biologic approach, the principles of Häupl and their applications to activator therapy had some detrimental consequences for the development of orthodontics in Europe.

Many orthodontists were convinced that only tissue-preserving treatments such as that provided by the activator should be used. The application of mechanical force was considered unbiologic and a technical error.

The convictions of European orthodontists were upheld by the research of Oppenheim, who published his investigations under the title *Crisis in Orthodontics* (1933). He noted the potential tissue-damaging side effects of heavy orthodontic forces. This strengthened the working hypothesis of Häupl, who decried the use of artificial, mechanically produced forces on oral tissues. For many schools throughout Europe the activator became the one universal appliance. Too often, however, its widespread use occurred in the absence of differential diagnosis and correct application. Some European orthodontists even considered active removable appliances with screws and springs dangerous to the teeth and investing tissues.

Schwarz (1952) indicated that activators worked by not only intermittently transmitting functional force stimuli but also applying light compressive forces such as those achieved with removable active plates. Reitan showed in his 1951 doctoral dissertation that no special histologic results evolved from the use of functional appliances; he also questioned the Roux "shaking of the bones" hypothesis, terming it speculative. Subsequent research by Benninghoff (1933) and Pauwels in general orthopedics and many investigators such as Weinmann and Sicher (1955), Moss, Petrovic, Moyers, McNamara, and Sander supported the Reitan attack on the "special quality of efficiency" claimed for activators by Häupl. They showed rather conclusively that each force application, whether induced by muscles or mechanical elements, alters the equilibrium of the tissues much as normal growth processes do and produces a strain on the tissues that can be considered a mechanical phenomenon.

The results of the foregoing research make alterations in the original treatment concepts necessary. The clinician can combine various therapeutic methods, either consecutively or simultaneously. None of these methods is able to produce a unique quality of reaction. As Reitan has shown, even the lightest force produces hyalinization changes in bone despite the claims of light wire fixed appliance proponents. Each appliance is able (assuming its correct application) to work with optimal and traumatic forces. All functional appliances take advantage of the interaction between mechanical function and morphologic design and use the common mechanisms of bone turnover rhythm, activation, resorption, and formation.

## FORCES

The forces employed in orthodontic and orthopedic procedures are compressive, tensile, and shearing (Figure 5-1). Mechanical appliances mostly use compressive forces and pressure strain. Tensile forces cause stress and strain in functional appliance therapy. They also alter the stomatognathic muscle balance. Both external (primary) and internal (secondary) forces can be observed in each force application.

External forces are the primary motivating influences harnessed by functional appliances. They include various forces acting on the dentition such as occlusal and muscle forces from the tongue, lips, and cheeks. A primary objective of functional appliances is to take advantage of natural forces and transmit them to selected areas to produce the desired change.

Internal forces are the reactions of tissues to primary forces. They strain the contiguous tissues, leading to the formation of an osteogenetic guiding structure (i.e., deformation and bracing of the alveolar process). This reaction is important for secondary tissue adaptation. The strain and deformation of the tissues result in remodeling, displacement, and all the other alterations that can be achieved by orthodontic therapy. The deformation of osseous tissues with removable functional appliances is advantageous for two reasons: (1) these appliances allow both the loading and unloading of the teeth and alveolar process, and (2) they may be used for treatment in the mixed or transitional dentition when the bony structures have good fibroblast turnover and bioelasticity.

### Differences

Quantitative differences are evident in force application, depending on the parameter and kind of application. A force can produce the desired orthodontic effect only if it has a certain duration, direction, and magnitude.

1. The duration of force in most functional appliance treatment is interrupted because the appliance is usually not worn constantly but only for 12 to 16 hours per day. The Hamilton and Clark full-time–wear appliances and bonded Herbst and Jasper jumper appliances are exceptions.
2. The direction of force (whether a stress or strain) for the movement of teeth should be consistent. Functional forces may stimulate tooth movement in one direction, but the forces of intercuspation and occlusion may drive the teeth in the opposite direction while the appliance is not being worn. Such "jiggling" effects should be eliminated if possible. This counterproductive activity does not occur with full-time–wear, bonded appliances.

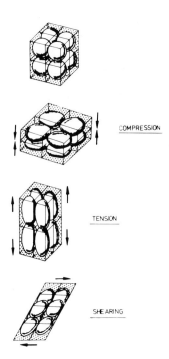

**Figure 5-1.** Various types of force. Each force application produces a deformation and strain in the tissues. The different types of force have different types of deformation as consequences.

3. The magnitude of force is small in functional appliance therapy. If the induced strain is too great, the patient has difficulty wearing the appliance. Application of heavy forces (e.g., headgear therapy) is not feasible for pure functional appliances. A combination of therapies is useful, however, if properly engineered.

## TREATMENT PRINCIPLES

Applied force may be compressive or tensile. Depending on the type applied, two treatment principles can be differentiated: force application and force elimination.

1. In force application, compressive stress and strain act on the structures involved, resulting in a primary alteration in form with a secondary adaptation in function. All active fixed or removable appliances work according to this principle (see Chapter 8).
2. In force elimination, abnormal and restrictive environmental influences are eliminated, allowing optimal development. The lip bumper and Fränkel buccal shields employ force elimination. Function is rehabilitated and followed by a secondary adaptation in form. During the elimination of pressure a tensile strain can arise as a result of the viscoelastic displacement of periosteum and the bone-forming response in affected areas. Tension can be more effective than pressure because most bony structures are designed to resist pressure but not tension.

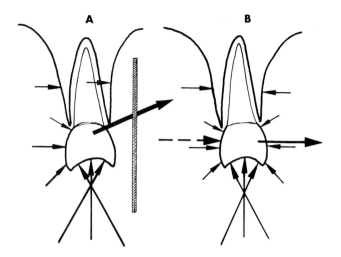

**Figure 5-2.** Various possibilities for tooth movement. Natural forces are effective on the teeth from all directions. To achieve tooth movements, one of these force components can be eliminated **A**, or an additional force can be used, **B**.

Oral and vestibular screening appliances work by eliminating pressure. The shields and pads of the Fränkel appliance, however, also are designed to develop periosteal pull, or tension, to enhance osteogenic response in the affected area.

Tooth movement may be achieved using either of these principles. The teeth move if the balance of the forces acting on them (e.g., occlusal, lip, cheek, tongue forces) is altered. Alveolar bone is pure, membranous bone that by its nature responds to the slightest change in balance. Balance can be altered by the application of a complementary artificial force of muscular or mechanical origin (the force application principle); if one of the components of the total force acting on the teeth in three planes is eliminated, the teeth respond to the reduced force by setting up a new balance (the force elimination principle) (Figure 5-2).

## APPLICATION

The alteration of the strain distribution in the bone and the induction of bone remodeling and tooth movement are possible with both of these fundamental treatment approaches. In addition to these physical force effects, functional appliances can incite sensory stimulations to trigger a neuromuscular response. If the posture of the mandible is altered, as by the construction bite produced by a functional appliance, neuromuscular adaptability to the new spatial skeletal relationship is possible only with the help of sensory input. Petrovic et al (1982d) have already shown the adaptive response of muscle to hyperpropulsion of the mandible in rats by means of foreshortening the lateral pterygoid muscle (LPM) to hold the forward posture. McNamara (1973) has described the reaction of condylar structures to muscle strain in the compensatory adaptability and reestablishment of the original muscle activity. This reactive process is not only biomechanic but also is a neurotrophic response, as described by Moss (1962).

## NEUROMUSCULAR RESPONSE

The success of functional appliance therapy depends on the neuromuscular response. Children with neuromuscular diseases such as poliomyelitis and cerebral palsy cannot be treated successfully with functional appliance therapy.

Functional methods apply mechanical forces and induce reactive muscle compensation. They also take advantage of growth and developmental processes occurring at the time of treatment, including osseous formation and tooth eruption. Biologic treatment, in its strictest sense, works by guiding and controlling natural processes and forces. In many cases, functional appliances can be considered biologic because of their force elimination and growth guidance functions. In addition to displaying "tissue kindness," or a tissue-conserving attribute, they also are more likely to achieve stability of treatment as perverted perioral muscle function is rehabilitated. Retention requirements are often minimal. If a relapse occurs after treatment, it is usually not as severe as one occurring after fixed appliances and heavy forces have been used to shift the teeth to a predetermined ideal occlusion, an occlusion that may be dentally perfect but is out of balance with environmental forces.

Functional appliance results are subject to problems of pubertal and postpubertal growth in which the mandible outgrows the maxilla. If the direction of growth is horizontal or an upward and forward rotational pattern of mandibular growth is evident, posttreatment stability in the lower anterior segment is threatened regardless of the appliance used. Functional appliance therapy, in addition to eliminating functional disturbances, should work with growth and development as much as possible. The orthodontic exhortation "to treat in the malposed area, at the right time, with the right force" also applies to functional appliance therapy. In many cases, faithfulness to this exhortation requires more than one treatment method—using functional and fixed appliances together—to attain the optimal achievable result. The goal of modern orthodontics is to make the appliances subservient to the achievable goals.

## FUNCTIONAL THERAPY BY FORCE ELIMINATION—SCREENING THERAPY

A number of appliances primarily influence the lip, cheek, and tongue muscles. They can guide stomatognathic function (as the Fränkel function regulator does) or work solely by eliminating unwanted muscle influence to permit undisturbed development of the dentition (as the vestibular screens designed by Kraus and Hotz do). The pure screening appliances are primarily designed to not so much change the form of the dental arches as eliminate abnormal perioral muscle functional effects on the developing dentoalveolar area. Unfavorable environmental influences are considered barriers to normal development. Over a long period, they can cause adaptation of orofacial structures and create true developmental malocclusions, hence the need for early interceptive therapy.

The application of protective barriers, or screens, in the

path of abnormal muscle forces also has been called *inhibitory treatment* because the purpose is to inhibit the deformation of the dentition by altering the functional balance. Screening therapy does not work, of course, in morphogenetic pattern–type deformities. The principle of interaction between form and function is based on the recognition that function significantly influences structure and that even the growth process depends to a certain extent on function. A basic tenet of this treatment approach is that normal function leads to normal structure and proportions whereas abnormal function leads to malformation and malocclusion. A change in function should therefore cause a change in structure. If an adverse reaction of the dentoalveolar area has already occurred by the time the patient is first seen, the objective of screening therapy is to reestablish normal function of the molding lip, cheek, and tongue muscles. The expectation is that subsequent development will correct the transient environmental assault on the integrity of the dentition. Some clinicians explain the use of vestibular screens using the functional matrix concepts of Moss (1962). The screen extends the capsular matrix to a more normal space, thus allowing the musculature to function over an artificial normal dentoalveolar shell until it can do so without the prosthetic replication. Meanwhile, the screen removes untoward deforming forces from the developing dentition, allowing the teeth and alveolar processes to move down and out to approximate the matrix provided by the acrylic screen. Proper morphology and function then combine to ensure the stability of the acquired relationship.

The reestablishment of normal growth and development after the elimination of unfavorable environmental influences can be achieved through the processes of metabolism and biologic functions (i.e., the ability to follow nature's pattern by maintaining the developmental rhythms and patterns controlled by phylogenetic factors). Disturbing environmental influences also are hindered by hereditary traits. Thus a normal stomatognathic system exists only if a normal expression of the hereditary pattern is untrammelled by environmental exigencies. However, to give a normal hereditary pattern the best chance to express itself or to correct the effects of environmental assault, interceptive therapy must start early so that it has the greatest adaptive opportunity and the most amount of growth with which to work. In addition to clinical examination, functional and cephalometric analyses indicate to the perceptive clinician the rules for planning, treating, and retaining the correction.

Appliances for this kind of treatment are not likely to produce iatrogenic damage because the elimination of dysfunction removes a hindrance to normal physiology. The therapeutic measures interrupt the abnormal reflex pattern and reestablish normal exteroceptive and proprioceptive engrams to ensure the inherently normal developmental pattern.

For example, in cases of habitual mouth breathing, both the anterior and posterior oral seals are not closed, the tongue is low and flat, and the contact of the tongue with the upper posterior teeth and palatal tissue is missing. By treating this nonphysiologic reflex pattern of habitual mouth breathing with a vestibular screen, the clinician provides a substitute for the anterior lip seal and aids the subsequent establishment

of the anterior lip seal with therapy. By eliminating the nonphysiologic reflex pattern, the clinician also derives the added benefit of an improved posterior oral seal.

## APPLIANCE CONSTRUCTION—THE VESTIBULAR SCREEN

The basic appliance for screening therapy is the vestibular screen (Figure 5-3). Common modifications include the lower lip shield, tongue crib, combination vestibular screen and tongue crib, and vestibular screen with breathing holes.

The effectiveness of this simple appliance depends on its correct construction. Made properly, it can be quite effective in eliminating dysfunction of the orofacial muscles; however, it must be made properly to achieve the maximal correction. Proper construction bites and models that have been mounted on straight line articulators are used in vestibular screen construction. An edge-to-edge bite is taken without consideration of the facial pattern. In activator therapy the mandible is guided into a predetermined position by the construction bite, with exact planning required to achieve this relationship. In contrast, the construction bite for screening treatment does not predetermine a precise mandibular forward posturing but requires only that the mandible be moved forward to the edge-to-edge relationship. After elimination of

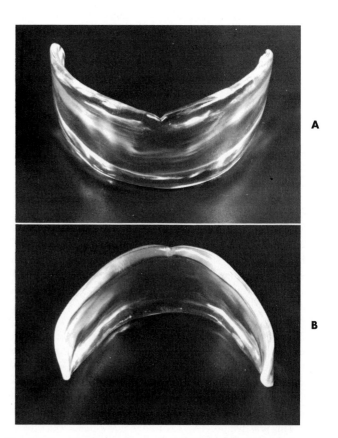

**Figure 5-3.** Vestibular screen. **A,** Labial view. **B,** Lingual view.

abnormal perioral muscle function the mandible should retract to its normal centric-relation balanced posture; the shield does not interfere with this process. A shield made with the teeth in habitual occlusion interferes with normal function. Of course, in open-bite cases a space exists between the incisal edges vertically, but the sagittal relationship approximates an end-on contact. After the wax construction bite is taken, it is chilled and replaced on the casts to check for accuracy. The casts must accurately reproduce the depths of the vestibular sulcus and labial fold for proper fabrication of the screen. Either a thermoplastic custom tray or a regular tray with peripheral wax buildup works quite well. The casts are then inserted in the wax bite and mounted on a straight line fixator before being sent to the laboratory for fabrication (Figure 5-4).

The vestibular shield extends into the vestibular sulcus to the labial fold. Care must be taken not to impinge on muscle attachments, the frenum, and other structures. The desired extension of the screen should be outlined in pencil on the models. This should approximate the configuration of a full denture periphery. The appliance extends vertically from the upper and lower labial fold and distally to the distal margin of the last erupted molar. If the acrylic is overextended, it is uncomfortable when the patient attempts to close the lips and impinges on the mucosa. A comfortable lip seal is most important. However, if the screen is too short, it will be inadequately anchored in the soft tissue and will tip, causing uncontrolled loading and movement of the upper incisors.

While the shield is in the mouth, the mandible, alveolar process, and teeth should be relieved. The appliance should not hinder the mandible's returning to its centric relation. Some clinicians believe the vestibular screen is contraindicated in Class II, division 1 malocclusions with deep overbites because of its tendency to tip the maxillary incisors lingually, deepening the bite and trapping the mandible in a retruded position. This is a legitimate concern if the appliance's role in inhibitory treatment is not considered during its construction.

If the screen is fabricated in the proper forward construction bite, the mandible can move only anteriorly from its retruded position. Lingual tipping of the teeth can be prevented if no contact occurs between the shield and incisor teeth.

The articulated models are covered with 2 to 3 mm of wax over the labial surfaces of the teeth to ensure that unwanted pressures are not created (Figure 5-5). If one dental arch is crowded and the other is relatively normal, the layer of wax on the crowded arch should be thicker. If expansion procedures have been performed before placement of the vestibular shield (as occurs in treatment of functional crossbite), the shield should be constructed following the same principles. The teeth and alveolar process are covered with wax, and the shield is fabricated in self-curing acrylic over the wax relief. The completed vestibular shield should be in contact only with the upper and lower labial folds (sulci terminali) during the anterior positioning of the mandible. The shield is fabricated without a holding ring, which might interfere with the desired lip seal.

The appliance should be worn at night and 2 to 3 hours per day when the child is not in school. During television time the patient should have little difficulty adjusting to the bulk. Lip exercises can make the appliance a potent tool because they teach the patient the importance of an adequate lip seal.

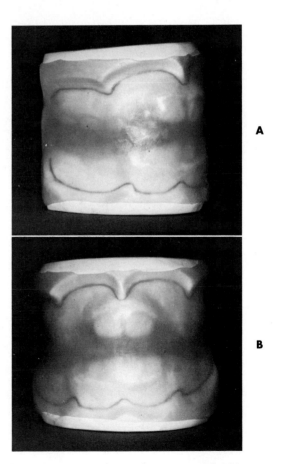

**A**

**B**

**Figure 5-5.** Casts in construction bite prepared for fabrication of a vestibular screen and covered with a wax layer. The extent of the appliance is marked. **A,** Lateral view. **B,** Frontal view.

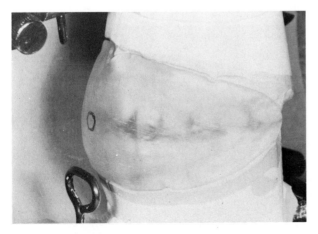

**Figure 5-4.** Vestibular screen in construction bite on the articulator.

Holding a piece of paper between the lips while wearing the vestibular shield is an exercise that assists in improving the lip seal.

The appliance is effective in eliminating abnormal sucking habits and lip dysfunction if it is properly made and worn. It helps establish a proper lip seal and indirectly influences the posture of the tongue. The shield interrupts contact between the tip of the tongue and lower lip, a vestige of the infantile suckling pattern. This leads to maturation of the deglutitional cycle and creates a somatic swallowing pattern. In most patients the vestibular screen can remove the maturation roadblock and establish normal tongue posture. Some patients, however, persist in thrusting the tongue even with the screen in place. This can be observed by the clinician because the acrylic is clear and the tip of the tongue shoves against the lingual surface of the screen. In such instances a lingual-restricting tongue screen also is needed and can be added to the vestibular screen with through-the-bite wire support. In most instances, as abnormal perioral muscle function is eliminated, autonomous improvement of the malocclusion occurs, especially within the dentoalveolar relationships.

Management of the appliance is simple. During the first few days the patient may experience some irritation in the vestibular sulcus or around the labial frenum. The acrylic should be carefully reduced and polished in these areas; care must be taken not to remove too much material, as in fitting a full denture. If a confirmed mouth-breathing habit with allergies is present, some patients may have difficulty sleeping with the appliance. In these cases, breathing holes can be made in the anterior part of the screen at the interincisal level.

As the patient wears the shield and shows progress holding the appliance well in the vestibule, the acrylic periphery can be reduced. The lower margin also can be trimmed 2 to 3 mm, enabling the achievement of a better lip seal. Lip seal exercises should continue, especially during television time. As one clinician tells his patients, "No tickie [lip exercise], no tellie."

The appliance only eliminates pressure. It cannot create a tension effect on the vestibular periosteum (as Fränkel [1973] claims for the function regulator) to enhance bone formation in this region. The most important factor in treatment is to have a soft-tissue seal of the screen with no strain in the peripheral portions (see Chapter 12).

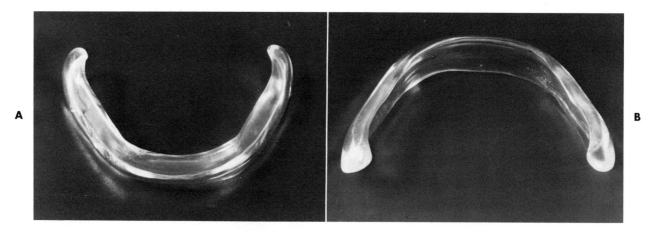

A                                                                      B

**Figure 5-6.**   Lower lip shield. **A,** Labial view. **B,** Lingual view.

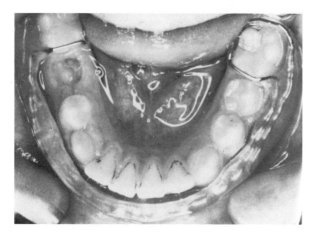

**Figure 5-7.**   Lower lip screen in the mouth. This type of shield stands away from the teeth.

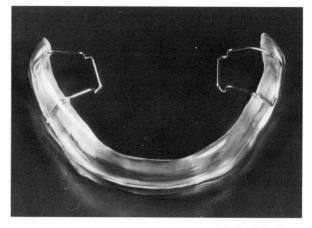

**Figure 5-8.**   Lower lip screen with Adams clasps to enhance stability.

Many variations of the basic screen are available. The shield can be modified to specific needs and morphology, eliminating pressure in particular areas; however, all such constructions should follow the principles previously elucidated.

## Lower Lip Shield

The lower lip shield is actually the lower half of a full vestibular shield (Figure 5-6). It is extended into the vestibular sulcus to the labial fold and the distal margin of the last molar. It is fabricated on a lower cast in which the wax relief has been placed in a similar manner as that used in constructing a full screen. The shield makes contact only in the depths of the lower vestibular sulcus. Although the appliance is made on the lower cast only, the occlusal relationship should be considered. It extends superiorly to the incisal third of the lower teeth. However, if this relationship disturbs the occlusion, the margin must be reduced.

No contact should occur between the shield and upper or lower incisor teeth, even in habitual occlusion (Figure 5-7). Patients can wear the shield without difficulty, and anchorage can be improved after eruption of the permanent first molars by adding reverse Adams clasps to these teeth (Figure 5-8). The lower lip shield has the added advantage of being wearable during the day both at school and home. Talking becomes quite normal after practice.

The lower shield eliminates the persistent and pernicious hyperactivity of the mentalis muscle, which forces the lower lip into the overjet space. The cardinal sign of a crinkling chin ("golfball chin") indicates the need for a screening device to prevent this malfunction from forcing the lower incisors lingually and increasing the protrusion of the upper incisors. The lip pads of the Fränkel appliance perform the same function. By guiding the lower lip into a more forward position and eliminating the lip trap, they enable dentoalveolar development to follow a normal pattern. The only indication for this type of appliance is the elimination of perverted lower lip function in Class II, division 1 malocclusions (or in Class I flush terminal plane situations in which a large overjet has already trapped the lip and the lower incisors are already lingualized and crowded—often with denudation of the labial mucosa). As soon as the overjet diminishes and normal lip seal is established (which can happen quickly, even with potentially incompetent lips), use of the shield is discontinued; however, if a residual hyperactivity of the mentalis muscle remains, the shield should be worn until this extraoral manifestation of abnormal function is eliminated. The clinician observes a spontaneous uprighting of the lower incisors in many of these cases, with resultant decrowding. If distal driving of the lower molars is needed to gain space, a lip bumper with muscle anchorage is indicated.

The shield alters the functional equilibrium of the orofacial musculature, moving the lower lip anteriorly and letting the lower incisors assume their normal, unrestrained positions. The tip of the tongue follows this movement and supports the newer, more normal labial position. Indeed, this support is probably a primary motivating factor in tipping the lower incisors to a more desired labial position. However, if the incisors are tipped labially before treatment, such tongue activity can create further undesirable procumbency. Tongue action has been observed with palatographic registration checks after lower screen insertion. A definite anterior posturing is evident in many cases (Figures 5-9 and 5-10). Thus lower vestibular shields are contraindicated in patients in whom already excessive labial tipping of the lower incisors exists.

## Tongue Crib (Oral Shield)

If the patient thrusts the tongue interdentally in either the anterior or posterior regions of the dental arches, a malocclusion can result. However, a tongue crib (Figure 5-11) with a removable or fixed appliance can inhibit this abnormal function.

The crib used with a removable appliance for an anterior open bite consists of a palatal plate with a horseshoe-shaped wire crib. The plate can be anchored with arrowhead or Adams clasps depending on the state of dental development. The malocclusion and age of the patient determine the crib's length (6 to 12 mm) and distance from the lingual surfaces of the upper incisors (3 to 4 mm). The crib is placed in the area of local tongue dysfunction and resultant malocclusion. It should neither touch the teeth nor disturb the occlusion. It can be made of 0.8-mm wire or acrylic. The tongue crib acts as an inhibitory appliance only; the acrylic construction should therefore not interfere with the autonomous improvement of the open bite.

The tongue crib is not exclusively a screening device. Some elements of the appliance incorporate features of the active plate. The labial bow not only helps retention but also can tip the upper incisors lingually. If the crib is placed at the gingival third, a proper adjustment can stimulate the eruption of these teeth, a movement needed in open-bite problems. The acrylic also can be interposed between the teeth, covering the occlusal surfaces of the upper molars, to prevent eruption of these teeth and enhance anchorage of the plate. This is espe-

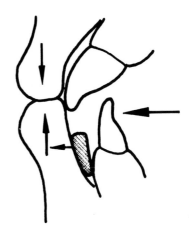

**Figure 5-9.** Effectiveness of the lower lip screen in the presence of labial movement. Lip seal is reestablished and contact between the tip of the tongue and the lower lip is interrupted without interference from anterior positioning of the tongue.

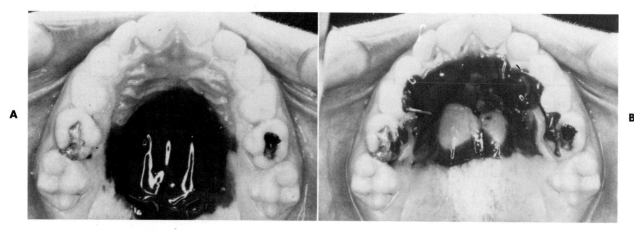

**Figure 5-10.** Side effect of the lower lip screen on tongue position. **A,** Palatogram without the appliance. **B,** Palatogram with the appliance in position. The dark field indicates contact of the tongue with the hard palate during swallowing.

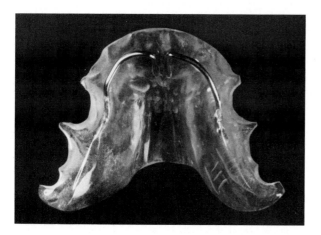

**Figure 5-11.** Tongue screen with a wire crib.

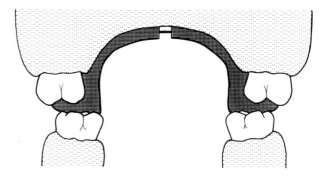

**Figure 5-12.** Acrylic plate extended occlusally to inhibit eruption of the posterior teeth.

cially beneficial in open-bite problems (Figure 5-12). The bite-blocking here can be 3 to 4 mm, which is usually beyond the postural vertical dimension in open-bite patients. In such cases a stretch reflex is elicited from the closing muscles that enhances the depressing action on the buccal segments and helps close the anterior open bite. The appliance also can incorporate an expansion screw to correct narrow upper arches. The appliance can thus combine inhibitory action through the screen with mechanic action through the jackscrew and labial bow (Figures 5-13 and 5-14).

The tongue crib also can be used with fixed appliances to eliminate tongue dysfunction. Circumferential clasps that snap above the molar buccal tubes can enhance anchorage of the removable palatal tongue crib. In addition, the crib can be combined with the vestibular shield using through-the-bite supporting and connecting wires.

**Posterior tongue crib.** Appliances such as posterior tongue cribs are used in cases of unilateral or bilateral open bite and true deep overbite (with infraclusion of molar segments). The posterior tongue crib consists of a plate attached to the teeth with clasps and supported by a labial bow (Figure 5-15). Multiple arrowhead clasps provide good retention. The plate is in contact with all teeth and trimmed in the area of the open bite to allow extrusion of the teeth. Thus the only contact with the teeth is above the greatest convexity of the lingual tooth surfaces. In the area of the open bite a crib intercepts the thrusting tongue. The wire framework extends sufficiently below the occlusal surface to prevent the tongue from thrusting into the interocclusal space during postural rest position (Figure 5-16). The crib is 2 to 3 mm away from the teeth and does not contact them. This type of plate also can be worn during the day and can be combined with the vestibular

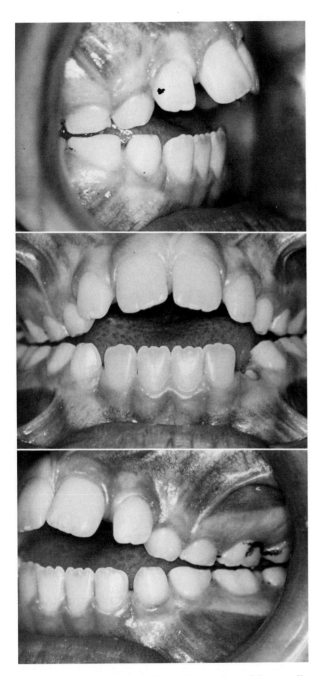

**Figure 5-13.** Anterior open bite with crowding of the maxillary arch in a 9-year-old patient.

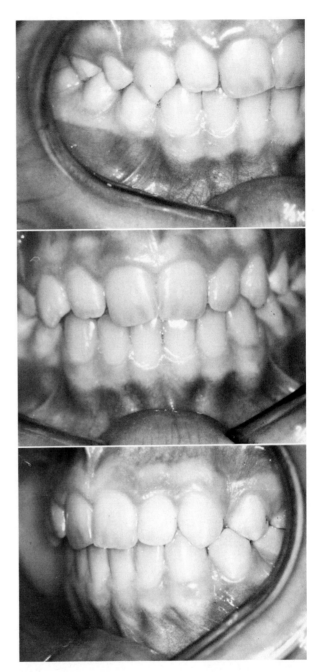

**Figure 5-14.** Same patient as in Figure 5-13 after orthodontic treatment and eruption of the permanent teeth.

screen. It needs no palatal acrylic but only the restricting crib construction formed from the through-the-bite wire elements if it is used with the screen.

## Combination Vestibular Screen and Tongue Crib

A tongue crib, or oral screen, can be attached to the vestibular screen in several ways. A wire or acrylic crib can be placed in the area of the open bite (Figure 5-17) and attached to the vestibular screen by a wire extending around the last

molar tooth. It also may be passed through the interocclusal space in the region of the canine and first premolar. In either instance, it should not touch the teeth, even in occlusion.

A crib also can be attached to the vestibular shield if tongue thrusting persists during wearing of the shield (Figure 5-18). This appliance is worn at night and for 1 to 2 hours during the day. If a tongue crib is used, the vestibular shield can be left open in the anterior region because the tongue action is controlled by the oral portion of the appliance. The appliance can then be worn during the day, prolonging its wearing time and potential effectiveness.

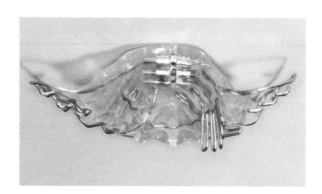

**Figure 5-15.** Palatal plate with lateral tongue crib.

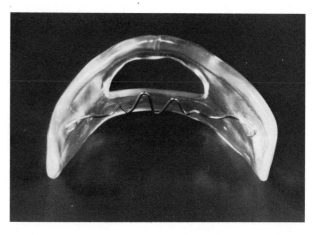

**Figure 5-18.** Combined vestibular screen (open anteriorly) and wire tongue crib.

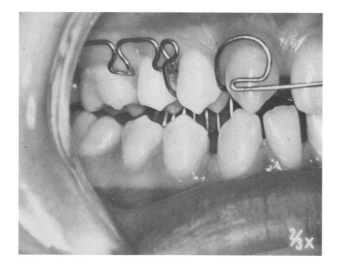

**Figure 5-16.** Palatal plate with lateral tongue crib in the mouth.

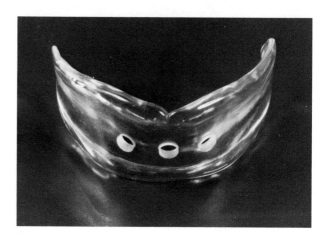

**Figure 5-19.** Vestibular screen with holes.

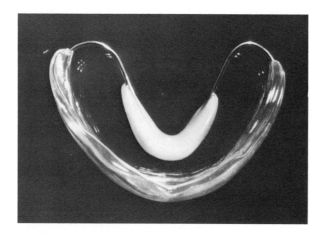

**Figure 5-17.** Combined vestibular screen with acrylic tongue crib.

## Vestibular Screen with Breathing Holes

The use of three small holes at the interincisal level in the anterior portion of the vestibular shield enhances wear for patients who have difficulty breathing through their noses (Figure 5-19). Habitual mouth breathers adjust better with this modification, although part of the adjustment is probably psychologic because the unmodified vestibular shield does not stop oral respiration. The holes can be gradually reduced after the patient becomes accustomed to the appliance, which stimulates nose breathing. However, any structural barriers to normal nasal breathing such as enlarged tonsils, adenoids, and turbinates must be eliminated. This task requires otolaryngologic teamwork. The mere removal of occluding epipharyngeal tissue does not ensure nose breathing. Many children continue to mouth breath through force of habit. In some cases the adenoids proliferate again. Thus the oral screen can be used at a critical time to break habits and assist in conversion of a mouth breather to a nose breather, preventing the need for later surgery. Lip seal exercises with vestibular screen wear must be encouraged.

## INDICATIONS FOR SCREENING THERAPY

Screening appliances are to be used only in the deciduous and mixed dentitions.

### Deciduous Dentition Indications

Screening appliances intercept and eliminate all abnormal perioral muscle function in acquired malocclusions resulting from abnormal habits, mouth breathing, and nasal blockage. Open-bite, narrow maxillary arch, and overjet problems are consequences of the prolongation of these habits. Nothing is gained by waiting for these habits to resolve. Open bites created by finger sucking and retained visceral deglutitional–pattern tongue function can be helped with vestibular screens. Self-correction of the malocclusion is frequently possible, as shown in Figure 5-20. A vestibular screen was placed in this 4-year-old-girl with a finger-sucking habit. By wearing the appliance at night and for 2 to 3 hours per day, she was able to break the habit. Improvement in the open bite occurred in 3 months.

Often, because of a lower tongue position and unopposed muscle forces of the buccinator mechanism on the maxillary buccal segments, a child's abnormal sucking habits cause not only an open bite but also an excessive overjet and a bilateral narrowing of the maxillary arch. This three-dimensional deformation disorients the proprioceptive and exteroceptive stimuli emanating from the normal occlusal relationship. The child seeks the best possible position for the teeth to chew. Narrow arches often produce a convenience shift to one side as the mandible swings anterolaterally and the condyle comes forward on the noncrossbite side. This kind of functional aberration is often revealed by occlusal wear patterns of the deciduous teeth, particularly the canines. In severe accommodative bites of this type the first step in treatment is the placing of an expansion plate. After the crossbite is corrected, the remaining open bite and dysfunction can be treated with a vestibular screen.

Vestibular screens also can be used in the deciduous dentition as pretreatment devices if an activator or active plate is going to be placed later. These simple appliances condition the young patient and usually have some success in reducing the severity of the malocclusion by screening the developing dentition from abnormal perioral muscle function.

For hyperkinetic children or those with potential behavior problems who exhibit persistent finger sucking and concomitant tongue thrust, the use of vestibular shields first is more likely to be successful and produce less psychologic trauma. One example of these benefits occurred in a 3-year-old boy with a severe open-bite malocclusion and bilaterally compressed upper arch (Figure 5-21). An older sister also had exhibited an open-bite malocclusion with a vertical growth pattern that had required extensive treatment at a later age. Because the patient had an intense finger-sucking habit and a crossbite in addition to the open bite and because of the unfavorable family history, treatment was begun at this early age. The unusual amount of anxiety in this patient necessitated reversing treatment objectives, and the neuromuscular dysfunc-

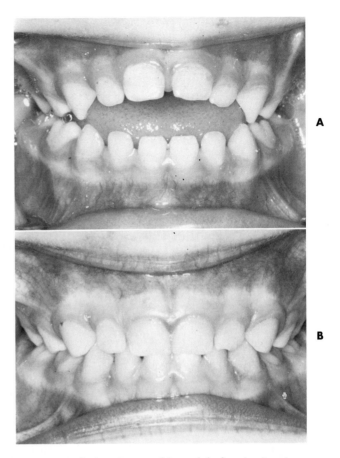

**Figure 5-20.** **A,** Anterior open bite and dysfunction in a 4-year-old girl. **B,** Same patient after 3 months of treatment with a vestibular screen.

tion was corrected first. The patient stopped the finger sucking on his own. The open bite and arch form improved within 5 months, but the crossbite persisted. Expansion treatment was then instituted.

A final indication for the vestibular screen in deciduous dentition is the patient with nasorespiratory problems. The use of a vestibular screen with breathing holes can help reestablish normal nose breathing in these cases.

### Mixed Dentition Indications

The mixed dentition places more limitations on the ways a screen can be used. Usually a combination screen with an additional method of therapy is necessary. In only a few malocclusion problems is the screening appliance capable of providing the sole form of treatment. These exceptional malocclusions result from local environmental factors, and their only symptoms are caused by abnormal perioral muscle function. Treatment in these cases aims to eliminate deforming muscle habit patterns, permitting normal development and eruption of the teeth. Thus screening therapy is causal and physiologic; the improvement of the malocclusion is caused by autonomous self-adjustment.

Screening therapy is not difficult to use for this age group;

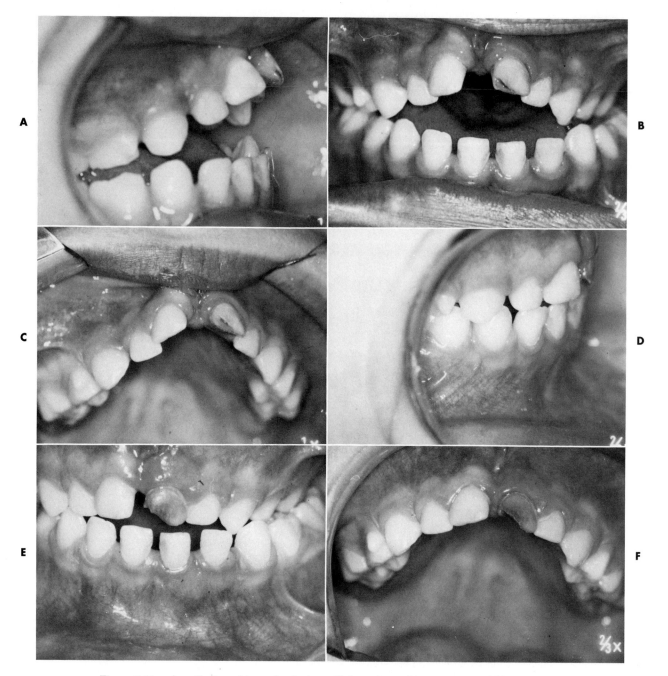

**Figure 5-21.   A** to **C,** Open-bite malocclusion with lateral crossbite in a 3-year-old boy. **D** to **F,** Same patient after 5 months of treatment with a vestibular screen. The open bite improved, but the crossbite persisted.

however, success depends on proper differential diagnosis. The correct functional and skeletal assessment criteria must be used. Postural rest position of the mandible is not influenced by such treatment; however, this is not a therapeutic objective in recently acquired malocclusions. The appliance is indicated in so-called functional retrusion cases in which an anterior postural rest position with the mandible closing up and back into occlusion under forced guidance by the teeth is evident. Usually an excessive overbite also occurs.

An example of the type of case amenable to successful treatment is a 9-year-old girl with an open bite, a tongue postural and sucking habit, and persistent mouth breathing (Figure 5-22). The growth direction was average. Abnormal function was eliminated after 1 year of vestibular screen therapy. In addition, the bite was closed, gingival tissue inflammation was improved, and mouth breathing was greatly reduced. The dentition was observed until eruption of the permanent teeth, and the result was stable without any retention.

Skeletal discrepancies cannot be altered by screening appliances alone. If the morphogenetic pattern and growth direc-

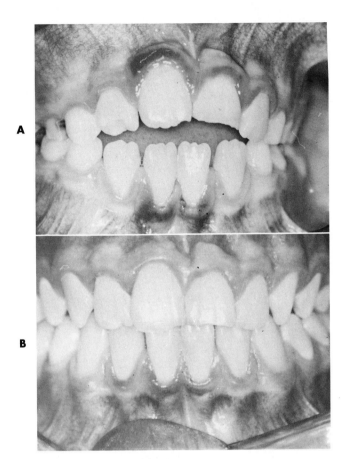

**Figure 5-22.** **A,** Dysfunction, disturbed nasal respiration, and open-bite malocclusion in a 9-year-old girl. **B,** Same patient after screening therapy and eruption of the permanent teeth.

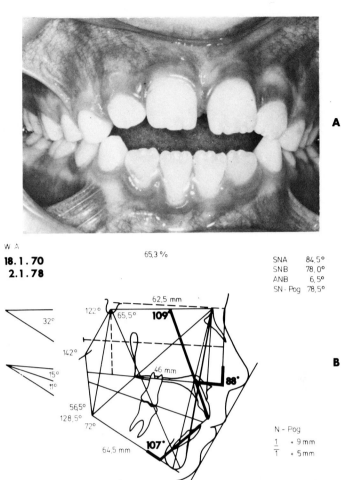

**Figure 5-23.** **A,** Open-bite malocclusion and horizontal growth pattern in an 8-year-old patient. **B,** Cephalometric tracing.

tion are abnormal, therapeutic alteration of local environmental conditions cannot prevent the expression of a dysplastic endogenous pattern. Screening therapy is contraindicated in such cases or should be used only with other methods. Indeed, screening therapy in the mixed dentition can often be used with other appliances (fixed or removable) if correction cannot be achieved by the screen alone. The elimination of abnormal environmental pressures in the mixed dentition is a proper treatment objective in a majority of cases. Thus the screen can be used in pretreatment, during treatment with other appliances, and as a posttreatment retention adjunct in dentofacial orthopedic therapy.

**Indications for pretreatment use of screening therapy.** Screening appliances in the mixed dentition can be used to eliminate abnormal perioral muscle function influences before other treatment is started. Rapid improvement usually occurs in the initial stages of treatment. However, if treatment progresses and improvement is minimal despite the elimination of abnormal perioral muscle function, the etiologic basis of the malocclusion may be caused by other nonenvironmental

factors requiring different approaches to treatment. The following provides an example of this scenario.

CASE STUDY

An 8-year-old boy (Figure 5-23) with an anterior open bite and abnormal tongue posture and function began treatment. The growth pattern was horizontal, and as is often the case, the dentition was biprotrusive. The mandible was orthognathic, but the maxilla was prognathic, with a long base and slight upward and forward inclination. Screening therapy was instituted, and the open bite and axial inclination of the incisor teeth improved, although the uprighting of the lower incisors was insufficient. The mandible grew 3.5 mm, and the sella-nasion-supramentale (S-N-B) angle increased. A retroinclination of the maxillary base that diminished the prognathic profile was observed, but no reduction in the subspinale-nasion-supramentale (A-N-B) angle was evident (Figure 5-24). No further improvement was achieved using inhibitory treatment, however. Indicated therapy included the uprighting of lower incisors with fixed tooth control mechanics. This is justifiable therapy—simple, noniatrogenic, and cost efficient.

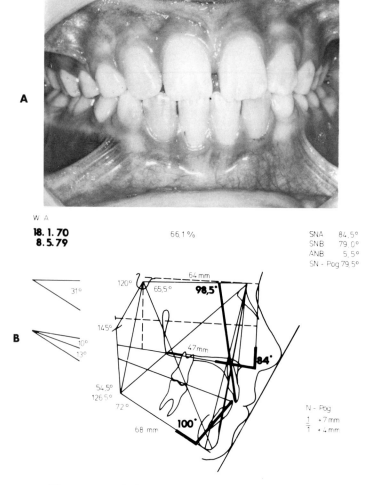

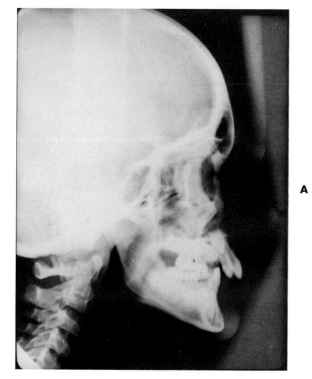

**Figure 5-24.** **A,** Same patient as in Figure 5-23 after 15 months of screening therapy. **B,** Cephalometric tracing.

Habitual mouth breathing in the mixed dentition can be treated using a vestibular shield with breathing holes. Before the screen is placed, however, the posture of the tongue should be examined. If the tongue is retracted with a humped dorsum and flat surface (as is common in Class II malocclusions), screening appliances can be used; however, if the tongue is flat and anteriorly postured, the screen is contraindicated because of the Class III tendency. The screen may actually worsen the anterior posturing of the tongue in such cases.

**Indications for combination with other appliances.** Some appliances such as the activator have shortcomings because of their bulk and limited wearing times during the day. In the presence of confirmed abnormal habit patterns (particularly tongue and lip problems), nocturnal wear may not be sufficient to eliminate abnormal pressures, and treatment response is subsequently slowed. Patients with tongue-thrust problems can wear plates with tongue cribs during the day to offset deleterious effects of tongue thrust and posture. Activators may then be worn at night.

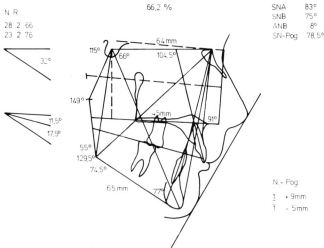

**Figure 5-25.** **A,** Lower lip dysfunction in an 11-year-old patient. **B,** Cephalometric tracing.

Part-time activator wear also is often insufficient to offset deforming action in patients with perverted lip habits in which the lower lip is cushioned to the lingual of the upper incisors during the day. In such instances a lower lip screen can be worn during the day, and the activator can be worn at night. As soon as the sagittal relationship improves and the lower lip is no longer trapped between the upper and lower incisors during function, screen wear can be discontinued and therapy completed with the activator and a short period of fixed appliance wear for final detailing if needed.

A 10-year-old boy with a Class II, division 1 malocclusion and associated lower lip habit is shown in Figure 5-25. His

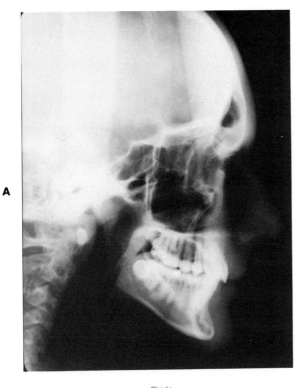

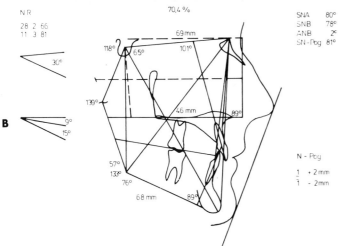

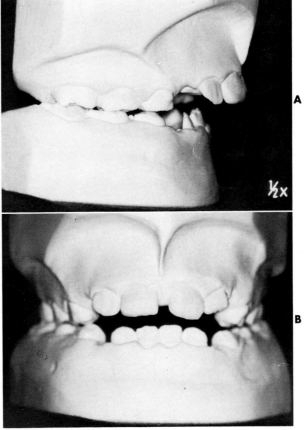

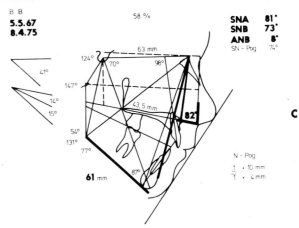

**Figure 5-26.** **A,** Same patient as in Figure 5-25 after treatment with a lower lip screen and activator and eruption of the permanent teeth. **B,** Cephalometric tracing 5 years later.

**Figure 5-27.** **A** and **B,** Combined treatment with a vestibular shield and lower lip screen in a 9-year-old girl. **C,** Cephalometric tracing.

growth pattern was horizontal, the mandibular ramus was long, the body was shorter and retrognathic, and the maxillary base was average and tipped upward and forward, exaggerating the discrepancy. The lower incisors were markedly tipped to the lingual as a result of hyperactive mentalis muscle function. The patient wore an activator at night and a lower lip shield during the day. The activator promoted horizontal growth while exerting an inhibiting influence on the maxilla. The lower incisors were tipped labially. The lower lip

screen eliminated the lip trap during the day and indirectly contributed to the labial tipping of the lower incisors. Figure 5-26 presents the patient's case after eruption of the permanent teeth and 1 year after retention; a balanced relationship occurred.

*Simultaneous use of two screening appliances.* Figure 5-27 shows a 9-year-old girl with an anterior open bite associated with poor tongue posture, thrust habit, and lip sucking.

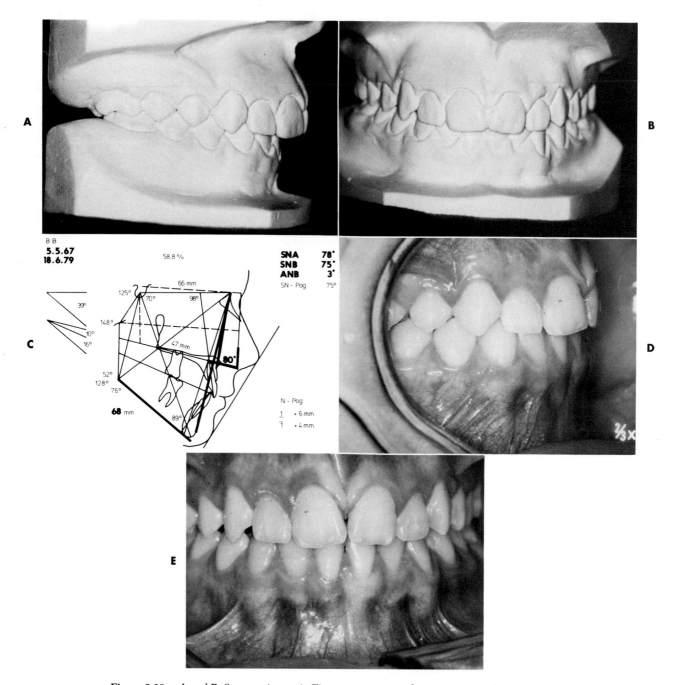

**Figure 5-28.** **A** and **B,** Same patient as in Figure 5-27 4 years after treatment and eruption of the permanent teeth. **C,** Cephalometric tracing. **D** and **E,** Patient 3 years out of retention.

The growth pattern was vertical and partially compensated by a slight down and back inclination of the maxilla (which was of average size and orthognathic). The mandible had a short ramus and body. Both upper and lower incisors were tipped slightly to the lingual side. Because of the combined lip and tongue dysfunction, a double shield (a vestibular screen with an oral tongue screen) was used during the night, and a lower lip screen was used during the day. A large mandibular growth increment was observed during treatment, with a reduction in the A-N-B angle partially caused by a decrease in the

sella-nasion-subspinale (S-N-A) angle. The vertical growth direction persisted. Despite this unfavorable pattern, treatment with the combined screens was possible because of the retroclination of the maxilla, which offset the vertical inclination of the mandible (Figure 5-28).

Even in extraction cases in which abnormal perioral muscle function is present, treatment may be started using a vestibular screen. Such a case is shown in Figure 5-29, *A,* a 7-year-old girl with an open bite and generalized crowding with abnormal muscle activity. A slight vertical growth ten-

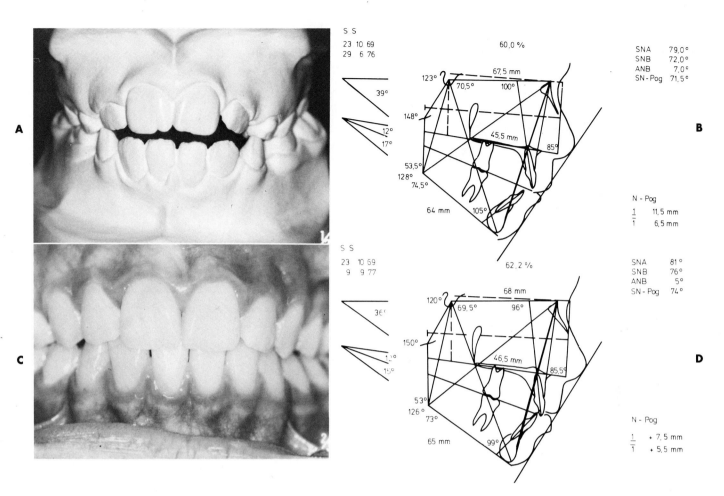

**Figure 5-29.** **A,** Open-bite malocclusion and crowding in the upper and lower dental arch in a 7-year-old patient. **B,** Cephalometric tracing. **C,** Same patient after serial extraction, screening combined with activator therapy, and eruption of the permanent teeth. **D,** Tracing after the screening therapy.

dency was apparent, and the mandibular ramus and body were both short. The lower incisors were labially tipped. A program of serial extraction was initiated, and a vestibular screen was fitted. The open bite closed after 1 year of treatment. Both the mandibular retrognathism and lower incisor inclination improved. Treatment was completed with an activator after removal of the four first premolars, and the spaces under activator influence were closed by guiding the eruption of the remaining posterior teeth and canines. The abnormal functional pattern did not reappear (Figure 5-29, *C*).

**Assessment of the indications for screening therapy.** The construction of the various types of screens is simple; however, they are effective only if used properly, with a correct diagnosis as a prerequisite. To determine the correct indications, the clinician should perform both functional and cephalometric analyses in addition to the general clinical examination.

*Cases with functional retrusion–type Class II relationships and functionally deep overbite problems.* Treating patients with functional retrusion–type Class II relationships and functionally deep overbite problems is often possible in the early mixed dentition period with screening appliances. If their mandibles are guided up and back from postural rest to habitual occlusion, they have excellent prognoses because of neuromuscular etiology and local tooth guidance factors. They frequently have associated hyperactive mentalis muscle malfunction. Many flush terminal plane relationships of the molars have been converted into Class II intercuspations by overclosure and tooth guidance, exacerbated by lower lip trap habits. In treating combined tongue and lip dysfunction, the clinician must assess the relationship of the dysfunction to the malocclusion. Screening therapy is successful only if the abnormal perioral muscle function is a primary etiologic factor in the malocclusion. Cephalometric analysis is usually required to confirm this diagnosis.

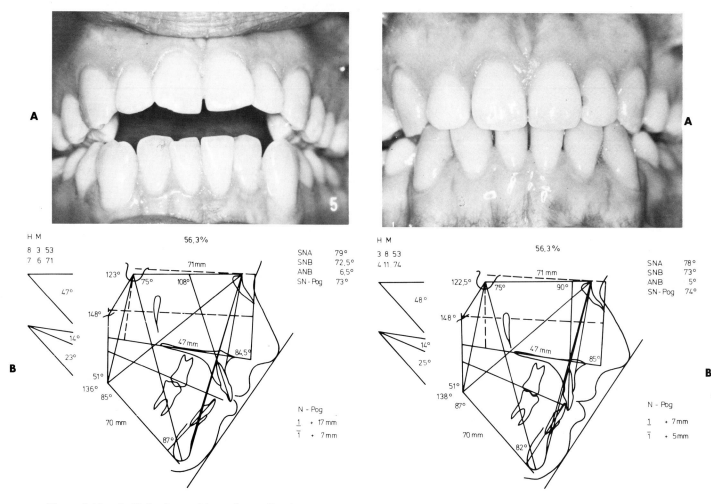

**Figure 5-30.** **A,** Skeletal open bite and crowding in an 18-year-old patient. **B,** Cephalometric tracing.

**Figure 5-31.** **A,** Same patient as in Figure 5-30 after extraction of four first premolars and active therapy. **B,** Cephalometric tracing.

*Need for cephalometric analysis to augment a functional analysis.* In skeletal dysplasia, screening therapy alone is inadequate and can be used only with other methods of treatment. The combined modalities eliminate associated, adaptive, and compensatory factors hindering treatment. The malocclusion must be identified as skeletal before a differential diagnosis can be made.

*Differential diagnosis between primary and secondary functional behavior.* Primary tongue dysfunction can result in localized malocclusions in the dentoalveolar region. Early treatment with screening therapy is indicated. Screening therapy is inadequate in secondary, or adaptive, tongue dysfunctions because the skeletal structures are involved. Depending on the severity of the skeletal dysplasia, screening therapy can be combined with other functional and fixed appliance methods. In very severe cases, however, even this combination is contraindicated. In secondary (compensatory) tongue dysfunctions, as in skeletal open-bite malocclusions, the growth pattern is usually vertical. This unfavorable growth vector can

be partially compensated by a down and back tipping of the maxillary base. The adaptation of the maxilla to a retroclined mandible can thus be therapeutically enhanced, but care must be taken not to create excessive incisor display. On the other hand, upward and forward inclination of the maxillary base can enhance the severity of the malocclusion. In such cases, in the presence of divergent rotation of the skeletal bases, the ultimate problem (as shown by Lavergne and Gasson [1982]) can be quite severe. Prognosis for any form of therapy is poor, and surgical intervention after growth completion may be the only way to correct the problems. Too many of these cases have been treated with ineffective functional and fixed appliance therapy for many years, with only partial correction and sometimes with iatrogenic damage in the form of apical resorption, elongated teeth, and sheared alveolar crests. In some cases, dentoalveolar compensation is feasible, with combined extraction of the first premolars and multiattachment fixed appliances to give the precise control needed. A careful cephalometric analysis is usually necessary to separate these cases and determine those amenable to or-

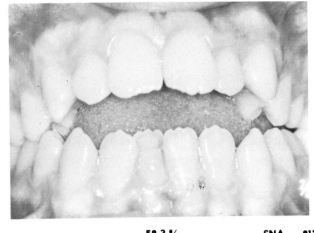

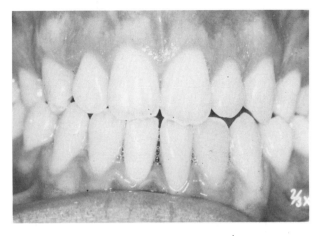

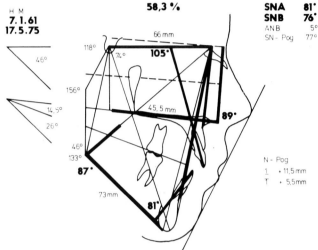

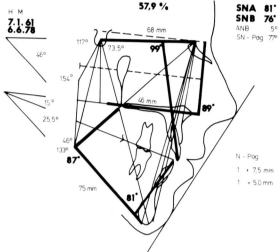

**Figure 5-32.** **A,** Skeletal open bite and crowding in a 14-year-old patient. **B,** Cephalometric tracing. The vertical growth pattern with forward inclination of the maxillary base is evident.

**Figure 5-33.** **A,** Same patient as in Figure 5-32 after extraction of four first premolars and active therapy. **B,** Cephalometric tracing. Difficulties in therapy resulted from the divergent growth rotations of the jaw bases.

thodontic treatment and those requiring combined orthodontic and orthognathic surgical assistance.

Three cases are presented here to demonstrate the limitations of functional appliance therapy in the treatment of openbite malocclusions. In each of these cases the correct diagnosis was not made initially.

CASE STUDIES

The first patient (Figure 5-30), an 18-year-old woman with an open bite, a vertical growth pattern, and crowding in both upper and lower arches, was treated for many years with functional appliances. The author first saw her at 18 years and recommended removal of four first premolars with insertion of full fixed appliances. The compensation of the vertical discrepancy was possible because only the mandible and not the maxilla was unfavorably inclined (Figure 5-31).

The second patient, a 14-year-old boy (Figures 5-32 and 5-33), exhibited a similar malocclusion, but dentoalveolar compensation was more difficult because of the upward and forward inclination of the maxillary base combined with a

down and back inclination of the mandibular base. The open bite could not be completely closed by orthodontic means alone, despite the combined use of extraction and fixed appliances, because of the significant divergence of the apical bases.

The third patient (Figure 5-34) was a 14-year-old girl who had an open bite with a horizontal growth pattern. The clinician removed the patient's four first premolars and initiated functional appliance treatment, which proved unsuccessful because both jaws were prognathic, the upper more than the lower. After the premolar extraction the general dentist, instead of closing spaces above by anchorage control and distalizing the maxillary teeth, moved the prognathic mandible in an anterior direction with the functional appliance to adapt it to the prognathic maxilla. The bite was later closed with full multibanded fixed appliance therapy because the patient was too old to begin functional treatment. (Figure 5-35).

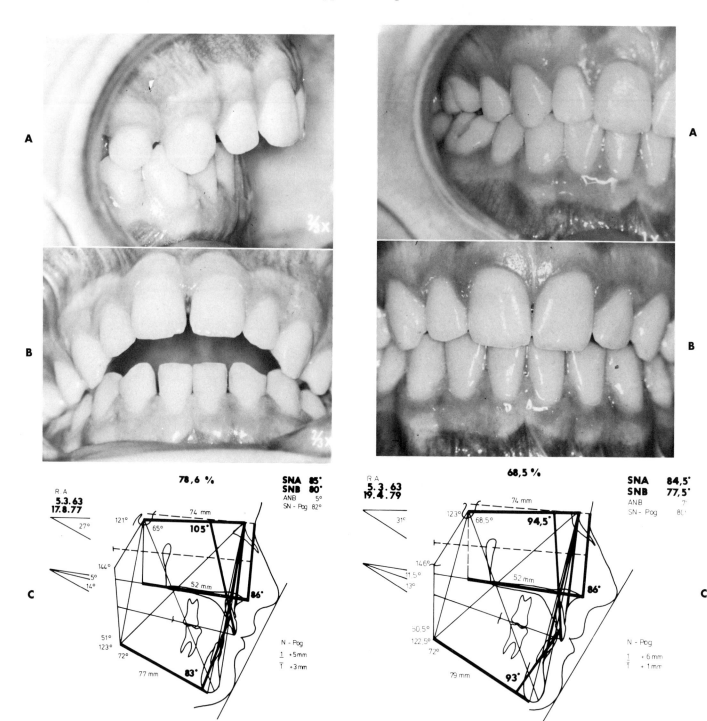

**Figure 5-34.** **A** and **B,** Open-bite malocclusion and horizontal growth pattern in a 14-year-old patient. **C,** Cephalometric tracing.

**Figure 5-35.** **A** and **B,** Same patient as in Figure 5-34 after active treatment. **C,** Cephalometric tracing.

*Differential diagnosis of overjet caused by skeletal or functional disturbances.* An excessive overjet can result from abnormal perioral muscle function and skeletal dysplasia. If lip dysfunction is the cause, the malocclusion is located in the dentoalveolar region. In cases of skeletal discrepancies the malocclusion is of a skeletal pattern–type origin; patients with these malocclusions have retrognathic mandibles and/or prognathic maxillas. Screening therapy is successful only in

cases of dentoalveolar disharmony. Cephalometric analysis enables the clinician to make the proper differential diagnosis for optimal dentofacial orthopedic therapy, as illustrated in the following case study.

### CASE STUDY
An 8-year-old girl (Figure 5-36) had an A-N-B angle of 10 degrees and a Class II malocclusion. The maxilla was pro-

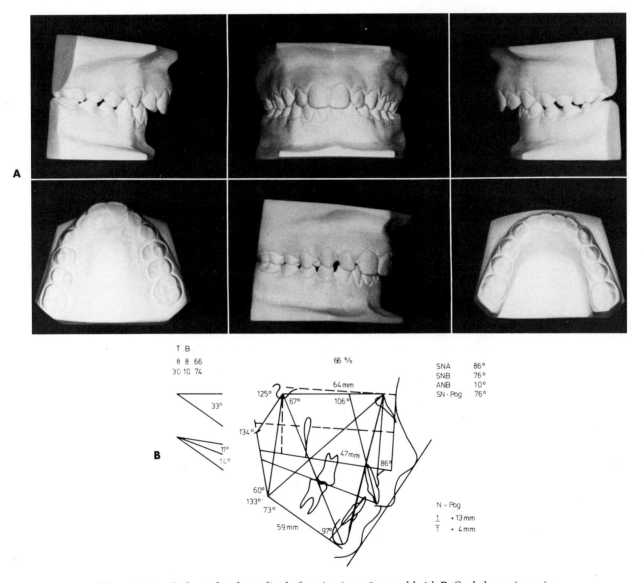

**Figure 5-36.** **A,** Secondary lower lip dysfunction in an 8-year-old girl. **B,** Cephalometric tracing. A skeletal discrepancy with an A-N-B of 10 degrees persisted.

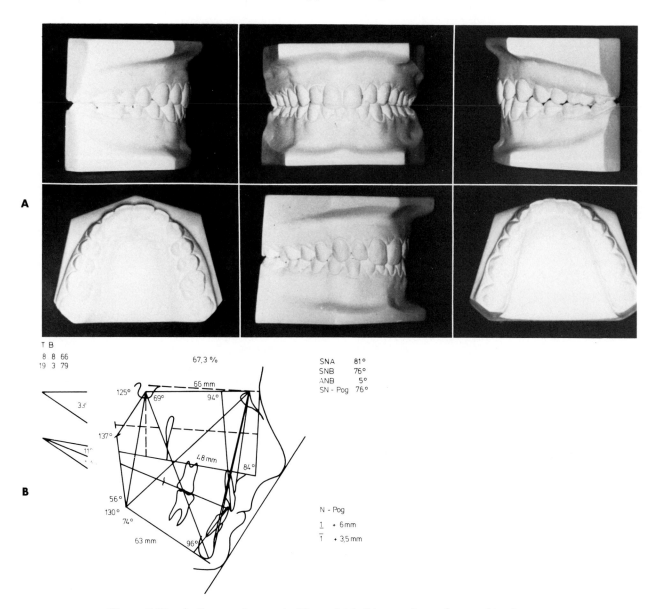

**Figure 5-37.** **A,** Same patient as in Figure 5-36 4½ years later after combined treatment. **B,** Cephalometric tracing.

gnathic, and the mandible was small and retrognathic. The upper incisors were tipped slightly labially and the lower incisors were proclined. In spite of the lip dysfunction, the overjet could not be influenced by a screening appliance because the malocclusion was caused by a skeletal disharmony. Not even the use of conventional functional appliances promised success because in addition to the retrognathic mandible, the prognathic maxilla had to be influenced by therapy.

This is a good example of a case that might benefit from combined extraoral force on the upper arch and the use of a functional appliance. As shown in Figure 5-37, the combined approach was successful with this patient. Many cases exist in which combined headgear-activator therapy can produce successful results not possible with functional appliances or headgear alone. Screening appliances can be combined with other methods by building screening elements into other appliances. The activator can have additional features (e.g., lip pads, buccal shields); Fränkel uses such features in his function regulator although other principles also are involved in pure function regulator therapy (see Chapter 12).

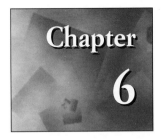

# Chapter 6

# Cephalometric Diagnosis for Functional Appliance Therapy

Thomas Rakosi

The determination of skeletodental relationships is not less important for functional appliance therapy than it is for fixed appliance treatment. Proper pretreatment assessment can mean the difference between successful and unsuccessful treatment. This assessment involves a number of diagnostic criteria; radiographic cephalometrics is an essential component of the diagnostic mosaic. Cephalometrics has been used (and misused) so much, however, that the editor of the *American Journal of Orthodontics* once remarked as he considered a stack of manuscripts submitted for publication, "We are surfeitted with cephalometrics. It is like Dukas' *Sorcerer's Apprentice:* the more I reject, the more the tide increases. Now I know what they mean by a numbers racket." This remark is a bit facetious, of course, but it holds more than a kernel of truth.

Cliques and cults have developed in cephalometric diagnosis much as they have in mechanotherapy. Arbitrary measurements on two-dimensional lateral head films can be made according to a Steiner, Tweed, quadrilateral, Schwarz, Bimler, Jarabak, or Ricketts analysis, to mention just a few of the popular combinations used routinely by orthodontists over the past 35 years. Treatment decisions have been and continue to be made on "current and choice" cephalometric criteria. The fact remains, however, that significant information is missing from many cephalometric analyses. Of particular concern is the lack of assessment of transverse dimensions. Most of the needed information regarding this "third" dimension can be gleaned from photographic and study cast analyses, however. Feeding inadequate data into a computer may enhance the clinician's image in the eyes of the patient, but it does not lend any more credibility to the lines, angles, and linear measurements arbitrarily chosen. The well-known computer acronym GIGO (garbage in, garbage out) applies.

This chapter presents and develops a cephalometric analysis that furnishes valuable information for functional appli-

ance use without becoming so complicated and lengthy as to discourage clinicians from attempting to use it. *An Atlas and Manual of Cephalometric Radiography* has been published by the author (1992b) and is widely used. It gives a general and detailed discussion of the use of cephalometrics in all phases of orthodontics and orthopedics. The most important cephalometric measurements have been chosen to assist the clinician in making a diagnosis and planning therapy with functional appliances. These measurements are practical tools that permit the assessment of ongoing treatment results, aiding therapeutic diagnosis and modifiability and attainment of the best possible treatment goals.

Because most functional appliance therapy is instituted in the mixed or transitional dentition stage (at 8 to 9 years), assessment criteria are adapted to this age period. However, they can be used equally well to follow the progress of each patient into the adult dentition.

Four major areas of emphasis exist in cephalometric diagnostic assessment for patients treated with functional appliances and functional appliance–headgear orthopedics:

1. Accomplishment of growth increments and the direction or vector of growth—These factors vary not only among individuals but also within an individual. Longitudinal studies by Graber et al (1967) reveal that changes often occur in the direction of growth, particularly during the prepubertal period. Although the vector occasionally becomes more vertical, it usually becomes more horizontal, giving the impression of following a logarithmic spiral (as has been noted by Moss). However, certain facial pattern characteristics permit prediction of growth direction probabilities for a particular time frame. The morphologic specifics, particularly of the mandible (where the greatest growth occurs), are vitally important in treatment.
2. Assessment of the magnitude of growth change—This assessment is as important as the determination of the growth direction of the dentofacial complex. Growth magnitudes can be small, average, or large. As Woodside (1969) has shown, at least 50% of all

This chapter is based largely on Chapter 5 of Graber TM, Neumann B: *Removable Orthodontic Appliances,* Philadelphia, 1984, WB Saunders.

cases exhibit growth spurts during the mixed dentition period. Because functional appliances are essentially deficiency appliances having their greatest use in Class II, division 1 malocclusions for patients with underdeveloped mandibles, the greater the amount of growth, the more favorable the therapeutic prognosis. In addition to static linear and angular cephalometric criteria, postural and functional assessment of the mandible is vitally important (see Chapter 4).

3. Inclination and position of the upper and lower incisors—When evaluating the inclination and position of the upper and lower incisors, the clinician should be able to forecast the probable reciprocal growth increments of the jaw bases. The stability of the cephalometric criteria and derived measure points must be good, and the measurements must be reproducible on a longitudinal and interobserver basis.

   The orientation of the incisors to the constructed facial plane can be validly assessed only if the plane is assumed to remain identifiable and stable during therapy. If mandibular basal growth exceeds that of the maxilla (as it does in most patterns) or if the upper terminus, or nasion, moves forward less than the mandibular symphysis, the plane angulation changes. The plane also moves anteriorly with growth, and this can alter the linear measurements of the upper incisors without any appliance effect on these teeth. The clinician must know the probabilities of growth direction, direction change, and increments in three dimensions in various parts of the face before projecting treatment procedures and consequences for the patient. The changes described here obviously create different therapeutic objectives for the upper and lower incisors.

4. Radiographic cephalometrics—Radiographic cephalometrics allows the identification and localization of anomalies and abnormalities of size, shape, and spatial relationship. It can differentiate between skeletal and dentoalveolar malocclusions and provides information on the combination of factors involved in both areas. This differentiation is important for the following reasons:

   a. Consideration of the etiology of malocclusions is important in treatment decisions. The consequences of abnormal perioral muscle function are generally restricted to the dentoalveolar region. For example, an open bite with a primarily dentoalveolar manifestation is usually the consequence of neuromuscular dysfunction. If it is combined with a vertical growth pattern, excessive anterior face height, or short posterior face height, the morphogenetic pattern is the probable primary causative factor.

   b. To determine the therapeutic possibilities for treatment, the clinician must know that in dentoalveolar malocclusions caused by neuromuscular dysfunction, a causal form of treatment is possible and likely to be successful through its elimination of abnormal environmental factors. In skeletally derived malocclusions, a causal type of treatment is possible only by

channeling basal growth patterns to provide the morphologic and functional changes needed to establish a normal structural and functional continuum.

If growth processes cannot be significantly influenced in a skeletal type of malocclusion, only a compensatory form of therapy can be performed; this usually entails adjusting the skeletal dysplasia by making dentoalveolar compromises (e.g., extraction, specific anchorage control, orthognathic surgery) in the most severely dysplastic jaw relationships. The clinician must perform a comprehensive cephalometric analysis to obtain this vital information before instituting a treatment regimen with fixed or removable appliances or functional or nonfunctional armamentaria.

## REFERENCE POINTS, LINES, ANGLES, AND METHODS OF EVALUATION

A large number of guidelines on the interpretation of cephalometric data are available from many clinicians and researchers around the world. Since the introduction of cephalometrics as a clinical orthodontic tool 65 years ago, more articles have appeared on this subject than any other in the orthodontic and dentofacial orthopedic literature; cephalometrics has played a dominant role in many thousands of theses written by orthodontic graduate students. Choosing an interpretation method from this formidable array is difficult for the uninitiated clinician. This chapter provides basic guidelines for accurate cephalometric analysis.

### Reference Points

Only some of the measurements that are of special interest are elucidated here with their interpretations and applications to functional appliance treatment. The following definitions are based on Rakosi's work (1992) (Figure 6-1):

| Code | Definition |
|---|---|
| 1. N | Nasion—most anterior point of the nasofrontal suture in the median plane, skin nasion (N) location at the point of maximal convexity between the nose and forehead |
| 2. S | Sella—midpoint of the sella (S), hypophysis cerebri (sella turcica); midpoint of entrance to the sella; midpoint of the hypophyseal fossa, a constructed radiologic point in the median plane |
| 3. Se | Midpoint of entrance to the sella—midpoint of the line connecting the posterior clinoid process and anterior opening of the sella turcica, at the level of the jugum sphenoidale, independent of the depth of the sella |
| 4. Sn | Subnasale—skin point where the nasal septum merges inferiorly with integument of the upper lip |

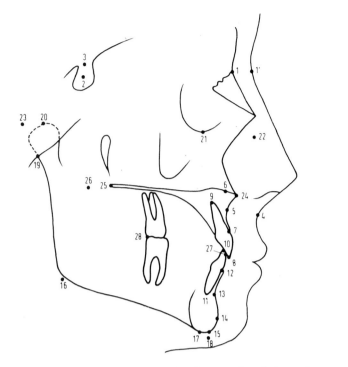

**Figure 6-1.** Reference points used in functional cephalometric analysis. (From Rakosi T: *An atlas and manual of cephalometric radiography,* ed 2, Philadelphia, 1992, Lea & Febiger.)

| | |
|---|---|
| 5. A | Point A, subspinale—deepest midline point in curved bony outline from the base to alveolar process of the maxilla (i.e., the deepest point between ANS and Pr), *subspinale* in anthropologic terms |
| 6. APMax | Anteriorly derived landmark for determining length of maxilla—determination by drawing of a perpendicular line from point A to the palatal plane |
| 7. Pr | Prosthion—alveolar rim of the maxilla; lowest and most anterior point on the alveolar portion of the premaxilla; in the median plane, between the upper central incisors |
| 8. Is (or 1) | Incisor superius—incisal edge of the maxillary central incisor |
| 9. Ap 1 | Apicale 1—apex of the maxillary central incisor |
| 10. Ii (or ī) | Incisor inferius—incisal edge of the mandibular central incisor |
| 11. Ap ī | Apicale ī—apex of the mandibular central incisor |
| 12. Id | Infradentale—alveolar rim of the mandible; highest and most anterior point on the alveolar process; in the median plane, between the lower central incisors |

| | |
|---|---|
| 13. B | Point B, supramentale—most anterior part of the mandibular base, most posterior point in outer contour of the mandibular alveolar process, in the median plane, *supramentale* in anthropologic terms, between infradentale and pogonion. |
| 14. Pog | Pogonion—most anterior point of the bony chin (symphysis), in the median plane |
| 15. Gn | Gnathion—according to Martin and Saller (1957), in the median plane of the mandible where the anterior curve in the outline of the chin merges into the body of the mandible; according to many authors, between the most anterior and inferior points of the chin; according to Craig, the point of intersection of the facial and mandibular planes; according to functional appliance analysis, the most anterior and inferior point of the bony chin—point determination by intersection of a perpendicular line dropped from Me-Pog to the bony outline |
| 16. Go | Gonion—constructed point forming the intersection of the lines tangent to the posterior margin of the ascending ramus and mandibular base |
| 17. Me | Menton—according to Krogman and Sassouni the most caudal point in outline of the symphysis; the lowest point of the mandible corresponding to anthropologic gnathion |
| 18. APMan | Anterior landmark for determining length of mandible—determination by drawing of perpendicular line from Pog to the mandibular plane |
| 19. Ar | Articulare—intersection of the dorsal contours of the processus articularis mandibulae and the inferior surface of the temporal bone as seen in lateral cephalometric projection, introduction by Björk (1947), for radiologic orientation |
| 20. Cd | Condylion—most superior point on the head of the condyle |
| 21. Or | Orbitale—lowest point on the radiograph of the orbit |
| 22. Pn/2 | Constructed point—point at bisect of the Pn vertical (dropped from Se-N at N') |
| 23. FH-R asc | Intersection—intersection of Frankfort horizontal and posterior margin of the ascending ramus |
| 24. ANS | Anterior nasal spine—pointed tip of the anterior nasal crest in the median |

plane corresponding to anthropologic acanthion

25. PNS    Posterior nasal spine—constructed radiologic point, intersection of the anterior wall of the pterygopalatine fossa and the floor of the nose, the dorsal limit of the maxilla

26. S'     Constructed point for assessing length of maxillary base—in posterior section a perpendicular line from Se to the palatal plane

27. APOcc  Anteriorly derived point for determining occlusal plane—middle of the incisor overbite in occlusion

28. PPOcc  Posterior point for determining occlusal plane—the most distal contact between the most posterior molars in occlusion

29. Ba     Basion—lowest point on anterior margin of the foramen magnum, in the median plane

30. Ptm    Pterygomaxillary fissure—projection onto the palatal plane, anterior wall representing the maxillary tuberosity outline, posterior wall representing the anterior curve of the pterygoid process corresponding to PNS

## Angular Measurements

Reference lines enable the clinician to make angular measurements on radiographs. The following angles are routinely determined (Figure 6-2):

| Code | | Definition | Mean value (degrees) |
|---|---|---|---|
| 1. | N-S-Ar | Saddle angle | 123 ± 5 |
| 2. | S-Ar-Go | Articular angle | 143 ± 6 |
| 3. | Ar-Go-Me | Gonial angle | 128 ± 7 |
| 4. | Sum | Sum of saddle, articular, and gonial angles | 394 |
| 5. | Ar-Go-N | Go 1, upper gonial angle | 52 to 55 |
| 6. | N-Go-Me | Go 2, lower gonial angle | 70 to 75 |
| 7. | S-N-A | Anteroposterior position of maxilla | 81 |
| 8. | S-N-B | Anteroposterior position of mandible | 79 |
| 9. | A-N-B | Difference between S-N-A and S-N-B | 2 |
| 10. | S-N-Pr | Anteroposterior position of alveolar part of premaxilla (prosthion) | 84 |
| 11. | S-N-Id | Anteroposterior position of alveolar part of mandible (infradentale) | 81 |
| 12. | Pal-MP | Angle between palatal and mandibular planes | 25 |
| 13. | Pal-Occ | Upper occlusal plane angle | 11 |
| 14. | MP-Occ | Lower occlusal plane angle | 14 |
| 15. | S-N-MP | Angle between S-N and the mandibular plane | 32 |
| 16. | Pn-Pal | Angle of inclination (/) between a perpendicular line dropped from Se-N at N¢ and the palatal plane | 85 |
| 17. | N-S-Gn | (Y-axis) Angle between S-N and S-Gn anteriorly | 66 |
| 18. | 1-SN | Angle between the upper incisor axis and S-N posteriorly | 102 |
| 19. | 1-Pal | Angle between the upper incisor axis and palatal plane anteriorly | 70 + 5 |
| 20. | 1̄-MP | Angle between the lower incisor axis and mandibular plane posteriorly | 90 ± 3 |
| 21. | ii angle | Interincisal angle between the upper and lower central incisor axes posteriorly | 135 |

## Linear Measurements

Reference lines also enable clinicians to determine linear dimensions on radiographs (Figure 6-3).

| Code | | Definition | Mean value (mm) |
|---|---|---|---|
| 1. | S-N | (Se-N) Anteroposterior | 71 |

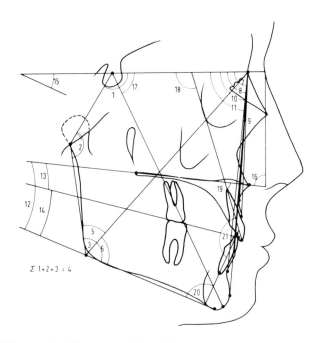

**Figure 6-2.** The most valid and frequently used angular measurements. (From Rakosi T: *An atlas and manual of cephalometric radiography,* Philadelphia, 1992, Lea & Febiger.)

extent of the anterior cranial base

2. S-Ar        Extent of the lateral         32 to 35
               cranial base
3. S-Go        Posterior face height
4. N-Me        Anterior face height
5. MaxBase     Extent of the maxillary
               base correlated with Se-N
6. ManBase     Extent of the mandibular
               base correlated with Se-N
7. R asc       Extent of the ascending
               ramus correlated with Se-N
8. S'-F Ptp    Distance from S' to the
               projection of the anterior
               wall of the pterygopalatine
               fossa on the palatal plane,
               an expression for antero-
               posterior displacement of
               the maxillary base
9. S-S'        Deflection of the maxillary    42 to 57
               base
10. 1 to       Distance from the incisal
    N-Pog      edge of the upper incisor to
               N-Pog
11. 1̄ to       Distance from the incisal
    N-Pog      edge of the lower incisor to
               N-Pog

## CEPHALOMETRIC ANALYSES

The various cephalometric evaluations can be divided into three groups: facial skeleton, jaw bases, and dentoalveolar relationships.

### Analysis of the Facial Skeleton

The first cephalometric analysis includes three angular measurements (saddle angle, articular angle, gonial angle) and four linear measurements (anterior and posterior face height, anterior and posterior cranial base length). Linear measurements are particularly important during treatment.

**Saddle angle (N-S-Ar).** The angle formed by joining these three points provides a parameter for assessment of the relationship between anterior and posterolateral cranial bases. The position of the sella turcica, the midpoint of the angle, is determined partly by growth changes in the area. Thus a large saddle angle usually signifies a posterior condylar position and a mandible that is posteriorly positioned with respect to the cranial base and maxilla—that is, unless the deviation in the position of the fossa is compensated by angular (articular angle) and linear (ramal length) relationships. A noncompensated posterior positioning of the mandible caused by a large saddle angle is very difficult to influence with functional appliance therapy (Figure 6-4).

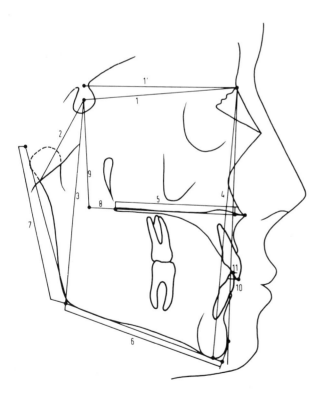

**Figure 6-3.** Linear measurements. (From Rakosi T: *An atlas and manual of cephalometric radiography,* Philadelphia, 1982, Lea & Febiger.)

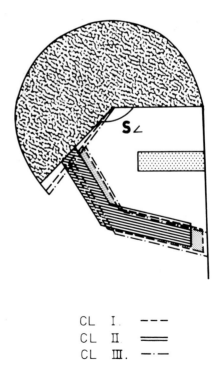

CL  I.   - - -
CL  II.  =====
CL  III. —·—

**Figure 6-4.** The saddle angle *(S)* is generally large in the retrognathic face but small in the prognathic face.

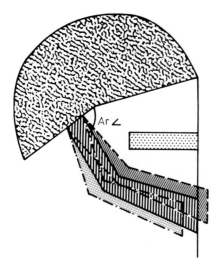

**Figure 6-5.** The articular angle *(Ar)* is large in the retrognathic face but small in the prognathic face.

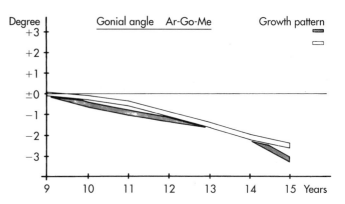

**Figure 6-7.** Growth increments of the gonial angle in horizontal and vertical growth patterns between the ninth and fifteenth years.

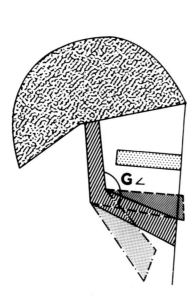

**Figure 6-6.** The gonial angle *(G)* is small with a horizontal growth pattern but large with a vertical growth pattern.

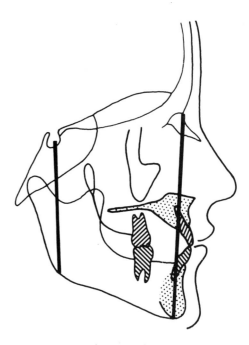

**Figure 6-8.** Posterior and anterior face height measurements. A ratio is established between these dimensions to assist in projecting sagittal growth direction probabilities.

**Articular angle (S-Ar-Go).** The articular angle is a constructed angle between the upper and lower parts of the posterior contours of the facial skeleton. Its size depends on the position of the mandible; it is large if the mandible is retrognathic but small if the mandible is prognathic. It can be influenced during orthopedic or orthodontic therapy; it decreases with anterior positioning of the mandible, closing of the bite, and mesial migration of the posterior segment teeth and increases with posterior relocation of the mandible, opening of the bite, and distal driving of the posterior teeth.

An alteration of this angle can be seen in some activator treatment results (Figure 6-5). In a study of 9-year-old children with horizontal growth patterns, the angle was found to be slightly smaller (on average 139.5 degrees) than it was in patients with vertical growth patterns (142.4 degrees). The growth increments between 9 and 15 years were −2.89 degrees with horizontal growth patterns and −2.49 with vertical growth vectors.

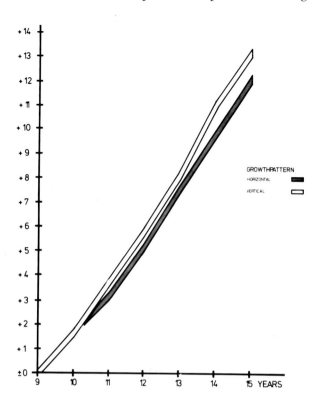

**Figure 6-9.** Growth increments of anterior face height (N-Me). The difference between horizontally and vertically growing faces is evident.

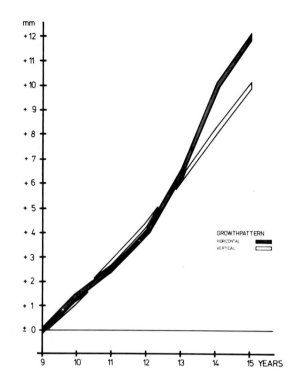

**Figure 6-10.** Growth increments of posterior face height (S-Go). The increments are larger in horizontally growing faces after 13 years.

**Gonial angle (Ar-Go-Me).** The angle formed by tangents to the body of the mandible and posterior border of the ramus is of special interest because it not only expresses the form of the mandible but also gives information on mandibular growth direction. If this angle is acute or small, especially in its lower component (the lower Go angle of Jarabak), the direction of growth is horizontal. This is a favorable condition for anterior positioning of the mandible with an activator.

In patients with large gonial angles, activator treatment is generally contraindicated. If this form of treatment is attempted, the appliance must be constructed in a way that takes the growth pattern into account (Figure 6-6). Functional appliances are used only as first measures to treat dentofacial dysplasia in these cases; comprehensive orthopedic or orthognathic surgery is generally performed later. In 9-year-old mixed-dentition children with horizontal growth patterns, the average angle is 125.5 degrees, with a lower angle of 69.5 degrees. In vertical growth patterns the angle increases to 133.4 degrees, with a larger lower angle of 78.3 degrees.

Between the ninth and eleventh year of growth the growth increment was −2.89 degrees with horizontal patterns and −2.42 degrees with vertical patterns (Figure 6-7).

**Anterior and posterior face height.** The measurement of anterior and posterior face height is a linear millimetric assessment. The posterior face height (S-Go) and anterior face height (N-Me) are measured on lateral cephalograms with the teeth in habitual occlusion (Figure 6-8).

Posterior face heights in the longitudinal study of 9-year-old children with horizontal growth patterns were longer on average (69.5 mm) than they were in children with vertical growth patterns (64.1 mm). The growth increment with the horizontal growth pattern between 9 and 15 years of age was 11.05 mm; it was 10.8 mm in the vertically growing group. The reverse ratio held true for anterior face height. In horizontal patterns the average was 103 mm with a growth increment of 12.18 mm as opposed to vertical measurements of 106.6 mm between nasion and menton with a total growth increment of 12.71 mm (Figures 6-9 and 6-10).

Clinicians can compare anterior and posterior face height and set up ratios to estimate growth direction according to the recommendations of Jarabak (1972):

$$\frac{\text{Posterior face height} \times 100}{\text{Anterior face height}}$$

A ratio of less than 62% expresses a vertical growth pattern, whereas a ratio of more than 65% increases the likelihood for a horizontal vector. At 9 years the average ratio in the horizontally growing group was 67.5%, increasing to 69.9% by 15 years. In the vertically growing group the posterior to anterior face height ratio was 60.1% at 9 years, increasing to 62.7% by 15 years. All measurements showed a general trend toward a more horizontal growth pattern.

Growth forecasting for early mixed dentition treatment with an activator should be done by comparing angular and linear measurements and morphologic characteristics of the

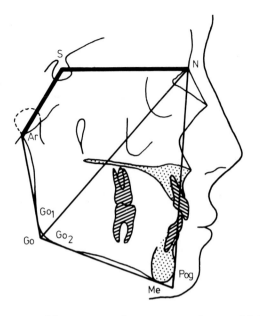

**Figure 6-11.** Measurements for anteroposterior cranial base length *(N-S and S-Ar)*.

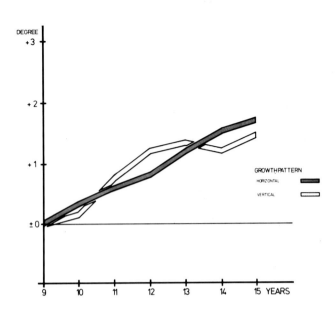

**Figure 6-13.** Growth increments of the S-N-A angle. Terminal growth is greater in horizontally growing patterns.

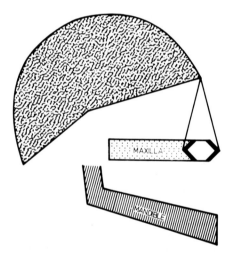

**Figure 6-12.** The S-N-A angle expresses the horizontal position of the maxillary base in relation to the cranial base.

mandible. The assessment of growth direction is important in functional appliance therapy; it helps determine whether functional appliances should be used and influences construction details, type of construction bite, and other factors. Periodic growth assessment during treatment is equally important for the plotting of midcourse corrections and alterations.

**Anterior cranial base length (Se-N).** The measurement of the anterior cranial base (Figure 6-11) can be performed using the center of the superior entrance to the sella turcica as a ref-

erence point instead of the center of the sella turcica fossa outline (as is usually done for cranial base establishment). The correlation of this criterion with the length of the jaw bases enables the assessment of the proportional averages of these bases.

In the longitudinal study group the average length of the anterior cranial base in 9-year-old children was 68.8 mm for horizontal growth patterns and 63.8 mm for vertical growth patterns. The incremental change between 9 and 15 years was 4.46 mm in horizontal patterns and 3.52 mm in vertical patterns.

**Posterior (lateral) cranial base length (S-Ar).** The magnitude of posterior (lateral) cranial base length depends on posterior face height and the position of the fossa (see Figure 6-11). Short posterior cranial bases occur in vertical growth patterns and skeletal open bites and give a poor prognosis for functional appliance therapy. In 9-year-old children with horizontal growth patterns the average length was 32.2 mm with an increment of 9.16 mm in the following 6 years as opposed to 30 mm with an increment of 4.47 mm in vertical patterns.

## Analysis of the Jaw Bases

The angles between vertical reference lines represent the sagittal relationship of parts (e.g., S-N-A, S-N-B), whereas angles between horizontal lines assist in the evaluation of vertical relationships (e.g., base plane angle, inclination angle). Linear measurements indicate the length of the maxillary and mandibular bases and ascending ramus. A morphologic assessment, particularly of the mandible, also is important in forecasting growth direction. Only selected measurements

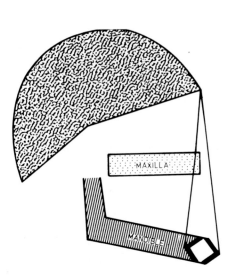

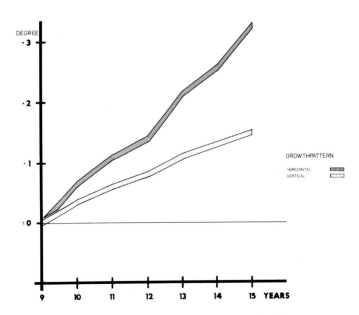

**Figure 6-14.** The S-N-B angle expresses the horizontal position of the mandibular base in relation to the cranial base.

**Figure 6-15.** Growth increments of the S-N-B angle. The greatest divergence in growth is apparent here as the mandible grows and is translated more anteriorly in horizontal growth patterns.

that are applicable in treatment planning for functional appliances are described in this overview.

**S-N-A.** The angle S-N-A expresses the sagittal relationship of the anterior limit of the maxillary apical base (Lundström's term for the junction of alveolar and basal bone) to the anterior cranial base (Figure 6-12). It is large in prognathic maxillas and small in retruded maxillas. In Class II, division 1 malocclusions caused by prognathic maxillas in which the S-N-A angle is larger than normal, the use of an activator is contraindicated.

McNamara (1981) points out in his study that the S-N-A angle does not vary much among the different types of malocclusions, nor does it change much with functional appliance treatment. The growth increments are small for this criterion, and the difference between growth direction types is insignificant (Figure 6-13).

| | S-N-A angle (degrees) | |
|---|---|---|
| *Growth direction* | *9 years* | *15 years* |
| Average | 79.5 | 81.28 |
| Horizontal | 79.73 | 81.57 |
| Vertical | 79.0 | 80.57 |

A moderate decrease of the S-N-A angle is possible through the use of conventional activator therapy. A larger decrease is possible with special activator construction as shown by the Clark twin block appliance.

**S-N-B.** The angle S-N-B expresses the sagittal relationship between the anterior extent of the mandibular apical base and anterior cranial base (Figure 6-14). With a prognathic mandible it is large, and with a retrognathic mandible it is small. Functional appliance treatment is indicated if the mandible is retrognathic and has a small S-N-B. This angle

provides information only on the anteroposterior position of the mandible, not on its morphology or growth direction. A posteriorly located mandible can be large or small; if it is small, the prognosis for anterior posturing in the mixed dentition is good because a larger growth increment can usually be expected.

The average angles and growth increments in horizontal face types are much larger (77.2 degrees at 9 years and 80.5 degrees at 15 years) than they are in vertical growth patterns (74.3 degrees at 9 years and 75.9 degrees at 15 years) (Figure 6-15). The favorable growth direction and greater increments of the mandible in horizontal patterns make successful treatment of these patients possible through anterior posturing of the mandible in functional appliance therapy.

**Base plane angle (Pal-MP).** The base plane angle between the maxillary and mandibular jaw bases also is used to determine the inclination of the mandibular plane (Figure 6-16). In horizontal growth patterns this angle is small (23.4 degrees at 9 years and 20.5 degrees at 15 years), whereas in vertical growth patterns it is larger (32.9 degrees at 9 years and 30.9 degrees at 15 years). The age-dependent decrease in this angle corresponds to the general trend toward a more horizontal growth pattern and expresses the logarithmic spiral type of growth described by Moss (1970), Graber, and others (Figure 6-17).

**Inclination angle.** The inclination angle gives an assessment of the inclination of the maxillary base (Figure 6-18). It is the angle formed by the Pn line (a perpendicular line dropped from N-Se at N') and palatal plane. A large angle expresses upward and forward inclination, whereas a small angle indicates down and back tipping of the anterior end of the palatal plane and maxillary base (Figure 6-19). This angle does not correlate with growth pattern or facial type. Func-

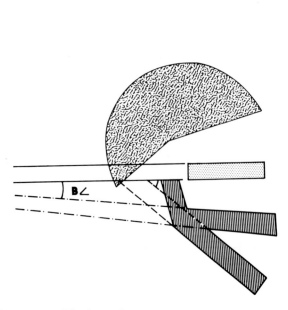

**Figure 6-16.** The base plane angle is small with a horizontal growth pattern but large with a vertical growth pattern.

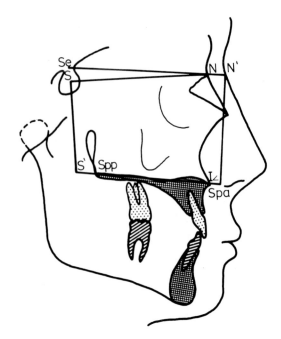

**Figure 6-18.** Inclination angle *(I∠)* perpendicular to the maxillary base plane from *N-Se* at *N'*.

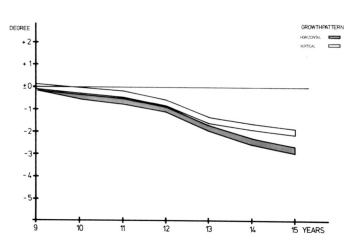

**Figure 6-17.** Growth increments of the base plane angle. The angle decreases more in horizontally growing faces.

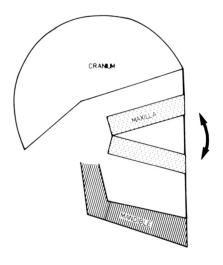

**Figure 6-19.** Retroclination and anteclination of the maxillary base. A broad range is possible.

tional and therapeutic influences can alter the inclination of the maxillary base, however (Figure 6-20). Hence the need for periodic assessment during active treatment.

**Rotation of the jaw bases.** The two previous measurements (base plane angle and inclination angle) are used to evaluate the rotation of the upper and lower jaw bases. These rotations are of special interest in treatment with functional appliances because they show whether such appliances are indicated and provide the criteria for appliance construction.

The rotation of the mandible is growth conditioned and depends on the direction and mutual relations of growth in-

crements in the posterior (condylar) and anterior (sutural and alveolar) facial skeleton. If condylar growth (and minimal increments of temporal fossa growth) proceeds at a greater rate, horizontal rotation results. If growth increments are balanced, parallel growth down the Y-axis occurs.

Björk (1962) differentiates the two processes involved in rotational growth of the mandible:

1. Remodeling of the mandible in the symphyseal and gonial areas—This remodeling is called *intermatrix rotation.* It is a function of the periosteal matrix (Moss) and often results in subsequent rotation. More apposition in

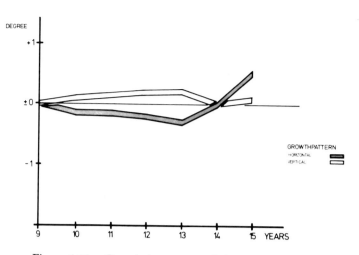

**Figure 6-20.** Growth increments of the inclination angle. In horizontally growing faces, terminal growth appears to increase this angle; in vertical patterns it remains constant.

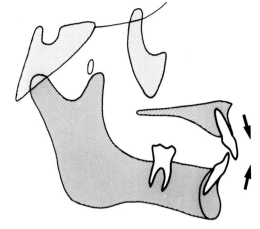

**Figure 6-21.** Convergent rotation of the jaw bases with closing of maxillomandibular basal angles.

the gonial area and resorption in the symphyseal area lead to horizontal rotation. Greater apposition in the symphyseal area and resorption in the gonial area causes vertical rotation.

2. Vertical or horizontal rotation of the mandible in its neuromuscular envelope—This rotation is called *matrix rotation,* or relocation of the functional matrix, according to Moss and Enlow (1962). Rotation observed cephalometrically is called *total rotation;* it consists of both intermatrix and matrix rotation.

Mandibular rotation is caused by both growth-dependent and functional influences. Functional orthodontic and orthopedic methods alter function and guide the growth process. For this reason the rotation of the mandible may be moderately influenced therapeutically.

The pattern of rotation of the maxillary base can be observed by sequential measurements of the inclination angle. Generally the inclination of the maxillary base is stable and no growth-dependent changes are seen. Environmental influences such as neuromuscular dysfunction, occlusal forces, gravity, and nasorespiratory malfunction (according to Linder-Aronson, Lowe, and Woodside [1986]) can modify this inclination. An upward and forward tipping of the anterior part of the maxilla is often observed in confirmed mouth breathers. A down and back tipping of the anterior part of the maxillary base is observed as a natural compensation in patients with vertically growing faces. The inclination can be influenced by both fixed orthopedic and functional therapeutic techniques. All techniques should be monitored during active treatment to prevent excessive gingival display.

**Mutual relationship of the rotating jaw bases.** Rotation of the mandible can decisively establish the vertical proportions of the facial skeleton. In horizontal rotation the anterior face profile is short, whereas in a vertically rotating mandibular pattern, it is long. A horizontal rotation indicates a predisposition toward a deep overbite; an excessively vertical rotation

indicates a tendency toward an open bite. The inclination of the maxillary base also is important to the occlusal relationship. Dentoalveolar occlusion or malocclusion depends on the combination of these rotations. The following types of rotations can be differentiated, as shown by Lavergne and Gasson (1982) in human implant studies:

1. Convergent rotation of the jaw bases—This rotation creates a severe, deep overbite that is difficult to manage using functional methods (Figure 6-21).
2. Divergent rotation of the jaw bases—This rotation can cause marked open-bite problems. In severe cases, orthognathic surgery is required for correction (Figure 6-22).
3. Cranial rotation of both bases—In this horizontal growth pattern a relatively harmonious rotation of both jaws occurs in an upward and forward direction. This rotation of the maxilla compensates for upward and forward mandibular rotation, offsetting a deep bite. The result is a normal overbite (Figure 6-23).
4. Caudal, or down and back, rotation of both bases—This rotation occurs in a relatively harmonious manner. The down and back maxillary rotation offsets the open bite created by down and back mandibular rotation (Figure 6-24).

Therapeutic control of the vertical dimension is usually more difficult than control of the sagittal dimension. If a causal therapeutic skeletal reconstruction is not possible, compensatory treatment is indicated. For example, if the vertical morphogenetic pattern cannot be altered, an occlusal adjustment must be achieved by retroclination of the maxillary base, often with tooth sacrifice. Orthognathic surgery is the ultimate corrective procedure if the magnitude of the malrelationship transcends orthodontic and orthopedic growth guidance procedures.

**Linear measurement of the jaw bases.** In the determination of indications for functional appliance therapy, not only

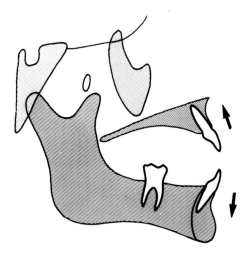

**Figure 6-22.** Divergent rotation of the jaw bases with opening of the basal angle.

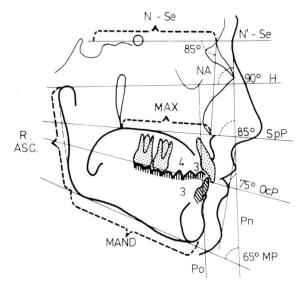

**Figure 6-25.** Proportional measurements of the jaw bases and ascending ramus.

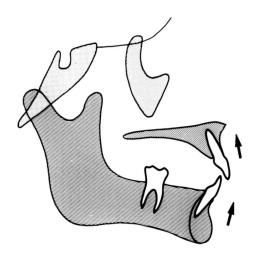

**Figure 6-23.** Cranial rotation of the jaw bases. Both bases rotate upward and forward.

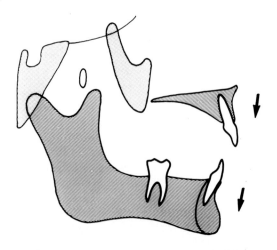

**Figure 6-24.** Caudal rotation of the jaw bases. Both bases rotate down and back.

the position but also the length of the jaw bases must be assessed. If the mandible is retrognathic, the clinician must decide whether its size is relatively small or large. This decision is important in the consideration of etiology and therapy for each patient. The length of the maxillary and mandibular bases and ascending ramus is measured relative to Se-N. Schwarz (1958) proposes measurements for this assessment in his roentgenostatic analysis (Figure 6-25). The ideal dimension relative to Se-N is calculated using the following ratios:

| | |
|---|---|
| N-Se:ManBase | 20:21 |
| Ascending ramus:ManBase | 5:7 |
| MaxBase:ManBase | 2:3 |

The evaluations result in two ideal dimensions, one related to the length of Se-N and the other to the mandibular base. Table 6-1 has been compiled to simplify the calculations.

***Extent of the mandibular base.*** The extent of the mandibular base is determined by measuring the distance gonion-pogonion (projected perpendicular to the mandibular plane) (Figure 6-26). Ideally the mandibular base should be 3 mm longer than Se-N until the twelfth year and 3.5 mm longer after the twelfth year. A length of 5 mm less than this average is considered within normal limits until 7 years, however, and a length of 5 mm more is normal until 15 years.

In the longitudinal study of children discussed earlier, basal length and growth increments were both higher in horizontal patterns than they were in vertical growth patterns. In horizontal patterns the average length at 9 years was 67.59 mm, increasing to 77.35 mm at 15 years. In vertical patterns the length at 9 years was 65.23 mm, increasing to 73.5 mm by 15 years (Figure 6-27).

***Extent of the maxillary base.*** The extent of the maxillary base is determined by measuring the distance between the posterior nasal spine and point A projected perpendicularly

| TABLE 6-1. · LINEAR MEASUREMENTS (MM) OF THE MAXILLARY AND MANDIBULAR BASES AND ASCENDING RAMUS | | | |
|---|---|---|---|
| **Mandible** | **Maxilla** | **Ascending Ramus** | **Ramus** |
| 56 | 37 | 40 | 22 |
| 57 | 38 | 40.5 | 22.5 |
| 58 | 39 | 41 | 23 |
| 59 | 39 | 42 | 23.5 |
| 60 | 40 | 43 | 24 |
| 61 | 40.5 | 43.5 | 24 |
| 62 | 41 | 44 | 24.5 |
| 63 | 42 | 45 | 25 |
| 64 | 42.5 | 45.5 | 25.5 |
| 65 | 43 | 46 | 26 |
| 66 | 44 | 47 | 26 |
| 67 | 44.5 | 47.5 | 27 |
| 68 | 45 | 48 | 27 |
| 69 | 46 | 49 | 27.5 |
| 70 | 46.5 | 50 | 28 |
| 71 | 47 | 50.5 | 28 |
| 72 | 48 | 51 | 29 |
| 73 | 48.5 | 52 | 29 |
| 74 | 49 | 53 | 29.5 |
| 75 | 50 | 53.5 | 30 |
| 76 | 50.5 | 54 | 30 |
| 77 | 51 | 55 | 31 |
| 78 | 52 | 55.5 | 31 |
| 79 | 52.5 | 56 | 31.5 |
| 80 | 53 | 57 | 32 |
| 81 | 54 | 58 | 32 |
| 82 | 54.5 | 58.5 | 32.5 |
| 83 | 55 | 59 | 33 |
| 84 | 56 | 60 | 33.5 |
| 85 | 57 | 60.5 | 34 |

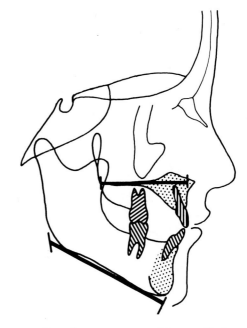

**Figure 6-26.** Length measurements of the mandibular and maxillary bases.

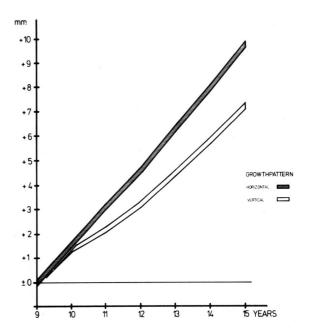

**Figure 6-27.** Growth increments of the mandibular base. The increments are greater for horizontal growth patterns.

onto the palatal plane. The evaluation of this dimension has two "ideal" measurements: one related to N-Se and the other to the length of the mandibular base.

The difference in length of the maxillary base between the two growth patterns studied was slight and the growth increment lower than were those of the mandibular base. As Johnston (1976) points out, the mandible outgrows the maxilla. In horizontal patterns the average length at 9 years was 44.56 mm, increasing to 48.6 mm in the 15-year-old sample. In vertical patterns the average length was 44.0 mm at 9 years and 47.16 mm at 15 years (Figure 6-28).

Because the growth potential of the mandibular base is greater than that of the maxillary base, the angle S-N-B increases, and A-N-B thus decreases. This observation corroborates the impression of many clinicians that the mandible is less retrognathic after 12 years. The recognition that the mandible outgrows the maxilla by as much as 5 mm is especially important to functional appliance proponents and, of course, to the Class II patients being treated.

*Length of the ascending ramus.* The measurement of the length of the ascending ramus is made by calculating the distance between gonion and condylion. The location of condylion

may be simplified by the construction of a Frankfort horizontal plane intersected by a tangent to the ramus. The point of intersection represents constructed condylion (Figure 6-29).

The Frankfort horizontal plane is constructed as follows: the distance between soft tissue nasion (N') and the palatal plane is bisected along the Pn line; from the point thus created, a straight line (H-line) is drawn parallel to the Se-N plane; this becomes the ideal Frankfort horizontal. This construction

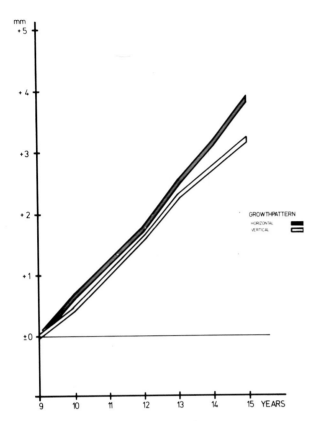

**Figure 6-28.** Growth increments of the maxillary base. The base length is greater in horizontally growing faces.

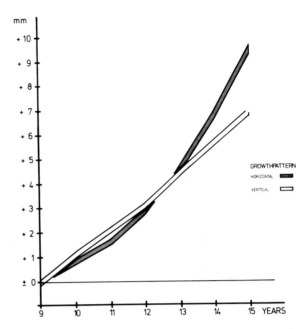

**Figure 6-30.** Growth increments of the ramus ascendens (condylion to constructed gonion). Greater growth increments are seen in horizontally growing faces.

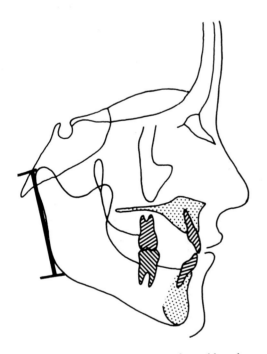

**Figure 6-29.** Measurements of ramal length.

should not be used for comparison with Frankfort plane measurements derived in other studies.

The length of the ramus is important in the determination of posterior face height and subsequent relation to anterior face height. The ramus tends to be longer in horizontally growing patterns, with an average length of 48.9 mm in 9-year-old children and 58.67 mm in 15-year-old adolescents; it is shorter in vertical patterns, with an average length of 44.47 mm in 9-year-old children and 51.7 mm in 15-year-old adolescents (Figure 6-30).

## Evaluation of the Length of the Jaw Bases

**Mandibular base.** If the length of the mandibular base corresponds to the distance N-Se (ManBase:N-Se + 3 mm), it indicates an age-related normal mandibular length and an average growth increment can be expected. If the base is shorter, the growth increment is probably larger. If it is longer, the growth increment may well be smaller. Forecasts can be improved by using two additional measurements—the lengths of the maxillary base and ascending ramus.

The correlation between the length and position of the mandibular base also should be examined. A retrognathic mandible may have either a short or long base. If the base is short, the cause of the retrognathism is probably a growth deficiency. If a favorable growth direction is present, the prognosis for functional appliance therapy is good. A mandibular base that is both long and retrognathic can result from two possibilities:

1. The mandible is in a functionally retruded (forced) position because of overclosure and occlusal guidance. In postural rest, it is anterior to habitual occlusion. Treatment is simple, consisting of elimination of the forced guidance and up and back path of closure in either the mixed or permanent dentition.
2. The mandible is morphogenetically "built" into the facial skeleton in a posterior position. The temporal fossa is posterior and superior. This discrepancy is not compensated despite the long mandibular base. The prognosis for functional appliance therapy in these cases is poor.

**Maxillary base.** Assessment of the length of the maxillary base has two ideal values: one related to the distance N-Se, the other to the length of the mandibular base. A deviation from the mandibular base–related norm indicates that the maxillary base is too long or too short. If the maxillary base corresponds to the mandibular base–related norm, the facial skeleton is proportionally developed, particularly if the ramal length also corresponds to these values. If the N-Se length does not relate to these three proportionate measurements, the facial skeleton is proportionate but either too large or small.

**Ascending ramus.** Evaluation of ramal length is performed similarly. If the ramus is too short in relation to the other proportions, a large amount of growth can be expected because the growth pattern is not vertical. In vertical growth patterns the ramus remains short. The morphologic characteristics of the mandible also should be studied to enhance the differential diagnosis.

**Morphology of the mandible.** Various facial types (orthognathic, retrognathic, prognathic) reflect to some degree the morphology of the mandible (Figure 6-31). In the orthognathic type of face the ramus and body of the mandible are fully developed, and the width of the ascending ramus is equal to the height of the body of the mandible, including the height of the alveolar process and incisors. The condylar and coronoid processes are almost on the same plane, and the symphysis is well developed.

In the prognathic type the corpus is well developed and wide in the molar region. The symphysis is wider in the sagittal plane. The ramus is wide and long, and the gonial angle is acute or small.

In the retrognathic facial type the corpus is narrow, particularly in the molar region. The symphysis is narrow and long, and the ramus is narrow and short. The coronoid process is shorter than the condylar process, and the gonial angle is obtuse or large.

The prognathic type of mandible grows horizontally. Even if an average or a slightly vertical growth direction is evident in the mixed dentition, shifting of the mandible to a horizon-

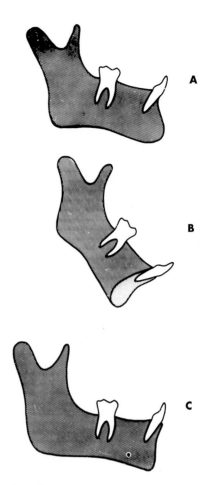

**Figure 6-31.** Morphogenetic types of mandible. **A,** Orthognathic. **B,** Retrognathic. **C,** Prognathic.

tal growth direction can be expected in the following years. In a retrognathic mandible, shifting of the growth pattern in the opposite direction is less likely and produces much less expressivity.

## Analysis of Dentoalveolar Relationships

An important part of the determination of the indications for and construction and management of functional appliances is assessment of the inclination and position of the incisors with respect to the anterior cranial base, their apical bases, and each other.

### Axial inclination of the incisors

*Upper incisors.* The long axis of the maxillary incisors (as viewed on lateral cephalograms) is extended to intersect the S-N line, and the posterior angle is measured (Figure 6-32). Until the seventh year this angle averages from 94 to 100 degrees. A year or two after eruption of the permanent teeth the inclination increases to an average of 102 degrees. Larger angles indicate incisor procumbency or labial crown tipping in Caucasian and Asian samples. Incisor protrusion requires lingual tipping, a therapeutic objective that can be achieved

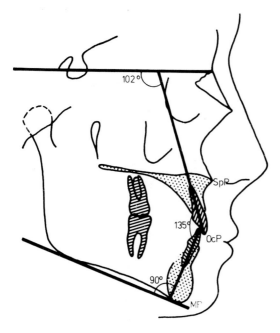

**Figure 6-32.** Axial inclination of the upper and lower incisors. Few normal groups have a 90-degree inclination of the lower incisors to the mandibular plane, however.

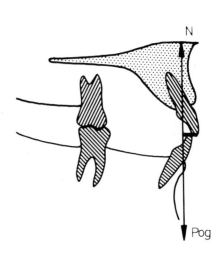

**Figure 6-33.** Linear measurements to assess the horizontal position of the upper incisors with reference to the facial plane.

quite successfully with removable appliances if adequate space is available. However, before deciding on the mode of movement of these teeth, the clinician must assess their positions.

*Lower incisors.* Measurement of the posterior angle between the long axis of the lower incisors and the mandibular plane is the classic method of assessing the axial inclination of these teeth. The ideal angle often stated is 90 degrees, but in most studies of heterogeneous samples, it is 4 to 5 degrees more. Between the sixth and twelfth years, it increases from 88 degrees for relatively upright deciduous incisors to 94 degrees on average for normal samples.

A smaller angle may indicate lingual tipping of the incisors, which is advantageous for functional appliance treatment. Classical activators are most effective in the sagittal plane and tend to tip the lower incisors labially.

If the lower incisors are already labially tipped, functional appliance treatment is more difficult. Anterior repositioning of the mandible and uprighting of the lower incisors become necessary; if possible, they should be moved in the opposite direction. This movement requires the use of a special appliance design in the lower anterior segment.

**Position of the incisors.** Linear measurements are the best assessors of the position of the incisors with respect to the profile. The most common assessment method is to measure the distance of the incisal edges to the line N-Pog, or the so-called facial plane (Figure 6-33).

The average position of the maxillary incisors is 2 to 4 mm

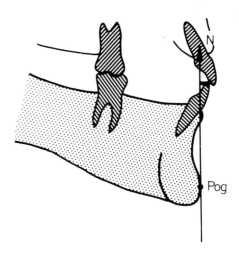

**Figure 6-34.** Linear measurements to assess the horizontal position of the lower incisors.

anterior to the N-Pog line. The lower incisors vary from 2 mm posterior to 2 mm anterior to this line. Orthodontic treatment seeks to achieve a similar relationship to this normal guideline. Uprighting of incisors that are tipped too far labially with respect to the N-Pog line is possible with removable appliances. However, adequate space must be available. If the labially malpositioned incisor already has a good axial inclination, bodily movement is required; this is possible only with fixed appliances and root torque.

The relationship of the lower incisors to the N-Pog line

**TABLE 6-2. • LINEAR MEASUREMENTS AND GROWTH INCREMENTS (IN MM) BETWEEN THE NINTH AND FIFTEENTH YEARS ACCORDING TO GROWTH PATTERN**

| Age (Yr) | Growth Pattern | S-N | S-Gn | S-Go | N-Me | ManBase | MaxBase | Ramus |
|---|---|---|---|---|---|---|---|---|
| 9 | Average | 64.4 | 108.6 | 66.8 | 104.5 | 66.5 | 44.9 | 46.6 |
| | Horizontal | 64.8 | 108.8 | 69.5 | 103.0 | 67.6 | 45.7 | 48.9 |
| | Vertical | 63.8 | 108.5 | 64.1 | 106.7 | 65.2 | 44.0 | 44.5 |
| 10 | Average | 64.9 | 110.8 | 68.2 | 106.3 | 67.9 | 45.4 | 47.5 |
| | Horizontal | 65.3 | 111.0 | 70.9 | 104.8 | 69.2 | 46.3 | 49.7 |
| | Vertical | 64.5 | 110.5 | 65.5 | 108.4 | 66.5 | 44.5 | 45.6 |
| 11 | Average | 65.4 | 113.0 | 70.1 | 108.2 | 69.2 | 46.0 | 48.5 |
| | Horizontal | 65.7 | 113.2 | 72.1 | 106.2 | 70.7 | 46.9 | 50.5 |
| | Vertical | 65.3 | 112.5 | 67.0 | 110.4 | 67.4 | 45.1 | 46.6 |
| 12 | Average | 66.1 | 115.3 | 71.8 | 110.4 | 70.4 | 46.7 | 49.8 |
| | Horizontal | 66.5 | 115.5 | 73.7 | 108.3 | 72.2 | 47.8 | 51.8 |
| | Vertical | 65.8 | 114.8 | 68.9 | 112.5 | 68.5 | 45.8 | 47.6 |
| 13 | Average | 66.8 | 118.0 | 74.0 | 112.7 | 72.0 | 47.4 | 51.4 |
| | Horizontal | 67.4 | 118.4 | 76.1 | 110.6 | 73.8 | 48.3 | 53.6 |
| | Vertical | 66.3 | 117.4 | 71.0 | 114.8 | 69.9 | 46.3 | 49.1 |
| 14 | Average | 67.5 | 120.5 | 76.1 | 115.0 | 73.4 | 48.0 | 53.3 |
| | Horizontal | 68.4 | 121.3 | 78.5 | 112.9 | 75.5 | 48.9 | 55.8 |
| | Vertical | 66.7 | 119.8 | 73.1 | 117.3 | 71.2 | 46.8 | 50.4 |
| 15 | Average | 68.2 | 123.3 | 78.0 | 117.6 | 75.1 | 48.6 | 55.3 |
| | Horizontal | 69.3 | 124.4 | 80.6 | 115.2 | 77.3 | 49.6 | 58.7 |
| | Vertical | 67.3 | 122.3 | 75.0 | 119.4 | 72.6 | 47.2 | 51.7 |

also helps determine the sagittal discrepancy (Figure 6-34). Incisors behind this line can be moved labially because space is available. Incisors anterior to the facial plane that must be moved lingually require additional space, which may be obtained only by extraction procedures. Not only the sagittal discrepancy but also the dental discrepancy (crowding) must be considered. Such decisions are important in the treatment plan and can be made only under the assumption that the reference line remains relatively stable. However, during the mixed dentition period, with its relatively greater mandibular growth increments, the lower terminus of the reference line drifts forward. This alters the relationship of the facial plane to the incisors, particularly the upper incisors, which appear closer to N-Pog because of this differential growth phenomenon. Thus the amount and direction of the growth spurt should be considered in the mixed dentition while the ideal position of the incisors at the end of treatment is being planned.

**Summary.** The salient points of cephalometric analysis for the use of functional appliance therapy can be summarized as follows:

Cephalometrics allows anomalies to be located and differentiations made between skeletal and dentoalveolar malocclusions. If the problem has both skeletal and dentoalveolar components, cephalometric assessment helps determine primary and secondary dysplastic structures and possible autonomous compensatory responses before treatment begins. Cephalometrics allows the determination of whether the jaw bases are anteriorly or posteriorly positioned, short or long. In the vertical plane the possible rotations of the maxillary and mandibular bases can be observed and the growth pattern delineated. While biomechanic factors of planned therapy are considered, the position and inclination of the upper and lower incisors are important from both a functional and an esthetic viewpoint.

Cephalometrics enhances the assessment of the influences of neuromuscular dysfunction on the dentition. This accurate assessment is vital for diagnosis and treatment planning with functional appliances.

## CEPHALOMETRIC EVALUATION OF TREATMENT PROGRESS IN THE MIXED DENTITION

One of the most important tasks of roentgenographic cephalometrics is the objective assessment of changes induced by therapy, growth, and development as treatment progresses. This assessment should be performed periodically. Even the best-developed treatment plan must be altered frequently, and continuing therapeutic diagnosis is the best approach to these alterations. Growth increment and direction, patient cooperation, and untoward treatment response are difficult factors to control. Early changes in treatment plans may make the difference between success and failure. In addition to the cephalometric criteria described at the beginning of this chapter, other complementary measurements can be used both during and after active treatment. Growth increments can be expressed in seven chronologic measurements (Table 6-2).

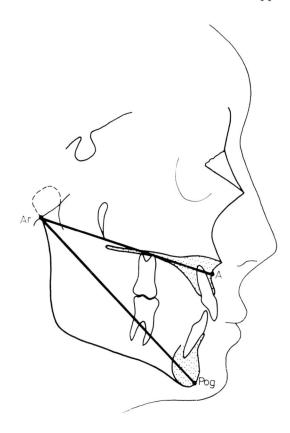

**Figure 6-35.** Measurements for evaluating treatment progress in activator cases (maxillary versus mandibular base horizontal change.) Condylion can be an alternative posterosuperior terminus if visualization of the temporomandibular joint is easy.

### TABLE 6-3. • EVALUATION OF GROWTH INCREMENTS DURING TREATMENT*

| Parameter | Length Before Treatment (mm) | | | Growth Increment (mm) | | |
|---|---|---|---|---|---|---|
| | Observed | Average | Difference | Observed | Average | Difference |
| S-N | 63 | 63.8 | −0.8 | 0 | 1.5 | −1.6 |
| S-Gn | 101 | 108.5 | −7.5 | 5 | 4.5 | +0.5 |
| S-Go | 60 | 64.1 | −4.1 | 4 | 2.9 | +1.1 |
| N-Me | 104 | 106.7 | −2.7 | 6 | 3.1 | +2.9 |
| ManBase | 64 | 65.2 | −1.2 | 3 | 2.2 | +0.8 |
| MaxBase | 44 | 44 | 0 | 1 | 1.2 | −0.2 |
| Ramus | 36 | 44.5 | −8.5 | 2 | 2.1 | −0.1 |
| Ar-A to Ar-Pog | 10 | | 14 | | | |

*The single measurements are compared with the average values from Table 6-2. Data for this table are based on observation of an 8-year-old child with a vertical growth pattern who was in treatment for 2 years.

Comparing measured growth with average values differentiated according to the morphogenetic pattern also is possible. These comparison methods assist in determining whether the growth increments and directions are high or low or favorable or unfavorable in the skeletal areas causing the greatest concern.

A special evaluation is available in activator cases. The distance Ar-Pog is measured and Ar–Point A is subtracted from it (Figure 6-35). Alternatively, condylion can be used as posterior terminus in these measurements. If the mandible is postured anteriorly, this coefficient increases. Table 6-3 illustrates one mode of evaluating growth increments during treatment.

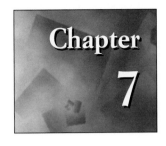

# Chapter 7

# Functional Analysis

T. M. Graber

A major reason for the development of functional appliances was the recognition that function affects the ultimate morphologic status of the dentofacial complex. The work of Wolff (1895) on form and function provided a major contribution to the nature versus nurture and heredity versus environment controversies. Koch's work on stress trajectories in the femoral head was complemented by Benninghof's study of stress trajectories in the midface. Both studies clearly demonstrate the response of bone to functional forces. Controversy still surrounds the exact contribution of function to bone size and shape, but no question remains that function plays an important role. In the craniofacial area particularly, in which membranous bone that is much more responsive to functional forces predominates, understanding of the actual and potential effects of these forces on the accomplishment of pattern change is essential. Alveolar bone is even more responsive to extraneous forces than are basal membranous structures.

When Petrovic was studying otospongiosis with Shambaugh at Northwestern University Medical School in Chicago some years ago, he concentrated on alveolar bone in his research because of its responsiveness; as the world of orthodontic research knows, this responsiveness so fascinated him that he switched from otolaryngology to orthodontics, providing the field with a wealth of information on the effects of function and malfunction on the dentofacial complex.

## THE MANY DEMANDS OF FUNCTIONAL ANALYSIS

Appraisal of the functional status of each patient is a priority before any form of orthodontic therapy is instituted. Because many functions occur in the stomatognathic system, a multiple assessment is necessary to analyze mastication, deglutition, respiration, speech, posture, and the status of each component involved in accomplishing functional activity. Much can be done with proper clinical examination, which is important for not only determining the current relationships among and past effects of each function on structure but also understanding the role this function or group of functions can be expected to play in the future. If function is ab-

This chapter is an updated version of Chapter 5 in Graber TM, Neumann B: *Removable orthodontic appliances*, Philadelphia, 1984, WB Saunders.

normal, the clinician must consider whether it should be altered and whether the change in forces produced can be used to help solve orthodontic problems. If one function (e.g., mastication) is changed, the clinician must assess its potential effect on other functions, which may then exert different forces on the dentofacial skeleton. Clinical study is somewhat subjective, however, and more exacting and reproducible objective criteria must be employed to provide data that are recordable and open to discretionary analysis by qualified observers and patients. Therefore part of the functional analysis should involve cephalometric, myometric, and dentitional measurements from study models and other tools. Most observers consider cephalometric and plaster cast records as static reproductions, but both have functional analysis potential if used correctly. Much can be learned from them about the dynamics of the stomatognathic system.

Thus functional analysis is of equal importance to the usual clinical examination and static, cephalometric, and study model analyses. It is especially significant in treatment with functional appliances because of the dynamic basis of therapy. The role of normal function for optimal growth and development of the orofacial complex has been demonstrated in many laboratory and clinical studies; the role of dysfunction in the etiology of some malocclusions has been similarly well established.

## Adaptability and Homeostasis—Fundamental Physiologic Phenomena

A good example of the adaptive capability and interrelationship between function and form is seen in Figure 7-1. A 5-year-old girl had a fractured mandible that was not mobilized sufficiently. The posterior condylar fragment became ankylosed. Nevertheless, a fibrous joint was formed between the fragments (pseudarthrosis) that permitted functional movement of the mandible. Because function was maintained, adaptive remodeling of the structural form occurred in this functioning area.

The adaptability of the condyle to various topographic and functional relationships during the growth period, which has been demonstrated by Petrovic and associates (see Chapter 2), is one of the basic principles of functional jaw orthopedics. Function is indeed the common denominator joining the individual parts of the orofacial system into a dynamic, integrated, purposive system. Disturbances in one part of this system do

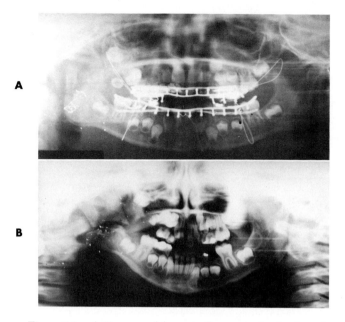

**Figure 7-1.** **A,** Fracture of the ascending ramus that has been insufficiently immobilized. The result is dislocation of the right condyle. **B,** Same patient 2 years later. Fibrous articulation (pseudarthrosis) is evident in the ascending ramus at the site of the original fracture.

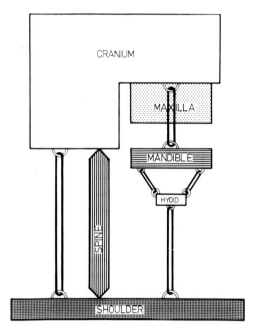

**Figure 7-2.** Prevertebral and postvertebral muscle chains. Each neuromuscular component interacts with the other muscle groups, balancing and stabilizing the head.

not remain isolated but affect the equilibrium of the whole system (Figure 7-2). This unique quality is important in not only etiologic considerations but also assessment of the effectiveness and various side effects of different orthodontic appliances. For example, observation shows that appliances directly influencing the muscles of the lips and cheeks (e.g., oral screens, the Fränkel function regular, the inner bow of a headgear face-bow) indirectly influence the position of the tongue.

## DIAGNOSTIC EXERCISES

Three diagnostic exercises are recommended for performance in the mixed dentition period to assess the possibilities for treatment with functional appliances:

1. Determination of the postural rest position of the mandible and interposed freeway space or interocclusal clearance
2. Examination of temporomandibular joint (TMJ) function or dysfunction and condylar movement in performing the stomatognathic system's tasks
3. Assessment of the functional status of the lips, cheeks, and tongue, with particular attention to the roles they play in dentofacial abnormalities

### Determination of the Postural Rest Position and Interocclusal Clearance

The initial task of functional analysis is the assessment of mandibular position as determined by the musculature. This position in the adult dentition is generally a centric relation that can be registered with a variety of gnathologic techniques. Gnathologic principles cannot be applied in the deciduous or mixed dentition, however, because occlusion is in a transitional stage and growing condylar structures have not yet reached their adult forms. Because a major determinant of adult shape is the functional pattern (originating from the postural rest position of the mandible), registration of this relatively unchanging neuromuscularly derived relationship is a priority. The functional pattern is more likely to be normal and less likely to be affected by skeletal abnormalities and neuromuscular compensations. In the postural rest position, synergistic and antagonistic muscular components are in dynamic equilibrium; their balance is maintained with basic muscle tonus. The rest position is the result of a myostatic antistretch reflex that responds only to the permanent exogenous force affecting the orofacial system (i.e., gravity). As a consequence the rest position depends on and alters with the position of the head. Thus natural head position (NHP) must be determined for each patient. Cephalograms should be taken in NHP.

The movement of the mandible from postural rest to habitual occlusion is of special interest for all functional analyses. It consists of two components: hinge (rotary) action and translatory (sliding) movement. The objective of examination is to assess not only the magnitude and direction of these movements but also the extent of action of each hinge or sliding component. During the closing maneuver from rest posi-

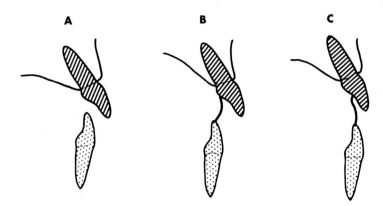

**Figure 7-3.** During closing from the rest position, several maneuvers can occur. **A,** A normal arc can progress into the occlusal position. **B,** In such a case the condylar action is primarily rotary. **C,** An abnormal and posteriorly deviated path can produce translatory condylar movement.

tion, two phases of movement can be observed (Figure 7-3)— the free phase from postural rest to the point of initial or premature contact and the articular phase from initial contact to the centric or habitual occlusal position.

Functional patterns without articular phases that produce free movement from rest to full occlusal contact are seen in only a few completely balanced occlusions. A slight sliding component (as much as 2 mm), particularly in the transitional dentition, is a normal phenomenon.

If the pattern is abnormal, the sliding may be caused by neuromuscular abnormalities, disturbances in dental interrelationships, or compensation of skeletal discrepancies. The abnormal pattern may combine components from one or more of these causes; therefore differential diagnosis is important for treatment planning.

The regimen for the examination is as follows:

1. Determination of the postural rest position with the head in NHP
2. Registration and measurement of the postural rest position
3. Evaluation of the relationship of rest position to occlusal position in the following dimensions:
   a. Sagittal
   b. Vertical
   c. Transverse

**Assessment of the postural rest position.** The rest position of the mandible depends on head and body posture as they are influenced by gravity. For this reason, postural rest position must be determined from a standard head position. The patient is seated upright, preferably with the back unsupported. The head is oriented with the patient looking straight ahead at eye level. Having the patient look directly into a mirror helps establish optimal head posture, a posture that can be replicated fairly easily. If this position seems too variable or the patient is not relaxed, the head can be positioned with the eye-ear plane (Frankfort) horizontal.

Several methods are available to determine the postural rest position of the mandible:

- Phonetic exercises
- Command methods
- Noncommand methods
- Combined methods

*Phonetic exercises.* The patient, who has assumed a relaxed upright body posture and is looking straight ahead, is asked to repeat selected consonants. The letter *m* is generally used to start and is repeated 5 to 10 times. *C* also can be used. Repeating or spelling the word *Mississippi* also is a good exercise. After the phonetic exercise the mandible usually returns to postural rest. The patient is instructed not to move the lips or tongue at this time, even while the dentist gently parts the lips to observe the interocclusal space and tongue position. This method is common in prosthetic dentistry but less satisfactory for children. In the mixed dentition, language habits vary and are not yet stabilized. For this reason, phonetic exercises are used less often as prime determinants and more often as checks on other methods.

*Command methods.* The patient is asked to perform selected functions; the mandible returns to the postural rest position after each function. Usually, having the patient lick the lips and then swallow produces the desired relationship because the mandible returns to postural rest within 2 seconds after the exercise. Phonetic exercises also are a command method in the strictest sense and can serve as a double determinant after the licking of lips and swallowing technique has been attempted.

*Noncommand methods.* In noncommand methods the patient has no idea of the parameter being examined. Careful observations are made as the patient talks, swallows, and turns the head while being questioned on a number of unrelated subjects.

*Combined method.* The combined method usually provides the best reproduction of the postural rest position in the mixed dentition. The patient performs a prescribed function (e.g., swallowing) and then relaxes. After instructing the patient not to move, the clinician gently palpates the submental muscles to assess whether they are relaxed. Tone is increased in opening or closing maneuvers.

The patient is asked to lick the lips, swallow, and then hold still. An intraoral examination is performed by gently parting the lips and observing the relationship of the canines. Normally the lower canine should be 3 mm below the upper in comparison with the occlusal position. An interocclusal space of 4 mm may be normal.

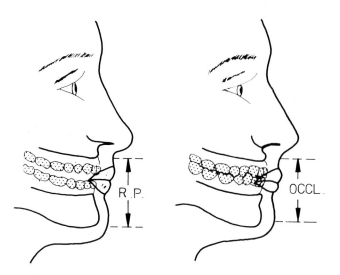

**Figure 7-4.** One direct extraoral assessment method enables the examiner to measure the difference between rest position (*R.P.*) and occlusal position (*OCCL.*) using lower face height from subnasale to gnathion or menton.

**Registration of the postural rest position of the mandible.** Various methods are recommended for producing the best record:

- Direct intraoral method
- Direct extraoral method
- Indirect extraoral method

***Direct intraoral method.*** In addition to the visual observation just described, the clinician can perform a direct intraoral procedure by using a plaster core registration similar to that sometimes used in prosthodontics. This registration is not feasible for children in the mixed dentition, however. Mensuration also is difficult, although millimetric calipers can be used to record the interocclusal space in the canine or incisor area.

***Direct extraoral method.*** Direct caliper measurements can be made on the patient's profile by measuring the distance from soft tissue nasion (at the bridge of the nose) to menton (on the lowest curvature of the chin). This measurement is done in both postural rest and habitual occlusion. The difference between the two measurements constitutes the interocclusal clearance (Figure 7-4). The disadvantages of this procedure are that the soft tissues reduce reliability and no record of the sagittal relationship is produced.

***Indirect extraoral method.*** The indirect extraoral method is the most common one used, and various techniques are available: roentgenography, cephalometry, electromyography, cinefluorography, and kinesiography (Figure 7-5). Cephalometric registration offers the most uniformly successful results. The clinician takes two or three lateral cephalograms under identical exposure and patient positioning conditions: the first in postural rest, the second in initial

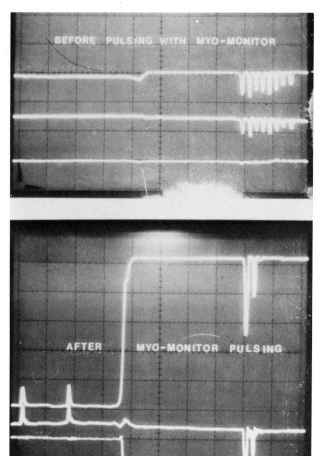

**Figure 7-5.** Kinesiographic registration of mandibular movements enables the examiner to assess the rest position of the jaw.

contact, and the third in full habitual occlusion (Figure 7-6). Two measurements can be performed on each head film. One records hinge movement of the condyle in the vertical plane. The second assesses sliding or translatory action in the sagittal plane. Comparison of the single movements permits an assessment of the path of closure of the mandible, which must be determined from rest to initial contact and initial contact to full occlusion. If a significant sliding component is observed from initial contact to occlusion, the abnormality must be recognized and recorded (Figure 7-7). Normally, condylar movement is both translatory and rotary beyond the rest position, but from postural rest to habitual occlusion, it should show little translation and primarily a rotary action (as the work of Blume [1952] and Boman [1952] has demonstrated). In contrast to the records observed in functional equilibrium and normal occlusion, a different set of values prevails and frequently a different path of closure is seen in Class II and III malocclusions (Figures 7-8 and 7-9).

Electromyographic, cinefluorographic, kinesiographic, and sirognathographic techniques for registering postural rest position require special equipment and are not necessary in routine private practice. They are largely confirmatory of the cephalometric registration.

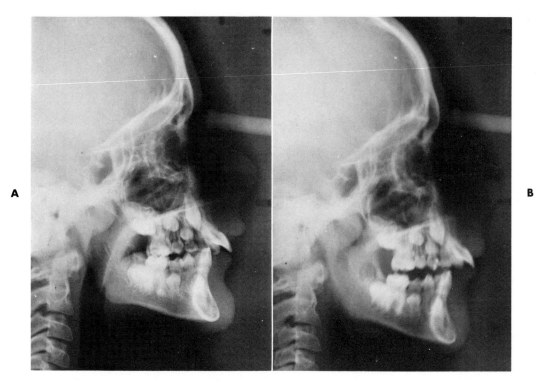

**Figure 7-6.** Cephalometric registration of the occlusal (**A**) and rest (**B**) positions.

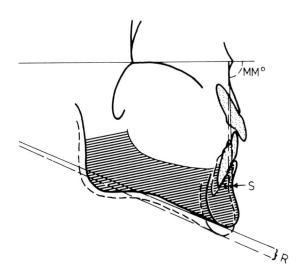

**Figure 7-7.** Comparison of occlusal and rest positions. The difference *(R)* represents rotary movement. In a similar manner the *MM* angle at rest and in occlusion can express the sliding or translatory component *(S)*.

**Evaluation of the path of closure from postural rest to occlusion in the sagittal plane.** Condylar movement from postural rest to occlusion can consist of pure hinge movement, hinge and anterior translatory displacement, and hinge and posterior superior translatory displacement.

*Class II malocclusions.* Treatment prognosis for functional appliance therapy depends on the analysis of relationships and the determination of the path of closure category:

1. In Class II malocclusions without functional distur-

bance the path of closure from rest to occlusion is straight up and forward, with a hinge movement of the condyle in the fossa. These are true Class II malocclusions (Figure 7-10).

2. In Class II malocclusions with functional disturbances a rotary action of the condyle in the fossa from postural rest to occlusion is evident. From initial contact to full occlusion, condylar action is both rotary and translatory up and backward (posterior shift). Thus the movement combines rotary and sliding components (Figure 7-11). As Boman (1952) and Blume (1952) showed in their re-

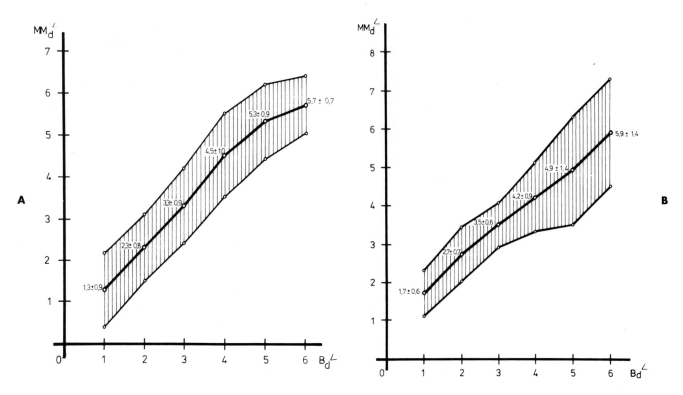

**Figure 7-8.** **A,** Average values of the rotary $(B_d)$ and sliding $(MM_d)$ components of movement from rest to occlusion in functionally correct or true Class II malocclusions. **B,** The same relationship in true Class III malocclusions.

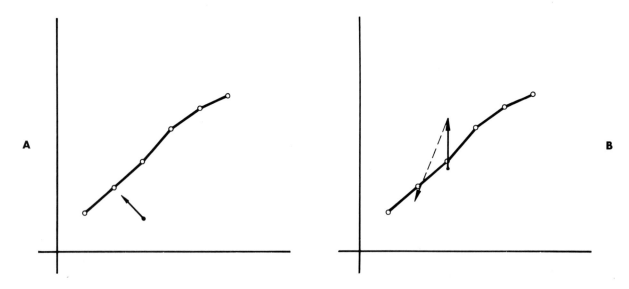

**Figure 7-9.** Average curve of the functional relationships and possible alteration of these relationships during treatment. **A,** In an abnormal path of closure the arrow moves in the direction of the curve after the functional disturbance has been eliminated. **B,** In a malocclusion with abnormal path of closure during treatment a functional disturbance arises because after improvement of the morphologic relationships, the rest position is not altered (arrow moves away from the curve). In the second phase of treatment or retention when the functional relationships are stabilized, a new rest position is established (arrow moves in the direction of the curve).

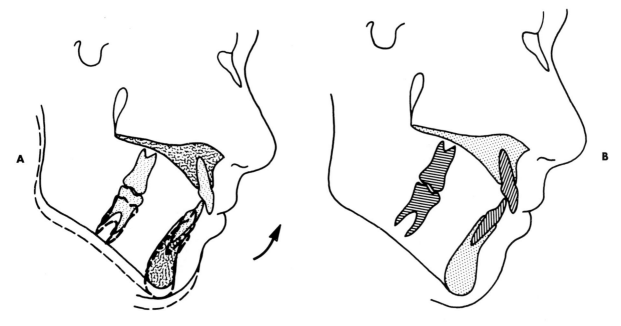

**Figure 7-10.**   Hinge movement from the rest (**A**) to occlusal (**B**) position in a functionally correct Class II relationship with a normal path of closure.

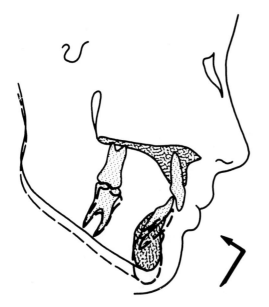

**Figure 7-11.**   Posterior translation or sliding into the occlusal position in an abnormal functional pattern with a deviated path of closure.

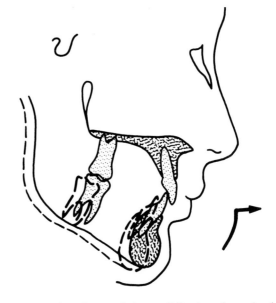

**Figure 7-12.**   Anterior translation or sliding into the occlusal position in a severe Class II malocclusion.

search, this type of activity is the most common, particularly in cases of excessive overbite. This functional type of Class II malocclusion appears more severe than it actually is sagittally.

3. In Class II malocclusions with functional disturbances in which the path of closure is up and forward from rest to initial contact (usually in the molar region), the mandible may be anteriorly displaced from initial con-

tact as the cusps guide the mandible into a forward position, with translatory movement of the condyle down and forward on the posterior slope of the articular eminence. The path of closure appears more up and forward than it is without tooth interference. This condition has been illustrated by Woodside (1984) in his research (Figure 7-12). This malocclusion is more severe than it appears with the teeth in occlusion. However, this variation of path of closure is least frequent for Class II malocclusions.

In functional Class II malocclusions the elimination of functional retrusion or protrusion leads to an improvement in the sagittal malrelationship. This improvement is a change in the spatial interrelation of parts and is not caused by growth and development. In Class II malocclusions with normal paths of closure the intermaxillary relationships still require alteration, but this alteration requires both a morphologic and a functional change to produce the desired sagittal correction. The original rotary condylar action from rest to occlusion is not changed, and the ultimate condyle-eminence relationship

is the same. However, the clinician works for dentoalveolar adjustment and optimal horizontal growth of the mandible under the influence of the activator. The clinician must assess the growth pattern by cephalometrics to be able to project a likely growth direction and probable incremental needs. In cases of posterior displacement combined with projected horizontal growth directions, the prognosis for Class II treatment is very good. If anterior displacement and a vertical growth vector are present, the prognosis is quite poor. Other combinations are possible—anterior displacement and horizontal growth direction or posterior condylar displacement with a vertical growth direction. In these two combinations the prognosis is not good; it can be improved or worsened depending on the age of the patient and the specifics of the facial pattern.

***Class III malocclusions.*** Hinge-type condylar function is often associated with Class III malocclusions with straight paths of closure (Figure 7-13). The possibility of successful functional appliance treatment of these problems exists only if the magnitude of the sagittal dysplasia is not too great and therapy is begun in the early mixed dentition. If the path of closure is up and back (an anterior postural rest position), the prognosis is even poorer. In Class III malocclusions with anterior displacement that creates an up and forward path of closure with combined rotary and translatory action of the condyle from postural rest to habitual occlusion, the prognosis is much better and treatment success is possible, even in the permanent dentition.

Functional therapy is the most efficient mode of treatment in the mixed dentition. However, functional analysis alone is not sufficient to determine prognosis because not all Class III malocclusions with anterior paths of closure are mandibular displacements with good prognoses. Sometimes a skeletal Class III relationship is partially compensated by labial tipping of the maxillary incisors and lingual tipping of the mandibular incisors. Because of the extreme tipping possible,

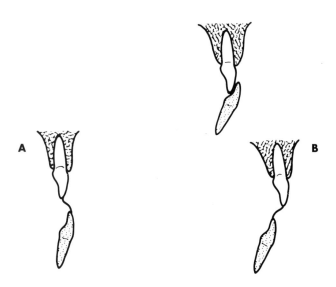

**Figure 7-13.** Various functional relationships in Class III malocclusions. **A,** Anterior rest position in a severe Class III malocclusion. **B,** Posterior rest position in a forced bite type of Class III malocclusion (i.e., pseudo–Class III).

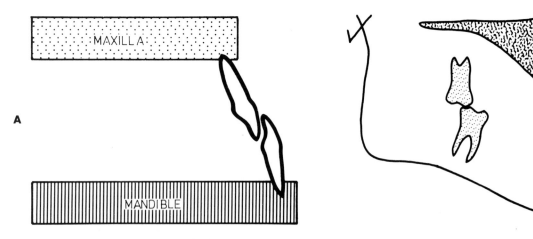

**Figure 7-14.** **A,** Pseudo–forced bite relationship with labial tipping of the upper incisors and lingual tipping of the lower incisors. This is a true Class III problem with a marked basal sagittal malrelationship. **B,** After uprighting of the incisors, the severity of the Class III relationship is quite evident.

an anterior sliding movement into occlusion can occur. Uprighting the incisors into their proper axial inclinations results in a severe Class III sagittal tooth relationship. Treatment of this type of malocclusion by orthodontic means is difficult because dentoalveolar compensation is not possible; the incisors are already overcompensated before treatment. Orthognathic surgery should be considered and discussed with the patient. This type of malocclusion is referred to as a *pseudo–forced* bite or displacement (Figure 7-14). The differentiation of a forced bite from a pseudo–forced bite is usually possible only with the aid of cephalometric analysis.

**Evaluation of the path of closure from postural rest to habitual occlusion in the vertical plane.** This evaluation is of special interest in the assessment of therapeutic potential in deep overbite cases. Two types of deep overbite can be differentiated (Figure 7-15):

1. The true deep overbite with a large interocclusal clearance is caused by infraclusion of the posterior segments. It often results from a lateral tongue posture or tongue thrust habit. Some Class II, division 2 malocclusions with adequate lip line relationships are good examples of true deep overbites. Treatment in the mixed dentition period requires the elimination of environmental factors inhibiting eruption of the posterior teeth. This is a valid and quite attainable functional appliance treatment objective.

2. The pseudo–deep overbite with a small interocclusal space already has normal eruption of the posterior segment teeth. Further extrusion is possible only to a moderate degree. The deep overbite is combined with over-eruption of the incisors. Some Class II, division 2 malocclusions that produce a "gummy" smile and poor lip line relation fall into this category. The amount of interocclusal clearance is a distinguishing criterion. The possibility of intruding incisors by using functional methods is questionable. The clinician usually must drive the maxillary molars distally to control the vertical dimension. Some extrusion is possible; it results in an increased anterior face height and reduced incisor overbite. All available intrusive mechanics on the incisor teeth using fixed appliances are usually indicated. Cephalometric

analysis is essential to disclose the morphogenetic pattern, growth direction, and precise areas of abnormal tooth position requiring therapeutic guidance.

The prognosis is good in a true deep overbite problem if a vertical growth pattern is present (Figure 7-16). In pseudo–deep overbite problems with horizontal growth patterns, the possibilities for correction with functional appliances are limited (Figure 7-17). In combined cases of true deep overbites and horizontal growth patterns or pseudo–deep bites and vertical growth patterns limited success can be expected (Figure 7-18).

In Class II malocclusions with deep overbites, functional treatment is sometimes advantageous for improving the sagittal relationship but not for controlling vertical dysplasia, and vice versa. A total of eight functional combinations between the vertical and sagittal relationship can be categorized (Table 7-1).

Generally in functional Class II problems with posterior displacement and functional deep overbite problems with large interocclusal spaces, functional appliances have good prognoses for successful therapy. The basic principle for functional treatment is the elimination of disturbing environmental factors and the promotion of optimal growth. In nonfunctional true Class II malocclusions and pseudo–deep overbite problems, therapy is more difficult regardless of the appliance used because of multisystem involvement and the need for neuromotor alteration.

**Evaluation of the path of closure from postural rest to habitual occlusion in the transverse plane.** Clinical examination of transverse functional relationships is easy to perform. It consists of observing the behavior of the mandibular midline as the teeth are brought together from rest position to habitual occlusion. Two types of crossbite cases with lateral shifting of the mandibular midline can be differentiated (Figure 7-19):

1. The first is a crossbite in which the midline shift of the mandible can be observed only in the occlusal position. In postural rest the midlines are coincident and well centered. The mandible slides laterally from rest position into a crossbite in occlusion. This is called a laterocclusion, or pseudo-crossbite, and is caused by tooth guidance. Treatment requires eliminating the disturbance in the intercuspation. This often is done by

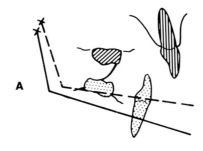
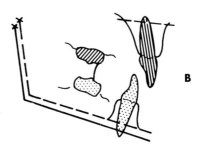

**Figure 7-15.** **A,** True deep overbite with a wide freeway space. **B,** Pseudo–deep overbite with a small freeway space.

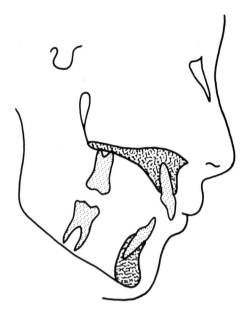

**Figure 7-16.**   True deep overbite with a vertical growth pattern. The prognosis for treatment of this overbite is good.

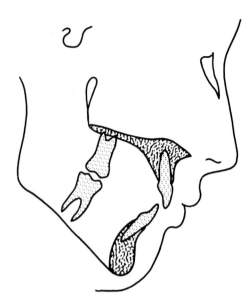

**Figure 7-17.**   Pseudo–deep overbite with a horizontal growth pattern. The prognosis for treatment is poor.

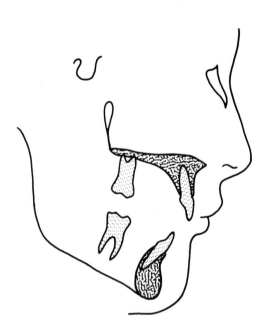

**Figure 7-18.**   True deep overbite with a horizontal growth pattern. The prognosis for treatment is fair.

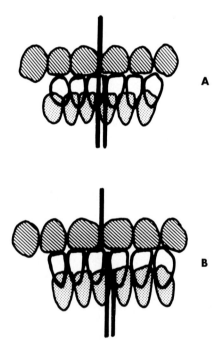

**Figure 7-19.**   Two functional types of crossbite. **A,** Midline shift occurs only in full occlusion. In rest position the midlines are well centered. The prognosis for functional appliance therapy is good. This crossbite is called *laterocclusion.* **B,** Persistence of the midline shift in rest position. The prognosis for treatment is poor. This crossbite is termed *laterognathy* (in rest and occlusion).

**TABLE 7-1. • CORRELATIONS BETWEEN SAGITTAL AND VERTICAL RELATIONSHIPS FOR THE PROGNOSIS OF FUNCTIONAL THERAPY**

| Type of Overbite | Displacement | Growth Pattern | Prognosis for Improvement in Condition | |
|---|---|---|---|---|
| | | | Deep Bite | Sagittal Relation |
| True | Posterior | Horizontal | + | ++ |
| True | Posterior | Vertical | ++ | + |
| True | Anterior | Horizontal | + | + |
| True | Anterior | Vertical | ++ | − |
| Pseudo | Posterior | Horizontal | − | ++ |
| Pseudo | Posterior | Vertical | + | + |
| Pseudo | Anterior | Horizontal | − | + |
| Pseudo | Anterior | Vertical | − | − |

+, Moderate; ++, good; −, poor.

widening the narrowed maxillary arch, thus improving function (Figure 7-20). The procedure also can be done in the permanent dentition, although some evidence suggests that prolonged crossbite relationships can lead to asymmetric jaw growth if allowed to continue for a number of years during the growing period (Egermark-Ericson, Thilander).

2. The second is a crossbite in which the midline shift is present in both occlusal and postural rest positions (e.g., a true asymmetric facial skeleton). This is sometimes referred to as *laterognathy* (Figure 7-21). Successful functional appliance treatment is not possible in such cases; in severe cases, surgery is the only alternative.

This first phase of functional examination thus provides significant information concerning the indications and contraindications for functional appliance treatment.

## Examination of the Temporomandibular Joint and Condylar Movement

The objective of this aspect of functional examination is to assess whether incipient symptoms of TMJ dysfunction are present. The examination is not as extensive for the general patient population as it is for patients with frank TMJ problems. However, initial TMJ symptoms are present in many 8- to 14-year-old children with various types of malocclusions. In a study of 232 children in this age group, 41% had various TMJ symptoms.

These symptoms are important for two reasons:

1. Through the early elimination of functional disturbances, some incipient TMJ problems can be prevented or eliminated. This is an indication for early orthodontic treatment.
2. During activator therapy the condyle is displaced or dislocated to achieve a remodeling of the TMJ structures and a change in muscle function. If the temporomandibular structures are abnormal at the start and hy-

persensitivity is a problem, the possibility of exacerbating the symptoms exists. Fortunately, this seldom happens; functional appliances often eliminate unfavorable sensory reactions in the process of posturing the mandible forward. This is an important requisite for the treatment of many adult TMJ cases. If TMJ problems are present in the deciduous dentition, forward posturing may be better achieved in a staged progression.

Early symptoms of TMJ problems include the following;

- Clicking and crepitus
- Sensitivity in the condylar region and masticatory muscles
- Functional disturbances (e.g., hypermobility, limitation of movement, deviation)
- Radiographic evidence of morphologic and positional abnormalities

Clicking is seldom noted at the initial examination. Crepitus can sometimes be observed during the opening movement (initial, intermediate, or terminal). More frequently, terminal clicking or crepitation occurs because of hypermobility or too-wide opening. Terminal crepitus is usually a sign of peripheral irregularity of the articular disk or unevenness of the condylar surface; this type of crepitus is amenable to correction. Crepitation during chewing is occasionally seen, especially in children with deep overbites. Similarly, crepitus can be observed during the closing maneuver in pseudoanterior crossbite patients and anterior functional displacement. In 51.5% of patients with initial TMJ symptoms, recognizable crepitus is present.

Tenderness to palpation in the condylar region could be found in only 5.3% of the cases reported in the study previously mentioned. The most characteristic symptom of initial functional disturbance of the TMJ was the palpatory tenderness of the temporalis and masseter muscles. The lateral pterygoid muscle (LPM) is probably implicated. However, palpation of the LPM is difficult and relatively unreliable. Nevertheless, in the previously discussed study, 52% of sub-

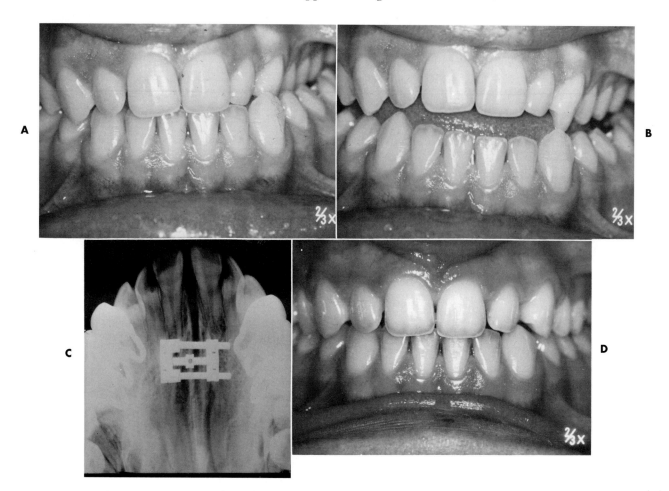

**Figure 7-20.** Functional crossbite (laterocclusion) in the permanent dentition. **A,** Midline deviation in occlusion. **B,** Well-centered midline in rest position. **C,** Palatal expansion or splitting. **D,** Improvement of the crossbite. A slight midline shift persists after palatal expansion.

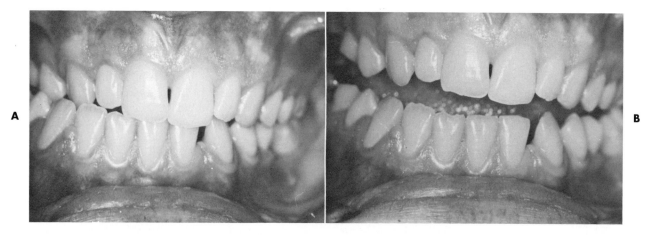

**Figure 7-21.** Laterognathy. **A,** A slight midline deviation occurs in occlusion and becomes worse in the rest position, **B.**

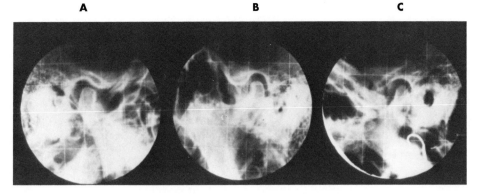

**Figure 7-22.** Three radiographic condylar findings. **A,** Anterior dislocation (right condyle). **B,** Eucentricity (left condyle). **C,** Posterior dislocation (left condyle).

jects reported tenderness in the right pterygoid; 59% reported tenderness in the left pterygoid.

Another possible TMJ abnormality in this age group is hypermobility, an opening of more than 45 mm in 6- to 8-year-old children and more than 49 mm in 10- to 12-year-old children. The problem is mostly habitual, but it can indicate a predisposition to later temporomandibular dysfunction (TMD). In the study, 50.5% of the subjects showed hypermobility. In 22% an anterior displacement of the condyle over the articular tubercle occurred. Another symptom is limited movement because of muscle spasm. This is seen only in isolated cases and is not a major concern. Deviation of the opening or closing movement sagittally or transversely can be seen in 24% of the cases studied in which TMJ symptoms occurred. In 11.5% an S opening occurred as the condyles moved forward or backward unevenly in the functional maneuvers. Deviation was most frequently accompanied by crepitus or clicking. Condylar dislocation was seen mostly with some form of functional deviation. In 36% of the dislocation cases, condylar deviation also occurred during opening and closing.

Neuromuscular involvement in TMJ problems was also observed in the lip and tongue areas. In children without TMJ dysfunction, 20.5% of the sample showed abnormal perioral activity; the percentages were significantly higher in children with TMJ symptoms (43%). Tongue dysfunction was seen in 12.4% of the sample without TMJ problems, compared with 21% in the TMJ problem group.

Radiographic evidence of structural abnormality in the TMJ in children is relatively rare. However, because morphology is difficult to interpret with even the best laminagraphs, the claims by some clinicians that flattening of the condylar surface and eminence frequently occurs are hard to verify. The relationship of the condyle to the fossa structures can be abnormal because of anterior or posterior displacement, as discussed earlier (Figure 7-22).

The greatest frequency of TMJ symptoms was seen in Class II malocclusions: 53% had some TMJ symptoms, whereas 68% had abnormal perioral muscle function. In addition, the TMJ cases usually had a deep bite and a horizontal growth direction of the mandible. This study confirms the observations made by Graber (1984) in his study of 374 TMJ patients. In the Rakosi TMJ study the frequency of TMJ symp-

toms also was high in Class III malocclusions with anterior displacements, crossbite conditions, and tongue dysfunctions.

**Clinical functional examination for the temporomandibular joint area.** The simplified clinical examination of the TMJ area consists of three steps:

1. Auscultation
2. Palpation
3. Functional analysis

*Auscultation.* A stethoscope is used to check for signs of clicking and crepitus. A stereostethoscope is better than the conventional instrument because it allows the operator to determine the magnitude and timing of abnormal sounds for each joint simultaneously.

The examination is performed by having the patient open and close the jaw into full occlusion. If clicking or crepitus is noted, the patient is instructed to bite forward into incision and then repeat the opening and closing movements. These movements are checked for any sounds with the stethoscope. Most often, sounds disappear in the protruded position.

*Palpation.* The condyle and fossa are palpated with the index finger during opening and closing maneuvers (Figure 7-23). The posterior surface can be palpated by inserting the little finger in the external auditory meatus. The condyles can thus be checked for tenderness, synchrony of action, and coordination of relative position in the fossae.

Palpation of the associated musculature is an important part of the examination. In TMJ patients, palpation of the muscles of the face, head, and neck is essential. Experience has shown that children with incipient TMJ symptoms almost always demonstrate some tenderness in the LPM. Palpation of this muscle is difficult but can be approximated by placing the forefinger behind the maxillary tuberosity, right above the occlusal plane, with the palmar surface of the finger directed medially toward the pterygoid hamulus (Figure 7-24).

In patients with early TMJ symptoms, unilateral tenderness commonly occurs. If hypersensitivity or pain is present on both sides, the condition is more protracted and palpation of other associated muscles is indicated. Tenderness in the superior head of the LPM is an important diagnostic clue because it

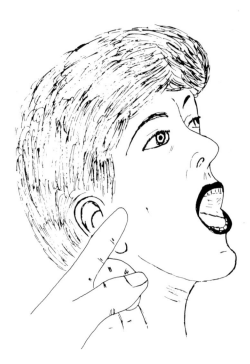

**Figure 7-23.** Assessment of the TMJ through palpation of the condyle during opening and closing movement.

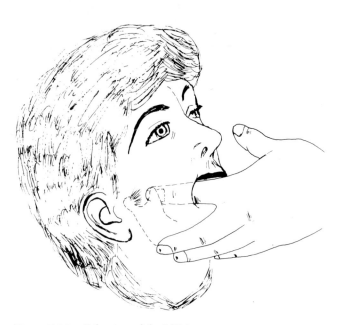

**Figure 7-24.** Palpation of the LPM area.

may indicate abnormal functional loading of the joint. This finding requires further study for possible etiologic factors.

*Functional analysis.* Dislocation of the condyles and discoordination of movements are early symptoms of functional disturbance. Palpation and inspection usually enable the clinician to make the necessary determination. In severe cases or in patients with TMJ disease, gnathologic registration may be useful. Myographic recordings also assist in this functional analysis. Simple electronic devices help measure the silent period of muscular contraction—a cardinal sign of dysfunction in many cases.

Functional movements of the mandible and condyles are carefully assessed. The extent of maximum opening is measured between the upper and lower incisors with a Boley gauge (Figure 7-25). In overbite cases this amount must be added to the measurement, whereas in open bite the distance separating the incisors on full occlusion must be subtracted. The direction of opening and closing movements should be registered graphically with curves (Figure 7-26). Premature contacts and deviations in sagittal and transverse directions are assessed.

Further dysfunctional signs are sought in the lips, tongue, and other structures. Lip dysfunction coexists significantly with incipient TMJ symptoms. Perioral neuromuscular abnormalities, crepitus, and tenderness of the LPM are important signs of early TMJ dysfunction. As a rule of thumb the diagnosis of incipient TMD can be made if two of these three signs are present.

Several specific measures can be employed to prevent functional TMDs:

1. Early care of deciduous teeth (especially the molars) for caries and interferences

2. Elimination of tooth guidance crossbites and unwanted translatory condylar movement in the deciduous dentition
3. Elimination of neuromuscular dysfunctions (especially those involving the lips) and habits that force the mouth open

If incipient TMJ signs already exist at the first examination of the patient, early orthodontic treatment is recommended, especially in the following conditions:

1. Class II malocclusions with excessive overjet, horizontal growth pattern, and lower lip cushioning to the lingual of the upper incisors (lip trap)
2. Deep overbite problems
3. Anterior open bite with associated abnormal lip, tongue, and finger habits
4. Crossbite conditions

In patients exhibiting clicking and functional disturbances, muscle exercises and interceptive appliance guidance (e.g., bite planes, the bionator) are recommended. This approach also is beneficial for patients who already have TMDs and thus require special examination and care.

## Assessment of Stomatognathic Dysfunction

Before functional appliance treatment is instituted, a thorough analysis of all possible dysfunctions is necessary. Dysfunction can be a primary etiologic factor in malocclusion. Many dysfunctions are acquired in the early stages of development. Neonates are capable of performing some vital functions—suckling, swallowing, and breathing—that are unconditioned reflex actions. Many functions learned during the first months or years of life (chewing, phonation, mimicry) are

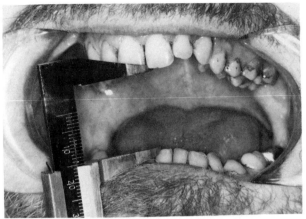

**Figure 7-25.** Measuring the amount of mandibular opening. A Boley gauge may be used. The distance is normally between 40 and 65 mm.

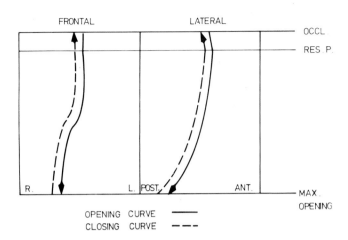

**Figure 7-26.** Closing and opening curves of the mandible (frontal and lateral views).

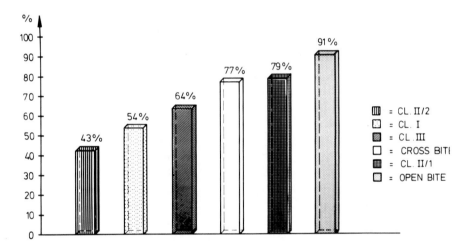

**Figure 7-27.** Frequency of abnormal sucking habits and perioral function in various malocclusions and normal (Class I) occlusion.

conditioned reflex actions developed from the unconditioned ones. Certain unphysiologic reflex actions develop concurrently with normal physiologic reflex activities. These include the dysfunctions of mouth breathing and bruxism. Some children seem predisposed toward certain dysfunctions they copy from their peers or parents. Children with psychologic or adjustment problems often use certain dysfunctions as escape or attention-getting mechanisms. If these parafunctional habits are prolonged, the potential for the dysfunction to cause or exacerbate a malocclusion grows. The deformation of structures is such that adaptive functional activity persists after the disappearance of the original inciting factor (e.g., thumb sucking, finger sucking). Adaptive dysfunction exacerbates the malrelationship that already exists. However, not all thumb, finger, tongue, and lip dysfunctions produce deformation of the teeth and supporting tissue that persists after cessation of the habit. In these cases, autonomous adjustment re-

stores the normal overbite and overjet. If a pattern-type predilection toward an abnormal sagittal or transverse malrelationship is already evident, the likelihood of persistence of dysfunction is enhanced by the deforming and adaptive perioral malfunction. A study of more than 2000 preschool-aged children confirmed this observation: 79% of children with Class II malocclusions had abnormal perioral habits; in Class III the percentage was 64%; in Class II, division 2, 43%; in open-bite problems, 91%; and in crossbite, 77%. However, 54% of the children without malocclusion had abnormal sucking habits (Figure 7-27).

Malocclusions acquired as a result of dysfunctions can usually be treated simply by eliminating the disturbing environmental influences, thus fostering normal development. Functional appliances serve well in this respect. In developmental malocclusions and those attributable to morphogenetic causes, causal functional rehabilitation is not possible.

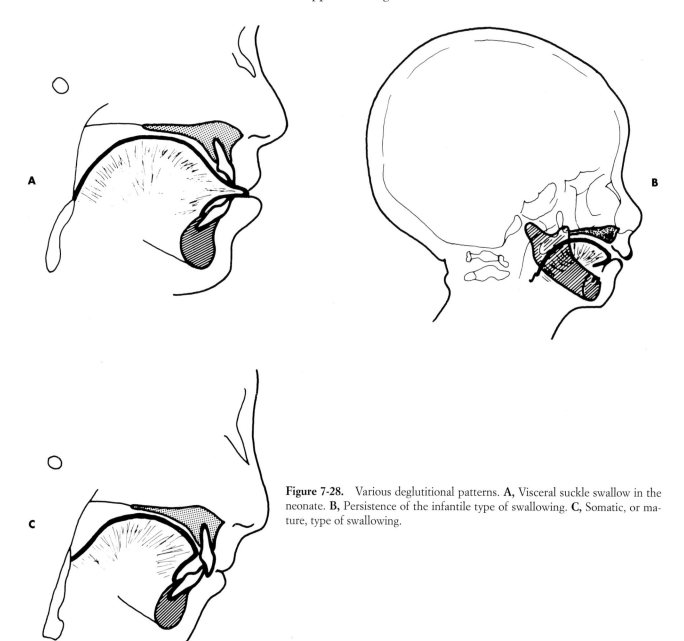

**Figure 7-28.**   Various deglutitional patterns. **A,** Visceral suckle swallow in the neonate. **B,** Persistence of the infantile type of swallowing. **C,** Somatic, or mature, type of swallowing.

Other therapies must be applied in such cases. In planning treatment with the help of functional analysis, recognizing these limitations ahead of time is essential.

Functional examination to ascertain dysfunctional aspects requires an assessment of the tongue, lips, cheeks, and hyoid musculature. Examination of the swallowing function usually involves all areas, although each muscle group can be studied separately. The primary means of examination are clinical observation and functional testing supported by cephalometric analysis. More sophisticated techniques of functional analysis (e.g., electromyography, cinefluorography, kinesiology, video imaging, magnetic resonance imaging [MRI]) are helpful but not usually available in private practice.

**Evaluation of the swallowing function.**   The first and most obvious step in functional assessment is to study the deglutitional cycle. In neonates the tongue is relatively large and located in the forward suckling position for nursing. The tip inserts through the anterior gum pads and assists in the anterior lip seal. This tongue position and coincident swallowing are termed *infantile* or *visceral.*

With eruption of the incisors at about 6 months, the tongue position starts to retract. Over a period of 12 to 18 months, as proprioception causes tongue postural and functional changes, a transitional period ensues. Between 2 and 4 years the functionally balanced, or mature, somatic swallow is seen in normal developmental patterns (Figure 7-28). Visceral swal-

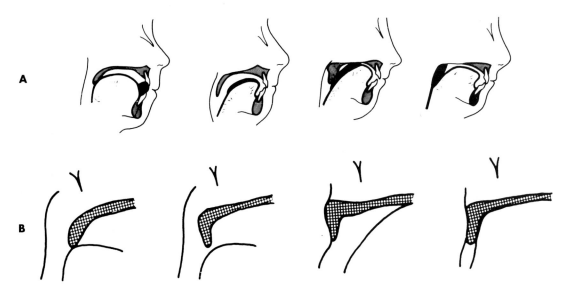

**Figure 7-29.** **A,** Four stages of the oral phase of swallowing. The change in tongue position as the food bolus is transported into the oropharynx during the deglutitional cycle is apparent. **B,** Function of the posterior seal in the four stages (velopharyngeal valving).

lowing can persist well after the fourth year of life, however, and is then considered dysfunctional or abnormal because of its association with certain malocclusive characteristics.

Several factors can account for the persistence of infantile swallowing patterns. Finger sucking, bottle feeding, mouth breathing, tongue sucking, and central nervous system developmental retardation can all contribute.

The symptoms of a retained visceral swallowing pattern usually include forward tongue posture and tongue thrusting during swallowing, contraction of the perioral muscles (hyperactive mentalis and orbicularis oris contraction), often excessive buccinator hyperactivity, and swallowing without the momentary tooth contact normally required. If all these symptoms are present, the pattern is called a *complex tongue thrusting problem.* A variety of malocclusions may accompany this dysfunction. Open-bite conditions often exist in both anterior and posterior regions. Elimination of the problem is usually more difficult in a complex tongue thrust, and a long period of retention is necessary to prevent the return of the visceral swallowing pattern if indeed it has been eliminated in the first place.

More amenable to interception is anterior tongue posture, or simple tongue thrust. This is largely a localized anterior tongue posturing forward during rest and active function with localized anterior open bite. Attendant muscle abnormalities are more adaptive than primary in such cases. The prognosis for functional therapy is usually good, and autonomous improvement can often be seen.

***Normal deglutition.*** In the normal mature swallow, no tongue thrust or constant forward posture occurs. The tip of the tongue is supported on the lingual of the dentoalveolar area; the contraction of perioral muscles is slight during deglutition, and the teeth are in momentary contact during the swallowing cycle. The objective of functional appliance ther-

apy is to establish this type of pattern for patients experiencing dysfunction.

Various means have been devised to analyze tongue function. Based on original work by Gwynne-Evans (1954), Ballard (1965), and Björk (1972), the deglutitional cycle may be divided into four stages (Figure 7-29):

*Stage 1*   The anterior third of the superior surface of the tongue is flat or retracted. The food bolus is collected on the flat anterior part of the tongue or in the sublingual area in front of the retracted tongue. The posterior arched part of the dorsum is in contact with the soft palate. The posterior seal is closed; swallowing cannot yet take place. The teeth and lips are not in contact.

*Stage 2*   The soft palate moves in a cranial and posterior direction. The palatolingual and palatopharyngeal seals are now open. The tip of the tongue moves up as the dorsum drops, creating a groove or depression in the middle third and permitting posterior transport of the bolus. Simultaneously a slight contraction of the lip muscles occurs while the lips are in contact; the anterior teeth approximate at the end of this stage. Symptoms of tongue thrust syndrome can be observed during this stage.

*Stage 3*   The superior constrictor muscle ring in the epipharyngeal wall (known as *Passavant's pad*) starts to constrict. It can be seen on lateral cephalograms or in cinefluorography as a bulge in the posterior wall. The soft palate assumes a triangular form; both tissues together form the palatopharyngeal seal, often referred to as the *velopharyngeal seal.* With the closing of the nasopharynx the posterior part of the dorsum of the tongue drops more; this allows the bolus of food to pass through the isthmus faucium. Simultaneously the anterior part of the tongue is pressed against the hard palate,

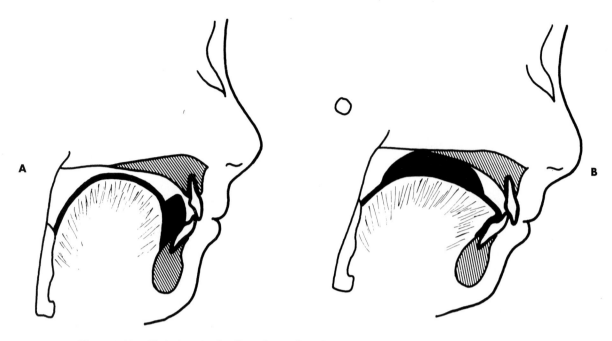

**Figure 7-30.** Variations in the first phase of swallowing. **A,** Collecting phase in front of the tongue tip. This is encountered more frequently. **B,** Collecting phase on the dorsum of the tongue. This variation is frequently caused by different food consistencies.

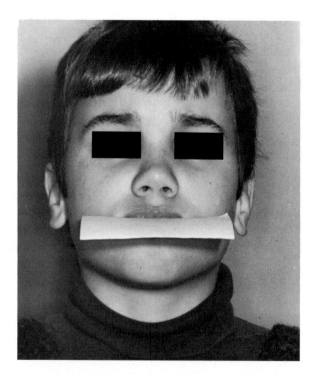

**Figure 7-31.** Lip exercises with a small piece of cardboard or paper.

which helps manipulate the bolus in a posterior direction. The teeth are in contact (usually slightly forward of full contact), and the lips are together. If tongue thrusting is present, the tongue has not retracted but has narrowed with the tip pressed forward to help in the anterior lip seal. A momentary negative atmospheric pressure is created.

*Stage 4*    The dorsum of the tongue now moves posteriorly and superiorly as the palatopharyngeal tissues move down and forward. The tongue pushes against the tensed soft palate, squeezing the residual food bolus out the oropharyngeal area. The terminal action may be likened to squeezing a tube of toothpaste.

This basic deglutitional cycle can be seen only in normal functional patterns with normal occlusions. During cinefluorographic examinations, many variations have been observed by the author.

In the first stage the food bolus is collected not only in front of the retracted tongue tip but also sometimes on the back of the protruded flat tongue. Such a variation is seen in the visceral type of swallowing and in Class III malocclusions in which the tongue position is habitually low. In the second stage the transfer of the food bolus can be performed by peristaltic-like movements of the tongue along its dorsum or by shovel-like movements of the tip of the tongue (Figure 7-30).

Cinefluorographic pictures also show that the basic position of the tongue is different in different malocclusions. The basic position is high or flat. In the flat posture the functional

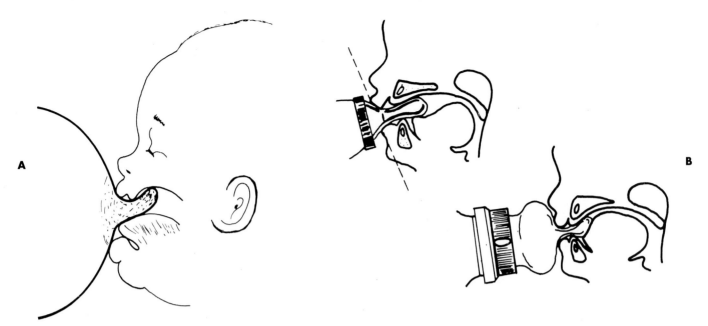

**Figure 7-32.** **A,** Normal position of the tongue in breastfeeding. **B,** Modified position of the tongue with various nipples in bottlefeeding. The lower jaw is usually forced open to a greater degree, increasing the buccinator pressure, particularly on the posterior segments of the maxillary arch. The normal plunger effect of the tongue in the natural nursing exercise is not possible.

pattern is more extensive because a longer path is necessary to achieve the palatolingual seal.

Of the four stages studied, the second stage shows the greatest intraindividual variations. Identical patterns in the second stage can be reproduced only if the examination is performed under the same conditions.

The type of therapy indicated depends on the problem. Usually the sequelae of abnormal swallowing patterns can be treated with oral screen types of appliances. The treatment of simple tongue thrust is causal and usually successful. In more complex tongue thrust problems (commonly referred to as *tongue thrust syndrome*), treatment can lead to improved morphologic relationships, but the atypical functional pattern often persists, necessitating prolonged retention.

Myofunctional therapy may be beneficial in helping to eliminate residual perioral muscle abnormalities. Lip exercises (e.g., holding a sheet of paper between the lips) can improve the seal (Fränkel) (Figure 7-31). These exercises are repeated several times a day. Children in school are asked to hold the lips together while in class; they can practice at home with small pieces of paper. Admittedly, influencing unconscious functions with conscious exercises is difficult.

Because of the diversity of tongue function during swallowing, tongue exercises are not recommended before or during treatment. During active treatment, tongue posture and function are controlled by the appliance. With an improved morphologic relationship the prognosis for establishing normal function is improved. If spaces are present, the tongue tends to find them and press into them; hence anterior space closure is advisable. If the visceral deglutitional pattern persists in the retention phase, supportive exercises can be prescribed to assist in establishing the somatic swallowing pattern. Success is questionable, however.

**Examination of the tongue.** Not only the function but also the posture, size, and shape of the tongue are significant. Such potential etiologic factors should be considered before any form of therapy is prescribed. Even in malocclusions with morphogenetic components the growth, posture, and function of the tongue are important. Flat, low-lying, anteriorly postured tongues are factors in the development of Class III malocclusions. Because similar tongue problems can occur within families, determining the precise roles of heredity and imitation is difficult; nevertheless, the role of tongue dysfunction is well documented in various types of malocclusions. The nursing mode can be vitally important. The nonphysiologic design of nipples on some baby bottles can force the tongue and cheeks to perform atypical and compensatory functions to extract the milk, eliciting adaptive responses of the associated dentoalveolar tissues that lead to characteristic malocclusions (Figure 7-32).

The work of Moyers (1964), Woodside (1984), and Linder-Aronson (1979) illustrates the possible role of nasal and pharyngeal blockage and compensatory tongue posture in malocclusions. Allergies also may be potent factors in the development of malocclusions. In the presence of excessive epipharyngeal lymphoid tissue, the tongue naturally postures forward to maintain an open airway. If the nasal passages are closed, mouth breathing with its attendant drop in mandibular and tongue posture must be practiced. The term *adenoidal facies* is often used in the literature to describe the appearance of this condition. Mouth breathing is only one possible adaptive response to respiratory difficulty.

Although the connection between speech disorders and malocclusions has not been determined exactly, the tongue does play a central role in phonation. Palatographic examinations by the author have shown compensations in articulation associated with severe malocclusions. Speech disorders also are observed in conjunction with less severe malocclusions. If good compensation is possible, the prognosis for functional therapy also is good.

*Tongue function.* The significance of tongue thrust and its role in the etiology of malocclusion have been evaluated by a number of authors. One school of thought (Ballard [1965], Tulley [1969], Milne [1970], Fränkel [1966], Subtelny and Sakuda [1964]) asserts that tongue thrust is the consequence of an abnormal morphologic relationship, an adaptive phenomenon. Other investigators (Andrew [1963], Hopkin [1967], McEwan [1959], Jann and Jann [1962], Baker, Pensa [1954], Kortsch, [1965]) consider the tongue a primary etiologic factor in malocclusion. Abnormal tongue posture and function can be primary factors as consequences of retained infantile deglutitional patterns or other abnormal oral habits, but they also may be strictly secondary or adaptive to unfavorable morphologic patterns. Functional appliance therapy is indicated if the role of tongue malfunction is considered a primary etiologic factor. However, if tongue function is adaptive to morphologic aberrations, its secondary or subordinate role does not take priority in treatment considerations. A correction of the basal dysplasia of skeletal parts often results in the establishment of normal tongue function. The object of the tongue function assessment is to make a differential diagnosis possible and determine the tongue's role in malocclusions.

*Tongue posture.* Some investigators hold that tongue posture is more important than tongue function (Mason, Proffit, 1974). The posture and shape can be flat or arched, protracted or retracted, narrowed and long, or spread laterally and shortened. Tongue posture is examined clinically with the mandible in postural rest position. Sagittal cephalometric registration of this relationship also is possible.

In a series of studies by the author (1963, 1975), tongue posture was compared at rest position and in habitual occlusion. From the basal tongue posture at rest position an assessment of three regions—root, dorsum, and tip—was made; this assessment disclosed the following:

- The root is usually flat in cases of mouth breathing and deep overbite caused by a small tongue; in all other cases, slight contact of the tongue usually occurs with the soft palate.
- In Class II, division 1 malocclusions and deep overbite the dorsum of the tongue is arched and high; in all other malocclusions a tendency exists for the tongue to flatten in accordance with the length of the interocclusal space.
- The tip of the tongue is usually retracted in Class II, division 1 malocclusions, but in other malocclusion categories a slight anterior gliding of the tongue tip occurs as the mandible moves into postural rest position.

Changes in the position of the tongue tip relate directly to mandibular malformations.

CEPHALOMETRIC EVALUATION OF TONGUE POSTURE. Clinical examination of the tongue and associated structures enables the clinician to make only a subjective evaluation of their status. Further complementary, exact, and reproducible study techniques are needed if important decisions such as those concerning glossectomy are to be made. Cephalometric analysis is exact, reproducible, and simple and can be employed in private practice. Use of a radiopaque coating (such as barium paste) on the tongue enhances visualization during palatography.

Assessment of tongue posture is made from a lateral cephalogram taken in postural rest and habitual occlusion.

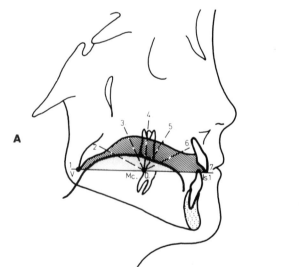
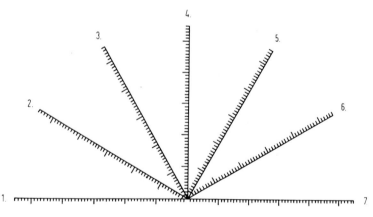

**A**    **B**

**Figure 7-33.** **A,** Means of assessing tongue position and morphology on cephalograms. **B,** Template for the assessment.

Exposure is adjusted to reveal the soft tissue. The size of the tongue can be measured on the occlusal film. A successful analysis depends on the proper use of correct mensurational data. A baseline, or reference line, for measurement should satisfy the following criteria:

1. The greatest possible area of the tongue should lie above the reference line because the two-dimensional radiograph does not show the anatomic borders and transverse dimensions of the tongue.
2. The baseline should be independent of variations in skeletal structures.
3. The relation of the baseline to the tongue should not change with changes in mandibular position.
4. The baseline should remain constant with changes in tongue position.
5. The anatomic and functional properties of the tongue should relate to the baseline.
6. The measurement should be easy to make and replicate.

Figure 7-33 shows the reference points and lines. *Is1* is the incisal margin of the lower incisors; *V,* the most caudal point on the shadow of the soft palate or its projection onto the reference line; *Mc,* the tip of the distobuccal cusp of the lower first molar. *Is1* and *Mc* are connected by a straight line extended to *V* to form the reference line. This line has the following features: (1) A relatively large part of the tongue as seen on the cephalogram normally lies superior to it, (2) skeletal relationships do not affect it, and (3) changes in tongue position do not influence it.

After the line is constructed, it is bisected between *Is1* and *V.* This point is called *O,* and a perpendicular is constructed from it to the palatal contour. A transparent template has been developed to help the clinician make the necessary measurements. The baseline of the template coincides with the constructed reference line, and the vertical line intersects the reference line at *O.* From point *O,* where three lines now meet, four more lines are constructed (as shown by the illus-

tration of the template). These seven lines form six angles of 30 degrees each. The lines can be marked in millimeters. Placing the template over the constructed lines permits the reading of the exact measurements.

Assessment of tongue size from occlusal cephalograms requires measurement of the distance between the superior tongue surface and the roof of the mouth. This is done along the seven constructed lines. These measurements indicate the relative size of the tongue. Only if the entire oral cavity is filled can a diagnosis of macroglossia be made. This diagnosis also must be supported by clinical evidence.

Measurements made from tongue templates can be expressed by graphs (Figure 7-34). The palatal vault may be represented by a horizontal line and the seven single measurements by a curve. The distances between the reference line and the seven points on the constructed curve provide a graph of the relationships of the superior surface of the tongue to the palatal vault and the soft palate to the tip of the uvula.

The posture of the tongue can be similarly evaluated by measurements taken on postural rest–position lateral cephalograms. To assess the posture and mobility of the tongue, the clinician can calculate the differences between rest and occlusal positions. The occlusal position is taken as zero, with changes in rest position expressed as positive or negative figures (positive if the tongue is higher in rest position, negative if it is lower).

Changes in tongue position are reflected mainly by the position of the tip of the tongue. The positions of the other parts of the tongue also are subject to change, although these changes are not relative to the mandible but occur in conjunction with it. Changes in tongue tip position relate closely to the different types of malocclusions. In Class II the tip of the tongue is more retruded in the rest position; in Class III, it lies further forward in rest position (Figure 7-35). Changes in tongue tip position presumably relate to mandibular malformation tendencies.

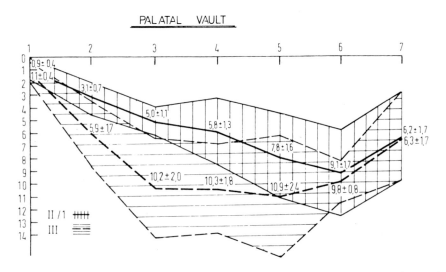

**Figure 7-34.** Average tongue position values with standard deviations in Class II and III malocclusions. A lower tongue position is common in Class III cases.

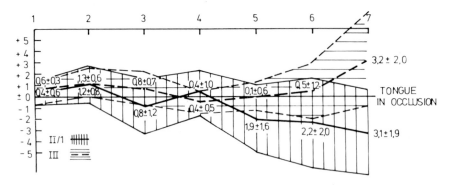

**Figure 7-35.** Average tongue mobility values with standard deviations in Class II and III malocclusions.

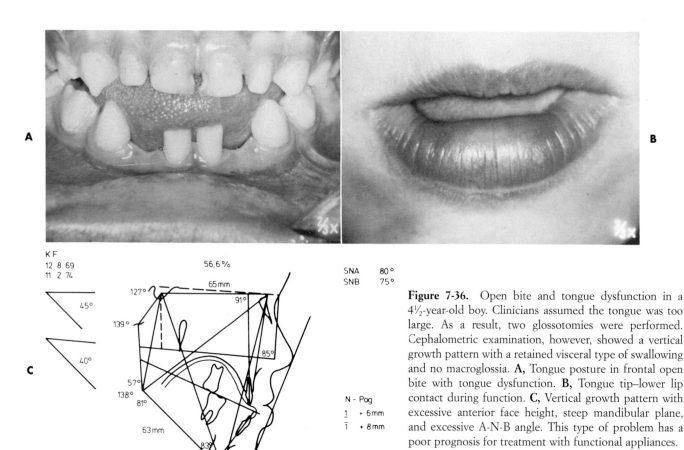

**Figure 7-36.** Open bite and tongue dysfunction in a 4½-year-old boy. Clinicians assumed the tongue was too large. As a result, two glossotomies were performed. Cephalometric examination, however, showed a vertical growth pattern with a retained visceral type of swallowing and no macroglossia. **A,** Tongue posture in frontal open bite with tongue dysfunction. **B,** Tongue tip–lower lip contact during function. **C,** Vertical growth pattern with excessive anterior face height, steep mandibular plane, and excessive A-N-B angle. This type of problem has a poor prognosis for treatment with functional appliances.

*Tongue size.* The size and shape of the tongue have many variations—bulky and short, narrow and long, and wide and long. Numerous clinical methods may be used to assess tongue size. The most common is to check whether the patient can touch the chin with the tongue tip. A positive result from this test is considered an indication of macroglossia. Glossectomies have actually been recommended on the basis of such overly simplistic tests. Both macroglossia (enlarged tongue) and microglossia (small tongue) correlate with certain

symptoms in the dentoalveolar area and the skeletal pattern that should be considered in evaluation.

In macroglossia the oral cavity is filled by the tongue mass. The mouth does not seem to have enough space, and the epipharynx is narrow. Indentations are evident on the tongue periphery, and spaces exist between the incisors, which are procumbent. The tongue is protruded, and usually an open bite is evident. True macroglossia often occurs with certain pathologic conditions such as myxedema, cretinism, Down syndrome, and hypophyseal gigantism. However, in children a definitive diagnosis of macroglossia cannot be made without cephalometric analysis. A skeletal open bite with tongue thrust can be mistaken clinically for a case of macroglossia. The 4½-year-old boy in Figure 7-36 provides an example of the problems that can be encountered in diagnosis. He had a Class III relationship, vertical growth pattern, and open bite. A glossectomy had been performed at 2 years and another at 4 years. Despite this, his tongue thrust and open bite persisted.

The obvious characteristic of microglossia, or hypoglossia, is a very small tongue. The protruded tongue tip reaches the lower incisors at best, and the floor of the mouth is elevated and visible on each side of the diminutive tongue. The dental arch reflects the small tongue size and is collapsed and reduced, with extreme crowding in the premolar area. A severe Class II relationship is usually evident. Third molars are usually impacted at the angle of the jaw. In cases of microglossia or aglossia (congenital absence of the tongue), severe functional disturbances also are present. The centrifugal force of the tongue is minimal or absent (Figure 7-37). These cases provide excellent examples of the dynamics of muscle balance and imbalance. The localized effects are extreme. In some cases, teeth from the posterior segments are tipped so markedly to the lingual that they touch each other in the midline. Despite this deformity and subsequent dysfunction, all evidence points to a relatively localized insult, with the effects limited mostly to the dentoalveolar area. The 35-year-old man in Figure 7-38 had a severe malocclusion associated with hypoglossia. Cephalometric analysis revealed a horizontal growth pattern, small gonial angle, and normally developed maxillary and mandibular bases. The bizarre dentoalveolar manifestations are evident from the anteriorly malposed and labially tipped upper incisors and the extreme repositioning and lingual tipping of the lower incisors.

The implications of this circumstance are of interest for not only determining etiology but also assessing the potential role of functional appliances that can screen, shield, or relieve the teeth and investing tissues from functional forces. Pathologic conditions teach much about physiology. In the case of hypoglossia the functional abnormality primarily affects the dentoalveolar region, not the basal skeletal structure. Oral and vestibular screens incorporated into functional appliances have similar capabilities. Fixed appliances also have primarily localized effects, which is the reason locating the malocclusion and correcting the sagittal dysplasia are so important before applying even simple inhibitory therapy.

*Tongue dysfunction.* The most common tongue dysfunctions involve selective outer pressure (pressing) and tongue biting. Tongue thrusting can be anterior, posterior, or combined. The consequences of the localization of aberrant pressures depend on the area of applied pressure:

1. Anterior open bite results from anterior tongue thrust and posture.
2. Lateral open bite and deep overbite result from lateral tongue thrust or postural spread that causes infraclusion of the posterior teeth.
3. Edge-to-edge incisal and cuspal relationships of the

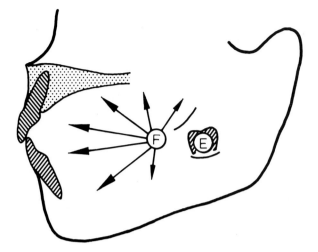

**Figure 7-37.** The centrifugal force of the tongue *(F)* and eruption potential of the teeth *(E)* are important natural forces that can be influenced and guided with functional appliances.

teeth in the buccal segments may indicate a combined thrust and anterior and posterior open bite occurring from a phenomenon called a *complex tongue thrust.*

The recognition of areas of excessive tongue pressure is important for not only determining the etiology of the associated malocclusion but also providing information needed to construct the screening or functional appliance. Depending on the dentoalveolar and skeletal relationships, abnormal tongue function and posture can be primary etiologic factors in malocclusion; these abnormal functions and postures include anteriorly relocated flat tongues and secondary adaptive and compensatory functions and positions resulting from skeletal dysplasia. In both cases the tongue dysfunction provides the anterior seal of the oral cavity.

Dentoalveolar anterior and posterior open-bite problems are usually attributable to abnormal tongue posture and function and usually respond successfully to functional appliance intervention in the mixed dentition. This also is true for cases of deep overbite in which lateral tongue spread during function and posture leads to infraclusion of the posterior teeth. The space is maintained by invagination of the peripheral portions of the tongue into the interocclusal space while the mandible is in the postural rest position. In such cases, a large freeway space is evident, and the deep overbite is functional.

A second type of overbite (called a *functional pseudo-overbite*) is caused by supraclusion of the incisors. In this case a small freeway space is apparent. Functional appliance intervention, particularly in the presence of developmental disturbances, is not indicated. Fixed appliances and orthopedic guidance are more likely to correct the problem. Surgery is the ultimate treatment.

In skeletal open-bite problems a genetically determined vertical growth pattern is present and often associated with marked antegonial notching. This type of case does not offer a favorable prognosis for orthodontic therapy. The inclination of the maxillary base also should be considered in the evalua-

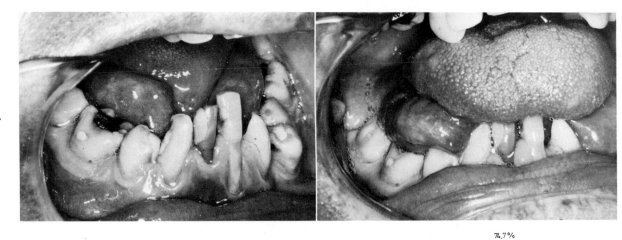

A

B

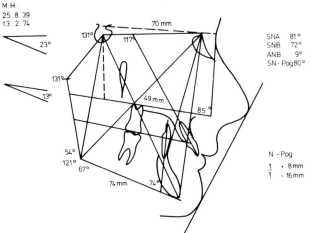

C

**Figure 7-38.** Hypoglossia in a 35-year-old man. **A,** The tongue is habitually in the floor of the mouth. **B,** Even when maximally protracted, the tongue barely clears the lingually tipped lower incisors. **C,** Dentoalveolar localization of the malocclusion in congenital hypoglossia. The tongue and adaptive lower lip malfunction combine to retract the lower incisors and tip the maxillary incisors labially.

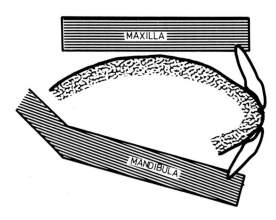

**Figure 7-39.** In horizontal growth patterns a tongue thrust habit can cause procumbency of both upper and lower incisors.

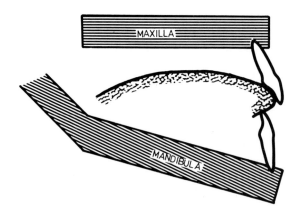

**Figure 7-40.** In vertical growth patterns a tongue thrust habit is more likely to cause labial tipping of the upper incisors and lingual tipping of the lower incisors.

tion of open-bite problems. An up and forward inclination enhances the open-bite relationship, whereas a maxillary base that is tipped down anteriorly compensates for it. The inclination of the maxillary base can be influenced both by functional factors and habits (good and bad).

The consequences of tongue posture and function abnormalities in the dentoalveolar region also depend on the skele-

tal pattern. In a horizontal growth pattern the forward tongue thrust or posture can result in bimaxillary protrusion. As the tongue presses against the lingual surfaces of both upper and lower incisors simultaneously, spacing in the incisor segments often occurs (Figure 7-39). In a vertical growth pattern the tongue thrust can open the bite, and the lower incisors may be tipped lingually. During the abnormal functional and pos-

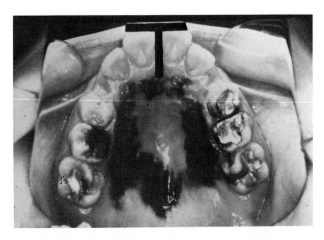

**Figure 7-41.** Palatogram with measurement of the distance between the tongue tip and incisal edges.

tural forward positioning, the tip of the tongue lies between the dental arches in contact with the lower lip, which the patient constantly sucks. Thus the incisors are tipped lingually (Figure 7-40).

PALATOGRAPHIC EXAMINATION OF TONGUE DYSFUNCTION. A complementary evaluation of tongue function is possible using palatography, a technique that permits tongue function to be observed during swallowing and speaking and allows the influence of various functional orthodontic appliances on the tongue to be evaluated. Originally, palatographic procedures were used only for assessment of speech disorders. Palatography may be applied in both direct and indirect methods.

In the direct method first described by Oakley Coles in 1872, gum arabic and flour were mixed and painted on the tongue. After selected functional exercises had been performed, the contacts on the palate and teeth were transferred onto the cast of the upper jaw with red ink.

The indirect palatographic technique was first used by Kingsley (1880). He prepared an upper plate of black india rubber and covered the tongue with a mixture of chalk and alcohol. The contacts seen on the palatal rubber plate were then transferred onto the cast as in the direct method.

The current direct method entails covering the superior surface of the tongue with a precise impression material (e.g., Imprex). A thin, even layer is applied to the tongue with a spatula. After functional exercises an instant (Polaroid) print is made of the palatal region with the help of a surface mirror. Evaluation of the palatogram is possible by direct measurements on the picture (Figure 7-41).

Speech assessment also is desirable for orthodontic diagnostics. The tongue, pharynx, velum, palate, and teeth play central roles in phonation. The movements of the tongue during speech are sophisticated and depend on local conditions. In malocclusions with malposed teeth, malposition of the tongue also may occur, impairing normal speech. Usually the tongue with its inherent flexibility is able to compensate for atypical morphologic relationships; this compensatory potential is an important diagnostic clue for the clinician es-

tablishing a treatment plan and prognosis for functional appliance therapy. The ability to compensate and adapt can be assessed from the palatographic record (Figure 7-42).

***Therapeutic requirements for various tongue dysfunctions.*** The variety of aberrations of tongue function requires a functional therapeutic approach tailored to the problem. The skeletal pattern is a conditioning factor. If the abnormal tongue function is the primary etiologic basis of the malocclusion, causal therapy can be instituted to eliminate it and restore the integrity of the teeth and investing tissues by means of functional appliances. This approach is likely to succeed in both anterior and lateral open-bite problems if the growth direction is horizontal or at least average. Other malocclusions have additional causative elements, and still others consisting of excessive overjet and sagittal discrepancies require control of not only these problems but also the tongue abnormality. In other words, more than one muscle or muscle group may be involved in the enhancement of a morphologic aberration; treatment planning should take this reality into account.

**Thumb- and finger-sucking effects.** One specific kind of malocclusion, which also is a consequence of abnormal function, requires combined treatment with active mechanical and functional appliances in the mixed dentition (Figure 7-43). Finger sucking can cause an open bite with simultaneous narrowing of the maxillary arch. Adaptive tongue function aggravates and prolongs the malocclusion. The patient often compensates for bilateral narrowing with a lateral shift to one side to gain maximal chewing surface contact. This functional type of crossbite, or convenience crossbite, is not skeletal in the initial stages but adaptive. Before functional appliance therapy begins, the maxillary arch should be expanded with a split palate jackscrew type of active plate. Sometimes a small wire crib can be incorporated to block the tongue in the crossbite area or at least create an exteroceptive engram that initiates tongue retraction. In some severe dysfunction cases, treatment may begin with the oral screen, and the active plate may be used later. This often occurs in the deciduous dentition.

In a skeletal open bite that progressively worsens because of a severe vertical growth pattern, successful causal therapy is not possible. Because tongue dysfunction in these cases is secondary to the primary morphogenetic basis, therapeutic demands are more rigorous. Fixed appliances, often with tooth sacrifice, offer a more effective treatment approach. In extreme cases, orthognathic surgery is the only viable alternative; it is performed after completion of growth. In the early mixed dentition, however, a partial improvement may be achieved by eliminating some of the dysfunction; this does not materially alter the growth pattern, which will require other therapeutic methods later (Figures 7-44 and 7-45). Nevertheless, a vertical growth pattern can be influenced by strong orthopedic forces (with or without repelling magnets) or specially designed activators. Heavy, vertical-pull, fixed orthopedics can alter the direction of mandibular growth while restricting buccal segment eruption, whereas activators can affect the inclination of the maxillary base. An analysis of the

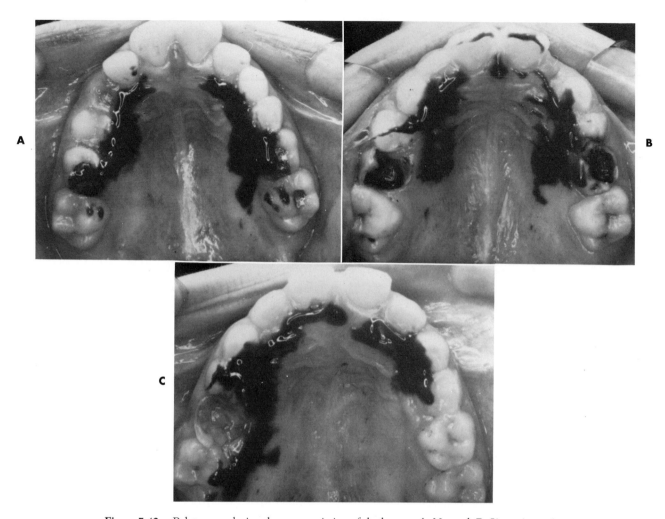

**Figure 7-42.**    Palatogram during the pronunciation of the letter *s*. **A,** Normal. **B,** Sigmatismus interdentalis (abnormal). **C,** Sigmatismus lateroflexus (abnormal).

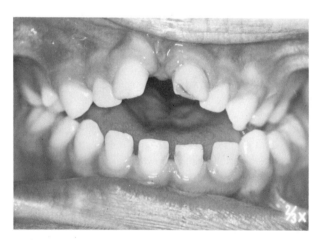

**Figure 7-43.**    Open-bite malocclusion with crossbite, a consequence of abnormal tongue posture and function. Frequently a prolonged finger-sucking habit is the instigating factor.

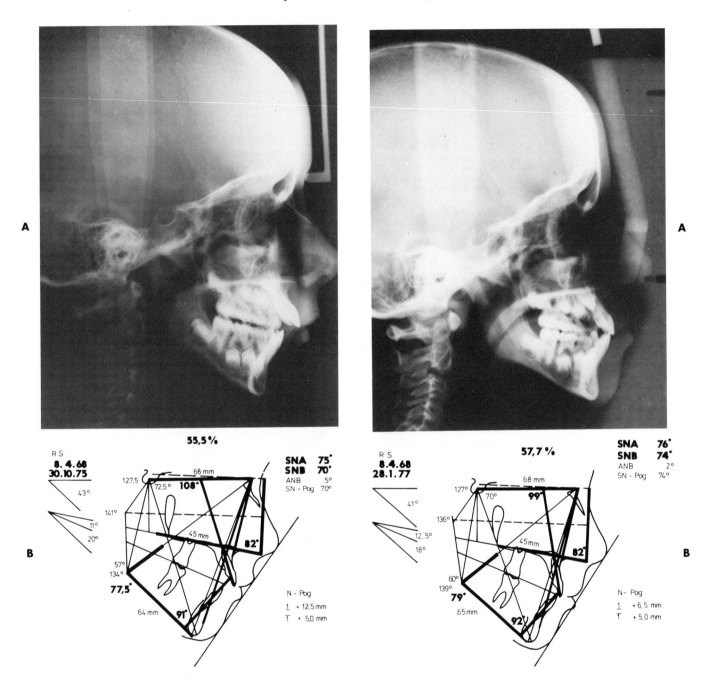

**Figure 7-44.** Open-bite malocclusion and vertical growth pattern in a 7½-year-old girl. **A,** Lateral cephalogram. **B,** Cephalometric tracing showing a somewhat favorable posterior-to-anterior face height ratio. In most cases of this type, supraeruption of posterior segments and a minimal or nonexistent freeway space are evident.

**Figure 7-45.** Improvement of the open-bite malocclusion in the same patient as in Figure 7-44 after elimination of the dysfunction. This result occurred despite the persistence of the vertical growth pattern. **A,** Lateral cephalogram. **B,** Cephalometric tracing. Significant dental compensation has been achieved.

growth pattern and a functional study also are needed to determine the therapeutic approach most likely to be successful.

**Examination of the lips.** The lips must be carefully examined as part of the functional assessment. External balancing muscle factors are as important as internal factors. The configuration of the lips should be studied in the relaxed position.

If the lips are trained, any patient can achieve a lip seal (at least under conscious effort); the clinician, however, wishes to know the lip relationship that commonly occurs:

1. If only a slight contact or a very small gap is evident between the upper and lower lips, the lips are competent.
2. If a wide gap is present or the lips (primarily the upper

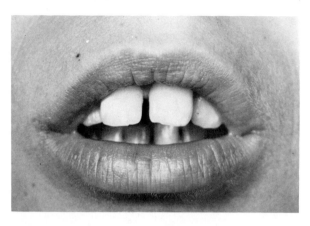

**Figure 7-46.** Incompetent lip posture associated with mouth breathing, excessive epipharyngeal lymphoid tissue, and other conditions.

lip) are too short, the lips can be considered incompetent. Improvement with orthodontic treatment and exercises is possible only in the early stages (Figure 7-46).

3. If the lips seem normally developed but the upper incisors are labially tipped, making closure difficult, Ballard (1965) and Tulley (1956) call the resulting phenomenon *potential lip incompetency*. The incisal margins interpose between the lips and rest on the lower lip, preventing the normal lip seal. The lower lip trap then enhances the already excessive overjet, tipping the incisors further forward into a dangerous zone in which any trauma may result in breakage. Hypermobility is possible in the incisor area as the lower lip pushes the upper incisors labially while often reclining and crowding the lower incisors. Early treatment of these problems is an important preventive measure (Figure 7-47).

4. If the lower lip is hypertrophic, everted, and redundant (i.e., with an excess of tissue), little can be done to improve the situation by orthodontic therapy.

Various methods are available for evaluating the lip profile. Photographs and lateral cephalograms can be used effectively.

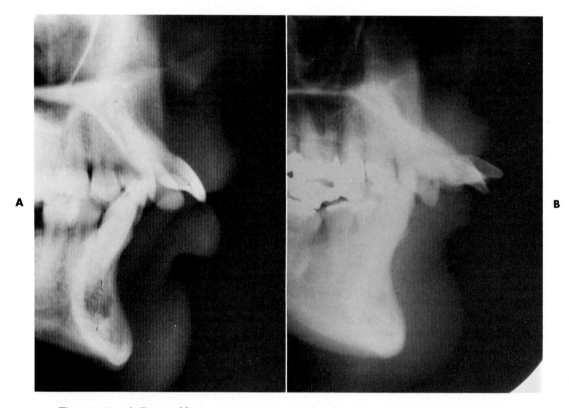

**Figure 7-47.** **A,** Potential lip incompetency associated with excessive overjet. The lower lip cushions to the lingual of the maxillary incisors, whereas the upper lip is short and hypofunctional. In trying to effect a lip seal during the deglutitional cycle, the mentalis muscle is hyperactive. **B,** Severe lip incompetency leading to mobility of the upper incisors. The strong hyperactive mentalis muscle is capable of forcing the upper incisors labially against the hypotonic upper lip. Constant jiggling of these teeth can cause periodontal involvement and ultimate bone loss.

*Schwarz analysis (lateral cephalogram).* Schwarz (1961) devised a quite useful analysis. For this method, three reference lines are constructed (Figure 7-48):

H line—corresponding to the Frankfort horizontal
Pn line—perpendicular to the H line at soft tissue nasion
Po line—perpendicular from orbitale to the H line

Between the two constructed perpendicular lines is the area Schwarz terms the *gnathic profile field (GPF)*. In normal proportions the upper lip touches the Po line, and the lower lip lies one third the width of the GPF posterior to it. The oblique tangential (T) line is constructed by joining subnasale (at the junction of the upper lip and nose) to soft tissue pogonion, the most anterior point on the profile curvature of the symphysis. In the ideal case the T line bisects the vermilion border of the upper lip and touches the anterior vermilion curvature of the lower lip.

*Ricketts lip analysis.* The reference line used by Ricketts (1958) is similar to the Schwarz T line but is drawn from the tip of the nose to soft tissue pogonion. In a normal relationship the upper lip is 2 to 3 mm and the lower lip 1 to 2 mm behind this line (Figure 7-49).

*Steiner lip analysis.* The upper reference point for the Steiner analysis is at the center of the S-shaped curve between the tip of the nose and subnasale. Soft tissue pogonion is the lower terminus. If the lips lie behind the reference line, they are too flat; if they lie in front, they are too prominent (Figure 7-50).

*Holdaway lip analysis.* The Holdaway lip analysis is a quantitative assessment of lip configuration. Holdaway (1983) measures the angle between the tangent to the upper lip from soft tissue pogonion and the N-B line, which he calls the *H an-*

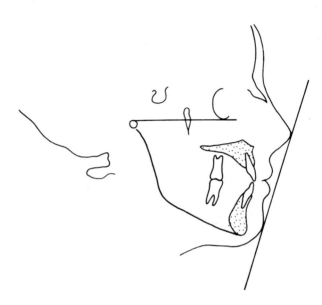

**Figure 7-49.** Reference line used by Ricketts for assessing the soft tissue profile.

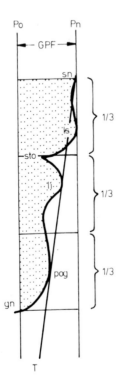

**Figure 7-48.** The gnathic profile field *(GPF)* permits assessment of the profile from the lateral cephalogram. *Po,* Perpendicular to the Frankfort plane at orbitale; *Pn,* perpendicular to the Frankfort plane at nasion; *sn,* subnasale; *ls,* labium superius oris; *li,* labium inferius oris; *sto,* stomion; *pog,* pogonion; *gn,* gnathion.

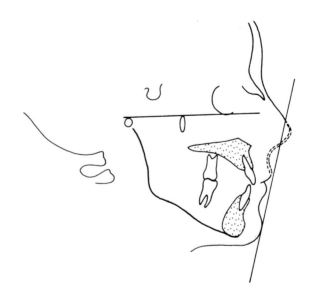

**Figure 7-50.** The Steiner lip analysis.

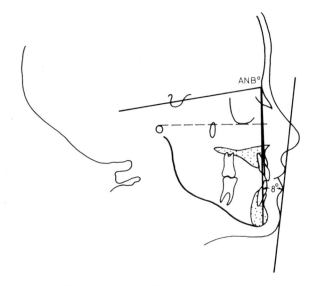

**Figure 7-51.** The Holdaway lip analysis.

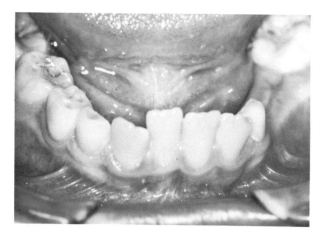

**Figure 7-52.** Crowding of the lower incisors caused by lip sucking or a confirmed hyperactive mentalis muscle.

*gle* (Figure 7-51). With an A-N-B angle of 1 to 3 degrees the H angle should be 7 to 8 degrees. Changes in the A-N-B angle reflect changes in the ideal H angle. Holdaway defines the ideal profile as follows:

A-N-B angle of 2 degrees, H angle of 7 to 8 degrees

Lower lip touching the soft tissue line that connects pogonion and the upper lip extended to S-N

Relative proportions of nose and upper lip balanced (soft tissue line bisecting subnasal S curve)

Tip of nose 9 mm anterior to the soft tissue line (normal at age 13 years)

No lip tension on closure

The upper lip is tense if the difference between the thickness of the soft tissue (A to S-N) and the thickness of the vermilion border of the upper lip is greater than ±1 mm (Holdaway, 1983). After the elimination of lip tension, each 3-mm retraction of the incisors results in a 1.0-mm retraction of the upper lip.

The length and thickness of the lips not only are age dependent but also correlate with various malocclusions. The following chart is based on examination of 12-year-old children:

| Parameter | Class I | Class II | Class III |
|---|---|---|---|
| Length of upper lip (mm) | 23.0 | 22.0 | 20.9 |
| Length of lower lip (mm) | 37.0 | 36.5 | 36.0 |
| Thickness of upper lip (mm) | 11.5 | 10.8 | 12.4 |
| Thickness of lower lip (mm) | 12.5 | 14.0 | 11.8 |

Differences among the various types of malocclusions disappear during orthodontic treatment.

***Dysfunction of the lips.*** A number of lip muscle abnormalities have been identified and characterized. The most common is sucking or biting of the lower lip, known as *mentalis habit* because of the crinkling "golf ball" ap-

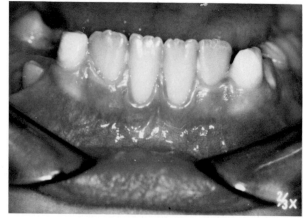
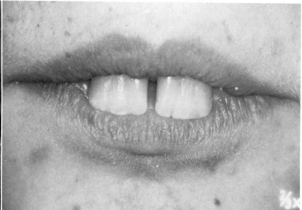

**Figure 7-53.** **A,** Retraction of the gingival margin. Dehiscence of this type is frequently seen with abnormal perioral muscle function (e.g., perverted lip habit), **B.**

pearance of the symphyseal tissue with excessive mentalis activity. In this type of dysfunction, contact usually occurs between the tongue and lower lip and can be observed during swallowing. Consequences of the combined muscle abnormality include the opening of the bite anteriorly and the lingual tipping of the lower incisors with crowding and labial malpositioning of the upper incisors. The pernicious lip trap thus works against the integrity of both the upper and lower dentitions (Figure 7-52). Retraction or dehiscence of the labial gingival tissue overlying the lower incisors can occur (Figure 7-53).

Upper-lip biting is a habit frequently seen in schoolchildren. It is a stress-strain relief syndrome. Tongue function can be normal, with the hyperkinetic behavioral activity and abnormal lip habit as the main pathologic factors. Of course, an inherent morphogenetic pattern type of Class II malocclusion can provide the overjet that requires lip compensation, which in turn exacerbates the original overjet.

As with tongue habits, lip sucking can be either a primary or a secondary factor. In cases in which it is the primary causative factor, overjet with labial tipping of the upper and lingual tipping of the lower incisors is evident, and only a slight skeletal sagittal discrepancy occurs. The lip habit enhances the original slight-to-moderate overjet. In cases in which it plays only a secondary role the original overjet is caused by a significant sagittal discrepancy, usually with mandibular underdevelopment. The inclination of the incisors can be normal. The lower lip cushions the gap between the upper and lower incisors, primarily as an adaptation to the morphologic malrelations. Lip activity may not be as intensive but may rather be more adaptive. Functional therapy is successful only in cases of primary dysfunction. In the case of secondary dysfunction, functional therapy is subservient to other orthopedic, orthodontic, or surgical methods.

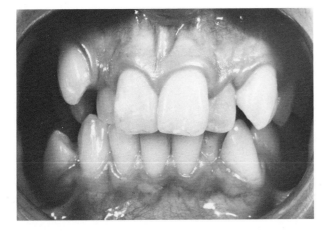

**Figure 7-54.** Crowding associated with habitual mouth breathing. This may not be a primary etiologic factor, however. Other concerns such as morphogenetic patterns and premature loss may be more important.

**Respiration.** The mode of respiration is of interest for several reasons:

1. Mouth breathing and disturbed nasal breathing can be considered etiologic factors or at least predisposing causes for some malocclusion symptoms. In 1968, Ricketts described the "respiratory obstruction syndrome," consisting of the following symptoms: visceral-type swallowing, predisposition to open bite, unilateral or bilateral crossbite, and slight deflection of the head. In examinations by the author a significantly high frequency of the following symptoms has been observed in patients with disturbed nasal respiration: Class II, division 1 malocclusion; narrowness of the upper arch; crowding of the upper and lower arches; and vertical growth patterns (Figure 7-54). The research of Lowe (1995) is particularly informative here.

2. If the patient has disturbed nasal breathing, treatment with some appliances is impossible. If the tonsils and adenoids are enlarged, with a compensatory anterior tongue posture, the patient cannot tolerate a bulky acrylic appliance in the oral cavity. Other appliances are available for use in cases of habitual mouth breathing (e.g., Clark twin block, Hamilton expansion activator) (Figure 7-55).

3. In mouth-breathing patients the lip seal is usually inadequate. The tongue has a low posture and disturbed function. If this condition persists after treatment, the result is not likely to be stable, with relapse as a consequence. If at all possible, establishing normal nasal respiration before orthodontic therapy is most advantageous. Unfortunately, in some patients with allergies or deviated nasal septums, this is not possible during the growth period.

**Conclusion.** Assessment of disturbed nasal function is not always easy. The case history data can give some idea of the frequency of ear, nose, and throat (ENT) diseases and mode of sleeping, habits, and allergies. The clinical examination should determine whether the lips are competent. Lip incompetency does not necessarily indicate mouth breathing but suggests the need for further investigation. Clinical examination with a mirror or cotton swab is not very reliable. However, the patient can be instructed to hold a sheet of cardboard between the lips or some water in the mouth to assess whether the patient can breathe through the nose without difficulty.

The presence and size of the adenoids and tonsils also can be estimated on lateral head films. Results of these films can indicate whether the nasopharyngeal passage is free or partially or totally obstructed. The work of Linder-Aronson (1992) and Woodside and Lowe (1995) shows the potential effects of epipharyngeal lymphoid tissue blockage and resultant tongue posture compensation and mouth breathing. Various ways of assessing the size of adenoids and tonsils are available. An arbitrary scale of small, medium, or large can be used in both the clinical examination and the lateral cephalogram (Figure 7-56). Spontaneous regression of epipharyngeal lymphoid tissue occurs with

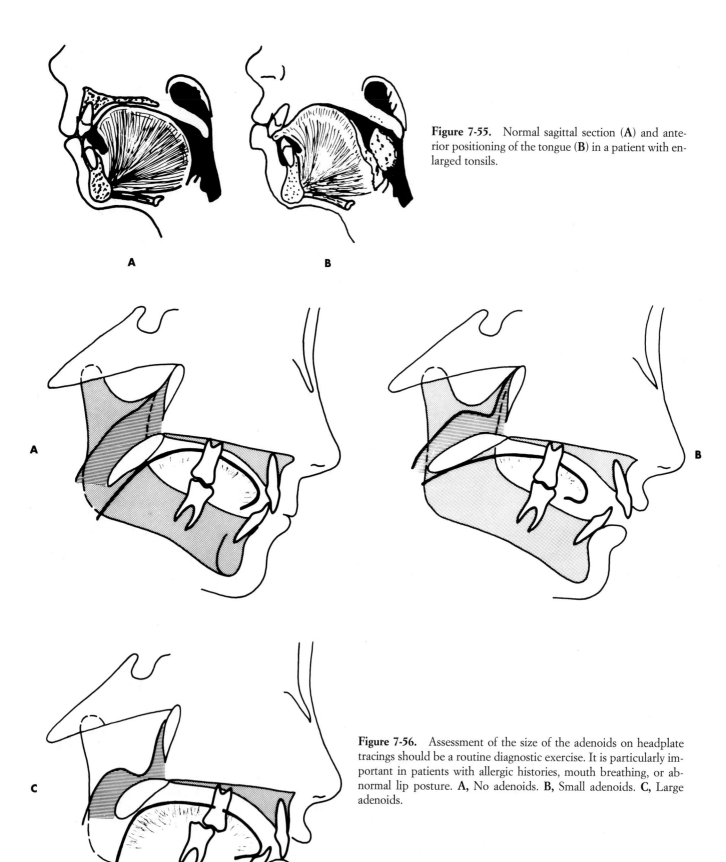

**Figure 7-55.** Normal sagittal section (**A**) and anterior positioning of the tongue (**B**) in a patient with enlarged tonsils.

**Figure 7-56.** Assessment of the size of the adenoids on headplate tracings should be a routine diagnostic exercise. It is particularly important in patients with allergic histories, mouth breathing, or abnormal lip posture. **A,** No adenoids. **B,** Small adenoids. **C,** Large adenoids.

development. At 10 years of age, 180% of the lymphoid tissue is present that will still be present at 18 years of age. Obstructive adenoids usually regress without surgical intervention.

Nasal respiratory resistance also can be measured using an indirect plethysmographic approach. In habitual mouth breathing, respiratory resistance is low, whereas in structurally conditioned mouth breathing, it is high. Holding a small piece of paper under the patient's nose while the patient is breathing also helps determine whether respiratory air is escaping from the nostrils. If the paper does not flutter, some obstruction is likely. Visualization of the nasal turbinates through the nostrils also is helpful. The diagnosis of mouth breathing is probably best made by the otolaryngologist, however, and a consultation is recommended if the problem is suspected.

The scope of functional therapy with respiratory problems can be summarized as follows:

1. In habitual mouth breathing with small respiratory resistance, functional therapy is indicated. Exercises can be prescribed. Holding a sheet of cardboard between the lips is one satisfactory means of enhancing lip seal.
2. If structural problems occur with excessive adenoid tissue and allergies, otolaryngologic consultation and possible treatment should be sought. If it is successful, orthodontic treatment can then begin.
3. If the structural conditions are unalterable, functional appliance therapy cannot be instituted. In such cases, only active fixed-appliance mechanotherapy is likely to produce the changes desired. Even then, the stability of the results is questionable unless autonomous improvement occurs.

## Significance of Functional Analysis in Treatment Planning with Removable Appliances

The importance of functional analysis in the examination of various types of malocclusions is universally recognized. Any treatment plan must begin with a sound functional analysis.

**Class II malocclusions.** The postural rest position of the mandible can be anterior or posterior to the habitual occlusal position. More frequently, it is anterior. If a large freeway space, mandibular overclosure, and deep bite are present, the prognosis with functional appliances is usually good.

Early TMD symptoms can frequently be seen in Class II malocclusions, especially in cases of deep overbite, horizontal growth pattern, and abnormal perioral muscle function. The dysfunction of the tongue should be evaluated, as should the lips, mentalis muscle, facial musculature, and suprahyoid and infrahyoid musculature; localized effects on dentoalveolar growth should be noted. Respiratory disturbances have potential interfering roles in the accomplishment of a normal growth and developmental pattern and should be eliminated (if possible) before orthodontic treatment.

**Class III malocclusions.** The postural rest position of the mandible can be anterior or posterior to the habitual occlusal position. If it is anterior, a true Class III malocclusion has oc-

curred. If it is posterior, a tooth guidance problem or forced bite (pseudo–Class III) is present; the lower incisors move past their maxillary counterparts in the closing maneuver, with the lingual surfaces of the lower incisors engaging the maxillary incisal margins as the posterior teeth are brought into contact. The path of closure and condylar position in the fossa should be examined carefully. The skeletal pattern also must be evaluated to differentiate between true and pseudo–Class III malocclusions.

Tongue posture and function should be assessed both clinically and cephalometrically. Functional appliance therapy is particularly indicated in pseudo–Class III malocclusions with normal tongue posture. A true skeletal Class III malocclusion does not offer a favorable prognosis for functional appliance therapy. Respiratory conditions also must be studied in treatment planning for this malocclusion category. Breathing disturbances and enlarged tonsils and adenoids seem to cause compensatory forward positioning of the tongue, with a flattening of the dorsum as unconscious reflex action keeps the airway open. The maxillary arch is thus unopposed by normal tongue support and can collapse both transversely and sagittally because of the effective low tongue posture.

**Open-bite malocclusions.** Open-bite malocclusions can be primary or secondary and, depending on the location of the dysfunction, anterior or posterior. In primary dysfunctions with abnormal muscle action as a major etiologic factor, the growth pattern is usually average or horizontal. If the growth pattern is mostly vertical, the dysfunction may be more secondary or adaptive. Functional appliances are likely to be successful in cases with primary dysfunction and at least an average growth pattern.

## Gnathologic Considerations

A gnathologic instrumental registration may be incorporated into the functional analysis in the permanent dentition, after active treatment, or in the assessment of TMD. In the mixed dentition (transitional period), with autonomous changes in sagittal and occlusal plane inclination, gnathologic assessment is not appropriate. Functional abnormalities may be determined by observing the path of closure, initial or premature contact, and any deflections occurring in the postural rest–to–habitual occlusal position stroke. The amount of interocclusal clearance also is a diagnostic criterion.

A differentiation between tooth-guided slides and skeletal problems that create the same habitual occlusions is necessary both before and after treatment. In dentoalveolar slides the cause is premature contact or abnormal intercuspation. Orthodontic tooth movement and equilibration can correct the problem. In skeletal slides a compensation may exist because of the mandible's sliding into a forced position; often an excessive overjet is compensated by an anterior sliding or posturing of the mandible, creating the so-called dual bite. This kind of problem requires a major assault on the multisystem involvement with orthopedic therapy, possible selective extraction, growth guidance over a fairly long time, and possibly surgical correction later.

The goal is the same for both functional and fixed multiattachment orthodontic appliances—a functional and stable occlusion. The same criteria are used in evaluating the result. The objectives for a normal Class I occlusion concerning position, inclination, and angulation of teeth are well expressed by Andrews (1972) in his "six keys of occlusion." Because these objectives are not always achievable with removable appliances alone, a combination approach may be necessary to achieve as many as possible. Bodily movement, changes in axial inclination and torque, correction of rotations, closure of spaces in a parallel fashion, and control of extraction sites usually require the precise control that only multiattachment fixed mechanotherapy can provide.

## APPLYING THE PRINCIPLES OF OCCLUSION

In treatment with removable appliances the principles of optimal static and functional occlusion should be considered as much as possible:

1. Eruption and axial inclination (particularly of the ca-

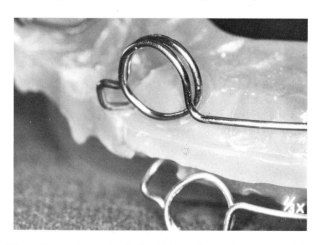

**Figure 7-57.** Loops on the labial bow of an activator control the axial inclination of the canines.

nine teeth) can be controlled. The erupting teeth can be guided into correct position by grinding and reshaping the acrylic guiding planes of the appliance. Control of the axial inclination of the canines is possible to a large degree through the use of loops on the labial bows of some activators concurrent with recontouring of the acrylic (Figure 7-57). By means of active plates (especially expansion plates) the axial inclination is subjected to certain forces to prevent buccal tipping of the crowns (Figure 7-58).

2. To control the lingual crown torque of teeth in the buccal segments, the clinician must consider the transverse curve of Wilson during therapy. In the course of expansion therapy a buccal crown torque or tipping can be created, with elongation of the canines and resultant traumatic occlusal interference and instability. This undesirable phenomenon can occur with both Haas' rapid palatal expansion technique and increases achieved by the jackscrew type of active expansion plate. Slow expansion during the mixed dentition is less likely to produce this iatrogenic reaction. However, the limitations of expansion therapy should be recognized at the proper time and other means employed if necessary to attain the treatment goal; therapy should be terminated if optimal bodily expansion and maintenance of normal buccolingual cusp contact with opposing teeth have been attained.

3. The curve of Spee can be concave, flat, or convex (Figure 7-59). Leveling it if it is abnormal is possible during the mixed dentition because eruption of the posterior teeth can be stimulated and guided by the functional appliance. After the eruption of the permanent

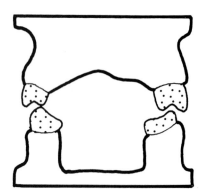

**Figure 7-58.** Overexpanded upper dental arch with disturbed occlusion.

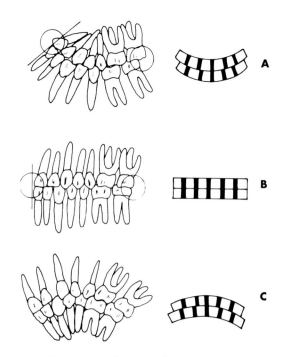

**Figure 7-59.** Variations in the curve of Spee. **A,** Concave. **B,** Flat. **C,** Convex.

teeth, control of the curve of Spee with removable appliances is more difficult. Leveling of the occlusal plane and control of the vertical dimension require the use of fixed multiattachment appliances.

4. Force application is interrupted during the use of removable appliances. The teeth can be moved into traumatic positions and then migrate back during static intervals. The clinician must be careful not to cause this "jiggling" during the use of removable appliances or must keep it to a minimum while correcting crossbite conditions.

5. After active treatment, some occlusal interferences may persist. Selective grinding and equilibrative procedures may be necessary. In such cases a gnathologic articulator may be beneficial for mounting the casts to observe possible areas of interference. In projection of the possible need for future equilibration, consideration of the growth direction during active treatment is necessary:

   a. In a horizontal growth pattern, selective grinding procedures should be employed in the molar region but not the incisal region because the bite can deepen and incisal guidance worsen during the terminal stages of mandibular growth, leading to incisor crowding. Final equilibration in this area should be postponed until growth has ceased.

   b. In a vertical growth pattern, equilibration can be done in the incisor region but should be postponed in the buccal segments. Molar guidance can worsen in the last stages of jaw growth, leading to a relapse into open bite. Correction by equilibration can be done to a moderate extent only in the postgrowth period.

6. Examination of the condylar guidance in the mixed dentition is important because of the information it can provide; however, condylar guidance is not stabilized during the transitional dentition period:

   a. The functional appliance directly influences condylar structures during the growing period. The condylar guidance can become flatter or steeper during orthopedic treatment. Asymmetry in the steepness of condylar guidance before treatment may be amenable to correction during activator therapy. In other cases the opposite condition is observed, and asymmetry results. This is especially true if a midline correction has been attempted using an incorrect construction bite for the activator.

   b. Before expansion treatment with active plates and particularly before treatment of crossbite, asymmetric condylar guidance is evident. Treatment can and should correct this condition in the TMJ and dentoalveolar area. Otherwise, the probability of later TMJ problems is substantial.

   c. A simple method of assessing condylar guidance in the mixed dentition has been developed. Sagittal measurement of the condylar guidance is performed using a condylar face-bow (Figure 7-60). The registration tray for the upper arch is modified and can be adapted to dental arches of various sizes. The

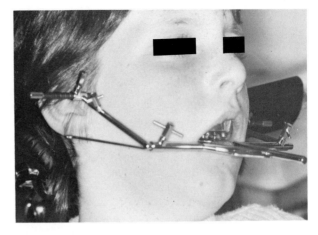

**Figure 7-60.** Face-bow for simplified extraoral registration in the mixed dentition.

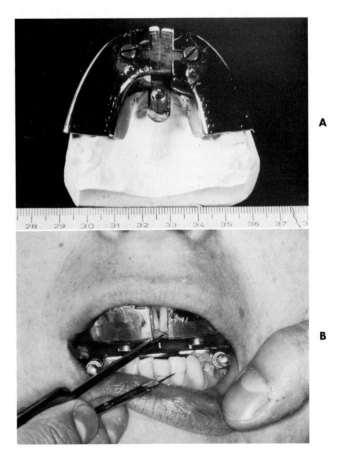

**Figure 7-61. A,** Adjustable tray for registration. **B,** Adjustable tray fixed in the mouth with impression material.

palate is left open (Figure 7-61). Fixation is achieved by impression material, and the tray is anchored dentally with triple support to eliminate any rolling or unwanted movement. The condylar guidance is

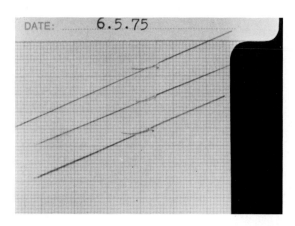

**Figure 7-62.** Triple registration of the condylar guidance.

registered three times on the Gerber registration chart on both left and right sides. The average is then computed for the evaluation (Figure 7-62).

Some gnathologic principles can thus be considered, even in the mixed dentition period and with removable appliance treatment:

1. The eruption and axial inclination of the teeth (particularly the canines) can be controlled.
2. The curve of Wilson can be controlled, particularly during expansion treatment.
3. The curve of Spee can be leveled during the eruption of the posterior teeth.
4. Occlusal trauma should be eliminated during orthodontic tooth movement.
5. The indications for and timing of equilibrative procedures should be anticipated and applied at the proper time.

## SUMMARY

Functional analysis relies on all diagnostic records and uses each in a special way. It is a philosophy of diagnostic interpretation. The orthodontist may be so used to employing the static set of plaster casts (related in habitual occlusion), lateral cephalograms (with the teeth in occlusion), panoral radiographs with the teeth in a manipulated incisal relationship to keep them within the focal trough, facial photographs (which usually record the teeth in occlusion and the facial muscles in repose), and intraoral photographs (which duplicate the interdental relationships on the study models) that a dynamic assessment of these records requires a new orientation.

Clinical examination is usually an appraisal of morphologic and interarch relationships for many clinicians—with some lip service paid to the appearance of the draping musculature. Many orthodontists do not put their patients through deglutitional, masticatory, and speech exercises. Many do not check the TMJ in various functional exercises and positions. Many do not really delve into the patient's history for information on these areas. Questions concerning finger sucking and tongue thrusting may be asked, but they are only part of the functional diagnostic mosaic.

A total approach is indicated for any form of orthodontic treatment but especially for functional appliance therapy. An appreciation of muscle function can be converted into therapeutic use of these same dynamic intrinsic forces. American orthodontists have become quite skilled in using extrinsic forces to achieve a predetermined norm of tooth-to-tooth relationship. Now, however, they also must enlist the intrinsic forces that may have caused or exacerbated the original malocclusion in the corrective process. Only then can optimal accomplishment and stability of results be achieved.

# Chapter 8

# The Activator

Thomas Rakosi

## DEVELOPMENT, CONSTRUCTION, AND MODE OF ACTION

Conventional orthodontics focuses on the dentoalveolar area. Moffett terms this the *second order of craniofacial articulation* because he considers the tooth socket an articulation, with the periodontal ligament providing the cellular elements to create the change (Figure 8-1).

Extending the effects of orthodontic guidance to the third order of articulation as classified by Moffett (i.e., the sutures and condylar joints) (1972), however, is not new. Historical evidence suggests that facial sutures were influenced as early as 1803 by Fox through the application of extraoral force. Therapeutic intervention in the condylar area and the temporomandibular joint (TMJ) involves the mandible rather than the maxilla. Because the mandible is the only freely functioning osseous structure on the body and is tied to its contiguous structures by 13 muscle attachments, its position in space, sagittally, transversely, and vertically, is relevant to the orthodontist. The possibility of influencing the mandibular position by altering the structure of the TMJ has intrigued orthodontists for many years.

In 1880, Kingsley introduced the term and concept of "jumping the bite" for patients with mandibular retrusion. He inserted a vulcanite palatal plate consisting of an anterior incline that guided the mandible to a forward position when the patient closed on it. This maneuver corrected the sagittal relationship without tipping the lower incisors forward. Clinical trials by Kingsley and others demonstrated the difficulty of holding the forward position of the lower jaw, and the technique is seldom used anymore—except as indicated by Hotz, whose *Vorbissplatte* was a modified Kingsley plate. Hotz used the appliance in cases of deep bite retrognathism, when the overbite was likely to cause a functional retrusion and the lower incisors were lingually inclined by hyperactivity of the mentalis muscle and lower lip. The modern Hawley biteplate, with an inclined plane behind the maxillary incisors, is frequently used in temporomandibular dysfunction (TMD) therapy. It is a direct descendent of the Kingsley plate.

Kingsley's ideas did influence the development of functional jaw orthopedics, however. The activator was originally used by Andresen (1908) with vertical extensions to contact the contiguous lingual surfaces of the mandibular teeth. Nevertheless, 85 years later the possibility of achieving a permanent forward positioning of the mandible is still controversial in some circles, despite treatment of many thousands of patients by this method. In many cases a forward

jumping of the bite has resulted in a dual bite after appliance removal (Figure 8-2). In these cases the patient habitually positions the mandible forward from a more retruded centric relation into a habitual occlusion that appears correct in the buccal occlusion but is actually a postural maneuver initiated by the protracting musculature to achieve full occlusion. This type of relationship can damage the TMJ. It causes jiggling of the teeth as the mandible drops back during excursive function associated with mastication. In other cases a jumping of the bite can be successfully achieved. These successful examples, however, involve functional retrusion problems with a forced retropositioning of the condyle in the fossa as a result of dominant retrusive activity of the posterior temporalis, deep masseter, and hyoid musculature associated with vertical overclosure and deep bite. Similar mandibular reposi-

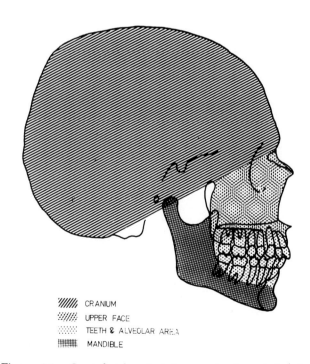

**Figure 8-1.** Craniofacial articulation—occlusal, periodontal, sutural, and condylar joints. Therapeutic measures can be performed with functional appliances in all these areas.

CRANIUM
UPPER FACE
TEETH & ALVEOLAR AREA
MANDIBLE

161

tioning also can occur sometimes after elimination of problems such as traumatic occlusion and crossbite, but this is not functional jaw orthopedics in the strictest sense, because functional jaw orthopedics permanently alters the position of the mandible by influencing and redirecting the growth processes. Among the pitfalls of activator therapy (accounting for dual bite) are improper diagnosis and case selection, which often lead to attempts to jump the bite in the wrong type of malocclusion.

A second postulate of Kingsley, associated with his original concepts, is often overlooked in current functional orthopedic therapy. The jumping of the bite should be performed without proclination of the lower incisors. Kingsley's requisite highlights a common dichotomy. The axiom requires no labial tipping of lower incisors, although the literature is replete with admonitions that activators can protrude these teeth. Too often this clinical fact means a failure of activator therapy, because the overjet is reduced by proclination of teeth instead of bodily anterior positioning of the mandible.

Impressed by Kingsley's concepts and appliances, Andresen developed a mobile, loose-fitting appliance modification that transferred functioning muscle stimuli to the jaws, teeth, and supporting tissues. The progenitor of the appliance

was a modified Kingsley plate that Andresen used as a retainer over summer vacation for his daughter after he removed fixed appliances used to correct a distocclusion. Seeing the continued improvement with this retainer, he called it a *biomechanic working retainer.* He used it after the removal of fixed appliances, not only as a way to stabilize the result achieved but also as a biomechanically functioning appliance, particularly during the summer holidays, when patients were gone for long periods.

Some years before Andresen started experimenting with his working retainer, Robin had created an appliance quite similar in its objectives. The *monobloc,* as he called it (because it was a single block of vulcanite), positioned the mandible forward in patients with glossoptosis and severe mandibular retrognathism who risked occluding their airways with their tongues. Robin noted that forward mandibular posture reduced this hazard and also led to significant improvement in the jaw relationship. The problem, usually associated with cleft palate, became known as the Pierre Robin syndrome. Despite the similarity of the two appliances, Andresen's inspiration came from Kingsley; he did not know of the Robin appliance.

When Andresen moved from Denmark to Norway, he became associated with Häupl at the University of Oslo. Häupl, a periodontist and histologist, was impressed with results obtained by Andresen's functioning retainer. He was particularly interested in its effect on the underlying tissues. He became convinced the appliance induced growth changes in a physiologic manner and stimulated or transformed the natural forces with an intermittent functional action transmitted to the jaw, teeth, and investing tissues. Familiar with the work of Roux, who subscribed to the shaking-the-bonding-substance-of-bone hypothesis, Häupl believed this was a clinical validation of the concept. By the time Andresen and Häupl teamed up to write about their appliance, they called it an *activator,* because of its ability to activate the muscle forces.

Some of Häupl's ideas have already been discussed in previous chapters. One point not mentioned is the importance of understanding the influence and limitations of the activator on the growth process. As to whether the activator promotes mandibular growth, the answer is qualified by the term *individual optimum.* The activator cannot create a large mandible from a small one, but it can help the patient achieve the optimal size consistent with morphogenetic pattern. Häupl considered this the goal of activator treatment. Even today, calculating this individual optimum is undeniably difficult. In the past the philosophy of treatment was to stimulate condylar changes by relocating the mandible anteriorly, thus achieving the desired occlusion. Growth prediction, direction, and timing were all vague concepts in clinical orthodontics at the time. That so many patients benefited from the activator is a tribute to these pioneers. Nevertheless, the purpose of the appliance is to influence the sagittal posture of the mandible; the reciprocal effect of the appliance on maxillary growth was essentially ignored for most of its history.

The original appliance combined an upper and a lower plate at the occlusal plane. Only one wire element was used—a labial arch for the upper anterior teeth (Figure 8-3). To

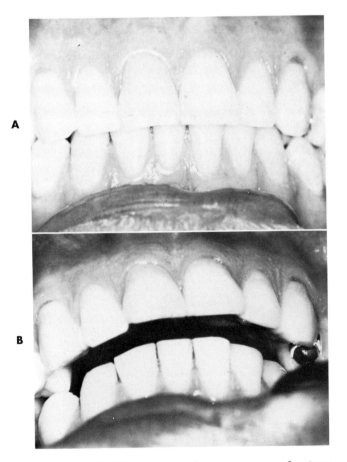

**Figure 8-2.** Dual bite can be a late consequence of activator treatment with a false indication. **A,** Habitual occlusion. **B,** Centric relation.

achieve expansion, the appliance was split in the center and a flexible coffin spring was incorporated (Figure 8-4). For more sophisticated use of the appliance, various springs were added later. Even jackscrews, a traditional form of appliance adjunct, were used, not primarily for expansion but for adjustment.

Andresen and Häupl, in cooperation with Petrik, produced the fifth edition of their book on functional jaw orthopedics in 1957. Many additional wire elements were described (Figure 8-5). Eschler (1952) had developed some modifications of the labial bow that improved intermaxillary effectiveness. One part was active, moving the teeth; the other was passive, holding the soft tissue of the lower lip away and thus enhancing the tooth movement desired. The principle of the bow's action influenced later developments; it eliminated un-

desirable soft tissue pressure while delivering force to precise tooth targets (Figure 8-6).

All the original appliances had a basic vulcanite or acrylic fabrication consisting of joined maxillary and mandibular components. Because the appliances were worn only at night, their bulkiness was not critical. However, subsequent modifications made to reduce the unwieldiness and bulk allow an increase in wearing time. Two types of modification can be differentiated:

1. Some appliances consist of one rigid acrylic mass for the maxillary and mandibular arches but with reduced volume or bulk.
   a. Some of these appliances are reduced in the anterior palatal region and are called *open activators.* Their goal is to restore exteroceptive contact between the tongue and palate, which is prevented by the classical activator (Figure 8-7). Patients prefer these appliances because they are reduced in the linguoincisal area and do not obstruct the oral cavity. However, the open activator has some disadvantages. The construction bite cannot be opened too far vertically because it impairs tongue function. If the vertical registration is too high, the tongue may thrust into the anterior interincisal gap, creating a postural and functional abnormality (Figure 8-8). A further disadvantage of the elastic open activator, introduced by Klammt in 1955, is the lack of support in the cutaway area of the appliance, especially if guidance of erupting teeth or expansion is necessary.
   b. These are appliances with reduced alveolar regions and with cross-palatal wires instead of full acrylic plates. They are supported or anchored dentally. Because of the toothborne anchorage, their uses (as introduced by Balters) are limited and their management can be difficult. Again, the labial bow eliminates abnormal muscle pressure by extending into the buccal vestibular area, opposite the canine and premolar regions (Figure 8-9).
2. Some appliances consist of two parts (upper and lower) joined with wire bows.

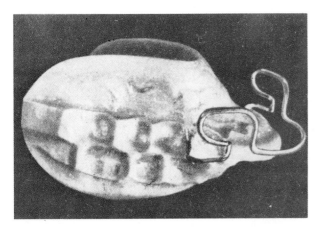

**Figure 8-3.** Original activator according to Andresen and Häupl.

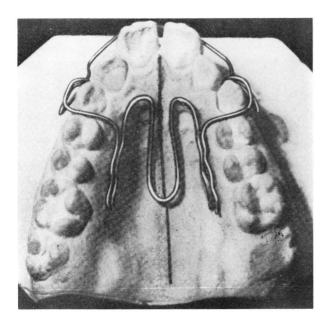

**Figure 8-4.** Coffin springs used for expansion.

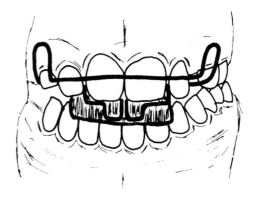

**Figure 8-5.** Additional elements for moving the incisors, used by Petrik.

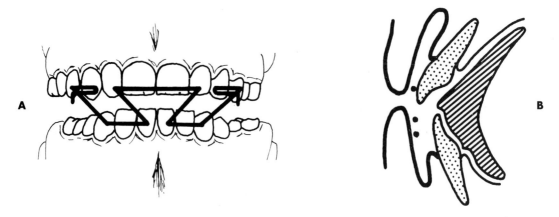

**Figure 8-6.** Combined labial bow according to Eschler. **A,** The upper part touches the teeth. **B,** The lower part holds the lip away from the incisors.

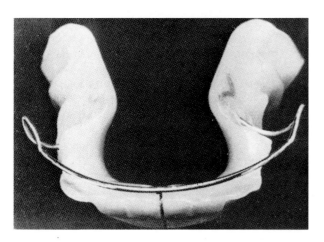

**Figure 8-7.** Open activator. The palatal acrylic is cut away.

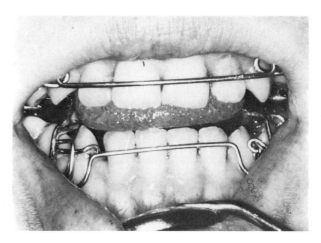

**Figure 8-8.** Tongue thrust habit that arose during the wearing of an open activator with a high construction bite.

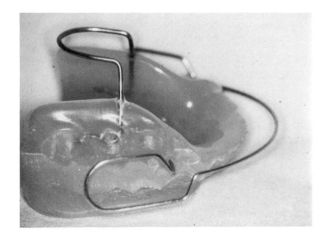

**Figure 8-9.** Balters' appliance—the bionator.

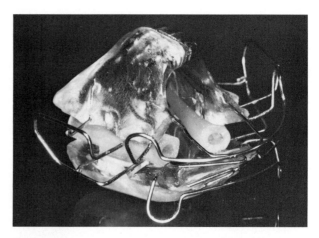

**Figure 8-10.** Elastic activator—the kinetor, according to Stockfisch.

a. The muscle impulses are reinforced by wire elements incorporated in the design. The flexibility or elasticity of the appliance permits mandibular movements in all directions (Figure 8-10). The Schwarz double plate is an earlier modification of this type. Stockfisch has developed a modern version with an elastic activator and a semidouble-plate appliance, which features latex tubing between upper and lower components to stimulate function.

The rigid one-piece appliance and the flexible two-piece joined by intermaxillary wiring have significantly different modes of action. The rigid activator does not permit muscle shortening, and therefore contractions that arise are isometric in nature. Isometric contractions develop higher tension than isotonic ones. A long-lasting tonic-stretch reflex contraction can be elicited by the proper appliance construction. The elastic construction permits muscle shortening, and less force magnitude is thus required. The momentary stretch in these flexible constructions produces a transient-phase reflex contraction.

The elastic activators are not bulky and do not impede the movements of the mandible. The patient can increase wearing time with relative comfort. However, the effectiveness of the appliance may be decreased because the isotonic contractions elicited are of lesser magnitude. Longer wearing time means increased efficiency. The flexible activator is also limited because taking the construction bite is possible only in an edge-to-edge relationship.

Recent modifications in design account for the morphogenetic pattern and growth direction prediction. The horizontal and vertical components of the construction bite vary depending on the goal of treatment, with different kinds of force activation.

## EFFICACY OF THE ACTIVATOR

According to Andresen and Häupl (1955), the activator is effective in exploiting the interrelationship between function and changes in internal bone structure. During the growth period an interrelationship also exists between function and external bone form. The activator induces musculoskeletal adaptation by introducing a new pattern of mandibular closure. The neuromuscular adaptation to the increased distance and change in direction is the basic requirement for reeducating the orofacial musculature.

The adaptations in the functional pattern caused by the activator also include and affect the condyles. Condylar adaptation to the anterior positioning of the mandible consists of growth in an upward and backward direction to maintain the integrity of the TMJ structures. This adaptation is induced by a loose appliance. The construction bite does not open the mandible beyond postural rest position (i.e., generally no more than 4 mm). Myotatic reflex activity is stimulated, causing isometric muscle contractions. This muscle force transmitted by the appliance moves the teeth. Thus the appliance works by using kinetic energy.

Although Andresen's and Häupl's original concept and working hypothesis have been discussed and practiced for 55 years, they are still controversial; some authorities accept some or all of their ideas, whereas others completely reject them.

Grude (1952) gives one explanation for the continuing controversy, suggesting that the activators' mode of action, according to the Andresen-Häupl concepts, can be observed only if the mandible is not displaced beyond postural rest position. If the construction of the appliance prevents the mandible from assuming this required position, the resultant mode of action is completely different. If the mandible opens beyond the 4 mm limit, the appliance does not work in the manner Andresen and Häupl suggest but instead works by stretching the soft tissues or relying on the viscoelastic properties of the muscles. Woodside used the latter technique, enlisting the stretch reflex and viscoelastic muscle force.

The following two statements by Grude can be accepted only with reservation:

1. An opening of 4 mm from the occlusal position does not induce the same muscle activation in every patient. A wide range of dimensions for interocclusal clearance exists. The distance varies not only among individuals but within the same individual from time to time.
2. The postural rest position is assessed when the patient is standing or sitting upright. The suspension of the mandible by the motivating musculature depends on such factors as head and body posture, the degree of wakefulness or sleep, and the intraoral vacuum. Alteration of the head posture causes a different gravity vector, resulting in a new relationship of parts and a new postural rest vertical dimension. Examination of sleeping patients wearing the activator has shown that these alterations are not decisive, but a clearance of some millimeters must be considered. Opening the mandible slightly or extensively creates different reactions and maintains a different force system. Between these two extremes are various transitional positions.

### Classification of Views

Within the literature, the writings of various authors can be classified into three groups, according to their different views:

1. Some authors (Petrovic, 1984; McNamara, 1973) substantiate the Andresen-Häupl concept that myotatic reflex activity and isometric contractions induce musculoskeletal adaptation by introducing a new mandibular closing pattern. Grude suggests that such adaptation is possible only with a small bite opening. In his experiments on skeletal adaptation, McNamara observed a progressive disappearance of the modified neuromuscular pattern. The stimuli from the activator and muscle receptors and periodontal mechanoreceptors promote displacement of the mandible. The superior heads of the lateral pterygoid muscles (LPMs) have the most important roles in this adaptation because they assist in skeletal adaptations. Petrovic came to similar conclusions based

on his extensive study of the condylar cartilage. A fundamental requirement for condylar growth stimulation is activation of the LPMs. An appliance rigidly holding the mandible in an anteriorly displaced position does not activate these muscles and so does not stimulate condylar growth (see Chapter 2). Nonfunctional splinting and minimal functional activity, particularly at night, do not increase the growth guidance. Petrovic and McNamara support the view that variations in the mode and direction of dislocation of the mandible are decisive factors in activator therapy.

2. A second group comprises authors (Selmer-Olsen, Herren [1953], Harvold [1974], and Woodside [1973]) who do not accept the theory that myotatic reflex activity with isometric muscle contractions induces skeletal adaptation. According to their views, the viscoelastic properties of muscle and the stretching of soft tissues are decisive for activator action. During each application of force, secondary forces arise in the tissues, introducing a bioelastic process. Thus not only the muscle contractions but also the viscoelastic properties of the soft tissues are important in stimulating the skeletal adaptation. Depending on the magnitude and duration of the applied force, the viscoelastic reaction can be divided into the following stages:

> Emptying of vessels
> Pressing out of interstitial fluid
> Stretching of fibers
> Elastic deformation of bone
> Bioplastic adaptation

The proponents of this explanation recognize only a modest skeletal adaptation in the vertical plane and no alteration in the sagittal.

Recent support for this thesis comes from Woodside. According to him, eliciting a stretch of the soft tissues primarily requires dislocating the mandible anteriorly or opening beyond the postural rest vertical dimension. Herren overextends in the sagittal plane, moving the mandible anteriorly into an incisal crossbite relationship. Woodside opens the mandible with the construction bite as much as 10 to 15 mm beyond the postural rest vertical dimension. The muscle tension, rising because of the stretching of the tissues, varies with the degree of mandibular displacement. The overextended activator, stretching the soft tissues like a splint, induces no myotatic reflex activity but instead applies a rigid stretch and creates a buildup of potential energy.

The rationale behind the Woodside theory is that the mandible normally drops open when the patient is asleep. If it is opened only 3 or 4 mm by the appliance, one of two things may happen: either the appliance may fall out, or it may be ineffective because the wider-open sleep position does not permit it to advance the mandible and thus the appliance does not elicit dental and possible skeletal adaptation. Woodside questions the amount of actual muscle contraction possible when the patient is asleep. The appliance will almost cer-

tainly stay in place with the wide-open construction bite, and the actual force likely to be directed at the teeth and jaws can thus be assessed. The extent to which this wide-open construction bite might cause deleterious maxillary vertical response has not been determined.

3. Between the two extremes a number of authors support a higher construction bite without the extreme extension advocated by Woodside. They use an opening of 4 to 6 mm, believing that the ultimate decision as to whether the force delivered is kinetic energy (isometric muscle contractions), potential energy (viscoelastic properties), or a combination of both depends on factors such as the nature of the malocclusion, the interocclusal clearance, head posture, state of mind, and level of consciousness.

Schmuth (1994), Witt (1981), and Witt and Komposch (1979) write of their experiences using activator construction bites that displace the mandible 4 to 6 mm below the intercuspal position. They have observed long periods of continuous pressure from the mandibular teeth against the activator. Thus the teeth are subjected to forces that act almost continuously. For this reason a vertical opening of more than 4 mm beyond habitual occlusion is not considered functional jaw orthopedics in the traditional sense.

Eschler (1952) defined techniques that open the vertical dimension beyond 4 mm in the construction bite as the *muscle-stretching method,* which works alternately with isotonic and isometric muscle contractions. He described the cycle: at insertion of the appliance the mandible is elevated by isotonic muscle contractions. When the mandible assumes a static position in contact with the appliance, isometric contractions arise. Because the mandible cannot reach the postural rest position, the elevators remain stretched. When fatigue occurs, the contracting muscles relax and the mandible drops. As soon as the muscles have recovered, the cycle begins again.

Ahlgren's electromyographic research (1970) shows that the activator functions as an interference, producing new contraction patterns in the jaw muscles. The innervation pattern can be adjusted after a while and the mandible repositioned forward.

## Synopsis

The various concepts can be summarized as follows: depending on the construction of the appliance, the activator can initiate myotatic reflex activity, induce isometric muscle contractions (sometimes also inducing isotonic contractions), or rely on the viscoelastic properties of the stretched soft tissues. According to the mode of action, two main principles apply. A third approach combines the two rationales.

1. According to the original Andresen-Häupl concept, the forces generated in activator therapy are caused by muscle contractions and myotatic reflex activity. A loose appliance stimulates the muscles, and the moving appli-

ance moves the teeth. The muscles function with kinetic energy, and intermittent forces are clinically significant. Successful treatment depends on muscle stimulation, the frequency of movements of the mandible, and the duration of the effective forces. Activators with a low vertical dimension construction bite function this way.

2. According to the second working hypothesis, the appliance is squeezed between the jaws in a splinting action. The appliance exerts forces that move the teeth in this rigid position. The stretch reflex is activated, inherent tissue elasticity is operative, and strain occurs without functional movement. The appliance works using potential energy. For this mode of action an overcompensation of the construction bite in the sagittal or vertical plane is necessary. An efficient stretch action is achieved by overcompensation and the viscoelastic properties of the contiguous soft tissues.

3. The third approach applies the modes of action of the preceding two. It can be called a transitional type of activator action, which alternately uses muscle contraction and viscoelastic properties of soft tissues. The appliances in this group have a greater bite opening than Andresen and Häupl recommend, but they do not overcompensate, as Woodside recommends. The stretch reflex resulting from activators in this group is seen as a long-lasting contraction. The intermittent forces induced by the contractions are less pronounced than those induced in the original construction. Eschler (1952) observed the occurrence of both isometric and isotonic contractions when this appliance construction was used.

All the modes of action depend on the construction bite's direction and degree of opening. By considering the individual characteristics of the facial skeleton, the individualized growth processes, and the goal of treatment, the clinician can make an appliance that works according to the desired mode of action.

## SKELETAL AND DENTOALVEOLAR EFFECTS OF THE ACTIVATOR

During craniofacial growth the activator can influence the third level of articulation, as outlined by Moffett (i.e., the sutures and TMJ). The construction bite determines the efficiency of its action. The activator also is effective in the dentoalveolar region, particularly during tooth eruption. The correct trimming of the acrylic contiguous to selected teeth is primarily responsible for the dentoalveolar effect.

1. As might be expected, any skeletal effect from the activator depends on the growth potential. Two divergent growth vectors propel the jaw bases in an anterior direction.
   a. The sphenoccipital synchondrosis moves the cranial base and nasomaxillary complex up and forward.
   b. The condyle translates the mandible in a downward and forward direction (Figure 8-11). The activator is most effective in controlling the lower vector, or the downward and forward growth of the mandible. This effect also can be designated as articular, because condylar growth is promoted or redirected. Johnston (1976) attributes this response to "unloading the condyle." If the mandible is positioned anteriorly, growth direction is more important than growth increments. Only the upward and backward growth of the condyle is capable of moving the mandible anteriorly.

Phylogenetic and ontogenetic peculiarities of the condylar cartilage affect the possibility of influencing condylar growth with functional orthodontic appliances. In contrast to primary cartilages (epiphyses, sphenoccipital synchondroses), condylar growth is regulated to a high degree by local exogenous factors. According to Moss (1962), Petrovic, Woodside (1984a), and others, condylar growth is an expression of a locally based homeostasis for the establishment and maintenance of a functionally coordinated stomatognathic system. As the research by Petrovic has shown, the LPM plays a decisive role in this growth. Forward posturing of the condyle activates the superior head of the LPM. In young people this induces a cell proliferation in the condyle and a growth response.

A favorable growth direction and incremental stimulation are necessary for treatment success. The activator can, to a limited degree, control the upper growth vector, supplied by the sphenoccipital synchondrosis, which moves the maxillary base forward. If the mandible cannot be positioned anteriorly, maxillary growth can be inhibited and redirected. Activators, particularly those of special construction, can influence the growth and translation of the nasomaxillary complex. Of course, maxillary growth also can be affected by extraoral force.

The activator also must assess and, if necessary, alter the vertical skeletal relationship. Changing the maxillary base inclination can compensate for rotations of mandibular growth vectors. A downward displacement of the maxillary base allows the maxilla to adapt to a vertical rotation of the mandible. If the rotation of the jaw bases during growth is unfavorable, activator therapy cannot be completed successfully. If the activator is constructed with a vertical opening of the bite only or with minimal sagittal change, the effect is primarily on midfacial development in the subnasal area. Both vertical maxillary growth and eruption of the teeth are restricted. Woodside believes that a small vertical opening restricts only horizontal midfacial development, whereas a wide vertical opening achieves the restriction by downward displacement of the midface area. A decrease in the sella-nasion-subspinale (S-N-A) angle can be observed unless the bite opening is extreme. In such cases the maxillary plane is then tipped up, and point A moves forward.

2. The dentoalveolar efficiency of the activator helps achieve a primary treatment objective. Teeth and bones

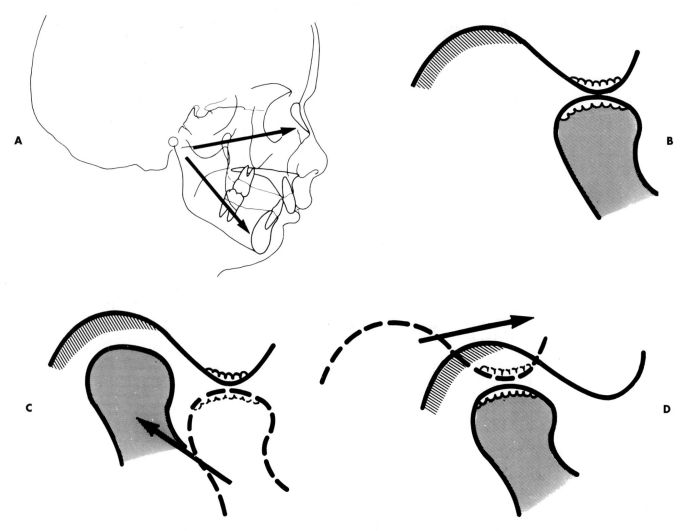

**Figure 8-11.**  **A,** Divergent growth vectors that move the jaw bases forward. **B,** The articular effectiveness of the activator moves the condyles into a forward-downward position. **C,** Adaptation to the new position through condylar growth. **D,** Adaptation to the new position by remodeling in the fossa.

fill in the space between the two divergent growth vectors. The dentoalveolar effect of the activator is to control tooth eruption and alveolar bone apposition. For this reason the activator is most effective if used in the early mixed dentition.

Various tooth movements have been observed during activator therapy, especially in the lower incisor area. Some authors have observed a forward displacement of the lower anterior segment (Björk, 1969) or a bodily displacement of the incisors (Jacobsson, 1967). Others have noted a labial (Richardson, 1982) or lingual (Moss, 1962) tipping of the lower incisors. These movements depend on the design of the appliance and the extension of the acrylic in the lower incisor area. With proper trimming of the appliance, different movements can be performed and the eruption of the teeth can be guided.

## FORCE ANALYSIS IN ACTIVATOR THERAPY

When the functional appliance activates the muscles, various types of forces are created—static, dynamic, and rhythmic.

1. Static forces are permanent and can vary in magnitude and direction. They do not appear simultaneously with movements of the mandible. The forces of gravity, posture, and elasticity of soft tissues and muscles are in this category.
2. Dynamic forces are interrupted. They appear simultaneously with movements of the head and body and have a higher magnitude than static forces. The frequency of these forces also depends on the design and construction of the appliance and the patient's reaction. Swallowing produces a dynamic force. Some clinicians tend to see only the active or dynamic force mechanisms of

the activator. However, the static forces also must be considered because of their constancy and duration.

3. Rhythmic forces are associated with respiration and circulation. They are synchronous with breathing, and their amplitude varies with the pulse. These trophic stimuli are quite important in stimulating cellular activity. The mandible transmits rhythmic vibrations to the maxilla. The applied forces are intermittent and interrupted. Force application to the teeth and mandible is intermittent. Removal of the activator from the mouth interrupts these forces.

Effectiveness of the activator during sleep depends on the frequency of movements, kind of construction bite, alterations in the interocclusal space and on muscle tone, and restlessness of the patient. According to Andresen and Häupl's original concept, the only forces operative in activator therapy are the natural ones, transformed and transferred by the activator to the jaws and teeth. However, recent modifications with different designs and the incorporation of additional elements (springs, jackscrews, pads, magnets) have allowed the active forces created to be used with the endogenous forces of the stomatognathic system. The appliance also can function by interfering with endogenous forces. Hence two principles are employed in the modern activator:

Force application—the source is usually muscular.
Force elimination—the dentition is shielded from normal and abnormal functional and tissue pressures by pads, shields, and wire configurations.

The types of force employed in activator therapy may be categorized as follows:

1. The growth potential, including the eruption and migration of teeth, produces natural forces. These can be guided, promoted, and inhibited by the activator.
2. Muscle contractions and stretching of the soft tissues initiate forces when the mandible is relocated from its postural rest position by the appliance. The activator stimulates and transforms the contractions. Whereas the forces may be functional (muscular) in origin, their activation is artificial. These artificially functioning forces can be effective in all three planes:
   a. In the sagittal plane the mandible is propelled down and forward, so that muscle force is delivered to the condyle and a strain is produced in the condylar region. A slight reciprocal force can be transmitted to the maxilla during this maneuver.
   b. In the vertical plane the teeth and alveolar processes are either loaded with or relieved of normal forces. If the construction bite is high, a greater strain is produced in the contiguous tissues. If transmitted to the maxilla, these forces can inhibit growth increment and direction and influence the inclination of the maxillary base.
   c. In the transverse plane, forces also can be created with midline corrections.

3. Various active elements (e.g., springs, screws) can be built into the activator to produce an active biomechanic type of force application.

The mode of force application, magnitude, and direction depend on the three-dimensional dislocation of the mandible, which is determined by the construction bite.

## CONSTRUCTION BITE

Proper activator fabrication requires the determination and reproduction of the correct construction or working bite. The purpose of this mandibular manipulation is to relocate the jaw in the direction of treatment objectives. This creates artificial functional forces and allows assessment of the appliance's mode of action. Before taking the construction bite, the clinician must prepare by making a detailed study of the plaster casts, cephalometric and panoral head films, and the patient's functional pattern.

### Diagnostic Preparation

Patient compliance is essential. Therefore the clinician must not only assess clinically the somatic and psychologic aspects of the patient but also determine the patient's motivation potential. Creating an "instant correction"—moving the mandible forward into an anterior, more normal sagittal relationship—may help motivate patients with Class II malocclusions. The patient sees the objectives of the correction to be made by the functional appliance and is more likely to work toward this goal than merely to realize the dental health and functional improvement (Figure 8-12). Video imaging also augments patient motivation. As Fränkel (1983) points out, performing this clinical maneuver at the beginning of treatment also indicates to the clinician whether the therapeutic goal is really an improvement. In some problems of maxillary protrusion and excessive vertical dimension and reduced symphyseal prominence, a forward positioning does not improve the appearance of the profile. Other therapeutic measures may be required.

**Study model analysis.** Before constructing the activator, the clinician must consider the following factors, based on the cast analysis:

1. First permanent molar relationship in habitual occlusion
2. Nature of the midline discrepancy, if any: if the midlines are not coincident, a functional analysis should be made to determine the path of closure from postural rest to occlusion; if the midlines change, a functional problem (amenable to correction in the appliance) is likely; dentoalveolar noncoincident midlines cannot be corrected by functional appliances.
3. Symmetry of the dental arches: Any asymmetries should be evaluated, because the activator may correct some of them (e.g., segmental open bite).

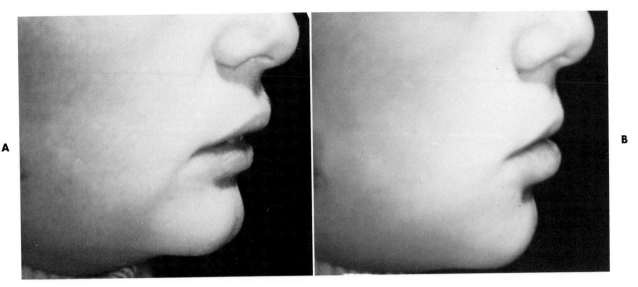

**Figure 8-12.    A,** Occlusal position. **B,** Construction bite position.

4. Curve of Spee: The curve of Spee should be checked to see whether it can or should be leveled by the activator; if it is severe and the premolars have already erupted, the activator will not be able to perform the necessary leveling.

5. Crowding and any dental discrepancies: These discrepancies are measured because with the cephalometric analysis they help determine the requirements and possibilities of lower incisor movement.

**Functional analysis.** Before the construction bite is taken, a functional analysis is performed to obtain the following information:

1. Precise registration of the postural rest position in natural head posture (because the vertical opening of the construction bite depends on this)

2. Path of closure from postural rest to habital occlusion (any sagittal or transverse deviations are recorded)

3. Prematurities, point of initial contact, occlusal interferences, and resultant mandibular displacement, if any (some of these can be eliminated with the activator, but some require other therapeutic measures)

4. Sounds such as clicking and crepitus in the TMJ (might indicate a functional abnormality or the need for some modification of appliance design)

5. Interocclusal clearance or freeway space (should be checked several times and the mean amount recorded)

6. Respiration (with allergies or disturbed nasal respiration, the patient cannot wear a bulky appliance; in such cases an open activator or twin block may be used, or the respiratory abnormalities may be eliminated first)

Epipharyngeal lymphoid tissue deserves particular attention. The size of tonsils and adenoids should be recorded, even if nasal breathing does not seem to be affected. If the tonsils are enlarged and the tongue has assumed a compensatory anterior position to maintain an open airway, the patient will not be able to tolerate the appliance. A consultation with an otolaryngologist may be needed first; possible removal of diseased or excessive epipharyngeal tissue should be considered in such cases.

**Cephalometric analysis.** The diagnostic tool of cephalometric analysis enables clinicians to identify the craniofacial morphogenetic pattern to be treated. The most important information required for planning the construction bite is the following:

1. Direction of growth—average, horizontal, or vertical (growth rotation tends to follow a logarithmic spiral)

2. Differentiation between position and size of the jaw bases (e.g., relation to cranium, sagittal apical base relationship)

3. Morphologic peculiarities, particularly of the mandible (may assist in determining the course of the development; in many cases in mixed dentition, form and function relationships aid in forecasting whether the growth pattern will be more horizontal or vertical in subsequent years)

4. Axial inclination and position of the maxillary and mandibular incisors (provide important diagnostic and prognostic clues for determining the anterior positioning the mandible requires and the details of the appliance design for the incisor area)

## Treatment Planning

The next step after accumulating and analyzing the diagnostic information is planning for the construction bite. The extent of anterior positioning for Class II malocclusions and posterior positioning for Class III malocclusions should be determined.

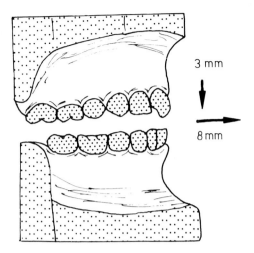

**Figure 8-13.** Construction bite in edge-to-edge relationship with slight opening.

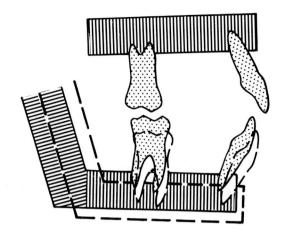

**Figure 8-15.** Anterior positioning of the mandible from the rest position.

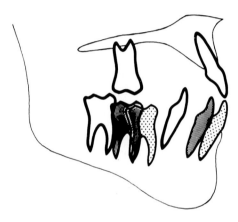

**Figure 8-14.** Anterior positioning of the mandible in two phases—first phase, *dark;* second phase, *dotted.*

**Anterior positioning of the mandible.** The usual intermaxillary relationship for the average Class II problem is end-to-end incisal. However, it should not exceed 7 to 8 mm, or three quarters of the mesiodistal dimension of the first permanent molar, in most instances (Figure 8-13). Anterior positioning of this magnitude is contraindicated if any of the following pertain:

1. The overjet is too large: In extreme cases, overjet can approach 18 mm. Anterior positioning then becomes a stepwise progression, accomplished in two or three phases (Figure 8-14).
2. Labial tipping of the maxillary incisors is severe: These incisors should probably be positioned upright first, if possible, by a prefunctional appliance.
3. An incisor (usually a lateral) has erupted markedly to the lingual: The mandible must be postured anteriorly to an edge-to-edge relationship with the lingually malposed tooth; otherwise, labial movement of this tooth will be impossible. Eschler (1952) termed the condition a *pathologic construction bite.* As with severely proclined upper

incisors, use of a short prefunctional appliance to improve alignment of lingually malposed teeth is advisable before starting activator treatment, thereby eliminating the need for the pathologic construction bite.

**Opening the bite.** Vertical considerations are as important as the sagittal determination and are intimately linked to it. Maintaining a proper horizontal-vertical relationship and determining the height of the bite are guided by the following principles:

1. The mandible must be dislocated from the postural resting position in at least one direction—sagittally or vertically. This dislocation is essential to activate the associated musculature and induce a strain in the tissues.
2. If the magnitude of the forward position is great (7 or 8 mm), the vertical opening should be minimal so as not to overstretch the muscles (Figure 8-15). This type of construction bite produces an increased force component in the sagittal plane, allowing a forward positioning of the mandible. According to Witt (1971), the approximate sagittal force that develops is in the 315 to 395 g range, whereas the magnitude of the vertical force approximates 70 to 175 g. The primary neuromuscular activation is in the elevator muscles of the mandible.
3. If extensive vertical opening is needed, the mandible must not be anteriorly positioned. If the bite opening exceeds 6 mm, mandibular protraction must be very slight (Figure 8-16). Myotatic reflex activity of the muscles of mastication can then be observed, as can a stretching of the soft tissues. A more extensive bite opening is possible in functionally true deep-bite cases. If the bite registration is high, both the muscles and the viscoelastic properties of the soft tissues are enlisted. The vertical force is increased, and the sagittal force is decreased. This type of construction bite is obviously not effective in achieving anterior positioning of the mandible, but it can influence the inclination of the maxil-

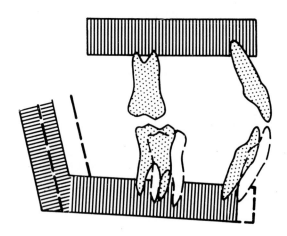

**Figure 8-16.** Opening the mandible below the rest position.

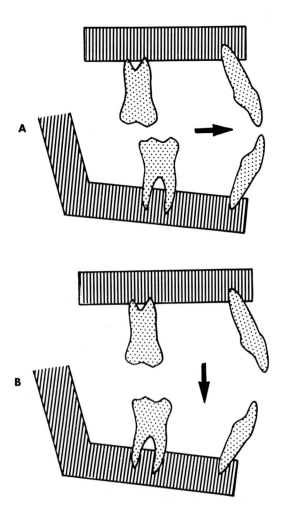

**Figure 8-17. A,** Sagittal force component, which arises during anterior positioning of the mandible. **B,** Vertical force component, which arises during opening of the mandible.

lary base. One possible indication for such a construction bite is a case with a vertical growth pattern. The vertical relationship, either deep bite or open bite, can be therapeutically affected by the activator. Disadvantages of a wide-open construction bite include the difficulty of wearing the appliance and adapting to the new relationship. Muscle spasms often occur, and the appliance tends to fall out of the mouth. The high construction bite also makes lip seal difficult if not impossible. The ultimate reestablishment of normal lip seal is essential in functional appliance therapy.

**General rules for the construction bite.** The assessment of the construction bite determines the kind of muscle stimulation, frequency of mandibular movements, and duration of effective forces (Figure 8-17).

1. In a forward positioning of the mandible of 7 to 8 mm, the vertical opening must be slight to moderate (2 to 4 mm).
2. If the forward positioning is no more than 3 to 5 mm, the vertical opening should be 4 to 6 mm.
3. The activator can correct lower midline shifts or deviations only if actual lateral translation of the mandible itself exists. If the midline abnormality is caused by tooth migration, no asymmetric relationship exists between the mandible and maxilla. An attempt to correct this type of dental problem could lead to iatrogenic asymmetry. Functional crossbites in the functional analysis can be corrected by taking the proper construction bite (Figure 8-18).

All preconditions for successful treatment with the activator, even small variations in mandibular position, can significantly alter activator force application.

Both experimental research and clinical experience have shown that an increase in muscle activation with overextended appliances does not increase the efficiency of the activator. According to Sander (1983), the frequency of maximal biting into a 6 mm-high construction bite is 12.5% of the sleeping time, whereas in an 11 mm-high construction bite, it is only 1.1%, and if this is increased to 13 mm, as prescribed by Harvold, it is only 0.8%.

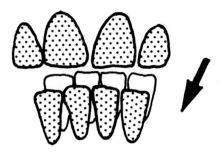

**Figure 8-18.** Correction of midline shift with the construction bite.

## Execution of the Construction Bite Technique

1. A horseshoe-shaped wax bite rim is prepared for insertion between the maxillary and mandibular teeth. It should have proper arch form and size and adequate width and be 2 to 3 mm thicker than the planned construction bite. It can be made for either the upper or lower arch occlusal surfaces. If the rim is first placed on the lower arch, however, the mandible can be guided into the desired anterior position required for treatment of the specific Class II malocclusion (Figure 8-19). If the operator chooses to place the softened wax bite rim on the upper arch, the mandible can be moved easily into the more retruded position required for the construction of a Class III activator.

2. Before taking the wax bite registration, the operator asks the patient to sit upright in a relaxed posture while gently guiding the mandible into the predetermined position. The operator guides but does not force the jaw to the desired sagittal relationship. The operator repeats this exercise three to four times while manipulating the patient's chin between thumb and forefinger. The patient is asked to repeat the exercise and then hold the forward position for a short time to set up an exteroceptive engram that can be replicated when the wax is placed between the teeth.

3. When the operator is relatively sure the patient can replicate the exercise, the softened wax bite rim is placed in the mouth as described in step 1. The wax should not be too soft. During the closing movement the operator controls the edge-to-edge incisal relationship and midline registration (Figure 8-20). The wax should be cut away from the labial of the central incisors so that the midlines can be observed and a correct reproduction of the incisal relationship established.

4. In the final step the wax is carefully removed from the mouth and checked on the upper and lower models. After it has been fitted on the casts, the margins are trimmed with scissors so that the operator can be sure the wax is close to all the cusps of the teeth. The hardened wax bite is then chilled and checked once again in the mouth.

The construction bite should be taken only after careful planning and must always be taken on the patient, not on the articulated models. A construction bite prepared on casts may have the following disadvantages:

- It may not fit.
- Asymmetric biting may have occurred on it.
- The patient may not be really comfortable and may be disturbed more frequently during sleep.
- The likelihood of unwanted lower incisor procumbency may be greater, because the appliance exerts undue stress on these teeth.

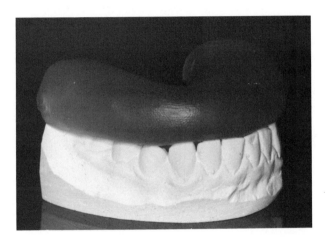

**Figure 8-19.** Wax rim on the cast.

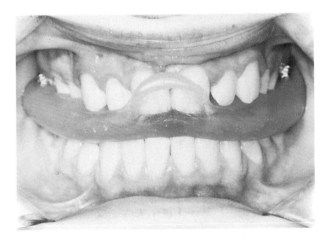

**Figure 8-20.** Wax rim in the mouth. When the bite is being taken, midline shift should be controlled.

## Technique for a Low Construction Bite with Markedly Forward Mandibular Positioning

The mandible is positioned anteriorly to achieve an edge-to-edge relationship parallel to the functional occlusal plane. In Class II functional retrusion cases that show posterior displacement from postural rest to habitual occlusion, the mandible can be positioned anteriorly to a greater degree than can be done in true Class II malocclusions, with a normal path of closure. A general rule is that the construction bite should always be at least 3 mm posterior to the most protrusive positioning possible. The mandible should remain within the limits of the interocclusal clearance and not exceed its postural rest position for the vertical registration.

When the mandible moves mesially to engage the appliance, the elevator muscles of mastication are activated. When the teeth engage the appliance, the myotatic reflex is activated. In addition to the muscle force arising during biting and swallowing, the reflex stimulation of the muscle spindles also elicits reflex muscle activity.

The activator constructed with a low vertical opening registration and a forward bite is appropriately designated the horizontal H activator (Figures 8-21 and 8-22). With this type of appliance the mandible can be postured forward without tipping the lower incisors labially. The maxillary incisors can be positioned upright, and the anterior growth vector of the

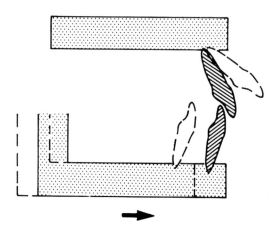

**Figure 8-21.** Effectiveness of the H activator—anterior positioning of the mandible, lingual tipping of the upper incisors. Only a modest influence on the maxillary base in the sagittal plane can be achieved.

maxilla is slightly inhibited. The maxillary base is not affected, however. As might be expected, this type of appliance is most effective if an anterior sagittal relationship of the mandible is the primary treatment objective. It is indicated in Class II, division 1 malocclusions with sufficient overjet.

**Class II caused by mandibular overclosure that results in a functional retrusion.** In some Class II malocclusions the activator can in effect jump the bite. An example is shown in Figure 8-23. The patient, a 10-year-old girl, was treated with a horizontal activator. The mandible was anteriorly positioned in postural rest but slid into a posteriorly guided functional retrusion position in habitual occlusion. With a large anterior positioning for the construction bite, the retrognathism was reduced and the upper incisors were tipped lingually into a more normal position. The lip trap was eliminated. A second activator was then constructed for maximal dentoalveolar effectiveness of the appliance. Judicious grinding helped guide the occlusion into a more favorable relationship. The active phase of orthodontic therapy was completed in 2 years (Figure 8-24).

**Additional indication for the horizontal H activator.** Class II, division 1 malocclusions with posterior positioning of the mandible caused by growth deficiency but with the likelihood of a future horizontal growth pattern are suitable candidates for treatment with the H activator. In these cases, planning for lingual tipping of the maxillary incisors and pretreatment

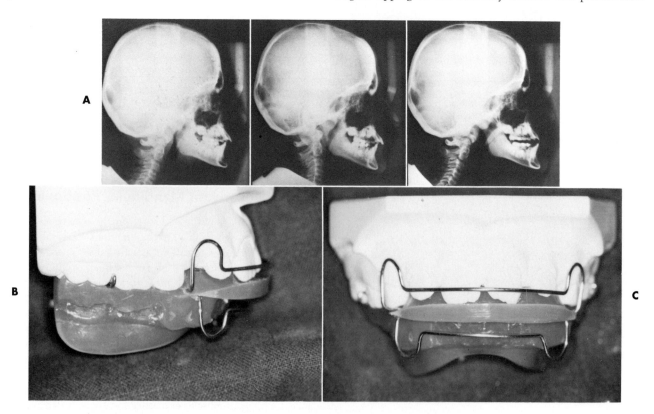

**Figure 8-22.** **A,** Anterior positioning of the mandible in construction of the H activator. *Left,* occlusion; *middle,* rest; *right,* construction bite. **B** and **C,** H activator, lateral and frontal views.

labial tipping of the lower incisors is advantageous. Treatment is more difficult in patients with labially inclined lower incisors, but posturing the mandible forward while simultaneously positioning upright the labially tipped lower incisors is possible.

Figure 8-25, which shows a 9-year-old girl with an average growth trend and retrognathic skeletal pattern, exemplifies this type of H-activator use. Only a slight skeletal discrepancy was apparent, with a subspinale-nasion-supramentale (A-N-B) difference of 3 degrees. The maxillary and mandibular bases

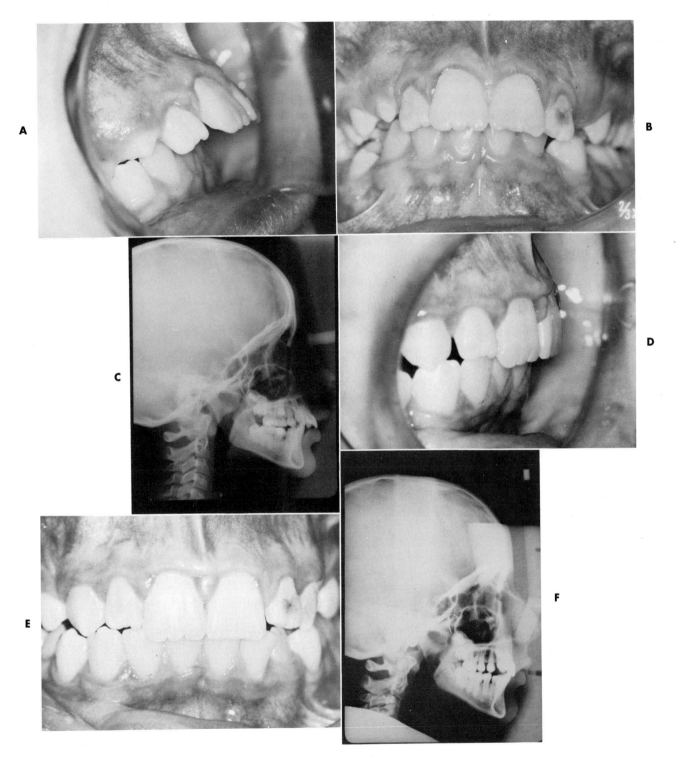

**Figure 8-23.**   Class II, division 1 malocclusion in a 10-year-old girl. **A** to **C,** Before treatment. **D** to **F,** After jumping the bite. The lingual tipping of the upper incisors is evident.

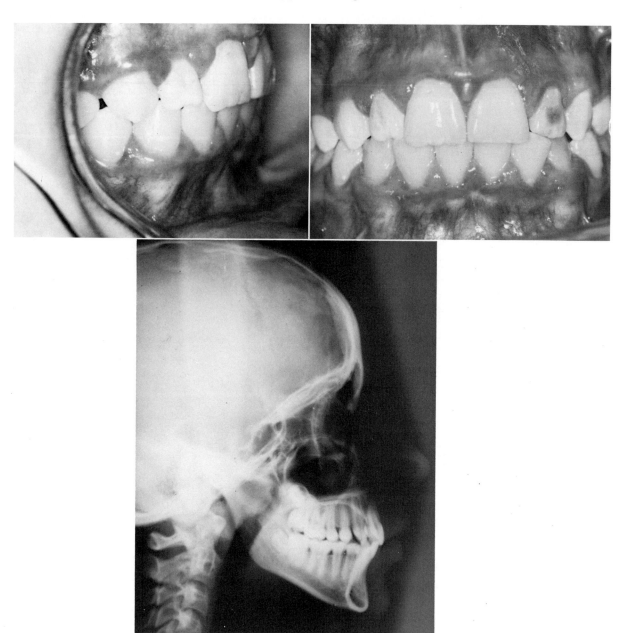

**Figure 8-24.** Same patient as in Figure 8-23 after seating of the occlusion.

were of average length; the ramus was short. The upper and lower incisors were inclined labially, with spacing between the uppers. The overjet was caused by the labial inclination and position (+8.5 mm anterior to the nasion-pogonion [N-Pog] plane) of the upper incisors. The lower lip was trapped between the upper and lower incisors in the excessive overjet. The lips were potentially incompetent, the swallowing somatic, and the respiration nasal. The mandible and symphysis were well developed. An important consideration was the likelihood of a horizontal growth direction shift in subsequent years.

A horizontal type of activator was prescribed. With an overjet of 6 mm and an overbite of 4.5 mm, the therapeutic objective was to create a slightly anterior position for the mandible and an upright position for the upper and lower incisors. The mandible was positioned only 5 mm anteriorly and opened 6 mm vertically with the construction bite to enable the muscles to push the incisors upright while leaving enough space for the labial acrylic cap to cover the lower incisors.

Active treatment lasted 3 years for this patient. Full-time treatment would have reduced this time significantly. The mandible assumed an anterior position with a growth increment of 3.5 mm (0.4 mm less than average). The ramal height growth was 6.0 mm, which was significant (3.4 mm above average). The basal relationship of articulare-subspinale (Ar-A) and Ar-Pog improved from 12 to 19 mm. Both the upper and

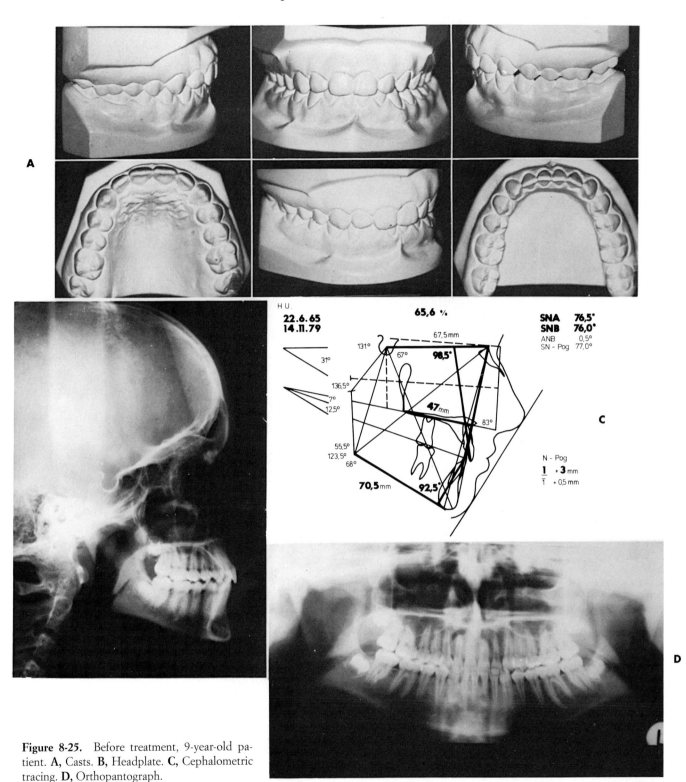

**Figure 8-25.** Before treatment, 9-year-old patient. **A,** Casts. **B,** Headplate. **C,** Cephalometric tracing. **D,** Orthopantograph.

lower incisors were positioned upright. Significantly, with a forward rotating growth direction, the growth pattern became more horizontal (Figure 8-26).

The indication for an anterior posturing of the mandible is not only an originally posterior position but also the likelihood of a favorable growth pattern—including direction and incremental change. The goal of functional appliance therapy is to influence favorably the growth of the mandible, achieving optimal growth direction and amounts, and to eliminate any dysfunction or posteriorly retruded habitual occlusion. A vertical growth pattern does not allow this type of therapy. Another type of appliance must be constructed.

## Technique for a High Construction Bite with Slightly Anterior Mandibular Positioning

In a high construction bite the mandible is positioned less anteriorly (only 3 to 5 mm ahead of the habitual occlusion position). Depending on the magnitude of the interocclusal space, the vertical dimension is opened 4 to 6 mm, a maximum of 4 mm beyond the postural rest–vertical dimension registration. The appliance induces myotatic reflexes in the muscles of mastication. Possibly the stretching of the muscles and soft tissues elicits an additional force, causing a response of the viscoelastic properties of the soft tissues involved. This greater opening of the vertical dimension in the construction bite allows the myotatic reflex to remain operative even when the musculature is more relaxed (i.e., while the patient is sleeping). The frequency of maximal biting into the appliance is less than with the H type of activator, however, as shown by

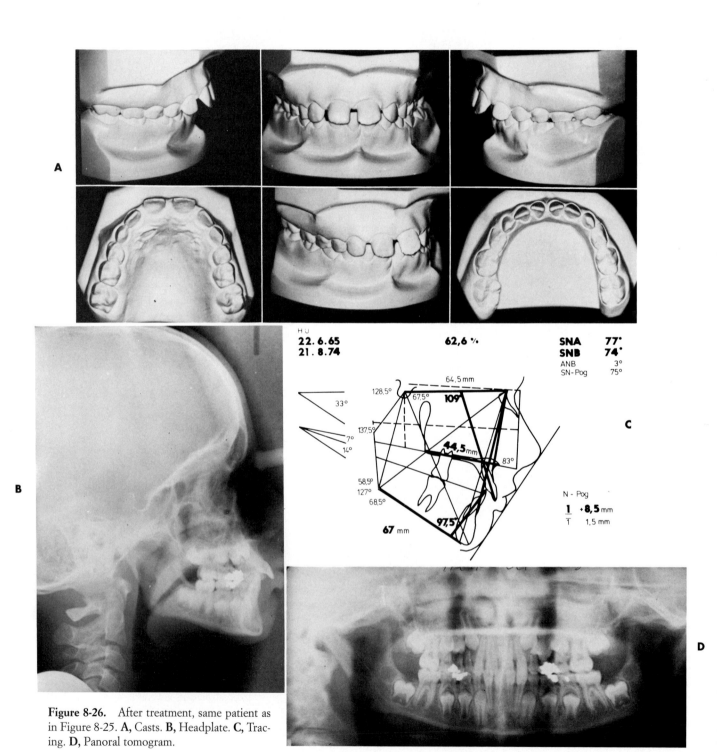

**Figure 8-26.** After treatment, same patient as in Figure 8-25. **A,** Casts. **B,** Headplate. **C,** Tracing. **D,** Panoral tomogram.

Sander (1983). The stretch reflex activation with the increased vertical dimension may well influence the inclination of the maxillary base. This appliance is indicated in cases with vertical growth patterns and can be properly designated as the vertical V activator (Figures 8-27 and 8-28).

The Class II, division 1 malocclusion with a vertical growth direction cannot be significantly improved sagittally by anterior positioning of the mandible. The mandible may be postured forward, but the danger of a dual bite is great, as the original experiences of Kingsley indicate.

The goal of activator treatment in this case is not just a minimal forward positioning of the mandible because of the vertical growth pattern but an actual adaptation of the maxilla to the lower dental arch. This goal can be only partially achieved by a retroclination of the maxillary base. This skeletal adaptation must be supported by dentoalveolar compensa-

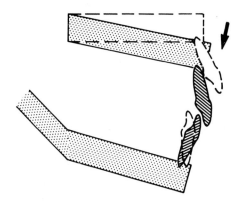

**Figure 8-27.** Effectiveness of the vertical activator—changed inclination of the maxillary base, slight anterior positioning of the mandible, dental compensation.

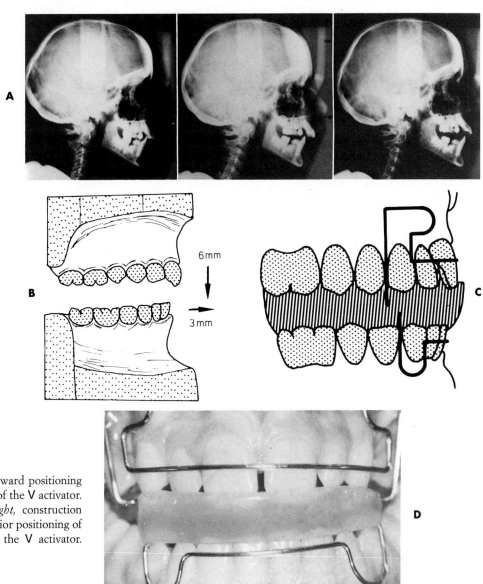

**Figure 8-28.** **A,** Forward-downward positioning of the mandible in construction of the V activator. *Left,* occlusion; *middle,* rest; *right,* construction bite. **B,** Opening and slight anterior positioning of the mandible. **C,** Schematic of the V activator. **D,** Activator in the mouth.

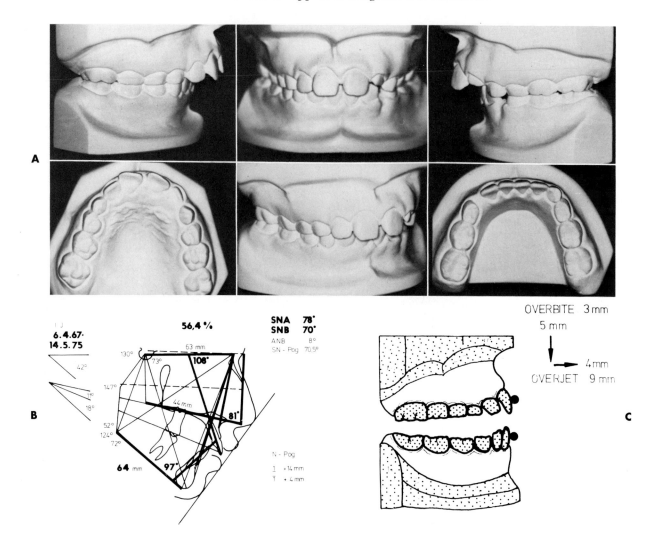

**Figure 8-29.** Before treatment, 8-year-old patient. **A,** Casts. **B,** Tracing. **C,** Construction bite position.

tion, which requires differential guidance of eruption of lower buccal segments, withholding of maxillary buccal segment eruption (as described by Harvold, 1974), lingual tipping of the maxillary incisors, and labial tipping of the mandibular incisors. Holding the upper incisors with a labially extended acrylic groove is necessary. The lower incisors can be supported on the lingual surfaces by acrylic and tipped labially until contact with the upper incisors is attained.

An example of this type of case is shown in Figure 8-29. The patient is an 8-year-old girl with a Class II, division 1 malocclusion and vertical growth pattern. Her posteroanterior height ratio was 56.4%, and the cranial base–mandibular plane angle was 42 degrees. The face was retrognathic, with an A-N-B angle of 8 degrees. The jaws were normally developed, but the ramus was extremely short. The upper and lower incisors were tipped labially. Because of the vertical growth pattern and the labial tipping of the lower incisors, the facial pattern was considered unfavorable for conventional activator therapy. However, some of the functional relationships could benefit from functional orthopedic guidance. The posterior position of the mandible could be slightly improved if

the abnormal retruding force of the musculature were eliminated. Retroclining the maxillary base could compensate somewhat for the vertical growth pattern. The upper incisors could be tipped lingually to compensate dentally for the Class II characteristics, although a further labial tipping of the lower incisors would be needed for complete compensation.

The treatment was performed with a vertical activator. The bite was opened 5 mm for the construction bite, but the anterior positioning of the mandible was only 4 mm. The upper incisors were tipped lingually with the labial bow and then supported with the acrylic cap (which extended over the labial). The acrylic was trimmed away on the incisal edges and on the lingual to permit maximal upper incisor lingual compensation. The lower incisors were held with the labial bow and supported lingually with the acrylic. The selective trimming of the activator in the maxillary arch stimulated intrusion in the buccal segments while permitting extrusion of the anterior teeth. The successful clinical result after 2 years of therapy is shown in Figure 8-30.

The posttreatment analysis showed an average growth increment, a slight anterior posturing of the mandible, and a de-

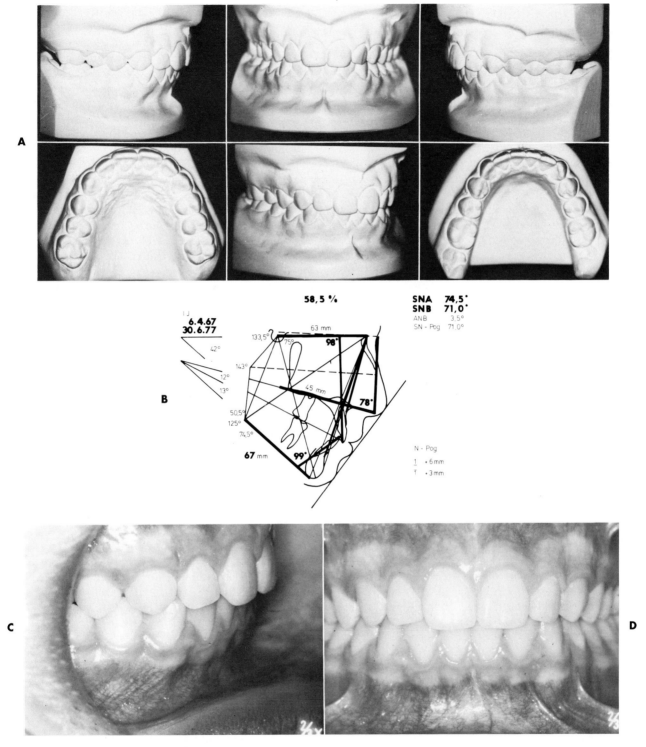

**Figure 8-30.** After treatment, same patient as in Figure 8-29. **A,** Casts. **B,** Tracing. **C** and **D,** Lateral and frontal views.

crease in the S-N-A angle, with further retroclination of the maxilla—a skeletal compensation for the sagittal malrelationship. Lingual tipping of the upper incisors and slight labial tipping of the lower incisors created a dentoalveolar compensation. Mandibular posterior segment eruption exceeded maxillary counterpart eruption. A study of the posttreatment cephalogram clearly indicates that the ideal incisor axial inclination could not have been achieved in vertically growing Class II malocclusions of this type. To do so would have left an excessive overjet and potential lip trap, and with the incisors unsupported by normal function, they would have been relatively more unstable.

## Technique for a Construction Bite without Forward Mandibular Positioning

A forward positioning of the mandible is not indicated in activator construction if a sagittal correction is unnecessary. Such appliances are used primarily in vertical dimension problems (deep overbite and open bite) and in selected cases of crowding (Figure 8-31).

### Vertical problems

*Deep overbite malocclusions.* Deep overbite malocclusions can be of either dentoalveolar origin or skeletal in nature.

In *dentoalveolar overbite* problems the deep overbite can be caused by infraclusion of the buccal segments or supraclusion of the anterior segment. Activators designed and trimmed to permit extrusion can be used to treat deep overbite cases with infraclusion of molars. Problems in this category are usually functionally true overbite cases, with a large clearance. Nevertheless, a retrusive sagittal relationship associated with the mandibular overclosure also can exist. The construction bite may be either moderate or high, depending on the size of the freeway space.

In deep overbite cases caused by supraclusion of the incisors, the interocclusal space is usually small. The activator should not be designed with a high construction bite in these cases. Intrusion of the incisors is possible to only a limited extent when an activator is being used. Any correction is attained by loading the incisal edges with an acrylic cover. Depression is relative rather than absolute, because the other teeth are free to erupt and accomplish the predetermined growth pattern. In such cases a successful result requires a significant increment of growth in the vertical direction.

The skeletal deep overbite malocclusion usually has a horizontal growth pattern, for which forward inclination of the maxillary base can compensate. Loading the incisors can achieve a slight forward inclination, as with supraclusion of the incisors. The acrylic cap engages these teeth while freeing the molars to erupt. With this therapeutic approach the construction bite should be high enough to exceed the patient's postural rest vertical dimension. This height enlists stretch reflex response and the viscoelastic properties of the muscles and soft tissues as they are stretched. The opening is beyond the 5 to 6 mm freeway space, in a construction similar to that prescribed by Woodside (1984). A dentoalveolar compensation is simultaneously possible by extrusion of the lower molars and distal driving of the upper molars with stabilizing wires.

*Open-bite malocclusions.* An anterior positioning of the mandible is not necessary or desirable if the skeletal relationship is orthognathic. The dentoalveolar open bite can be treated by properly trimming the acrylic of the appliance. These procedures are described in Chapter 9. The bite is opened 4 to 5 mm to develop a sufficient elastic depressing force and load the molars that are in premature contact. Properly constructed activators that follow this principle can influence the vertical growth pattern in these cases. A precondition for successful therapy, however, is a retroclination of the maxillary base with a restriction of the patient's vertical growth pattern. This literally requires the clinician to "close the V" between upper and lower maxillary bases, depressing the posterior maxillary segments with the activator in a manner analogous to that of orthognathic surgery. In surgical open-bite cases the posterior segments are impacted, allowing autorotation of the mandible. Dellinger's magnetic vertical corrector is most effective in these cases. If divergent rotation of the bases is apparent, the treatment of open-bite malocclusions with the activator is not possible.

**Arch length deficiency problems.** Malocclusions with crowding can sometimes be treated with activators. In the mixed dentition period, problems of anchorage with regular expansion plates can occur. The activator can accomplish the desired expansion because it is anchored intermaxillarily.

The appliance works in a manner similar to that of two active plates with jackscrews in the upper and lower parts. The construction bite is low because jaw positioning and growth guidance by selective eruption of teeth are not desired. The treatment objective is expansion using an appliance stabilized by intermaxillary relationships (Figure 8-32).

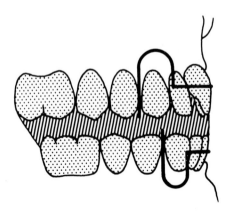

**Figure 8-31.** Activator with vertical opening only and no anterior positioning of the mandible.

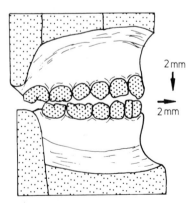

**Figure 8-32.** Construction bite with slight forward–downward positioning of the mandible.

The force application from this type of appliance is reciprocal, an advantage in situations in which the demands are usually bilateral (Figure 8-33). With the same appliance a reciprocal force also can be developed in the sagittal plane. If the incisors are lingually inclined and the molars must be moved distally to increase arch length, the protrusive force loading the incisors can be directed onto the stabilizing wires that fit in the contact embrasures, producing a molar distalization response.

An example is shown in Figure 8-34, a 9-year-old girl with a retrognathic face but a balanced skeletal pattern and an A-N-B angle of only 2 degrees. The length of the mandibular base was slightly deficient, about 3 mm below average in relation to the cranial base. (A deficiency of 3 mm at this age does not indicate a significant growth deficiency.) The maxillary base was 41 mm, but greater growth increments could be expected in this area. The growth direction was assessed as hor-

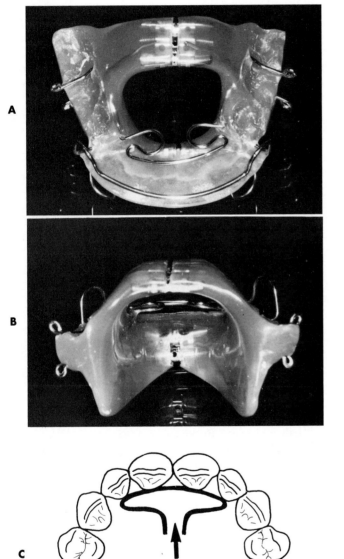

**Figure 8-33.** Activator with two jackscrews. **A** and **B,** Frontal and oral views. **C,** Reciprocal effectiveness in the sagittal and transverse planes.

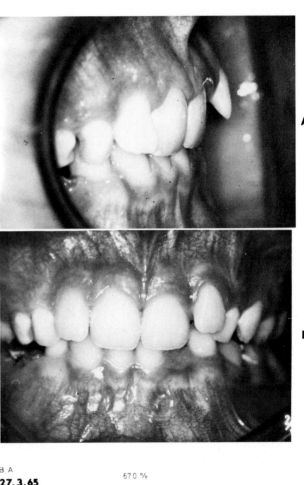

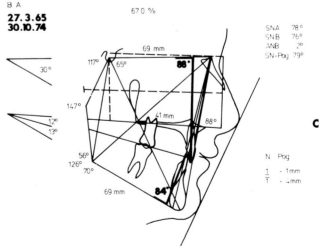

**Figure 8-34.** Before treatment, 9-year-old patient. **A** and **B,** Lateral and frontal views. **C,** Tracing.

izontal. The overbite was not extremely deep, and a slight compensation in the vertical relationship stemming from the small forward inclination of the maxillary base was noted. The upper and lower incisors were tipped lingually. A crowding condition existed in both dental arches, with an overall pattern of Class II, division 2–type problems as indicated by the position of the upper incisors and the Class II molar relationship.

Diagnostic records indicated that expansion of the dental arches transversely and sagittally was therapeutically desirable. Because exfoliation of deciduous teeth in the buccal seg-

ments would be a future problem, perhaps accelerated by a conventional expansion plate, an activator was recommended. Another reason for activator treatment was the sagittal malrelationship. Because the vertical dimension was essentially normal, only a slight opening of the construction bite was made for the activator.

The objective of treatment in this case was not to activate the muscles and contiguous soft tissues but to provide sufficient long-term anchorage to accomplish the arch width and length expansion. Hence the force enlisted did not come from the muscles but was provided by two expansion screws in the transverse direction with maxillary lingual protrusion springs and stabilizing wires in the anteroposterior dimension. Allowing the acrylic to contact the lower incisors on the lingual created the labial tipping of the lower incisors. The upper and lower labial bows did not contact the teeth but helped eliminate labial tissue strain and assisted in labial movement of the anterior teeth by force elimination similar to that of the lip pads used on the Fränkel appliance.

The treatment, active until the eruption of the permanent teeth, improved the retrognathic profile. The growth rate for the maxillary base was high. Posttreatment measurements showed normal proportional relations between the maxillary and mandibular bases and the cranial base. The horizontal growth pattern and inclination of the maxillary base were not altered. The axial inclinations of the upper and lower incisors were improved, and the Class II relationship was corrected. The primary objective of correcting the crowding with transverse and sagittal expansion was accomplished (Figure 8-35).

## Construction Bite with Opening and Posterior Positioning of the Mandible

The construction bite's sagittal change depends on the malocclusion category and treatment objectives. In Class III the goal is a posterior positioning of the mandible or maxillary protraction. The construction bite is taken by retruding the lower jaw (Figure 8-36). The extent of the vertical opening depends on the retrusion possible.

**Tooth guidance or functional protrusion Class III malocclusions.** The assessment of a possible forced bite is relatively easy. The mandibular incisors approximate prematurely in an end-to-end contact, and the mandible slides anteriorly to complete the occlusal relationship. The vertical dimension is opened far enough to clear the incisal guidance for the construction bite. This eliminates the protrusive relationship with the mandible in centric relation. An edge-to-edge bite relationship can be achieved with the posterior teeth still out of contact.

The prognosis for pseudo–Class III malocclusions is good, especially if therapy begins in early mixed dentition. At this stage the skeletal manifestations are not usually severe; the malocclusion develops progressively. If holding the mandible in a posterior position and guiding the maxillary incisors into correct labial relationships are possible, a good incisal guidance can be established. If done in early mixed dentition, the maxilla adapts to the prognathic mandible, creating a balance.

An example of this type of situation is shown in Figure 8-37, a 7-year-old boy with the maxillary incisors already

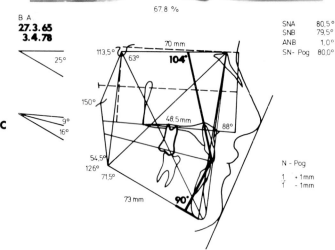

**Figure 8-35.** After treatment, same patient as in Figure 8-34. **A** and **B**, Lateral and frontal views. **C**, Tracing.

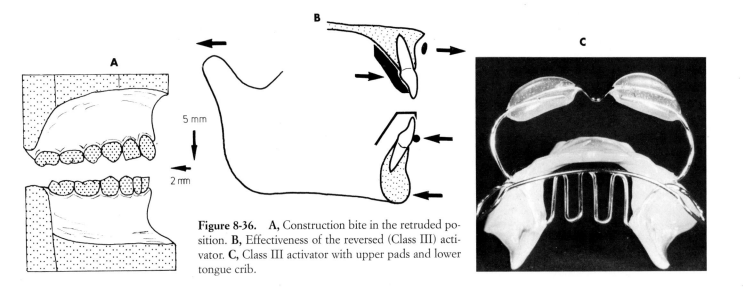

**Figure 8-36.** **A,** Construction bite in the retruded position. **B,** Effectiveness of the reversed (Class III) activator. **C,** Class III activator with upper pads and lower tongue crib.

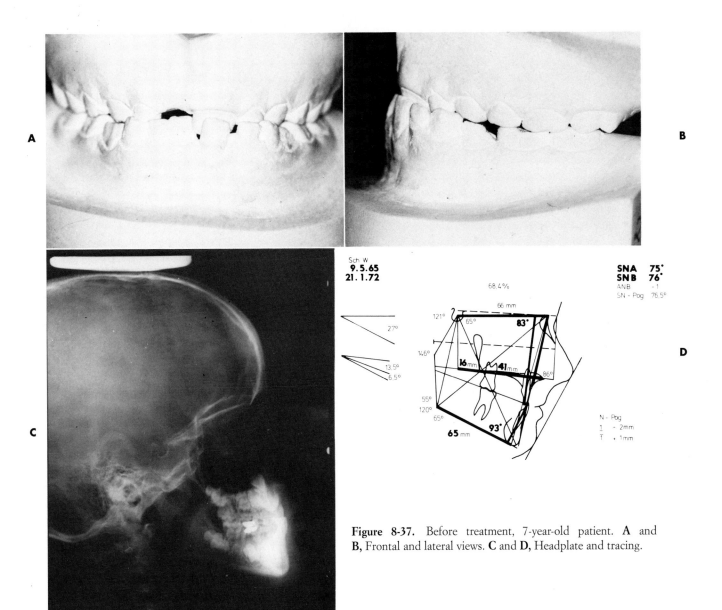

**Figure 8-37.** Before treatment, 7-year-old patient. **A** and **B,** Frontal and lateral views. **C** and **D,** Headplate and tracing.

erupted in a lingual crossbite relationship. The profile was retrognathic and the jaw bases short. The A-N-B angle was −1 degree. As might be expected, the growth pattern was horizontal and the gonial angle extremely small. The maxillary incisors were tipped lingually, a favorable characteristic in Class III therapy.

Therapy consisted of the activator rocking open the mandible to a more posterior position, allowing the condyle to drop back in the fossa. At the same time the maxillary incisors were tipped labially to provide the proper incisal guidance. Concurrently, force was eliminated in the upper arch with maxillary lip pads to allow the fullest extent of the growth potential in this seemingly deficient area during the eruption of the incisors. The construction bite was opened only 3 mm to permit retrusion of the mandible to an edge-to-edge incisal contact. The mandible was held in this posterior position with the labial bow and an acrylic cap on the lower anterior segment. The acrylic was relieved on the lingual of the lower incisors, and the maxillary incisors were supported with close contact.

During treatment, posterior positioning of the mandible could be observed. The S-N-A angle increased, and the A-N-B angle changed to + 2 degrees. The articular angle increased because of the posterior positioning of the mandible. The mandibular plane opened slightly, and the maxillary incisors were tipped labially (Figure 8-38).

**Skeletal Class III malocclusion with a normal path of closure from postural rest to habitual occlusion.** Treatment with functional appliances is not always possible or desirable. The opening of the vertical dimension for the construction bite depends on the possibility of achieving an end-to-end incisal relationship. If the overjet is large, the construction bite requires a larger opening. Indications for functional treatment of true Class III problems are limited. Usually only combined therapy such as with fixed and removable appliances and maxillary or-

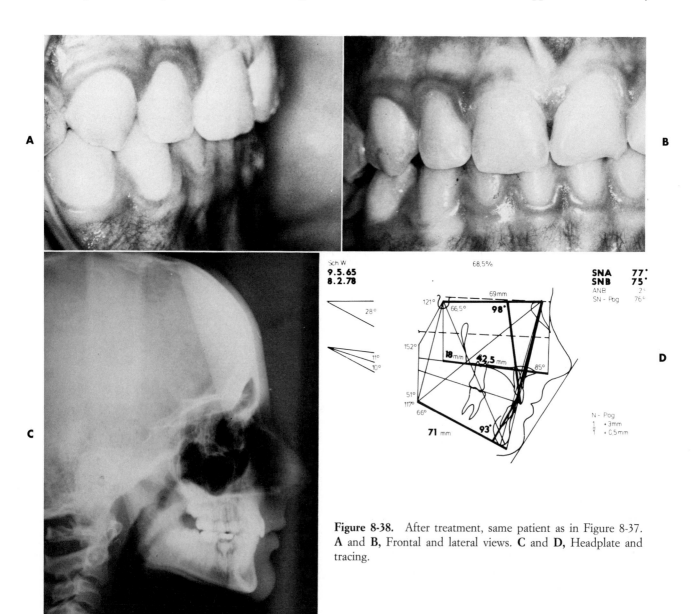

**Figure 8-38.** After treatment, same patient as in Figure 8-37. **A** and **B**, Frontal and lateral views. **C** and **D**, Headplate and tracing.

thopedic protraction is likely to be successful. Even then, orthognathic surgery is always possible to achieve proper sagittal and transverse relationships. However, if treatment is initiated in the early mixed dentition, improvement can be achieved. If the bite can be opened and incisal guidance established, adaptation of the maxillary base to the prognathic mandible can be expected to a certain degree. Correct incisal guidance prevents anterior displacement of the mandible during treatment.

An illustration of the type of case that responds to activator guidance is shown in Figure 8-39. The patient was a 7-year-old boy. The profile was retrognathic, with a midface concavity. The maxilla was small and retrognathic; the mandible, of normal size. The A-N-B angle was − 3 degrees in habitual occlusion. The path of closure was normal, with no anterior tooth guidance. Cephalometric analysis indicated an average growth pattern. Both maxillary and mandibular incisors were lingually tipped. Assessment showed that this was a true Class III, with the major problem being a deficient maxilla.

Therapy was started with an activator. The bite was opened, and establishing an end-to-end bite relationship was then possible. This required a 5 mm open construction bite. The acrylic portion of the appliance contacted the maxillary incisors to move them labially. As noted in the cephalometric analysis, the original axial inclination was favorable for labial tipping. Lip pads were placed in the vestibular region to stimulate all apical base improvement possible in the maxilla. The lower incisors were held with a labial bow and acrylic cap. Lingual tipping of these incisors was not considered necessary, although the inclination was not ideal. The buds of the lower first premolars were removed to assist in the compensation with a potential dentoalveolar adaptation.

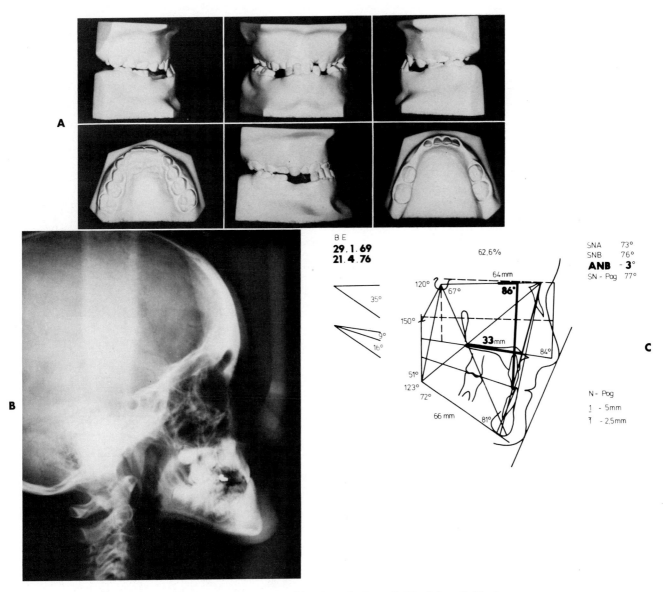

**Figure 8-39.** Before treatment, 7-year-old patient. **A,** Casts. **B,** Headplate. **C,** Tracing.

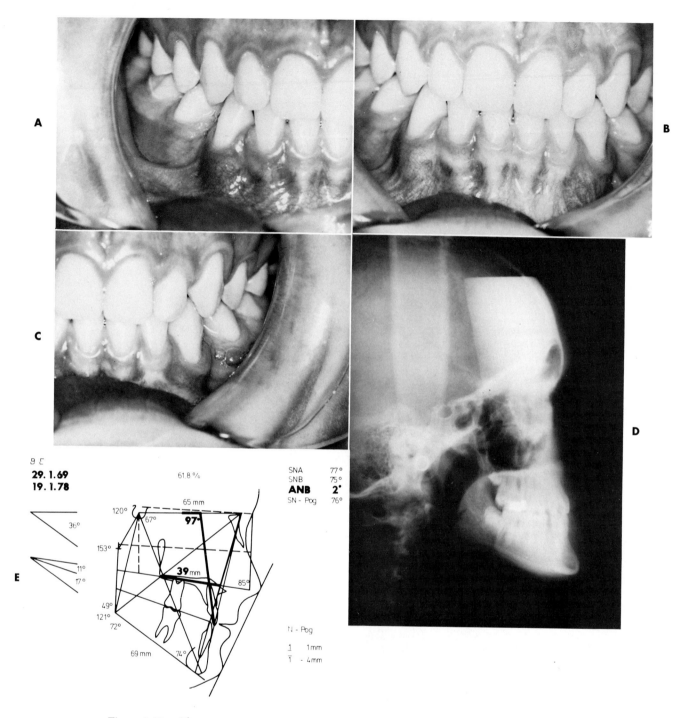

**Figure 8-40.** After treatment, same patient as in Figure 8-39. **A** to **C,** Frontal and lateral views. **D** and **E,** Headplate and tracing.

After 1 ½ years of treatment, definite posterior positioning of the mandible and stimulation of the maxillary apical base were evident. Before treatment the maxillary base had been 11 mm too short in relation to the mandibular base. After this first phase of activator guidance, the discrepancy was reduced to 5 mm. The A-N-B angle was improved by 2 degrees. The upper incisors were tipped labially, and the lower incisors were markedly lingual (probably as a result of the enucleation of the lower first premolars). When permanent tooth eruption occurred, the treatment objective was to close spaces in the lower arch with fixed appliances, lingual root torque on the lower incisors, and other methods (Figure 8-40).

As important as the proper construction bite registration is, the full effectiveness of the activator can be achieved only with proper trimming of the acrylic at the appropriate time. The details of trimming are discussed in Chapter 9.

# Chapter 9

# Fabrication and Management of the Activator

Thomas Rakosi

## PREPARATION

Several preliminary steps are required before the conventional activator appliance is constructed. After the construction bite is taken, evaluated on the patient, and rechecked on the working models, the working models are mounted on a fixator. Some clinicians prefer to send the models and wax bite separately to the laboratory and allow the technician to mount the models. However, if the models and wax bite are shipped in the construction bite on the fixator, damage to or deformation of the bite is less likely to occur in transit. Because the mounting of the models is a critical step in the fabrication process, great care must be taken to safeguard the construction bite.

The design of the appliance is dictated by a series of diagnostic measurements and decisions. The different categories of Class II malocclusion as determined by cephalometric and functional analyses demand structural modifications in the activator for their treatment. Proper fabrication of the appliance saves chair time and helps ensure greater patient compliance.

The fabrication of the activator demands proper communication with the technical laboratory. The extension of the acrylic body and flanges is drawn on the upper and lower working models with an indelible pencil. The wire elements also should be drawn on the models. A detailed prescription form is then filled out for the laboratory technician; these forms are supplied by most laboratories, which are anxious to ensure the appliance is made properly and works correctly. A detailed drawing of the construction can be made separately or rendered on the diagram provided by the laboratory. If the appliance is complicated, this is an important step (Figure 9-1). The working models, bite, and fixator should be wrapped in foam rubber for their protection during shipping.

## LABORATORY PROCEDURES

The activator consists of a combination of acrylic and wire components. An important part of the fabrication process is the accurate transfer of the construction bite onto the activator. Despite all the technical advances in materials (e.g., rapid-set, self-curing acrylics; soft acrylics; good separating media; ad-

vanced wire formulas) the success or failure of an appliance often depends on the accurate replication of the clinically determined correct sagittal and vertical posturing of the mandible. More appliance failures are caused by improper construction bites and improper fabrication than any other cause.

If the clinician has not already mounted the working models in the construction bite and placed them on the fixator, this should be the technician's first step. If any doubt arises that the relationship is correct, the technician should call the referring doctor, discuss the problem, and possibly make arrangements for a new construction bite to be taken. The fixator (Figure 9-2) allows the upper and lower parts of the activator to be made separately; both parts can later be united in the correct construction bite.

### Preparation of the Wire Elements

After mounting the casts, reading the detailed instructions on the prescription, and checking the markings on the casts, the technician bends the wire elements. The usual design for the conventional activator requires an upper and lower labial bow.

**Labial bow.** The primary wire elements of the activator are the upper and lower labial bows. They consist of horizontal middle sections, two vertical loops, and wire extensions through the canine–deciduous first molar embrasure into the acrylic body. The horizontal section contacts the labial surfaces of the four incisors. Depending on the vertical dimension (deep overbite or anterior open bite), the wire crosses the incisors above or below the area of greatest convexity (Figure 9-3). The bow can be either passive or active depending on the prescription. The passive labial bow influences the soft tissues without touching the teeth, similar to the action of screening appliances.

The vertical U-shaped loops of the upper labial bow start with a 90-degree bend at the lateral incisor–canine embrasure, form gentle continuous curves above the gingival margin, and pass freely through the canine–first deciduous molar or premolar embrasures to anchor in the lingual acrylic. The wire approximates the mesial marginal ridge of the first deciduous molars in case it is needed to exert a distalization force vector on these teeth (Figure 9-4).

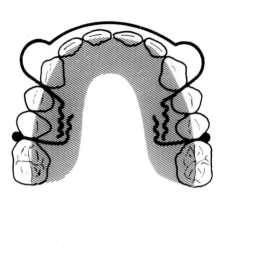

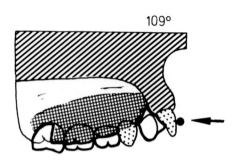

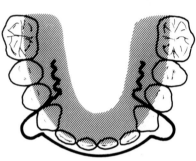

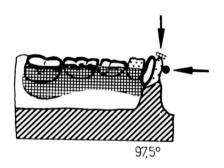

**Figure 9-1.** Construction diagram of the activator.

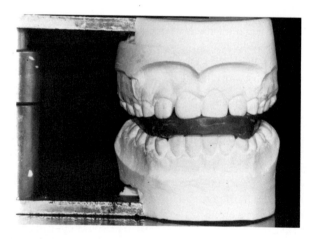

**Figure 9-2.** The casts are trimmed in the construction bite relationship on the fixator and mounted sideways.

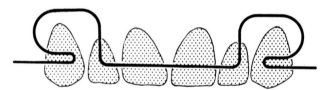

**Figure 9-3.** Labial bow with loops for the canines; the bow contacts the incisors in the incisal third.

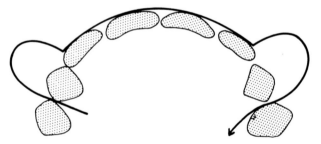

**Figure 9-4.** Labial bow activated for distal driving of the premolars (right).

The lower labial bow is similar in configuration to the upper. However, the middle horizontal portion is longer because the bend for the vertical loops starts more distally in the mesial third of the canines. The wire returns in the canine–decidous first molar or premolar embrasure, making the U-shaped vertical loop somewhat narrower.

The gauge of the wire is different for active and passive labial bows. For the active bow the spring-hardened type of stainless steel wire is 0.9 mm thick; for the passive bow, it is only 0.8 mm thick.

**Additional elements.** Depending on the prescription, additional spurs or elements may be required. These elements are formed during preparation of the wire elements. (The needs and designs of these wire elements are described in Chapter 8.)

## Fixation of the Jackscrews and Wire Elements

The jackscrews are first attached to the cast. The magnitude of the required opening is determined according to palatal configuration and type of malocclusion. A groove must be sawed in the midline of appliances with screws in the up-

per and lower casts. Screws are affixed in this groove with sticky wax (Figure 9-5). The wire elements are then fixed on the labial surfaces of the teeth. The areas that are to be free of acrylic are isolated with a layer of wax.

## Fabrication of the Acrylic Portion

The activator consists of upper, lower, and interocclusal parts (Figure 9-6). In the upper and lower parts the dental and gingival portions can be differentiated; the gingival portion can be extended posteriorly (especially in the lower cast). If the construction bite is high, as it is in a vertical activator, the extension of the flanges is greater than for a horizontal type of activator that positions the mandible more anteriorly. This extension is important to enhance the retention of the appliance (particularly for the vertical activator) because patients requiring this type of appliance habitually have open mouth postures (Figure 9-7).

The flanges for the upper part are 8 to 12 mm high in the gingival area and cover the alveolar crest. The palate is not

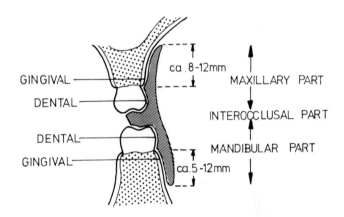

**Figure 9-6.** Acrylic parts of the activator.

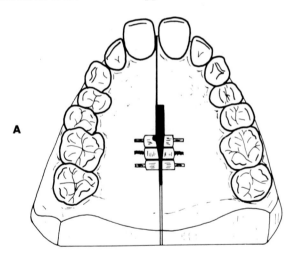

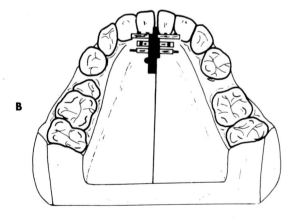

**Figure 9-5.** Jackscrews fixed on the casts in the upper (**A**) and lower (**B**) arch.

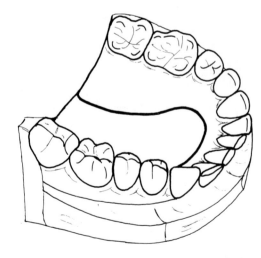

**Figure 9-7.** Lingual extension of the appliance in the lower molar region.

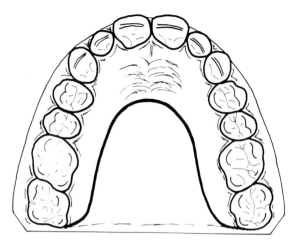

**Figure 9-8.** Limits of the appliance's base acrylic in the upper jaw.

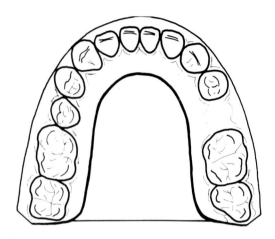

**Figure 9-9.** Limits of the appliance in the lower jaw.

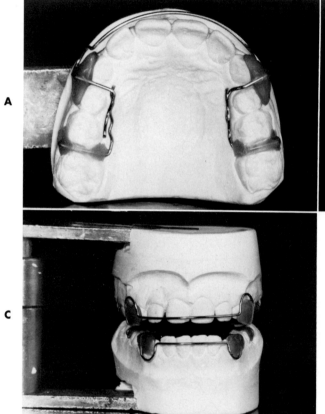

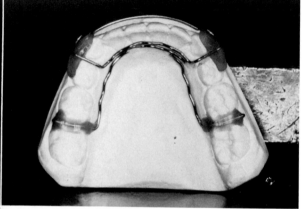

**Figure 9-10. A,** Upper cast prepared with wire elements. **B,** Lower cast prepared with wire elements. **C,** Casts with wire elements in the fixator prepared for molding the acrylics.

covered (Figure 9-8). If the acrylic plate is thin, it does not encroach on the tongue space; however, acrylic that is too thin may cause excessive appliance flexibility. A palatal bar may be used to increase rigidity. The bar is similar to that used in the standard bionator appliance and is constructed of 1.2-mm thick stainless steel. It is used only for appliance stabilization. The lower acrylic plate is generally 5 to 10 mm wide, although it is sometimes wider in the molar area, with flanges of 10 to 15 mm (Figure 9-9).

Appliance fabrication is almost always performed by tech-

nicians; nevertheless, a brief outline is given here of the acrylic fabrication technique:

1. Before the acrylic portion is constructed, the casts are placed in a water bath for 20 minutes, dried, and isolated.
2. After the wire elements have been fixed and the acrylic-free areas covered with baseplate wax, the upper and lower portions are molded from self-curing acrylic.
3. The casts are placed on the fixator, and the upper and

lower portions are joined with endothermic acrylic at the interdental area (Figure 9-10).

4. The Dentaurum fixator allows simultaneous acrylic application in the interocclusal part from both lingual and buccal sides.

5. After polymerization the appliance is ground and polished. It is not trimmed in the laboratory; any necessary trimming for specific tooth guidance is done later by the clinician with the patient in the chair.

6. The appliance is shipped to the clinician with a copy of the original prescription.

## MANAGEMENT OF THE APPLIANCE

After the appliance has been returned and checked to ensure the instructions were followed, a trimming plan is developed; each grinding procedure needed and the expected movement are noted in the diagnostic record. Trimming is done with the patient in the chair, which permits frequent spot checks to assess whether the acrylic guide planes are functioning as desired. Some clinicians prefer that the patient wear the appliance for a week with no grinding to allow the patient to get used to it. The trimming plan is then implemented according to the written outline.

The importance of communication with patients and guardians cannot be overemphasized. Time spent in establishing a high level of patient compliance is well spent. Videotapes, demonstrations, and patient information booklets are all beneficial. Most important, however, is the doctor-patient relationship and the sincere interest and enthusiasm of all staff members in maintaining a high level of patient motivation during treatment.

The patient must know the way to place the appliance in the mouth before leaving the office. The appliance is usually worn 2 or 3 hours during the day for the first week. During the second week the patient sleeps with the appliance in place and wears it 1 to 3 hours each day. The appliance is checked by the clinician after 3 weeks to evaluate whether the trimming is accurate and the activator is working as desired. Guide plane contact areas are usually shiny if they are functioning properly; they can be reshaped and corrected as needed. If the patient has difficulty wearing the appliance for the whole night, more daytime wear is required to compensate until full nighttime wear is routine. The sealing or addition of self-curing soft acrylic to the lower flanges sometimes improves retention during the early accommodative stages.

If the patient is wearing the activator without difficulty and following instructions, checkup appointments should be scheduled every 6 weeks. During these office visits the clinician should maintain rapport with the patient, reinforce motivation, and perform the following procedures:

1. All guide planes that have been ground and all areas in contact with the teeth should be observed for shiny surfaces that indicate whether the appliance is being worn correctly and is working properly.

2. Reshaping of acrylic guide areas may be required after initial trimming to improve function; it also may be needed during the course of treatment to ensure continued tooth movement (particularly in the upper arch) if retrusion or distalization is desired. Maxillary change is usually minimal at best, however. If the permanent teeth are erupting, reshaping also may be necessary.

3. Acrylic contact guide planes often must be resealed or recontoured to maintain the proper functional activation on the desired teeth by adding self-curing soft acrylic in a thin layer. Clinical examination of the acrylic inclined planes for shiny spots helps determine the amount of sealing to be done.

4. The labial bows and any additional wire elements must be checked for action and possible deformation. Constant motion of the appliance in the mouth may change wire configurations and occasionally fatigues wires sufficiently to cause fracture. The active bow should touch the teeth. The passive bow should position away from the teeth but remain in contact with the soft tissues. The guiding and stabilizing wires are activated by the patient's biting into the appliance.

5. The lip pads should be checked for possible irritation in the sulcus area. They may require reshaping. They should not contact the alveolar process or teeth.

6. In expansion treatment the jackscrews are normally activated by the patient at 2-week intervals. The clinician should check this activation for too-frequent or infrequent activation. Too much activation prevents the appliance from fitting properly. The activation interval may need to be changed.

7. The construction bite position may require occasional alteration. This can be performed by various methods:

   a. In the direct method an acrylic layer is ground away on the dental surface of the lower plate and new self-curing acrylic is added to position the mandible as desired. This method is required if the clinician chooses to advance the mandible in steps instead of all at once.

   b. In the indirect method, new impressions are taken, a new construction bite is made, and the casts are mounted in the laboratory. Acrylic modification is performed on the newly mounted casts on the fixator.

   c. The upper and lower portions of the activator can be separated interocclusally and then rejoined in the new construction bite position by endothermic acrylic.

# Chapter 10

# Trimming of the Activator

Thomas Rakosi

## PRINCIPLES OF THERAPEUTIC TRIMMING FOR TOOTH GUIDANCE

In activator therapy, stimulation of the functional activity of the perioral musculature with loose appliances to guide the movement and eruption of selected teeth can best be achieved by grinding away areas of the acrylic that contact the teeth. After the activator has been fabricated in the laboratory, it is placed in the patient's mouth to assess the fit and correctness of the construction bite. Normally the acrylic is interposed between the upper and lower occlusal surfaces of the buccal segments and provides a negative reproduction of tooth surface anatomy. If forward posturing alone is desired, a tightly fitting appliance serves as a handle on the dentition to hold the mandible in the planned protraction. However, merely holding the mandible in a forward position is not adequate to achieve the proper relationship of teeth in three dimensions. Selective guidance of the eruption of teeth and development of arch form is necessary, as are the elimination of all functional retrusive muscle activity and the encouragement of the best possible condylar growth adaptation to a more correct sagittal relationship. Carefully planned grinding and trimming of the activator in the tooth contact area improves its effectiveness in the dentoalveolar region. Trimming should help achieve a loosely fitting appliance that is manipulable by the patient but maintains the correct sagittal relationship while stimulating or restricting selective eruption and movement of anterior and posterior teeth.

The principles of force application in the trimming process are determined by the type, direction, and magnitude of force created by the loosely fitting activator:

1. Intermittent force application allows dynamic and rhythmic muscle forces to act in concert; the appliance thus works by kinetic energy.
2. The direction of the desired force is determined by selective grinding of the acrylic surfaces that contact the upper and lower teeth. After proper grinding the desired force acts on predetermined areas of the teeth and applies pressure in the direction of needed tooth movement. Any surfaces that might impede this movement are relieved or cut away.
3. The magnitude of the force delivered can be estimated by determining the amount of acrylic contact with the tooth surfaces. If the force is delivered to a small portion of the tooth surface, it is greater than if broad contact occurs between the acrylic and a larger tooth surface. Acrylic surfaces that transmit the desired intermittent force and contact the teeth are called *guide planes.*
4. After the activator has been carefully evaluated for proper fit in the patient's mouth, an exact plan of required tooth movement is developed. Approximate trimming can be done on the plaster casts, but the final grinding must be done in the mouth. Any undercut acrylic surfaces that might interfere with planned tooth guidance must be removed. The need for trimming can be assessed with an explorer (Figure 10-1) or by observing the shadows created on the acrylic by undercut surfaces (Figure 10-2). Because some adjustment and "give" should be expected during appliance wear in the first couple of weeks, final trimming is not done until the second visit (in most cases) to achieve the best possible efficiency. The acrylic areas that contact the teeth are likely to become polished and shiny; the area of force delivery can thus be well identified. Careful grinding can be performed to direct the force more accurately.

Because of the variability of behavioral activity and difference in maturity levels, the grinding procedure is sometimes varied. Because a tightly fitting appliance adapted to the teeth is more easily accommodated in the early stages, the first stage of trimming usually does not fully establish the loose functional fit desired. A few contacts are left to stabilize the appliance until the patient adjusts. Then the remainder of the planned trimming is done on the second or third visit. This gives the patient time to adjust to the forward posturing of the mandible; the loose appliance is more acceptable but still protracts the mandible. If expansion is needed to correct a very narrow maxillary arch, the appliance may be squeezed between the buccal segments, exerting light force for the whole treatment period as expansion occurs.

Trimming should be done in stepwise progression. Single tooth movements are analyzed to assess their compatibility with the contiguous teeth. The planned grinding procedure is written and each trimming procedure is noted as it is performed. Through systematic and careful therapy, tooth movement in vertical, sagittal, and transverse directions is possible.

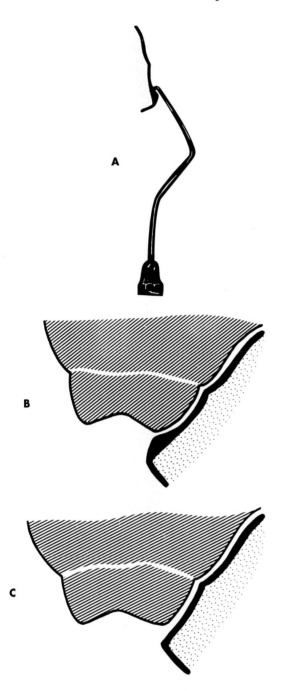

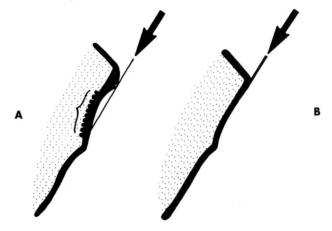

**Figure 10-2.** Shadow test. **A,** Before trimming. **B,** After trimming.

## Intrusion of Teeth

Intrusion of incisors can be achieved by loading the incisal edges of these teeth (Figure 10-3). If they are ground properly, they become the only loaded or contacting surfaces, with no other contact between the incisors and acrylic, even in the alveolar area. If the simultaneous use of an active labial bow is indicated, the contact between the bow wire and incisors is below the area of greatest convexity or on the incisal third (Figure 10-4). This location does not interfere with intrusive movement of the incisors and may actually stimulate it. Such intrusive loading is indicated in deep overbite cases.

Intrusion of molars is performed by loading only the cusps of these teeth (Figure 10-5). The acrylic detail is ground away from the fossas and fissures to eliminate any possible inclined-plane (oblique) stimulus to molar movement if only a vertical depressing action is desired. This allows the activator to deliver greater forces. If larger occlusal surfaces are loaded, reflex mouth opening occurs more frequently, resulting in less effective depressing action by the appliance. Molar depression and loading are indicated in open-bite problems if minimal or nonexistent interocclusal clearance is apparent.

## Extrusion of Teeth

Extrusion of incisors requires loading their lingual surfaces above the area of greatest concavity in the maxilla and below this area in the mandible. Although extrusion generally is not very effective because of dental anatomy, it can be enhanced nonetheless by placing the labial bow above the area of greatest convexity (Figure 10-6). Such extrusion modifications are indicated for open-bite problems, particularly those caused by chronic finger sucking in which the incisors are relatively intruded.

Extrusion of molars can be facilitated by loading the lingual surfaces of these teeth above the area of greatest convexity in the maxilla or below this area in the mandible (Figure 10-7). Molar and premolar extrusion is indicated in deep-bite problems. The trimming of the activator for molar extrusion can be performed at the same time for all molars. Dental an-

**Figure 10-1.** Evaluating activator trimming. **A,** Evaluation with an explorer. **B,** Undercut surface in the acrylic. **C,** Acrylic surface after trimming.

## TRIMMING THE ACTIVATOR FOR VERTICAL CONTROL

Two movements occur in activator therapy—intrusion and extrusion. The activator provides only limited intrusion; some teeth are selectively prevented from erupting, whereas others are free to erupt and are stimulated to do so by acrylic planes. Selective extrusion in the mixed dentition is an important and valid treatment objective that can affect both vertical and horizontal tooth relationships if done properly.

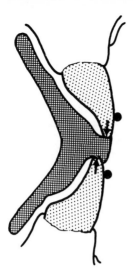

**Figure 10-3.** Intrusion of the incisors through acrylic capping.

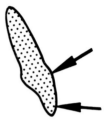

**Figure 10-4.** Labial bow position for intrusion (incisal third) or extrusion (gingival third) of the incisors.

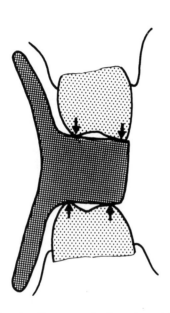

**Figure 10-5.** Acrylic contact for intrusion of the molars.

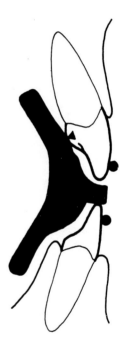

**Figure 10-6.** Extrusion of the upper incisors through placement of the labial bow below the area of greatest convexity.

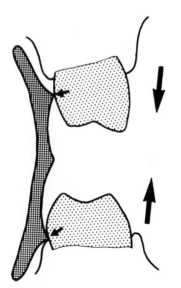

**Figure 10-7.** Acrylic contour for extrusion of the molars.

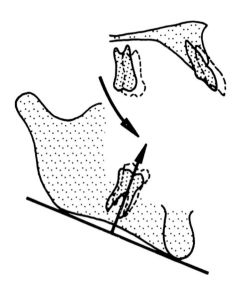

**Figure 10-8.** The eruption pathway of the molars should be considered in selective trimming.

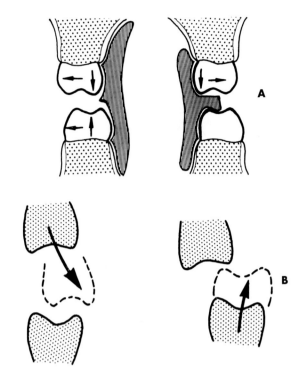

**Figure 10-9.** Selective trimming. **A,** Both molars are extruded simultaneously (*left*); only the upper molar is extruded (*right*). **B,** Selective eruption of the upper molars for correction of a Class III relationship (*left*); selective eruption of the lower molars for correction of a Class II relationship (*right*).

choring of the appliance is unnecessary because it is sufficiently stabilized in the alveolar regions by the acrylic extensions. Simultaneous extrusion of the buccal segment teeth in the upper and lower jaws does not allow adequate control. The teeth can overerupt and move mesially. The subsequent reduction of the deep bite may be more rapid but less desirable from a sagittal point of view. As Balters has recommended for the trimming of the bionator and Clark has suggested for the twin block, controlled differential eruption guidance must be employed for the best interdental and occlusal plane relationships. Particularly in the case of a flush terminal plane relationship, proper selective grinding can convert an impending Class II or III malocclusion into a Class I interdigitation.

## Selective Trimming of the Activator

During selective trimming procedures, only the upper or lower molars are extruded. After these teeth have erupted sufficiently, the eruption of the antagonists can be controlled. Thus both sagittal and vertical relationships can be influenced.

If selective grinding is being planned, the path of eruption of the molars must be considered. The lower molars erupt in an upward and slightly forward direction; the upper molars erupt down and forward and display a greater mesial migration component if left unattended (Figure 10-8). If the eruption of the maxillary molars is inhibited and the eruption of the mandibular molars is stimulated in Class II malocclusions, the upper molars remain in their mesiodistal position with respect to the basal structures but the lower molars improve their sagittal relationship (Figure 10-9). This phenomenon is particularly important in flush terminal plane relationships in which an end-to-end bite exists until the deciduous molars are shed and the differential migration to fill the leeway space is completed. The resultant improvement of sagittal relationships through differential eruption and the maintenance of

the upper molars in a distal relationship can cause a mandibular vertical rotation that initially accentuates the mandibular retrognathism. This result can be useful, however, in cases with horizontal mandibular growth directions and deep overbites. In cases with vertical growth patterns and tendencies to open bite, the distal position of the molars can be altered before final eruption. After the lower molars have erupted, the distal surfaces of the upper second deciduous molars may be sliced, permitting the upper molars to migrate slightly to the mesial, closing the bite and reducing the mandibular retrognathism; care must be taken not to create a Class II malocclusion in the process.

If eruption of the upper molars is stimulated and lower molar eruption is inhibited, the upper molars move mesially. This reaction can be used to help correct relatively mild Class III malocclusions. The mesial positioning of the upper molars results in a closing of the bite and a more horizontal growth vector, which is not favorable in most Class III malocclusions. For vertical growth patterns and open-bite cases, however, this phenomenon is favorable because the alveolodental compensation reduces the apparent dysplasia. Distal driving of the upper molars (with a Kloehn headgear) opens the bite more; more vertical eruption of upper molars also can be elicited if desired. In such cases, mesial movement is impeded by spurs from the acrylic body of the appliance.

More sophisticated methods of trimming can be used to control not only eruption of the molars but also the dental anchorage of the appliance. Dental anchorage assumes greater importance in modifications of the activator as acrylic bulk is reduced in the alveolar and palatal regions. (The method of trimming these skeletonized activators is described in Chapter 11.)

## TRIMMING THE ACTIVATOR FOR SAGITTAL CONTROL

Specific goals of protruding or retruding the incisors and changing the molar sagittal relationship mesially or distally can be achieved through judicious appliance control. Protrusion and retrusion of incisors can be accomplished only through grinding of the acrylic and guide planes and adjustment of the labial bow wires. If the labial bow touches the teeth, it can either tip them lingually or retain them in posi-

tion. In these cases, it is called an *active bow*. If it is positioned away from the teeth and prevents soft tissue contact, it is termed a *passive bow* (Figure 10-10).

The active bow may contact the incisors on the gingival third of their labial surfaces to promote extrusion in open-bite cases or may contact the incisal third to inhibit extrusion in deep overbite cases. Bow placement may be either gingival (to reduce tipping while lingualizing these teeth) or incisal (to accentuate tipping of severely protruded incisor crowns if adequate space is available) in incisor retrusion. Thus the axial in-

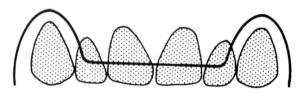

**Figure 10-10.** Upper labial bow.

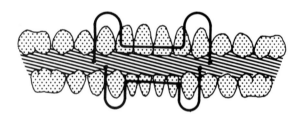

**Figure 10-11.** Upper and lower labial bows.

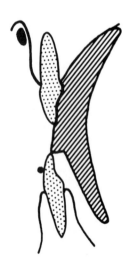

**Figure 10-12.** Placement of lip pads in the upper labial fold for a Class III malocclusion.

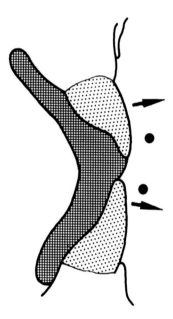

**Figure 10-13.** Protrusion of the incisors through loading of the whole lingual surface.

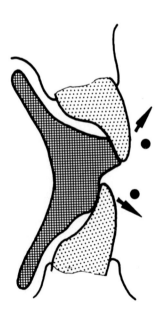

**Figure 10-14.** Labial tipping of the incisors through loading of the incisal third of the lingual surfaces.

clination of the incisors is subject to some control. The labial bow does not work as a spring force, however. It is fabricated from a relatively thick (0.9 mm) wire and activated only when the mandible closes in the construction bite position. All wire modifications in the activator are of a thick nonspring construction and work according to the same principle.

By relieving the pressures and muscle strains placed on the dentition by the lips and checks, the passive bow permits labial and buccal movement of selected teeth. The conventional activator in which the bow does not extend distally to the canines primarily permits labial tipping or holding of the maxillary and mandibular incisors. Some appliances are therefore constructed with an upper and a lower labial bow (Figure 10-11). The only exception is the Class III activator, which has lip pads similar to those of the Fränkel appliance instead of a labial bow (Figure 10-12).

## Protrusion of Incisors

The incisors can be protruded by loading their lingual surfaces with acrylic contact and screening away the lip strain with a passive labial bow or lip pads. Loading can be achieved by either of two methods:

1. The entire lingual surface is loaded (Figure 10-13). Only the interdental acrylic projections are trimmed to avoid opening spaces between the teeth. This method allows the incisors to be moved labially with a low magnitude of force because the applied force is spread over a large surface. Some tipping can be expected despite total acrylic contact in the beginning of treatment.

2. The incisal third of the lingual surface is loaded (Figure 10-14). This variation results in labial tipping of the incisors with a greater degree of force because the contact surface is small. If the incisal third is loaded, the axis of rotation is closer to the apex of the incisors.

Incisor protrusion also can be accomplished using auxiliary elements:

1. *Protrusion springs*   Continuous or closed springs of fairly heavy wire (0.8 mm) are activated only when the teeth are closed into the appliance (Figure 10-15).
2. *Wooden pegs*   Small wooden pegs are inserted with minimal projection into the lingual acrylic. The wood swells when wet; the pegs thus project more and exert a small amount of increased force when the teeth are fully seated in the activator (Figure 10-16). The protrusion springs or wooden sticks usually contact the incisors in the middle or gingival third of the lingual surfaces (Figure 10-17). The labially tipped incisors can then be partially uprighted by an active labial bow that contacts the incisors at their incisal third. However, significant torque and bodily movement are not possible with an activator.
3. *Guttapercha*   Guttapercha may be added to the lingual acrylic; however, this traditional approach has been superseded by the use of thin layers of soft acrylic applied where desired. The self-curing acrylics (e.g., Coe-Soft) are ideal for use not only behind the teeth but also in the alveolar crest portion. They also may be used in moving the maxillary centrals and supporting alveolar bone labially as the permanent teeth erupt in Class III malocclusions.

## Retrusion of Incisors

The acrylic is trimmed away from the backs of the incisors to be retruded. The active labial bow, which contacts the teeth during functional movements, provides the force for moving these teeth.

The acrylic can be completely ground away from behind the incisors and alveolar process (Figure 10-18). If the labial bow touches the teeth in the incisal margin region, the center

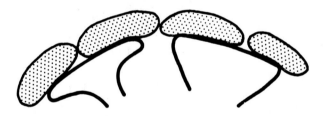

**Figure 10-15.** Protrusion springs for labial tipping of the incisors.

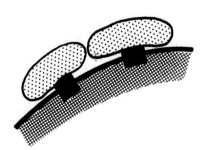

**Figure 10-16.** Protrusion of the incisors using wooden sticks.

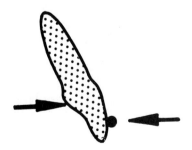

**Figure 10-17.** If the protrusion spring is placed gingivally, the labially tipped incisor can be uprighted with an incisally placed labial bow.

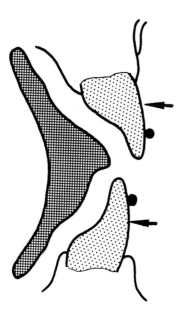 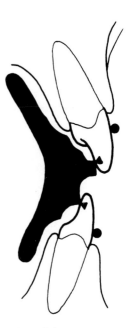

**Figure 10-18.** Retrusion of the incisors can be achieved by grinding the acrylic away from the backs of these teeth.

**Figure 10-19.** Retrusion of the incisors can be encouraged by placing a fulcrum in the cervical region.

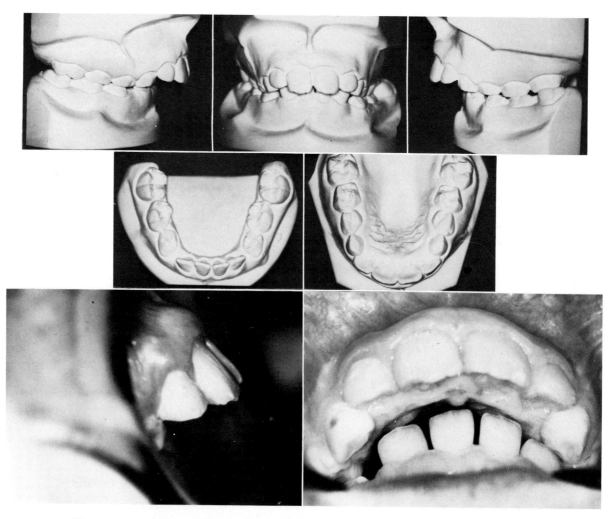

**Figure 10-20.** A 9-year-old boy before treatment. Excessive overjet and lingually inclined lower incisors are caused by a lip trap habit. A narrow maxillary arch and unilateral crossbite are evident.

of rotation approaches the apex. If the labial bow contacts the gingival third of the incisors, the centrum is moved coronally toward the junction of the apical and middle thirds. The gingival position can elongate the incisors depending on the degree of labial convexity. This type of effect is desirable only in open-bite cases in which both retrusion and elongation are desired. In labially inclined incisor problems with deep bites, every attempt should be made to minimize extrusion of the incisors while they are being axially uprighted.

If an axis of rotation in the middle third of the incisors is desired, the acrylic is trimmed away only in the coronal region, leaving a cervical contact point or fulcrum. The labial bow contacts the incisal third of the labial surfaces, providing some motivational force and preventing incisor extrusion during retraction (Figure 10-19). Vertical control is essential during incisor retraction. An important task of the activator is

to control the axial inclination of the lower incisors. This inclination cannot be managed with simple single movements such as retrusion and intrusion. The status of the malocclusion and design of the appliance must be considered.

**Design of the activator for the lower incisor area.** The design of the appliance in the lower incisor area is particularly important. The conventionally made appliance loads the lingual surfaces of the lower incisors and tips these teeth labially because of the reciprocal intermaxillary reaction built into the construction bite and design of the nighttime wear appliance. This movement is desirable if lingual inclination of the lower incisors has occurred because of hyperactive mentalis function and lip trap habits.

Figure 10-20 shows a 9-year-old boy with a Class II, division 1 malocclusion and retrognathic profile but no severe skeletal

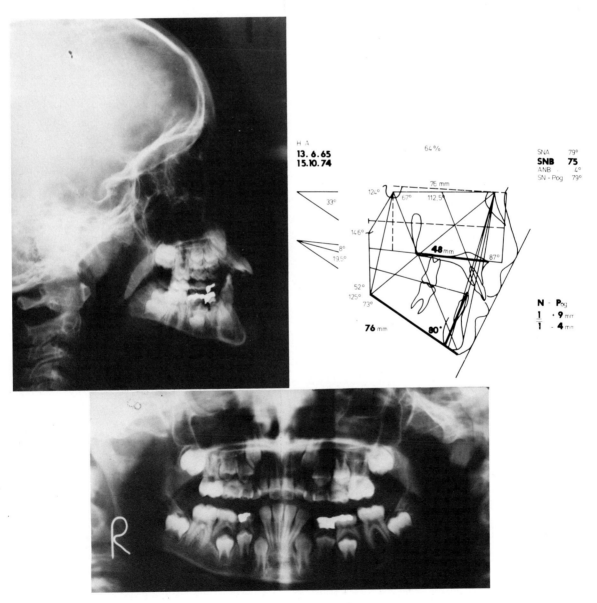

**Figure 10-20, cont'd**

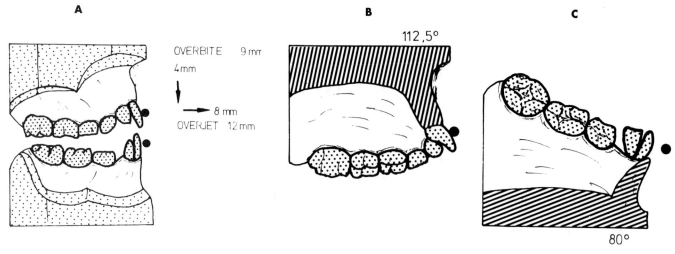

OVERBITE    9 mm

4 mm

8 mm

OVERJET   12 mm

112,5°

80°

**Figure 10-21.** **A,** Casts in the construction bite for the patient in Figure 10-20. **B,** Active upper labial bow. **C,** Passive lower labial bow.

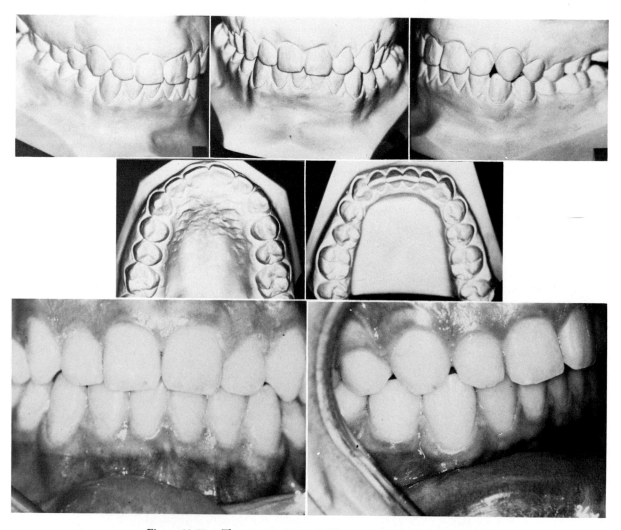

**Figure 10-22.** The same patient as in Figure 10-20 after treatment.

malrelationship. The growth pattern was horizontal, with short jaw bases and a wide symphysis. The large overjet was caused by a confirmed lip trap habit and perioral malfunction; the maxillary incisors were tipped labially some 9 mm in front of the line between nasion and pogonion (N-Pog line). The upper dental arch was narrow because of excessive buccinator mechanism pressures, leading to a convenience bite swing and crossbite of the first molars on the right side.

Treatment was begun with an expansion plate to align the upper dental arch and correct the crossbite. An activator was later employed. Because the overjet was 12 mm, the construction bite was positioned in steps, with the first bite 8 mm anterior to habitual occlusion (Figure 10-21). The overbite was 9 mm but was opened only 4 mm. Because of the very deep bite, the lower incisors were loaded lingually and capped with acrylic to prevent eruption. The lower labial bow was passive. The acrylic was ground away from the lingual of the upper incisors, including the alveolar area, and only the incisal edges were supported to prevent elongation during retrusion. The upper active labial bow contacted the

teeth on the incisal third. The acrylic was trimmed for extrusion in the molar area. A stabilizing spur was added mesially to the upper molars to exert a distalizing component as these teeth erupted. The results achieved after 2½ years of treatment and 1½ years of retention are shown in Figure 10-22.

The patient had a high growth increment, especially in the mandibular area (2.3 mm more than average), and the facial profile became orthognathic with a pronounced horizontal growth vector. Despite this, the overbite improved because of molar extrusion and retarded incisor eruption that leveled the curve of Spee. The lower incisors were tipped labially, somewhat reducing the overbite. This reduction occurred in spite of the incisal acrylic cap over these teeth because the addition of self-curing soft acrylic on the contiguous lingual surfaces exerted both a labial and an intruding component. With extrusion of the upper incisors controlled, the usual extrusive tendency was nullified during incisor retraction. The appliance design impeded the usual extrusion expected with lingual tipping of incisor teeth. The uprighting of the upper and lower incisors helped improve the overjet, as did the labial

**Figure 10-22, cont'd.** Superimposition of cephalometric tracings before and after treatment.

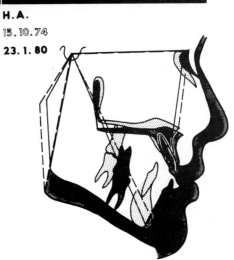

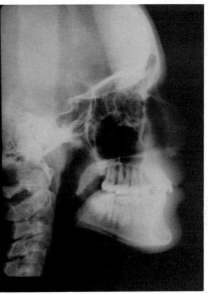

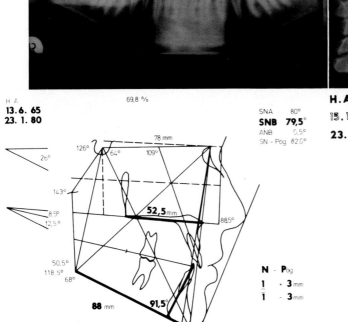

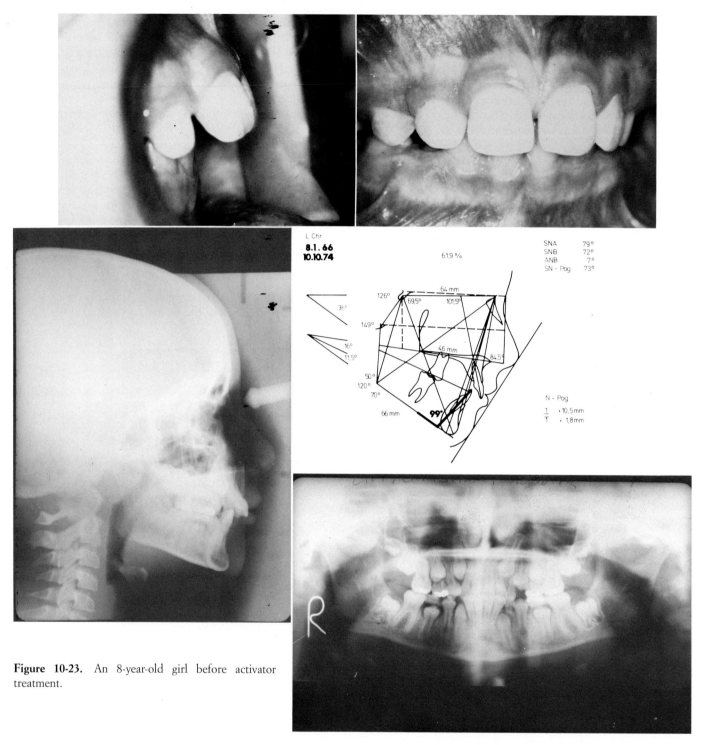

**Figure 10-23.** An 8-year-old girl before activator treatment.

movement of the lower incisors, which also opened space for the canines.

On the final cephalogram the lower incisors were 3 mm behind the N-Pog line; the upper incisors were 3 mm ahead of it. The satisfactory result was caused by not only the movement of the incisors but also the growth-conditioned forward positioning of the mandible and resultant displacement of the N-Pog line.

If the lower incisors are tipped labially before treatment is started for a Class II, division I malocclusion, conventional activator therapy is contraindicated. Further protrusion of the

incisors not only worsens the axial inclination and lip line profile but also prevents the successful correction of the sagittal Class II malrelationship. Such a result is unstable, and the following consequences are possible:

- Because the lower incisors are excessively procumbent, they may contact the lingual of the maxillary incisors, eliminating the overjet before the buccal segment sagittal malrelationship is completely corrected.
- If the mandible cannot be adequately postured anteriorly, dental compensation of an original skeletal discrep-

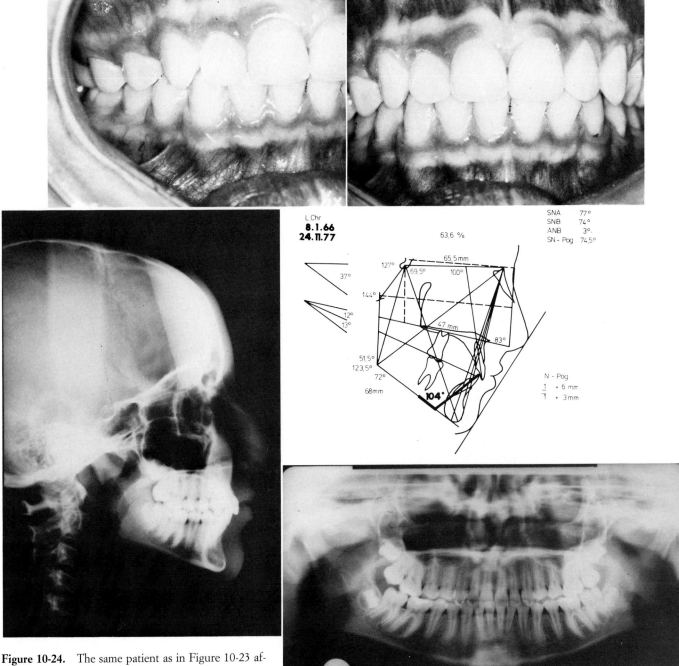

**Figure 10-24.** The same patient as in Figure 10-23 after 3 years of treatment.

ancy occurs. This is acceptable only in cases of vertical growth patterns. In average or horizontal growth vectors, it is a poor treatment regimen for the mixed dentition period.

- If the mandible continues to grow anteriorly after appliance therapy (as is likely), outgrowing the maxilla, crowding of the lower incisors is likely, particularly in horizontal growth patterns. Seemingly positive results after termination of activator wear deteriorate rapidly.

Figure 10-23 shows the pretreatment records of an 8-year-old girl with a retrognathic face and an average growth pattern. The mandible was in a posterior position but of aver-

age length. The ramal height was very small (43 mm). The maxilla was slightly retrognathic but had a long base. Despite the good axial inclination of the upper incisors, they were 10.5 mm ahead of the N-Pog line. The lower incisors were labially inclined at almost 100 degrees.

Conventional activator treatment was started. Because of the full Class II molar relationship, activated springs were used to assist in distalizing these teeth. The upper incisors were held with an acrylic cap to prevent their being tipped lingually while activating the labial bow. The lower incisors were loaded lingually; the lower labial bow was passive.

A good clinical result was achieved after 3 years of treatment (Figure 10-24). Cephalometric analysis showed an improve-

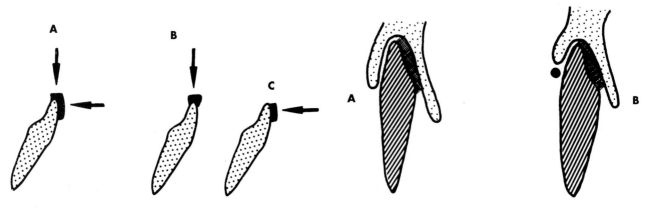

**Figure 10-25.** Acrylic groove or cap holding the incisors. **A,** Incisally and labially. **B,** Incisally. **C,** Labially.

**Figure 10-26.** Acrylic groove. **A,** Holding the incisors. **B,** Uprighting them with a labial bow.

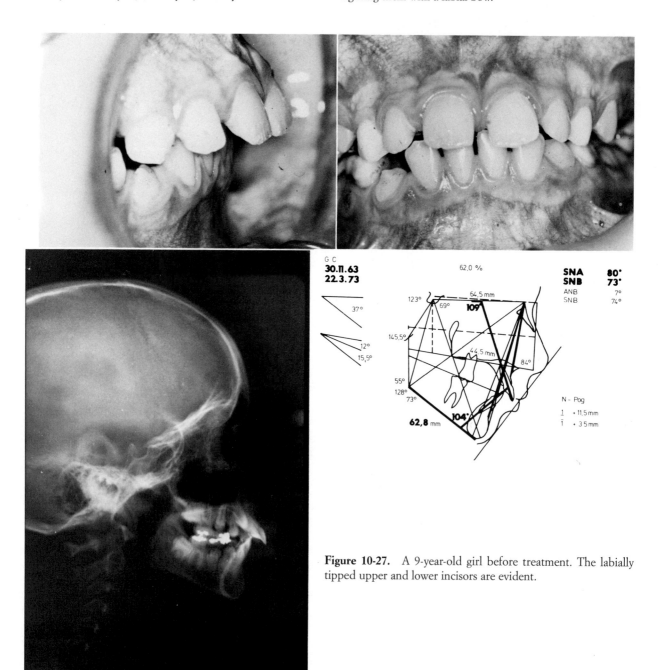

**Figure 10-27.** A 9-year-old girl before treatment. The labially tipped upper and lower incisors are evident.

ment of sagittal skeletal relationships, with a 4-degree reduction of the A-N-B angle to 3 degrees. The growth increments of the mandibular and maxillary bases were low (−1.9 mm and −2.5 mm below average, respectively), whereas that of the ramus was average. The basal relationship articulare-pogonion (Ar-Pog) to articulare-subspinale (Ar-A) improved from 13 to 20 mm. The axial inclination of the lower incisors worsened, tipping forward to 104 degrees. The result was not considered stable because a greater growth increment of the mandibular base was likely to occur in the next several years, with consequent lower incisor uprighting and crowding.

Based on the previous case and the observations made, several design factor changes can be suggested for these problems. Depending on the axial inclination and position of the incisors, three possibilities for treatment are available:

1. Labial tipping of the lower incisors
2. Holding of the incisors in their initial positions
3. Uprighting of the lower incisors while positioning of the mandible anteriorly

If proclining of the lower incisors is desired, it can be done by loading the entire lingual surface or only the incisal third. The labial bow is passive. In open-bite cases, no incisal groove is provided, whereas in deep bite cases a flat acrylic rim that only lightly touches the incisal edges discourages extrusion. If the incisors are to be held in their positions, the acrylic should be trimmed only interdentally and contact the teeth lingually, with an acrylic cap extending to the labial of the incisors (Figure 10-25).

If a retrusion or an uprighting of the incisors is required during anterior positioning of the mandible, the design of the lower incisor area should be managed in a more sophisticated manner (Figure 10-26). No contact should occur between the teeth and acrylic on the lingual, not even during functional movements of the mandible. An acrylic labial cap that contacts the labial incisal holds the incisors. In deep overbite cases the incisal edges are loaded only from the labial side, creating a lingual movement component through the inclined-plane action while preventing extrusion. The incisal edges are not loaded in open-bite cases. The labial bow is active, moving the incisors lingually and extruding if possible.

### CASE STUDY
A 9-year-old girl with very proclined incisors (104 degrees) began treatment. She had a skeletal Class II relationship with a retrognathic mandible. The mandibular base was extremely short, and the maxillary base was of average length. The growth pattern was average. In addition to proclination of the lower incisors, labial tipping of the uppers was evident (Figure 10-27).

A horizontal type of activator was constructed with an opening of 4 mm in the construction bite to enable retrusion of the upper and lower incisors. This could be performed easily because of the spacing between the teeth. The incisors were capped on the labial with acrylic, and the acrylic was ground away on the lingual, alveolar, and dental areas. The molars were extruded with guided eruption. The lower incisors were uprighted more than the uppers. The upper molars were guided distally with stabilizing wires at the mesial embrasures.

After 4½ years of treatment and retention the Class II relationship had improved, with the mandible positioned more anteriorly. The growth increment of the mandibular base was average, whereas that of the maxillary basal growth was +2.5 mm above average. For this reason, not only the sella-nasion-supramentale (S-N-B) but also the sella-nasion-subspinale (S-N-A) angles increased. The basal relationship of Ar-Pog to Ar-A improved only from 10 to 15 mm. The growth pattern became horizontal. In spite of the somewhat unfavorable reaction of the maxillary base to therapy, the lower incisors were uprighted during the anterior positioning of the mandible from 104 to 95 degrees (Figure 10-28).

**Design of the activator for the upper incisor area.** Some variations in activator design in the upper incisor area have already been described. In deep overbite cases the incisal edges are loaded with the acrylic rim. In open-bite cases, the acrylic is ground away to enable the teeth to be extruded. For protrusion the lingual surfaces are loaded.

A special design for the upper incisor area is required for retrusive movements and in the construction of the vertical activator. Retrusion of the upper incisors requires that the acrylic be ground away and the labial bow be active. During retrusion the incisors are extruded. In deep overbite cases, however, extrusion is undesirable; construction demands labial acrylic capping with incisal contact. This creates an oblique guide plane at the labioincisal, effectively guiding the incisors lingually while not allowing them to erupt (Figure 10-29). The acrylic is ground away on the lingual to the labioincisal margin and inclined plane previously described. The labial bow is active. The incisors are thus moved lingually along the path dictated by the acrylic guide plane on the incisal margin, with extrusion resulting.

In the vertical activator the design for the upper incisor area is similar to that required for retrusion and deep overbite cases. However, some differences in design exist:

1. The labial acrylic cap is extended to the area of greatest convexity at the junction of the incisal and middle thirds of the labial surface (Figure 10-30).
2. The acrylic is completely ground away on the lingual of the incisors and away from the palatogingival tissue contiguous with the incisor alveolar support area.
3. The labial bow contacts the teeth on the gingival third.

This design has a twofold objective: it should influence the axial inclination of the teeth and affect the inclination of the maxillary base in vertical growth patterns. (This inclination change is possible because of the vertical force created by the high construction bite.)

**Movements of the posterior teeth in the sagittal plane.** The buccal segment teeth can be moved mesially or distally by the activator. Although large mesiodistal bodily movements are not possible with the activator, modest movements of these teeth can be achieved in Class II or III malocclusions. If

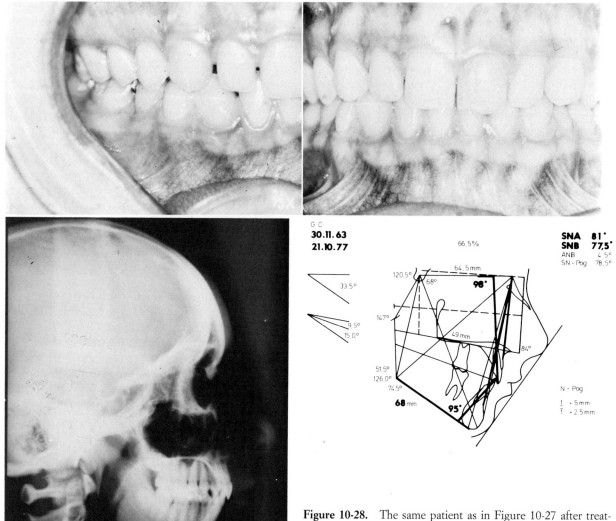

G C
30.11.63
21.10.77

66.5%

SNA  81°
SNB  77,5°
ANB    4.5°
SN - Pog  78.5°

33.5°

120.5°    64.5mm
68°    98°

147°    49mm    84°

9.5°
15.0°

51.5°
126.0°    N - Pog

74.5°    $\frac{1}{}$ · 5 mm
68 mm    95°    $\frac{}{1}$ · 2.5 mm

**Figure 10-28.** The same patient as in Figure 10-27 after treatment. Lower incisors were successfully uprighted.

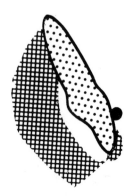

**Figure 10-29.** Extension of the acrylic labially on the upper incisors and grinding in the dental area lingually. The labioincisal cap guides the incisors lingually. The labial bow is active.

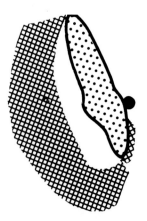

**Figure 10-30.** Design for an upper vertical activator. The acrylic is extended labially to the middle third of the labial surface and lingually over the whole dentoalveolar and palatal area.

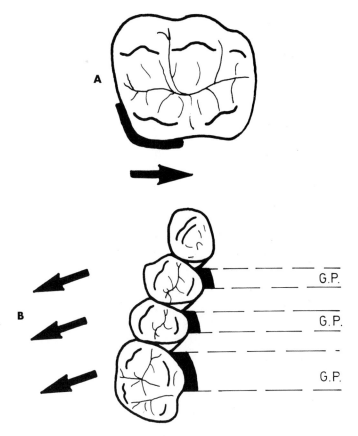

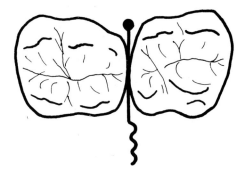

**Figure 10-32.** Stabilizing wire. This type of wire also is used for distalizing the molars and preventing their mesial movement.

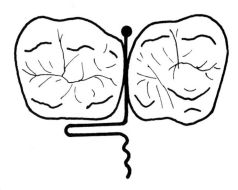

**Figure 10-31.** Distal movements of the molars. **A,** Loaded area. **B,** Guide planes.

**Figure 10-33.** Active open spring used to effect sagittal tooth movement.

activator therapy begins in the early mixed dentition, the permanent first molars should be sagittally controlled by the appliance. During eruption the premolars also can be guided toward their desired positions by grinding the activator properly. The molars can be moved mesially or distally according to the way the guiding acrylic planes are made to contact the teeth.

For distalizing movements the guide planes load the molars on the mesiolingual surfaces (Figure 10-31). The guide plane extends only to the area of greatest convexity in the mesiodistal plane. A distalizing movement is indicated for the maxillary arch in Class II nonextraction problems. The extent of this movement is limited with activator use. Guiding the eruption of the teeth is an important part of treatment. Additional elements can be incorporated in the activator to increase the distalizing effect.

Stabilizing wires or spurs are rigid (0.9 mm) projections from the lingual acrylic that contact the mesial surface of the first permanent molars interproximally (Figure 10-32). Mesial movement can be prevented using these wires. If treatment is begun with a headgear or lip bumper and continued with an activator, stabilizing wires should be used to prevent mesial migration of the first molar teeth. The stabilizing wires also implement distalizing eruption guidance for the first molars. This guidance can be accomplished with a slight activation of the wires, bending them distally or using the reciprocal force

created by a protruding adjustment on the maxillary incisor teeth if needed. Distalizing guidance of maxillary molars also is possible with active open springs (Figure 10-33).

Occasionally, particularly in first premolar extraction cases, distalizing of the canine teeth is needed. This can be done with various design elements:

1. Originally the labial bow was modified to move the canines distally (Figure 10-34). The lateral, U-shaped bends of the bow were connected with the horizontal middle portion by loops. This design had one major disadvantage: activating both the loops for distalizing the canines and the middle portion of the bow for retruding the incisors at the same time was difficult.

2. The use of guide wires for this purpose has been suggested (Figure 10-35). These wires work independently of the labial bow. They are rigid (0.8 to 0.9 mm) and contact the mesial surfaces of the canines. They have a U-shaped outline to permit their adaptation.

3. Another variation in canine retraction is the use of retraction springs (Figure 10-36). These springs contact the canines mesiolabially over a large surface. They can be pulled back or activated by a parallel movement, enabling the canines to be moved back with only a slight tipping. The springs are active wires 0.6 mm in diameter.

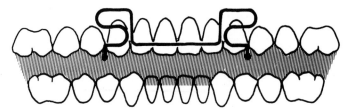

**Figure 10-34.** Labial bow with loops for the canines used to effect distalization.

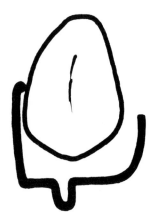

**Figure 10-35.** Guiding wires developed by Petrik move the canines distally.

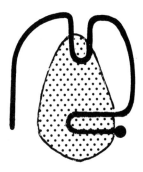

**Figure 10-36.** Retraction spring for the canines. These active springs are 0.6 mm in diameter.

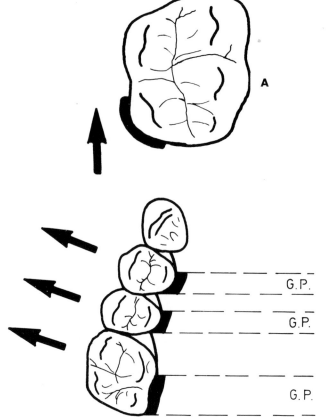

**Figure 10-37.** Mesial movements of the molars. **A,** Loaded area. **B,** Guide planes.

Mesial movement of buccal segment teeth is accomplished by having the acrylic guide planes of the activator contact the teeth on the distolingual surfaces. The guide planes extend only to the greatest lingual circumference in the mesiodistal plane (Figure 10-37). A mesial movement of the posterior teeth is indicated only in the upper dental arch in Class III malocclusions without crowding.

In Class II malocclusions the guiding planes for the lower posterior teeth are ground not for mesial movement but for expansion or extrusion. A mesial force component is already present because of the reciprocal intermaxillary anchorage created by the construction bite and the influence of the stretched retractor muscles on the anteriorly positioned mandible. A mesial driving of the lower teeth could aggravate the labial inclination of the lower incisors (Björk, 1951).

**Movements of the teeth in the transverse plane.** If the construction bite is shifted to one side, an asymmetric action is created in the transverse plane (Figure 10-38). This action is a contralateral reciprocal force that may be needed for the alignment of an asymmetric narrow maxillary arch on one side and a narrowness of the mandibular arch on the other. Such treatment cannot be controlled very well, however, and alignment of asymmetric dental arches is better achieved with other appliances.

The activator may be trimmed to stimulate expansion of the buccal segment teeth, although the opportunities are limited compared with those available with active plates, jackscrews, and other design elements. To achieve transverse movement, the lingual acrylic surfaces opposite the posterior teeth must be in contact with the teeth (Figure 10-39). If a higher level of force is required in one dental arch or tooth area, this can be achieved by adding a thin layer of self-curing soft acrylic. More effective expansion is obtained by using expansion-type jackscrews and trimming the appliance to enhance the expansion. The expansion screw is placed in the anterior intermaxillary portion of the appliance to achieve a symmetric force application (Figure 10-40). This construction is quite bulky, however, and pushes the tongue posteri-

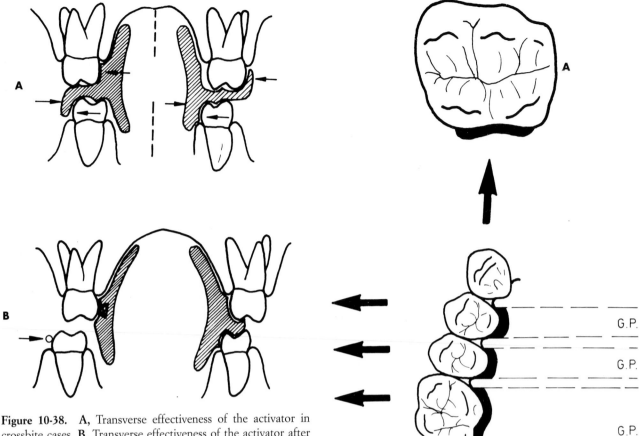

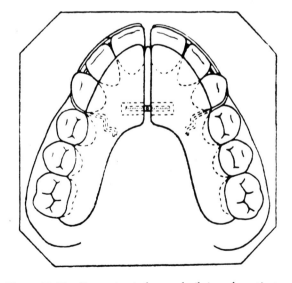

**Figure 10-38. A,** Transverse effectiveness of the activator in crossbite cases. **B,** Transverse effectiveness of the activator after anchoring the appliance on one side and moving the teeth on the opposite side with pegs and springs or the addition of soft acrylic.

orly. The appliance also can be made with two eccentrically placed jackscrews in the upper and lower portions (see Chapter 6). The anterior acrylic portion can then be partially cut out.

Single teeth also can be moved laterally. If a crossbite condition is apparent for one or more teeth, the malocclusion can be corrected with two springs and corresponding grinding of the appliance (Figure 10-41). The upper molar is moved buccally with a closed-loop spring, and the lower molar in buccal crossbite is moved lingually with a frame loop. The acrylic is ground away on the lingual of the lower molar. Transverse mesiodistal movements for single teeth in the incisor region can be achieved using guide wires or rigid-wire elements; such movements are often needed to close existing spaces.

## Guidelines

Although single-tooth movements have already been discussed, in activator therapy only combined movements are done simultaneously on anterior and posterior teeth. Before selective grinding of the activator begins, a treatment plan should be formulated, listing the areas to be trimmed and the reason for each grinding procedure. For the general categories of malocclusions, general trimming procedures can be described, although individual variation may be necessary for specific problems.

**Figure 10-39.** Transverse movement of the molars. **A,** Loaded area. **B,** Guide planes.

**Figure 10-40.** Expansion jackscrew built into the activator.

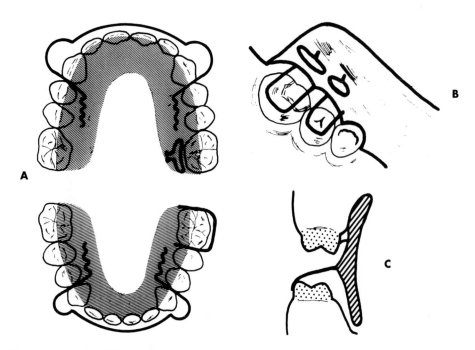

**Figure 10-41.** Modification for the crossbite correction of single molars. **A,** Protrusive spring in the upper and closed loop in the lower molar areas. **B,** Both springs from above. **C,** Springs in cross section.

### Activator trimming in Class II malocclusions

*For incisors.* In some cases, if the upper incisors are to be retruded and the labial bow is active, acrylic capping is necessary to prevent extrusion from occurring with the retrusion. If the lower incisors are to be protruded and the labial bow is passive, a number of modifications may be necessary in the acrylic design, depending on the requirements of holding or retruding the lower incisors or preventing eruption. As in a deep bite case, acrylic capping is used when possible to prevent excessive labial inclination of these teeth.

*For posterior teeth.* The upper posterior teeth may need to be moved posteriorly or withheld from mesial movement by guide planes and stabilizing wires. The acrylic is trimmed away next to the lower posterior teeth to guide eruption and level the curve of Spee. The lower teeth tend to move mesially as they erupt, however, and this movement is expected to make a small contribution to correction of the sagittal malrelationship. The eruption of the upper teeth should be prevented as much as possible to reduce the rocking open of the mandible, which increases the retrognathism. Selective grinding of the acrylic so that the guide planes contact the mesiolingual cusp surfaces of the buccal segment teeth enhances the Class II correction. Stabilizing wires or spurs also may assist in the distalizing process as the first molar teeth erupt (Figure 10-42).

### Activator trimming in Class III malocclusions

*For incisors.* The upper incisors are loaded for protrusion, and the labial bow is passive. If the upper incisors are in the process of eruption, they can be guided labially along acrylic guide planes or through the addition of a thin layer of self-curing cold acrylic lingual to the teeth. Lip pads may be used instead of a labial bow to stimulate basal maxillary development. The lower incisors should be retruded. The acrylic on the lingual of the lower incisors is ground away, and a labial acrylic cap is placed. The lower labial bow is active. The acrylic does not touch either the lingual of the lower incisors or the alveolar crest. The lower anterior portion of the activator can be completely trimmed away or left open because no force application is required in this area. The activator cannot influence the flat position of the tongue often seen in Class III malocclusions. Although omitting the anterior portion of the acrylic and leaving the space open makes the appliance less bulky, the incorporation of a wire crib for tongue control is recommended in some cases.

*For posterior teeth.* The guide planes for the upper posterior teeth are trimmed for mesial movement. Eruption is encouraged in a down and forward direction. The lower posterior teeth have guide planes trimmed to contact the mesiolingual cuspal surfaces for posterior vector stimulus as these teeth erupt. Eruption is kept to a minimum (Figure 10-43).

### Activator trimming in vertical dysplasia–type malocclusions

*Deep overbite malocclusions.* The incisor area is trimmed for intrusion, and the molar area is trimmed for extrusion. The labial bow is active and contacts the teeth at their incisal third.

*Open-bite malocclusions.* The incisor area is ground away for extrusion, and the molar area is ground away for intrusion. The labial bow is active and contacts the incisor teeth at their gingival third.

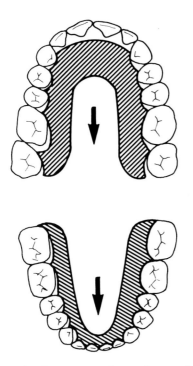

**Figure 10-42.** Plan for trimming the acrylic interdental projections for distal driving of the upper teeth and mesial movement of the lower in Class II malocclusions.

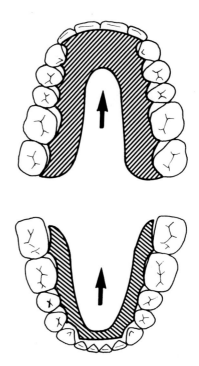

**Figure 10-43.** Plan for trimming for mesial movement of the upper teeth and distal driving of the lower in Class III malocclusions.

## SUMMARY

Both skeletal and dentoalveolar changes can be achieved in activator functional appliance therapy. However, the functional method has its limitations. The best time to approach most malocclusions is in the mixed dentition. The activator can solve many problems that become more severe if left unattended. The restoration of normal function is a major contribution to improvement in the morphofunctional interrelationship. If treatment objectives require more orthodontic guidance, functional appliance therapy can continue or fixed or removable appliances may be used in the permanent dentition. Sometimes combination therapy is indicated (even in the mixed dentition) as the activator is combined with expansion plates and extraoral force.

The construction bite varies for different types and degrees of abnormality. Depending on timing, technique, and trimming, significant facial and occlusal changes can be achieved. In addition to the elimination of abnormal perioral muscle function, growth guidance is the major contribution of functional therapy. The correction of functional retrusions (Class II), protrusions (Class III), and lateral functional shifts is simple with the activator. The trimming technique permits guidance of eruption and individual tooth movements. Occlusal changes can be seen in all three planes. In the sagittal plane the mandible can be repositioned, incisors can be protruded or retruded, and buccal segment teeth can be moved mesiodistally. In the vertical plane, routine objectives include guiding the inclination and growth direction of the maxillary base and extruding teeth. In the transverse plane the clinician can correct a functional crossbite, expand the dental arches, and correct single tooth crossbites.

The limitations of functional appliance therapy should be recognized. First, it should not be considered a stand-alone regimen, a method for full correction of all malocclusions. The elimination of abnormal perioral muscle function and the guidance of growth and eruption of teeth are important treatment objectives, but other facets of malocclusion respond better to other biomechanics and can be used separately or with the activator and its modifications. The degree of success in treating skeletal problems depends on growth timing, direction, and magnitude. Dentoalveolar changes are best accomplished during the eruption of teeth.

The functional appliance is quite effective in treating mandibular retrognathism in patients with horizontal growth patterns. It is less effective in influencing maxillary prognathism or vertical growth patterns; it is contraindicated in some instances and requires special modification in others. It is inappropriate for achieving extensive bodily movement, torque, rotation, and intrusion of teeth.

The clinician must consider the special characteristics of each malocclusion before fabricating the activator because the appliance should be designed for the individual. The construction bite, grinding technique, function and placement of the labial bow, and possible need for other design features are all subject to discretionary diagnosis and treatment planning. The degree of protrusion or opening for the construction bite, anchorage of the appliance, and relationship of teeth to the appliance are all prime considerations.

A popular and effective modification of the classic activator is the bionator, introduced by Balters (1943) and subsequently modified by other clinicians. Because of its special design and anchorage considerations and unique trimming technique, it is discussed in Chapter 11.

# The Bionator—
# a Modified Activator

Thomas Rakosi

## PRINCIPLES OF BIONATOR THERAPY

The bulkiness of the activator and its limitation to nighttime wear have deterred clinicians interested in attaining the greatest potential of functional growth guidance. During sleep, function is obviously minimal or nonexistent; hence using the term *functional appliance* to describe an activator is not completely correct in the strictest sense. In response to this criticism, the appliance has been made less bulky and more elastic, modifications that improve the efficiency of the activator and facilitate daytime use.

The bionator is the prototype of a less bulky appliance. Its lower portion is narrow, and its upper has only lateral extensions, with a crosspalatal stabilizing bar. The palate is free for proprioceptive contact with the tongue; the buccinator wire loops hold away potentially deforming muscular action; the appliance may be worn all the time, except during meals. Balters (1960) developed the original appliance during the early 1950s, at the same time that Bimler (1964) was working (in the same direction) with a skeletonized activator. Although the theoretic principles of Balters' appliance are based on the works of Robin, Andresen, and Häupl, it is different from the activator.

According to Balters, the equilibrium between the tongue and circumoral muscles is responsible for the shape of the dental arches and intercuspation (Figure 11-1). The functional space for the tongue is essential to the normal development of the orofacial system. This hypothesis supports the early function and form concepts of van der Klaauw and the later functional matrix theory of Moss. For Balters the tongue (as the center of reflex activity in the oral cavity) was the most important factor in treatment. A discoordination of its functions could lead to abnormal growth and actual deformation. The purpose of the bionator was to establish good functional coordination and eliminate these deforming, growth-restricting aberrations.

Balters thought the position of the tongue should be considered carefully in planning therapy because it was responsible for certain types of malocclusions. For example, posterior displacement of the tongue could lead to a Class II malocclusion; low anterior displacement could cause Class III malocclusion; narrowing of the arches with resultant crowding (particularly of the maxillary arch) was the result of diminished outward pressure during both postural rest and function, as opposed to the forces from the buccinator mechanism on the outside; and open bite was the consequence of hyperactivity and forward posturing of the tongue.

Nevertheless, despite its initial similarity to the functional matrix theories of Moss, which came later, Balters' concept had a significant difference. Balters believed that only the role of the tongue was decisive. Using lateral wire configurations to relieve the forces of the surrounding neuromuscular structures, he took only secondary consideration of the neuromuscular envelope. According to the research of Winders in 1958, however, the tongue exerts three to four times as much force on the dentition as does the buccal and labial musculature; these findings would seem to support Balters' thesis, if resting

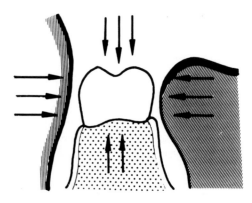

**Figure 11-1.** In the transverse plane, muscle forces influence the position of the teeth; in the vertical plane, occlusal forces do this.

force and other factors (tissue rigidity, the elastic index, atmospheric pressures, intercuspation) are not considered.

Convinced of the tongue's dominant role, Balters designed his appliance to take advantage of tongue posture. He constructed it to position the mandible anteriorly, with the incisors in an edge-to-edge relationship, which he considered important for natural bodily orientation. Because the forward posturing of the mandible enlarged the oral space, bringing the dorsum of the tongue into contact with the soft palate, and helped accomplish lip closure, the appliance was designed to help patients learn normal functional patterns.

The principle of treatment with the bionator is not to activate the muscles but to modulate muscle activity, thereby enhancing normal development of the inherent growth pattern and eliminating abnormal and potentially deforming environmental factors. In light of this, the bionator falls between simpler screening appliances and the activator.

Unlike the construction bite of the activator, that of the bionator cannot make allowances for facial pattern and growth direction by variations in vertical opening as the mandible is postured forward. The bite cannot be opened and must be positioned in an edge-to-edge relationship. If the overjet is too large, however, the forward posturing can be done step-by-step but will still not open the bite. Balters reasoned that a high construction bite could impair tongue function and the patient could actually acquire a tongue-thrust habit as the mandible dropped open and the tongue instinctively moved forward to maintain an open airway.

Because no allowance is made for the vertical component except in guiding eruption of the posterior teeth, the indications are reduced for this appliance. Myotatic reflex activity with isotonic muscle contraction is stimulated, and the loose appliance works with kinetic energy. Unlike the Harvold-Woodside–type activator, the viscoelastic properties of muscles and soft tissues and the stretch reflex response are not employed in the vertical dimension. The labial bow and palatal bar directly influence the behavior of the lips and tongue. The appliance can create sagittal and vertical dentoalveolar changes with certain sucking habits. Nevertheless, the main consideration still is to influence the function of the tongue, in contrast with the Fränkel appliance, whose main aim is to influence the outer neuromuscular envelope. With the onset of normal function, desired changes then occur. Researchers now know that abnormal tongue function can be secondary, adaptive, or compensatory because of skeletal maldevelopment, but Balters did not consider this in the original version of his appliance.

The main advantage of the bionator lies in its reduced size, which allows it to be worn day and night. The appliance exerts a constant influence on the tongue and perioral muscles because of the screening effect of the labial bow and its lateral extensions (which hold off muscle contact with the dentoalveolar area, particularly in the usually narrowed maxillary arch of Class II, division 1 malocclusions). Because unfavorable external and internal muscle forces are prevented from exerting undesirable and restrictive effects on the dentition and supporting structures for a longer time, the bionator's action is faster than that of the classic activator. Constant wear results in more rapid sagittal adjustment of the musculature to the forward mandibular posture because the mandible retracts only during eating (or a small percentage of the time).

The main disadvantage of the bionator lies in the difficulty of correctly managing it. This difficulty stems from the simultaneous requirements of stabilization of the appliance plus selective grinding for eruption guidance. Normalization of function can occur only if the inherent growth pattern is normal in the first place, with no environmental influences to prevent accomplishment of that pattern. In the case of skeletal disturbances, however, the effectiveness of the Balters bionator is very limited, as it is for any functional appliance. The various activators can be modified for different growth directions (the H or V activator constructions). A correct differential diagnosis is essential for successful bionator treatment, and treated cases must be functional-type retrusions with relatively normal skeletal potential and sufficient growth increments to permit a favorable change. A further potential disadvantage, shared with other skeletonized activators (the Bimler appliance particularly), is the vulnerability to distortion, which occurs because far less acrylic support exists in the alveolar and incisal region. Of course, the bionator can be modified (as other functional appliances have been) to satisfy some of these criticisms.

## BIONATOR TYPES

Three basic constructions are common in the bionator: the standard, the open bite, and the reversed, or Class III.

## Standard Appliance

The standard appliance (Figure 11-2) consists of a lower horseshoe-shaped acrylic lingual plate extending from the distal of the last erupted molar around to the corresponding point on the other side. For the upper arch the appliance has only posterior lingual extensions that cover the molar and pre-

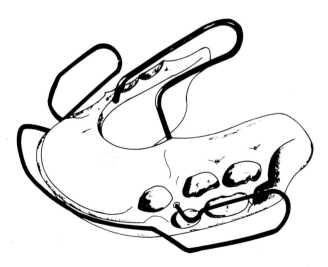

**Figure 11-2.** The Balters bionator basic appliance.

molar regions. The anterior portion is open from canine to canine. The upper and lower parts, which are joined interocclusally in the correct construction bite relationship, extend 2 mm above the upper gingival margin and 2 mm below the lower gingival margin. The upper anterior portion is kept free to prevent interference with tongue function. However, tongue function is controlled by the edge-to-edge incisal contact relationship, leaving no space for thrusting activity. If establishing this relationship is possible, no acrylic capping of the lower incisors is done. If some space exists between the upper and lower incisors in the construction bite, acrylic can be extended to cap the lower incisors. This does not hinder the potential procumbency of these teeth, however, because the labial wire does not contact them and the capping is only partially successful in preventing labial tipping—a limitation of the bionator, particularly if lower incisors are already labially inclined.

The function and posture of the lips and cheeks are guided by two wire constructions, the palatal bar and the labial bow with buccal extensions. The palatal bar is formed of 1.2 mm hard stainless steel wire extending from the top edges of the lingual acrylic flanges in the middle area of the deciduous first molars (Figure 11-3). The palatal bar lies approximately 1 mm away from the palatal mucosa and runs distally as far as a transpalatal line between the distal portions of the maxillary permanent first molars to form an oval, posteriorly directed loop that reinserts on the opposite side.

The crosspalatal bar stabilizes the appliance and simultaneously orients the tongue and mandible anteriorly to achieve a Class I relationship. The forward orientation of the tongue, according to Balters, is accomplished by stimulating its dorsal surface with the palatal bar. This is the reason for the posterior curve of the palatal bar.

The labial bow, made of 0.9 mm hard stainless steel wire (Figure 11-4), begins above the contact point between the canine and deciduous upper first molar (or premolar). It then runs vertically, making a rounded 90-degree bend to the distal along the middle of the crowns of the posterior teeth, and extends as far as the embrasure between the deciduous second molar and the permanent first molar. Making a gentle down and forward curve, it runs anteriorly at about the same position with respect to the buccal surfaces of the lower posterior teeth as far as the lower canine. From there, at a sharp angle it extends obliquely upward toward the upper canine, bends to a level line at approximately the incisal third of the incisors, and extends to the canine on the opposite side. It ends in mirror-image form on the opposite side and inserts into the acrylic. The labial portion of the bow should be approximately the thickness of a sheet of ordinary writing paper from the incisors.

This position of the wire produces a negative pressure, with the wire supporting lip closure. In the course of treatment, however, the wire should move the incisors upright and provide extra space when the dental arch is widened. The posterior portions of the labial bow are designed as buccinator loops, screening muscle forces in the vestibule (Figure 11-5). The loops are sufficiently far from the teeth to allow for expansion but not far enough to cause discomfort to the cheeks. The buccinator loops screen the buccinator muscles, and the lingual acrylic parts prevent both the cheeks and tongue from interposing in the interocclusal space. Thus stimulating selective eruption is possible with proper trimming.

## Open-Bite Appliance

The open-bite appliance (Figure 11-6) is used to inhibit abnormal posture and function of the tongue. The construction bite is as low as possible, but a slight opening allows the interposition of posterior acrylic bite blocks for the posterior teeth, to prevent their extrusion. To inhibit tongue movements, the acrylic portion of the lower lingual part extends into the upper incisor region as a lingual shield, closing the anterior space without touching the upper teeth. The palatal bar has the same configuration as the standard bionator, with the goal of moving the tongue into a more posterior or caudal position.

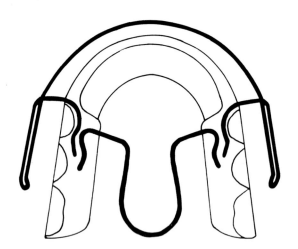

**Figure 11-3.** Palatal bar of 12 mm hard stainless steel for the basic appliance.

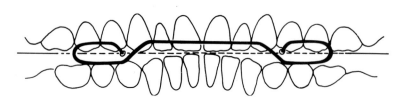

**Figure 11-4.** Labial bow of 0.9 mm hard stainless steel for the basic appliance.

The labial bow is similar in form to that of the standard appliance, differing only in that the wire runs approximately between the incisal edges of the upper and lower incisors (Figure 11-7). The labial part of the bow is placed at the height of correct lip closure, thus stimulating the lips to achieve a competent seal and relationship. The vertical strain on the lips tends to encourage the extrusive movement of the incisors, after eliminating the adverse tongue pressures.

## Class III or Reversed Bionator

The Class III or reversed bionator–type appliance (Figure 11-8) is used to encourage the development of the maxilla. The construction bite is taken in the most retruded position possible, as is done with the Fränkel function regulator, to allow labial movement of the maxillary incisors and simultaneously exert a slight restrictive effect on the lower arch. The bite is slightly opened, creating about 2 mm of interincisal space for this purpose. The lower acrylic portion is extended incisally from canine to canine. This extension is positioned behind the upper incisors, which are stimulated to glide anteriorly along the resultant inclined plane. The acrylic is trimmed away behind the lower incisors about 1 mm to prevent tipping the lower incisors labially.

The palatal bar configuration runs forward instead of posteriorly, with the loop extending as far as the deciduous first molars or premolars (Figure 11-9). From this point the wire extends back to the upper margin of the acrylic posterior to the distal surface of the permanent first molar, where it enters the acrylic with a right-angle bend. The tongue is supposedly stimulated to remain in a retracted position in its proper functional space. It should contact the anterior portion of the palate, encouraging the forward growth of this area.

The labial bow runs in front of the lower incisors rather than in front of the upper incisors, as occurs in the standard appliance (Figure 11-10). It emerges from the acrylic in the same manner as in the standard appliance, but the labial part runs along the lower incisors without a bend in the canine region. The wire touches the labial surfaces lightly or stands away at a distance of the thickness of a sheet of paper.

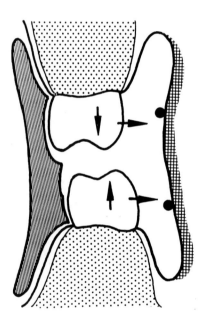

**Figure 11-5.** Buccinator loop in the deciduous molar region. The loop screens excessive force of the muscle.

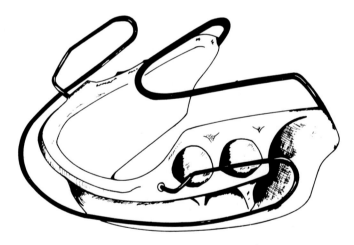

**Figure 11-6.** The open-bite bionator appliance.

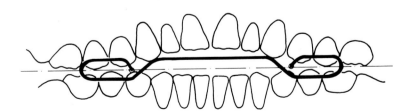

**Figure 11-7.** Labial bow for the open-bite appliance. It crosses the interincisal area.

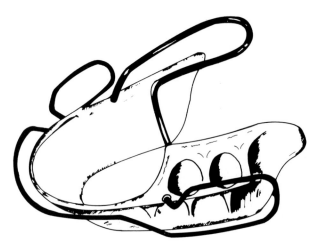

**Figure 11-8.** The reversed bionator appliance for Class III malocclusions.

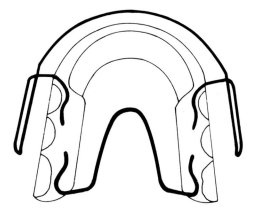

**Figure 11-9.** Palatal bar for the reversed appliance. The loop extends anteriorly to the canine–deciduous first molar embrasure.

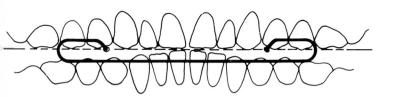

**Figure 11-10.** Labial bow for the Class III reversed appliance.

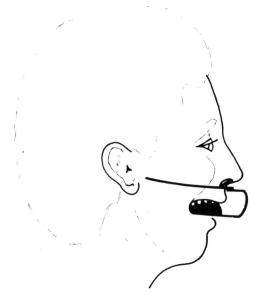

**Figure 11-11.** Assessment of the articular plane before impression-taking. It should parallel the alar-tragal line.

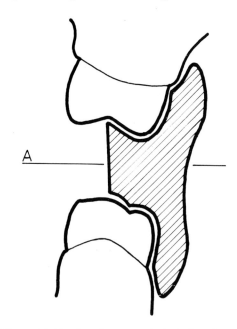

**Figure 11-12.** Loading area. *A,* Articular plane.

## TERMINOLOGY USED IN TRIMMING THE BIONATOR APPLIANCE

Because the volume of the appliance is reduced, its anchorage is more difficult than that of the activator. The trimming of the appliance must be selective because of the simultaneous requirements of anchorage. To elucidate these problems, Balters introduced the following terms:

1. *Articular plane*—This plane extends from the tips of the cusps of the upper first molars, premolars, and canines to the mesial margin of the upper central incisors. Running parallel to the alar-tragal line, it is important for the assessment of the mode of trimming (Figure 11-11).

2. *Loading area*—The palatal or lingual cusps of the deciduous molars (or premolars) and permanent first molars are relieved in the acrylic part of the appliance. The grinding away of acrylic here enhances the anchorage of the appliance (Figure 11-12).

3. *Tooth bed*—Some parts of the loading areas are trimmed away to the articular plane. Acrylic surfaces prepared in this manner are termed the *tooth bed* (Figure 11-13).

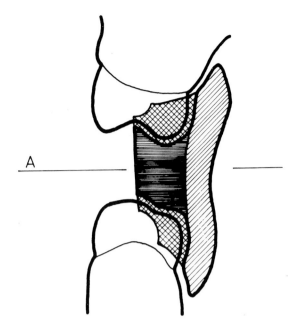

**Figure 11-13.** Tooth bed. Acrylic is trimmed to a thin cap over the opposing teeth. *A,* Articular plane.

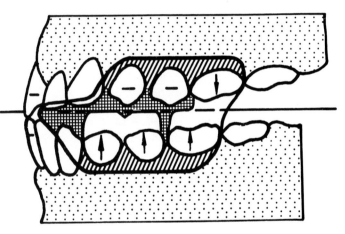

**Figure 11-14.** Nose in the lower first molar region (acrylic interdental projection).

4. *Nose*—Between the tooth beds, interdentally, acrylic fingerlike projections called *noses* may be fabricated (Figure 11-14). These extensions act both as guiding surfaces and sources of anchorage for the appliance in the sagittal and vertical planes.
5. *Ledge*—Depending on the tooth movements desired, the appliance acrylic is trimmed and the nose reduced. A reduced plastic extension placed only on the occlusal third of the interdental area is called a *ledge* (Figure 11-15). The nose is mostly on the mesial margin of the first permanent molars, whereas the ledge is between the premolars, or deciduous molars.

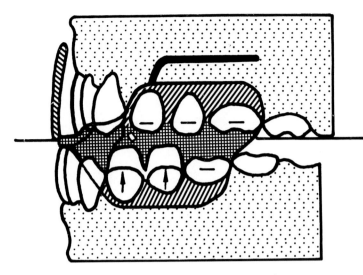

**Figure 11-15.** Ledge between the lower premolars.

## ANCHORAGE OF THE APPLIANCE

Because the bulk, volume, and extension of the appliance are reduced, special requirements exist for anchorage. When treatment with the bionator begins, trimming all the guiding acrylic planes simultaneously for all the areas is not possible. Some acrylic surfaces are used to stabilize the appliance; others can be ground as needed to effect the desired stimulus for tooth movement. The second stage of treatment requires alternating the loaded or stabilizing areas with areas being trimmed for tooth guidance. Stabilization or anchorage of the appliance is obtained from the following areas:

1. Incisal margins of the lower incisors, by extending the acrylic over the incisal margin as a cap
2. Loading areas, because the cusps of the teeth fit into the respective grooves in the acrylic
3. Deciduous molars, which can always be used as anchor teeth
4. Edentulous areas, after premature loss of the deciduous molars
5. Noses in the upper and lower interdental spaces
6. Labial bow, which if correctly placed, prevents posterior displacement of the appliance

## TRIMMING THE BIONATOR

The anchorage of the bionator permits an anterior posturing of the mandible, which is determined by the construction bite. As on the activator, trimming of occlusal surfaces on the bionator is essential to allow certain teeth to erupt further while fully erupted teeth are prevented from further eruption through contact with the acrylic. Balters' terminology refers to simulation of eruption as *unloading* or *promotion of growth* and prevention of eruption as *loading* or *inhibition of growth.* Trimming of the acrylic tooth beds and elimination of the influence of tongue and cheeks allow the teeth to erupt until they reach the articular plane. Once there, they should

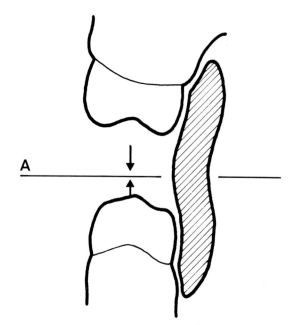

**Figure 11-16.** Unloading of the upper and lower molars for extrusion. *A,* Articular plane.

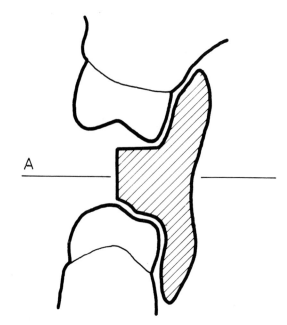

**Figure 11-18.** Loading of the upper and lower molars, with expansion effect for the uppers. *A,* Articular plane.

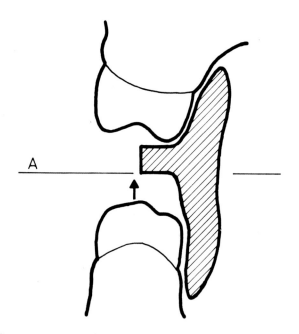

**Figure 11-17.** Loading of the upper molars and unloading of the lower molars. *A,* Articular plane.

be prevented from erupting further so that the loading can be accomplished by the addition of self-curing acrylic as needed. The appliance can be trimmed or ground periodically until the teeth reach the desired relationship with the articular plane. Because of the need to anchor the appliance, this pro-

cedure cannot be performed in all areas at the same time. Thus periodic loading and unloading of the same area are necessary. This means that the same tooth can function as an anchor and later be allowed to erupt.

The difficulty in managing the classic bionator is the alternate loading and unloading of certain areas. On one visit acrylic is added to load a specific tooth. On the next visit it may be ground away in the same area. Especially in cases of deep overbite, adequate space is necessary to allow for the full eruptive potential of the teeth. Deciduous teeth, if present, are used as anchors. The types of anchorage, according to Ascher (1968), are as follows:

| *Dentition* | *Anchorage* |
| --- | --- |
| 1, 2, III-V, 6 | IV, V—upper and lower |
| 1, 2, III-V, 6 | V and space after IV |
| 1, 2, II-6 | alveolar process—IV, V |
| 1, 2, III, 4-6 | 6 and alveolar process |

If deciduous molars are present, anchorage is not difficult. If the premolars are already erupting, however, a change in the loading and unloading areas is necessary.

Because the method of trimming or selective grinding on the bionator is similar to that used on the activator, only the main differences are described here:

1. To allow extrusion of the posterior teeth, some acrylic is always left interdentally at the level of the occlusal (articular) plane, forming the so-called tooth bed (Figure 11-16). The upper and lower molar regions

should be trimmed first. Then the lower premolars are trimmed while the molars are loaded. Finally the upper premolars are stimulated while the lower premolars and molars are loaded. Care must be taken to ensure that the lingual acrylic surfaces do not interfere with eruption (Figure 11-17).

2. The acrylic projections between the teeth (the noses) are left untouched or replaced with self-curing acrylic. Their roles are similar to those of the stabilizing spurs of the conventional activator—they exert a distalizing influence on the permanent first molars. Instead of the noses, guiding wires of 0.8 to 0.9 mm can be used. These are fabricated of stainless steel, as with the activator. Guide wires are especially important if space opening is required or if treatment has been begun with extraoral force. The noses in the areas of the lower molars must be well defined to prevent the mandible from dropping back.

3. The occlusal surfaces of the bionator are trimmed to facilitate transverse movement. However, on closure the cusp tips should remain in contact with the tooth bed. In cases of open bite the posterior teeth are fully loaded for intrusion (Figure 11-18).

## CLINICAL MANAGEMENT OF BIONATOR TREATMENT

For maximal beneficial effect the bionator must be worn day and night. The time interval between office visits is 3 to 5 weeks, depending on the state of eruption of the teeth.

The labial bow should be checked to ensure it touches the teeth only lightly if at all. The buccinator loops should be away from the deciduous first and second molar areas but should not irritate the cheek mucosa. If expansion is required, the loops can be activated. In the final stages, minor spaces can be closed by active retraction of the bow.

In accordance with the plan of anchorage and growth promotion, the loading and unloading of acrylic areas or planes should depend on whether tooth movement is to be stimulated or retarded. Any modifications should be performed on the first molars initially, the lower premolars (if present) secondly, and the upper premolars thirdly—alternating the unloading and loading for anchorage purposes to stabilize the appliance.

During the first phase of treatment the occurrence of rapid horizontal and vertical changes in mandibular position is common. This first change is a muscular adaptation to the new position, with a shortening of the lateral pterygoid muscle (LPM) (as shown by Petrovic et al, 1972). The rapid changes lead to an open bite in the posterior segments. Articular and dentoalveolar adaptation occurs in the second stage following neuromuscular adaptation. The dentoalveolar changes in the deciduous molar area are often insufficient; thus the posterior open bite in this area persists until the premolars can be guided into full occlusion, under the corrective stimulus of the appliance.

## INDICATIONS FOR BIONATOR THERAPY

Opinions about the clinical usefulness of the bionator as Balters envisioned and used it vary widely. Some clinicians believe the appliance is less effective than the activator; others hold that it can be used in every type of malocclusion. No doubt exists, however, that those who use it without the proper diagnostic study and indications or the proper clinical acumen experience many failures or only partial successes.

The main objective of the appliance, according to Balters, is to establish a muscular equilibrium between the forces of the tongue and outer neuromuscular envelope. The form and shape of the dental arches depend on this functional equilibrium. Changes in the equilibrium can lead to deformities that appear in the growth period. The consequences of these dysfunctions may be localized primarily in the dentoalveolar area, which is why the bionator is so effective in this region, as research by Janson (1982) has shown. Although many cases exist in which treatment with the bionator alone is possible, in most instances a combination of various therapeutic measures is needed to produce the best result. This is not all bad, however.

Special tooth movements (e.g., rotations, torquings, bodily movements for space closure, distalizations for opening space) cannot be performed with the bionator, any more than they can be with the conventional activator, even though the wearing time is doubled. Other mechanisms are available to satisfy these treatment objectives. The treatment of Class II, division 1 malocclusions in the mixed dentition using the standard bionator is indicated under the following conditions:

1. The dental arches are well aligned originally.
2. The mandible is in a posterior position (i.e., functional retrusion).
3. The skeletal discrepancy is not too severe.
4. A labial tipping of the upper incisors is evident.

The bionator is not indicated if the following is true:

1. The Class II relationship is caused by maxillary prognathism.
2. A vertical growth pattern is present.
3. Labial tipping of the lower incisors is evident. Anterior posturing of the mandible with simultaneous uprighting of the lower incisors cannot be performed with the bionator.

Cases of deep overbite also can be successfully managed with the standard bionator, after grinding away of the acrylic is performed to permit uninhibited eruption of the buccal segment teeth. This means a step-by-step trimming in the area of the molars and premolars. The best treatment time is during the eruption of the premolars. However, treatment will be successful only if the deep bite is caused by infraclusion of the molars and premolars, which is caused primarily by lateral tongue posture or thrust. Treatment will not work if the overbite is caused by supraclusion of the incisors. In buccal segment infraclusion the freeway space is usually large, which is a good precondition for both the bionator and the activator. In cases with a strong horizontal growth pattern the bionator is not indicated for treatment of deep overbite.

Malocclusions with crowding should not be treated with the bionator, despite the buccal segment expansion that might be achieved because of the buccinator loops. Cases with crowding can be better managed with a specially modified activator or after eruption of the premolars with active plates. Of course, fixed appliances provide the best individual tooth control in such cases.

Open-bite cases can be handled with the open-bite bionator, in which the buccal segment teeth are loaded for all possible intrusive stimulus. The bionator is particularly successful in open-bite cases that result from abnormal habits such as finger sucking, retained infantile deglutitional patterns, and aberrant tongue function. Open-bite problems with skeletal etiology require other methods of treatment, however.

Although Balters recommended his reverse-type bionator for Class III–type malocclusions, other clinicians have had only limited success.

The appliance is designed to load the mandibular teeth and unload the upper anterior alveolar portion, where growth stimulation is desired, especially during eruption of the incisors. The objective envisioned by Balters was a functional loading of this maxillary lingual area by increased tongue function. He thought this could be stimulated by guiding the tongue forward with the palatal bar. This in turn would move the incisors and supporting alveolar process labially. Studies by Rakosi et al (1977), however, have shown that the palatal bar usually only flattens the dorsum of the tongue and does not move it anteriorly. Whether the loop is opened anteriorly or posteriorly is of no consequence, according to cinefluorographic records made on patients. The reversed appliance seems to tip the maxillary incisors labially but does not stimulate basal bone forward movement. Thus the only indication for this type of appliance is in pseudo–Class III problems in which the upper incisors are tipped lingually, causing an anterior mandibular displacement on closure from postural rest to habitual occlusion.

## BIONATOR AND TEMPOROMANDIBULAR JOINT CASES

A special use for the bionator, which has been quite successful, is in temporomandibular joint (TMJ) problems. This success is especially noteworthy in adult patients. A majority of TMJ problems have coincidental bruxism and clenching during the rapid eye movement (REM) period of sleep. Wearing a bionator at night tends to relax the muscle spasms that occur, particularly those of the lateral pterygoid muscle (LPM). The design of the appliance for this purpose is similar to that of the standard appliance, except the construction bite need not move the mandible as far forward. The main purpose is to prevent the riding of the condyle over the posterior edge of the disk, which causes the clicking. By checking clinically, first in habitual occlusion and then in a forward-postured mandible, the operator can determine how far forward the mandible must be brought to eliminate the clicking on the opening maneuver. The clicking usually disappears in these cases when the mandible is opened in the forward posture. This means that the condyle no longer rides over the posterior disk margin, onto the retrodiscal pad. Such action is ultimately damaging to both the disk and the pad, causing problems such as objective pain, dysfunction symptoms, and headaches. The bionator maintains the forward position, preventing deleterious parafunctional effects at night. The construction bite also is opened slightly, and lower incisors can then be capped. No grinding is done; thus when the acrylic is worn, it grasps or loads both upper and lower buccal segments, guiding the mandible forward during the clenching or bruxing activity. Bionator therapy, with local heat applications and muscle relaxants, can provide dramatic and almost immediate relief. In many instances, adult Class II patients learn an accommodative forward position as the muscles adapt. The apparent reason for this adaptation is the foreshortening of the protracting muscles of the mandible, not a stimulus of growth or morphologic changes in the condyle. However, the patient must wear the appliance indefinitely as a splint at night for this to happen.

## SUMMARY

The bionator is effective in treating functional or mild skeletal Class II malocclusions in the mixed and transitional dentitions, provided that the appliance is chosen after a careful diagnostic study, it is made correctly and managed properly by loading and unloading different areas as indicated during the eruption of the premolars, and the patient complies in both daytime and nighttime wear. A special indication is in the treatment of TMJ patients who have bruxism and clenching, clicking, and crepitus. Such problems are amenable to bionator therapy, and relief of the objective symptoms is dramatic.

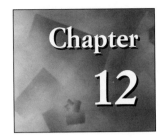

# Chapter 12

# The Fränkel Function Regulator

T.M. Graber

The philosophy of traditional functional appliances and their indications, use, and success have been discussed in previous chapters.

Essential diagnostic procedures have been discussed in detail to help the clinician assess the original malocclusion and determine whether it is a suitable case for a functional appliance. The biologic basis of the workings of these appliances has been extensively studied and validated in the first two chapters. The American clinician no longer doubts that a potent tool exists to be used for the right case at the right time. However, major questions remain: Which functional appliance should be used? Are they all the same? What are the criteria for appliance selection and use? Which is preferable—nighttime or full-time wear? Should a classical Andresen activator, Bimler appliance, Stockfisch kinetor, Balters bionator, or Herren, Clark twin block, or Hamilton wide open-bite activator be used? What about the Fränkel appliance?*

For answers to some of these questions a full appreciation of the concepts of Fränkel and the appliances he uses is imperative. Fränkel has had a greater impact on American orthodontics than has any other proponent of functional appliances. His visits to the United States in the past 20 years have been extremely successful as judged by the great numbers of orthodontists who have attended his courses under the aegis of the American Association of Orthodontists, Kenilworth Research Foundation, G.V. Black Institute for Continuing Education, University of Chicago, Ann Arbor Orthodontic Study Club, and University of Detroit. His appearances on the annual program of the American Association of Orthodontists have drawn large audiences, as did his pre-Congress course in San Francisco at the AAO-WFO meeting in May 1995. From American orthodontists, trained with fixed multiattachment appliances and taught that European methods were inferior or socioeconomic compromises, this is quite a tribute. Fränkel, a meticulous scientist and consummate clinician, has passed the major test—he has provided strong proof of his method's effectiveness. Plaster study models illustrate its capabilities. Serial radiographic cephalometric records also substantiate that success, as do facial and intraoral radiographs.

*Credit is gratefully given to Rolf Fränkel for most of the illustrations in this chapter.

As is often the case, the disciple is not immediately able to duplicate the results attained by the master. Teaching a new way of approaching orthodontic problems and correcting them cannot be done in a series of 2-day courses or 45-minute lectures to national meetings. Self-teaching is effective if a computer or learned teacher provides feedback, but most American clinicians have not benefited from firsthand guidance. Using a Fränkel appliance for the first time may be likened to learning to use a sailboard. Anyone who has climbed on one of these fascinating and challenging crafts knows what it feels like to be dunked in the water a number of times before mastering the art of sailing. This effort has resulted in disappointment for many sailboard users. Similarly, some practitioners have published articles questioning the effectiveness of the Fränkel appliance. The experiences of these practitioners can be compared to those of the sailboard neophyte with no firsthand lessons who has nearly drowned trying to stay on the board and then decides to write about the experience after the first 50 unceremonious dunkings. The practitioner's situation is even worse than this. The sailboard novice can at least assume that the board is made properly and balanced and will work well in the right hands. For the Fränkel appliance user who is untrained in taking a construction bite and then sends impressions to a laboratory that does not know the way to fabricate the appliance properly, the chance of success is poor. The additional continuing challenge of maintaining patient compliance with an appliance that requires considerable effort to wear in the beginning weeks, an appliance that makes normal speech very difficult at first, also militates against the achievement of treatment goals. As with any misused orthodontic appliance, even iatrogenic response is possible, and labial tipping of lower incisors or actual labiogingival dehiscence from improperly made lip pads may result.

Because of the problems encountered by many beginning Fränkel appliance users (who often turn to other, less demanding functional appliances), this chapter primarily addresses those aspects of function regulator (FR) management that are most crucial for success—the different philosophies, the construction of the Fränkel appliances (FR I, II, III, IV), the construction bite, laboratory proceedings, the mode of action of the various FR modifications, the clinical handling of the appliance, and successful treatment considerations.

## FRÄNKEL PHILOSOPHY

The larger part of the Fränkel appliance is confined to the oral vestibule (Figure 12-1), unlike the structure of conventional activators. The buccal shields and lip pads hold the buccal and labial musculature away from the teeth and investing tissues, eliminating any possible restrictive influence from this functional matrix (Figure 12-2). In this way, the Fränkel appliance resembles the bionator.

Fränkel thinks this active muscle and tissue mass (the buccinator mechanism and the orbicularis oris complex) has a potential restraining influence on the outward development of the dental arches, particularly during the transitional period of development. Abnormal perioral muscle function can exert a deforming action that prevents full accomplishment of the optimal growth and developmental pattern. This approach differs from the conventional "push-out-from-within" action of other removable appliances, which expand without relieving external muscle forces and force the new dentoalveolar morphology to adapt. Fränkel conceives his vestibular constructions as an artificial "ought-to-be" matrix that allows the muscles to exercise and adapt. Implicit in this protection from constant neuromuscular constriction of the dentition, particularly mesial to the deciduous second molars, is the possibility of expansion; if the buccinator-mechanism pressures are screened from the dentition, significant expansion may occur in the critical intercanine dimension. This relieves the crowding often seen in the lower anterior segment, which often leads to the removal of four first premolars in fixed multiattachment mechanotherapy. Fränkel shows extensive long-term data to support this working hypothesis in the form of plaster casts before and well after treatment and in anteroposterior cephalograms showing significant apical base expansion relative to controls. The autonomous improvement and stability associated with this treatment are striking for an appliance that does not even touch the affected teeth.

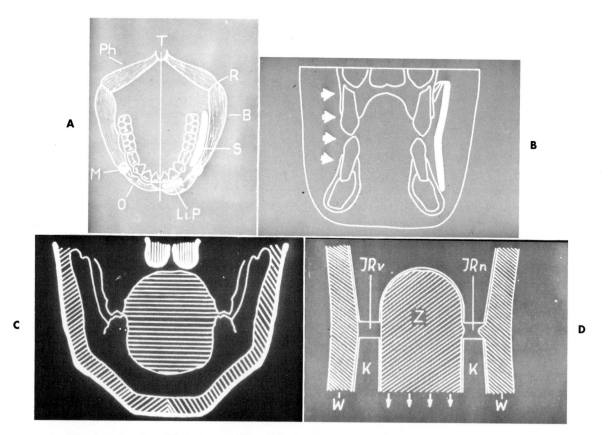

**Figure 12-1.** **A** and **B,** Screening effect of the buccal shields and lip pads, holding off the buccinator mechanism and orbicularis oris pressures. The continuous band of muscles, anchored at the pharyngeal tubercle (*T*), passes around the pharynx through the constrictor muscles to the pterygomandibular raphe (*R*) and continues anteriorly through the buccinator (*B*) and orbicularis oris (*O*) to form a continuous restrictive band. *Ph,* Pharyngeal musculature; *S,* shield; *M,* corner of mouth; *LiP,* lip pad. **C,** Counterbalancing effect of the tongue if the dorsum is in contact with the palate. On swallowing, a negative atmospheric pressure is created that sucks the cheeks into the interocclusal space, **D,** to help maintain the interocclusal space at postural resting position before the mandible drops at the end of the deglutitional cycle. *W,* Cheeks; *K,* dentoalveolar area; *JRv,* interocclusal space; *JRn,* interocclusal space with cheek invagination. (Courtesy Rolf Fränkel.)

A prime factor in its success is that the Fränkel appliance is an exercise device, stimulating normal function while eliminating the lip trap, hyperactive mentalis, and aberrant buccinator and orbicularis oris action. To achieve these objectives requires full-time wear, not just nighttime wear when asleep. Daily functional exercise is vitally important for Fränkel appliance success. To Fränkel (and other proponents of daytime-wear functional appliances, such as the Clark twin block), *functional* means continuously repetitive and frequent activity, which is not possible during sleep only.

The concept is not new: Kraus, a pioneer in "screening" therapy from Czechoslovakia, espoused the same philosophy in his book in 1956. Simple oral screens have been used for years, and the Mühlemann-Hotz propulsor has some of the same features as the bionator, albeit to a very limited degree. The routine expansion achieved after proper buccal-shield and lip-pad construction has been amply demonstrated, and long-term assessment of posttreatment results shows a noteworthy stability not seen with conventional fixed appliance expansion procedures. Expansion can undoubtedly be

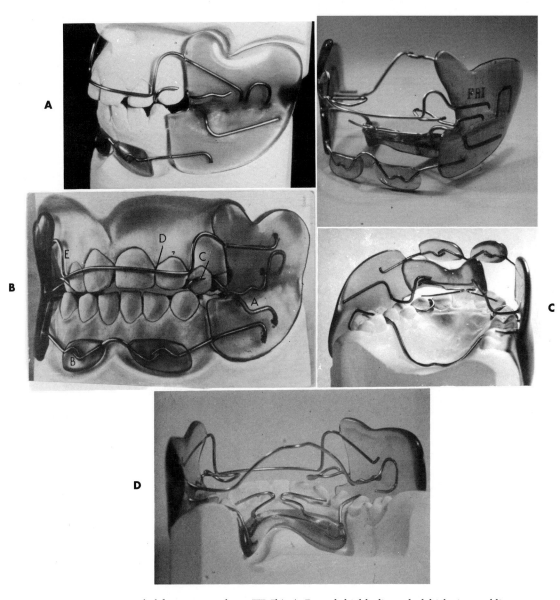

**Figure 12-2.** Fränkel function regulator (FR Ib). **A,** Buccal shields, lip pads, labial wire, and lingual appliance components on and off the plaster casts. **B,** Shields (*A*), lip pads (*B*), canine clasp (*C*), labial arch (*D*), and labial arch loop (*E*) identify the major vestibular components. **C,** Appliance in place on the maxillary cast. The palatal bow, molar occlusal rests, and canine clasps are visible on the left. The appliance is locked on the maxilla as the palatal bow and canine clasps pass through the embrasures mesial to the permanent first molar and first premolar. **D,** Lingual acrylic pad, lingual wires, and crossover hanger wire, in addition to the wire configurations mentioned, on the mandibular cast.

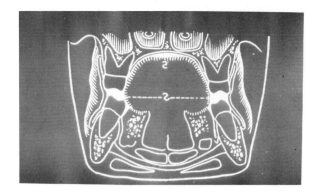

**Figure 12-3.** Contiguity of buccal musculature and tongue to the teeth and supporting structures. The lingual inclination of the mandibular buccal segments is evident. Abnormal perioral muscle function allows the tongue to drop and tips the maxillary buccal segments lingually. Mandibular width is seldom affected, however. (Courtesy Rolf Fränkel.)

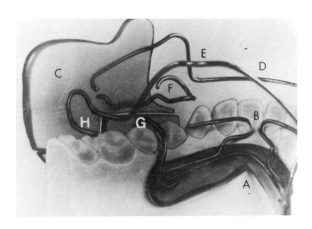

**Figure 12-4.** FR Ia mounted on the lower cast. Lingual pad (*A*), passive lingual springs (*B*), shield (*C*), labial wire (*D*), palatal bow (*E*), canine clasp (*F*), crossover hanger wire (*G*), and molar rest (*H*).

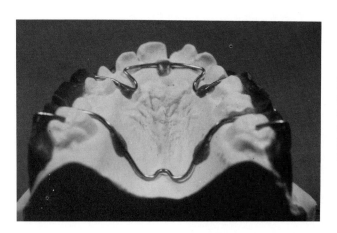

**Figure 12-5.** FR II under construction (occlusal view). Palatal and lingual incisor wires are anchored in the embrasures mesial to the permanent first molars and first premolars or deciduous first molars if present. This is essential to ensure proper FR action. For proper seating below the marginal ridge, disking (or notching) of the deciduous teeth at the embrasure is usually necessary.

achieved from within and without, but the adaptation of the contiguous musculature to the vestibular artificial functional-matrix constriction with appropriate exercises clearly indicates that musculature plays a significant role in determining the arch form and size (Figure 12-3).

The analysis of the effects of buccal shields and lip pads in the previous paragraphs does not discuss the role of the tongue. Fränkel does not altogether ignore it. He holds that the tongue plays a significant role in the ultimate outward progression of the teeth and investing tissues. He also thinks, however, that its effect has been overstressed to the exclusion of the equally important buccal musculature. Much of tongue function may be compensatory or adaptive to dentoalveolar morphology and not necessarily the primary cause of the existing malocclusion.

As might be expected in an analysis of functional appliances, Fränkel emphasizes the form-function relationship. He calls for an understanding of the physiology of deglutition. Normally, with anterior lip seal and a posterior oral seal provided by the tongue and soft palate during the deglutitional process, a negative atmospheric pressure occurs within the oral cavity. The cheeks are actually sucked into the interocclusal space as the mandible returns to postural rest position in the terminal phase of the swallowing process (*JRn,* Figure 12-1). The effect is both a constricting influence on the dentoalveolar process and a prevention of eruption of the buccal segments by virtue of the interposed cheek tissue. The partial vacuum created inside the arch momentarily creates greater external pressure, offsetting the intrinsic force potential of the tongue. The FR buccal shields prevent the pressure of the buccinator mechanism from being exerted on the dentoalveolar area both during deglutition and at rest. The net effect is outward expansion to the "ought-to-be" acrylic shield functional matrix. Worn at a critical time in dental development, with maximal eruption in the direction of least resistance, the FR can induce optimal downward and outward movement of both teeth and investing tissues, as numerous studies have demonstrated.

Another difference between the Fränkel FR and conventional activator therapy is the manner in which the anteroposterior correction is achieved. Fränkel is not the only clinician to criticize the tendency for the conventional tooth-borne acrylic mass of the classic Andresen appliance (and the Herren, Harvold-Woodside, Hamilton, and L.S.U. modifications) to procline the lower incisors excessively. Björk pointed this out long ago. The loose-fitting appliance cannot be prevented from contacting the teeth in the anterior and posterior segments as the patient moves it up and down. At the very least the activator tends to rest on the lower incisors at night, when the mouth is partly open. To prevent this undesirable occurrence, Fränkel designed his appliance to impede all tooth contact in the lower arch. The forward posturing for the construction bite is achieved by lingual wire loops of the FR Ia or by a relatively thin acrylic pad that contacts the infradental mucosa only behind the lower anterior segment in the FR Ib or II (Figure 12-4). The pad serves more as a proprioceptive signal and pressure-bearing area for maintenance of mandibular propulsion than as a physical barrier to the return to the original sagittal relationship. The design and construction of the vestibular acrylic and wire configuration augment this proprioceptive trigger to maintain forward posturing.

An important part of the Fränkel technique is the fact that the FR is anchored to the maxillary dental arch in a positive manner. The priority for appliance use is that this objective be achieved in the mixed dentition through wires between the contacts at the mesial of the permanent maxillary first molars and the distal of the deciduous maxillary canines (Figure 12-5). The teeth *must* be separated to allow the wires to pass through the contacts below the occlusal surfaces. This separation may require disking of the distal surfaces of the deciduous canines and second molars. Simply allowing the wires to rest on these embrasures from the occlusal is inadequate and allows the same undesirable effect of lower incisor labial tipping common to the conventional activator. Added to this is the potential for damage to the labial gingival tissue by the lip pads as the appliance bobs up and down during the day. Recent articles on the subject demonstrate that this can cause the appliance to fail. Indeed, its failure stems from blatant misuse and is a reflection of the clinician who has ignored this axiom but nevertheless writes up the results. Unfortunately, this type

of misinformation has led to a marked reduction in use of the Fränkel appliance in the United States.

As Woodside, Rakosi, and Clark have shown in their chapters in this book, freeing the lower posterior teeth from acrylic or wire restraints while holding the bite open allows the unrestricted upward and forward movement of these teeth, contributing to both vertical and horizontal correction of the malocclusion. Maxillary molars are prevented from downward and forward movement by the FR appliance, which is anchored on the maxillary arch. Some expansion is possible, of course. The differential eruption can be expected to contribute 1 or 2 mm toward the usual 6 to 7 mm needed for establishment of correct sagittal interdigitation.

The labial wire of the Fränkel appliance rests on the maxillary incisors, but it is not activated or "pinched up," as is often done with a Hawley appliance to close spaces. This action tends to tip the incisors excessively to the lingual and their apices labially if the teeth rock on the lingual alveolar plate. It may even restrict full mandibular horizontal growth as the bite is deepened and the upper anterior segment exerts a retruding effect on the lower incisors and mandible at full closure when the appliance is not worn. The Fränkel appliance does have a restraining effect on the maxillary teeth and arch, although McNamara's research (1981) indicates that this is minimal. Lee Graber (unpublished study, 1993) however, has shown that in selected cases the FR actually has a headgear effect, holding back the maxilla's downward and forward progression. Incisors can be tipped lingually and spaces closed if needed by pre–functional appliance treatment with fixed or removable appliances; this is preferred to activation of the FR labial wire.

Fränkel has stressed another theoretic action of the buccal shields and lip pads. In addition to preventing deforming muscle action and permitting the teeth to erupt down and outward, the shields and pads can be extended into the depth of the vestibule, putting the tissue under tension without creating irritation. This tension conceivably exerts a pull on the contiguous periosteal tissue of the maxillary bone (Figure 12-6). Experiments by Enlow, Hoyt, and Moffett have shown that periosteal pull can elicit increased bone activity in contiguous osseous structures. If periosteal pull works, the maxillary basal bone is widened as the thin alveolar shell over the erupting teeth proliferates laterally. Anteroposterior (AP) cephalograms of many of Fränkel's cases do, indeed, show apical-base widening. The working hypothesis is valid, but experimental work thus far has not verified this effect. In a research project on primates sponsored by the National Institutes of Health (NIH) at the American Dental Association (ADA) Research Institute by Graber et al (unpublished study, 1988) the buccal shields have been clearly shown to stimulate *bodily* buccal movement of posterior teeth and buccal plate activity far beyond the activity observed in controls (Figure 12-7). As far as periosteal pull is concerned, however, the effect seems to be temporary, confined to the first 2 weeks of appliance wear. The degree to which the significant expansion is caused by periosteal pull or relief of the restraining effect of the musculature is conjectural at this point. Again, the vestibular constructions serve as a base for oral gymnastics—prescribed exercises

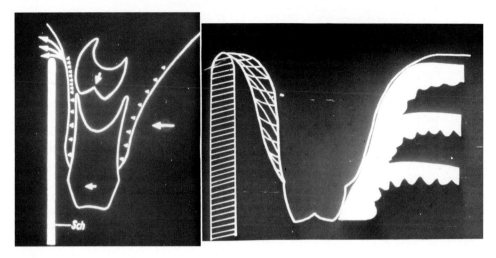

**Figure 12-6.** Relief of the buccinator mechanism forces on the dentoalveolar area. The shield extends to the depths of the vestibule, exerting pressure on tissue attachments to the alveolar bone. In addition to relieving the external pressure, particularly when it is strongest (during deglutition), the shields exert an indirect tension on the periosteum overlying the bone. Experiments have shown that this enhances osseous proliferation and results in more bodily tooth movement of both erupted and unerupted teeth, with changes in the buccal and lingual bony surfaces.

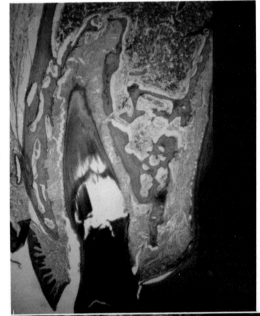

A

**Figure 12-7.** Experimental results of studies on squirrel monkeys by Graber et al. Buccal shields extended into the maxillary vestibular depths from Fränkel-type appliances pinned to the palate substantiate Fränkel's clinical claims. The histologic section, **A,** shows the erupting tooth, with resorption on the contiguous buccal plate and deposition on the lingual alveolar process and external surface of the buccal plate. This response is illustrated better in **B** and its diagram, **C.** The section of the buccal alveolar crest clearly shows the resorptive processes contiguous to the buccal surface of the tooth, with lamellar deposition at the crest and on the buccal surface, in animals wearing buccal shields. It also shows bodily eruption of the premolar tooth.

B

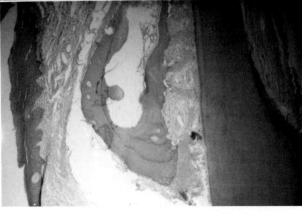

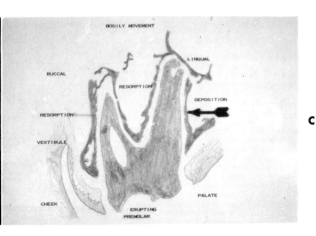

C

performed by the patient each day—to accomplish maximal benefit. Lip-seal exercises are a most important part of patient management (as is stressed later). Primates cannot be trained to do this, which may be the reason that some research fails to mention the total effect possible on the periosteal tissue. One phase of the unpublished ADA study is on 50 patients with Class II, division 1 malocclusion in the mixed dentition. The results obtained with Fränkel appliance wear confirm the claims by Fränkel and McNamara and others.

## VISUAL TREATMENT OBJECTIVE DIAGNOSTIC TEST (FR-VTO)

At the initial clinical examination a simple but important maneuver can give the operator an excellent clue as to whether the Fränkel appliance or any functional appliance that postures the mandible forward will improve the facial appearance and profile. First the patient is asked to swallow and then lick the lips and relax. Sometimes a few syllables are repeated to achieve a relaxed mandibular position and an approximation of postural rest. Then the patient is instructed to close the teeth in habitual occlusion, again licking the lips first, and to keep the teeth lightly together with the lips relaxed. These two profile relationships are carefully studied and may be photographed to obtain an instant print. The pa-

tient is then asked to posture the mandible forward into a correct sagittal relationship, or construction bite, reducing the overjet. A photograph of this profile may be compared with the original snapshot depicting the teeth in occlusion (Figure 12-8). If this clinical exercise makes the facial balance look better, the functional appliance will probably be beneficial. For good patient management, operators should give the photographs to the patient and parent to show the significant improvement in the facial profile and motivate the patient toward an achievable treatment goal. If the profile is not improved by forward mandibular posturing or is actually made worse, other forms of treatment are probably needed. This may occur in patients with excessive anterior face height, procumbency of the lower incisors, deficient symphyseal development, and very steep mandibular planes. Obviously a cursory visualization is no substitute for a comprehensive cephalometric analysis to determine the best possible appliance. Patients with anteriorly rotating growth patterns, functional retrusion, deep overbites, and excessive interocclusal clearances with a normally positioned maxillas are good candidates. Previous chapters on principles of functional appliances, cephalometric and functional diagnosis, Class II treatment, and deep overbite discuss the indications and contraindications for functional appliance treatment. Because essentially the same criteria apply to Fränkel appliance treatment, details are not repeated here.

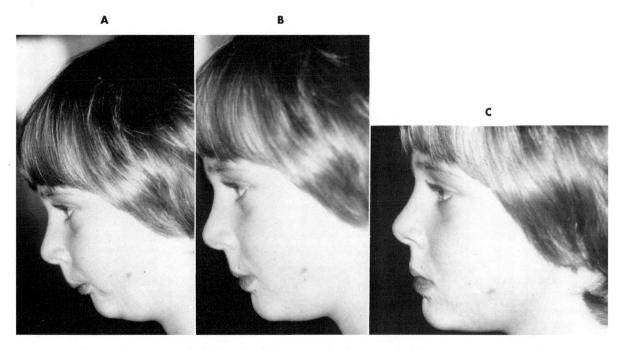

**Figure 12-8.** A marked Class II, division 1 malocclusion with full occlusion, **A,** 3 mm of mandibular protraction, **B,** and 6 mm of cuspal advancement into a Class I buccal segment relationship, **C.** The dramatic change produced provides a visual treatment objective (VTO) for potential Fränkel appliance users. If the profile is not improved by this maneuver, some other appliance may be needed.

## CONSTRUCTION BITE AND FABRICATION OF THE FRÄNKEL APPLIANCE

The primary use of functional appliances in the United States has been as a deficiency appliance and a deterrent to abnormal perioral muscle function. Therefore most cases are Class II, division 1 malocclusions. To a lesser degree the activator has been used in Class II, division 2 and open-bite problems. The same case-selection constraints apply to the Fränkel appliance. Rolf and Christine Fränkel (1989) have presented dramatic evidence of the efficacy of the FR III in Class III and the FR IV in properly chosen cases of skeletal open bite, findings that were also reported in the *American Journal of Orthodontics and Dentofacial Orthopedics.*

Fränkel has designed four basic variations of the FR appliance. The FR I is for correction of Class I and Class II, division 1 malocclusions. The FR II is for Class II, division 1 and 2 cases. The FR III is for Class III problems. The FR IV is used for open bites and bimaxillary protrusions. This section of the chapter, devoted to appliance construction, primarily addresses the FR I and III. Variation for the FR II and IV is minimal. Classic nonextraction treatment is described; this does not mean that the FR cannot be used in extraction cases, with some appliance changes. Fränkel has illustrated a number of successful extraction cases. However, the more sophisticated uses of the FR are beyond the scope of this book.

On first impression the Fränkel appliance appears complicated and possibly fragile to both operator and patient. Fränkel's design demands precise fabrication and minimal compromises during construction, which may discourage some clinicians. However, such precision and care result in few subsequent adjustments needed during active therapy other than advancing the lip and lingual pads and correcting appliance distortions. Laboratories with well-trained and competent staff can now make appliances according to prescription—a situation that did not exist in the early days of FR use in the United States. Many of the early failures were caused by improper fabrication.

### FR I

Three FR I appliance modifications actually exist. However, the original FR Ia, with a lingual wire loop instead of an acrylic lingual mandibular pad, is now seldom used (Figure 12-9). Perhaps the best use of the FR I has been in Class I cases with minor crowding and delayed development of the basal bony and dental structures. Fränkel recommends the FR Ia for Class I deep-bite cases with protruded maxillary and retruded mandibular incisors. Although the appliance is occasionally used for Class II, division 1 malocclusions in which the overjet does not exceed 5 mm, the lingual-acrylic construction of the FR Ib is generally preferred now (see Figures 12-2 and 12-4).

The vestibular shields are unique components of the Fränkel appliances (see Figures 12-1, 12-2, 12-4, 12-6, 12-9, and 12-10). The labial lip pads, or pelots (as Fränkel calls them), are analogous to some of the lip bumpers used with various fixed appliances in the United States to eliminate lip trap and hyperactive mentalis muscle function, but their placement and fabrication must be extremely precise. As Figure 12-2 shows, in addition to connecting wires between the shields and pads, the Fränkel appliance also features a maxillary labial bow with canine loops.

Instead of the bulky acrylic of most activators that covers the palate, the FR has a palatal bow shaped like a coffin spring with the open end facing anteriorly. The buccal extensions of

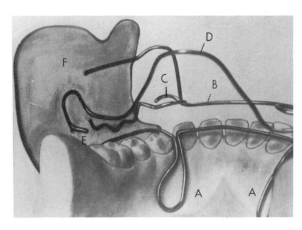

**Figure 12-9.** FR Ia on the mandibular cast. Wire loops (*A*) instead of the acrylic lingual pad, are used to posture the mandible forward. Other parts identified are the maxillary labial wire (*B*), maxillary canine clasp (*C*), palatal wire (*D*), maxillary molar occlusal rest (*E*), and buccal shield (*F*). The hanger wire (passing between the upper and lower occlusal surfaces) is an extension of the lingual loops (*A*). It is passive and does not contact the upper or lower posterior teeth.

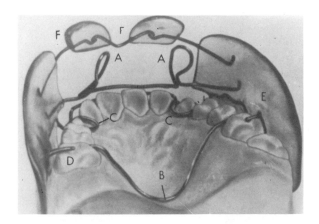

**Figure 12-10.** FR Ia mounted on the maxillary cast. Identified are the mandibular lingual posturing loops (*A*), transpalatal wire (*B*), canine clasps (*C*), occlusal rest (*D*), buccal shield (*E*), and lip pads (*F*). The palatal and canine wires pass through the notched proximal embrasures in direct contact with the maxillary first molar and first premolar–canine area. This locks the appliance on the maxillary dentition and is essential for proper use.

the loop pass through the embrasures between the permanent first molars and deciduous second molars and are anchored on each side in the buccal shields (Figure 12-10). These lateral extensions must extend below the occlusal surfaces of the embrasures to lock the appliance on the maxillary arch and prevent a free float. As noted earlier, the locking of the FR appliance on the maxillary arch is accomplished largely by this firm insertion in the embrasure. Special elastic separators are available to create sufficient space; however, if they are difficult to place, the distal convexity of the deciduous upper second molar may have to be disked or notched. Therefore separating the molar and canine embrasures, even before taking the impressions, and then replacing the heavy separators are recommended steps.

For the FR, the ends of the palatal bow can be bent back to terminate on the maxillary first molars as occlusal rests (see Figure 12-10). The maxillary canine loops also project from the lingual part of the shield into the canine–deciduous first molar embrasure, wrapping around the lingual of the canines and terminating on their labial surfaces. The loops assist in anchoring the appliance on the maxilla and guiding the erupting canines into place. They also exert mild distal pressure on the deciduous first molars to prevent these teeth from coming forward (see Figures 12-2, 12-4, and 12-10).

On the mandible a lingual bow with U loops may extend to the floor of the mouth to fit against the lingual tissue below the incisors, as in the FR Ia (see Figure 12-9), or an acrylic pad may replace these wires, as will be discussed in reference to FR Ib (see Figures 12-2 and 12-4). The objective in each case is to provide a proprioceptive signal to the mandible so it remains in the forward position when the appliance is worn to correct a Class II condition. The mandible is held forward by the protracting muscles and not the appliance itself (although the ends of the lower loops do contact the apical base lingual tissue). This bilateral foreshortening of the lateral pterygoid muscles (LPMs) is quite important for all functional appliances and may lead to permanent changes in the muscle. The lingual wire that joins the loops, crossing the lower incisors at their cingula, does not exert any pressure on the incisors. In rare instances in which the proclination of the incisors is desirable, the wire can be activated for this purpose.

To hold this new position, the mandible is stabilized against the maxillary teeth by cross-occlusal wires at the first molar–canine-premolar embrasures, as previously described. The interproximal wires are aided by a passive labial bow on the maxillary incisors. The cross-palatal coffin-spring type of stabilizing wire provides rigidity for the appliance because it has no palatal acrylic (see Figure 12-10). The occlusal supports between the mesiobuccal and distobuccal cusps of the first molars keep the FR I from being dislodged superiorly, which would force the periphery of the shields into the sulcus tissue and allow the crosspalatal wire to impinge on the tissue. These supports also prevent upper molar eruption; the lower molars, however, are free to erupt mesially in Class II corrections, as with the Clark twin block (see Chapter 13).

The buccal shields (see Figures 12-1, 12-2, 12-4, 12-9, and 12-10) are contiguous to the buccal surfaces of the molars and premolars, extending as deeply into the vestibular limits as the tissue and patient comfort allow while still maintaining a slight tension. To relieve pressures from the buccinator mechanism, the buccal shields stand away from the maxillary dentition and basal alveolar bone. As shown earlier, the aim is to allow all possible alveolodental development and needed bodily expansion of the teeth in the buccal segments (see Figure 12-1). The extension of the peripheral portions of the shields into the vestibular depths creates a slight tension on the connective tissue fibers in the sulci (see Figure 12-6). The objective is to stimulate periosteal pull with an intermittently outward force aided by lip seal exercises. The working hypothesis, as previously noted, is that this unidirectional pull enhances basal bone development and allows the teeth to erupt bodily into a more buccal position.

Like the buccal shields, the lip pads (see Figure 12-2) work by eliminating abnormal perioral muscle activity, particularly of the hyperactive and potentially deforming mentalis muscle. By intercepting the lip trap, with the lower lip cushioning to the lingual of the maxillary incisors, lip pads control the deforming muscular activity in both arches (Figure 12-11). Fränkel has suggested that a periosteal pull occurs labially from the lip-pad pressure in the anterior vestibular depth that exerts a bone-growth stimulus, reducing the pronounced mentolabial sulcus. (This has not been demonstrated in primate studies, however.) The lip pads serve another function. They form the labial boundary of the mandibular posturing trough. With the lingual loops (or acrylic pad in the FR Ib), they maintain the mandible in its forward construction bite for Class II correction.

**FR Ib.** The FR Ib has largely replaced the FR Ia. With the exception of substituting a lingual acrylic pad for the lower anterior wire loops to maintain forward mandibular posture, it is essentially the same appliance (see Figures 12-2 and 12-4).

In the FR Ib, instead of a single wire crossing the lingual surfaces of the lower incisors, two passive recurved springs rest gently above the cingula. The skeletal wires that help form the lingual acrylic pad penetrate the buccal shields, passing between the upper and lower occlusal surfaces in the deciduous molar region. Care must be taken to prevent the cross-occlusal wires from contacting any teeth when the appliance is fully seated. Fränkel suggests the use of this appliance in Class II, division 1 malocclusions with a deep bite and an overjet that does not exceed 7 mm. As is true of most functional appliances, the prognosis with the FR Ib is better if the molars do not exceed an end-to-end sagittal cuspal relationship. Construction is simpler than it is for the FR Ia, and patients generally become accustomed to the lingual acrylic pad more easily than they do to the U-loops. The preliminary clinical procedures and laboratory fabrication of the FR Ib are described next.

***Separation.*** Experts recommend that separators be placed in the maxillary canine–deciduous first molar and deciduous second molar–permanent first molar contact areas before the impression-taking procedure. If this is done 5 to 7 days before the impressions are taken, the need for disking or notching is reduced. Special heavy elastic separators are available for this

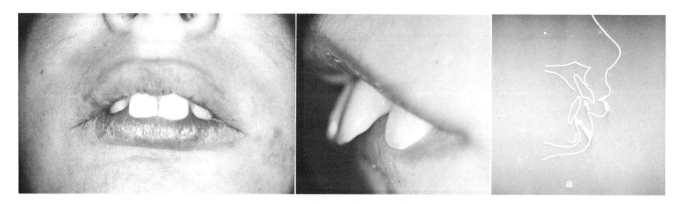

**Figure 12-11.**  Deforming activity of the lip trap, with the lower lip cushioning to the lingual of the maxillary incisors during function. Under these conditions, normal lip seal is not possible. Not only are the maxillary incisors moved forward against a hypotonic upper lip, but the hypertonic lower lip and hyperactive mentalis muscle exert a lingualizing and crowding effect on the lower anterior segment.

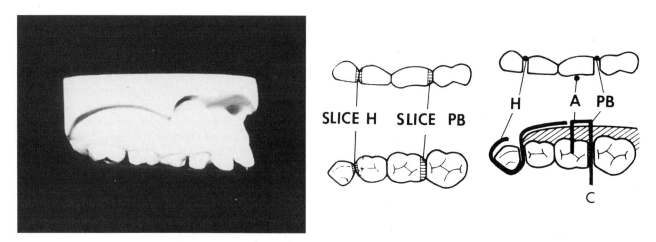

**Figure 12-12.**  Space between the maxillary first molar and deciduous second molar and at the canine–deciduous first molar embrasure is essential before placing the FR appliance. If separators do not create sufficient room to anchor the appliance on the maxillary arch, the proximal areas can be "sliced" or disked (as shown in the drawing). Care must be taken, however, not to injure any permanent teeth. Slice *H* is for the canine clasp; *PB* for the palatal bow. On deciduous dentitions the maxillary molar rest (*A*) is bent mesially to overlie the deciduous second molar.

purpose. As already emphasized, the appliance must be anchored on the maxillary arch when placed or as soon as possible thereafter (see Figures 12-5 and 12-10). The separators usually provide sufficient room in the embrasures for seating of the palatal loop extension and canine loop crossover wires without cutting away tooth structure. However, mixed-dentition treatment often necessitates slicing the distal contact of the deciduous upper second molars and the mesial marginal ridges of the deciduous upper first molars to ensure proper locking of the appliance on the maxilla in the critical period of initial adjustment (Figure 12-12). An occlusal rest is then placed on the deciduous upper second molars.

*Impression taking.* As with other functional appliances, impression taking with the FR Ib is critical. Indeed, the technique is more demanding, because the impressions should re-

produce the whole alveolar process to the depths of the sulci, including the maxillary tuberosities.

In his various trips to the United States, Fränkel has stressed the importance of impression-taking and construction-bite procedures more than any other phase of management, having frequently found mistakes in these areas. With the need for total extension of the coverage, care must be exercised not to distort the soft tissues and muscle attachments. The metal flanges of the impression trays should not reach too far into the sulci (Figure 12-13). Rimming the trays with a soft utility wax or similar compound permits individualizing the trays for a more faithful reproduction. The consistency of the impression material should allow for a good but *thin* peripheral roll, displacing the tissue gently and reproducing the muscle attachments (see Figure 12-13). The idea is to reproduce the resting vestibular sulcus and not overextend or distort the

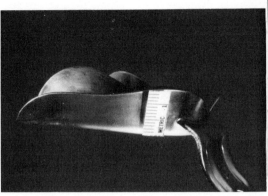
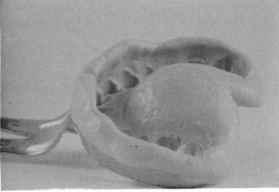

**Figure 12-13.** The proper tray should not be overextended because this distorts the musculature and muscle attachments. A distance of 15 mm from the bottom of the tray to the top is about as far as the tray should extend. A relatively thin peripheral roll is needed on the impression to prevent distortion of the contiguous tissue.

tissues. Preformed disposable Styrofoam trays are usually inadequate. One of the more successful techniques uses a thermal-sensitive acrylic tray that can be softened in hot water (175° F), fitted to the model, and then inserted and adapted to the individual morphology. A custom tray also can be fabricated based on the study models, if desired. The proper tray choice, beading, and impressions improve the detail needed while reducing the amount of cast trimming.

***Construction bite (Figures 12-14 and 12-15).*** Current opinions on the placement of the mandible for functional appliances vary. Procedures differ in both the degree of vertical opening and amount of forward posturing of the mandible. As with all physiologic phenomena, adaptation is likely for a range of vertical and horizontal positionings. Figure 12-14 shows one way, suggested by Fränkel, that allows complete visualization of the incisor relationship for correct midline and vertical opening. The following procedure is based on the author's experiences with the Fränkel appliances:

For minor sagittal problems (2 to 4 mm) the practitioner takes the construction bite in an end-to-end incisal relationship, as with the bionator, exercising extreme care to prevent the obvious strain of facial muscles. The balance between protractor and retractor muscles must not be disturbed. A good clinical practice is to have the patient hold the mandible in the desired forward position, with midlines correct, for 3 to 5 minutes and repeat the maneuver of moving the mandible forward several times (Figure 12-16). Use of a practice construction bite, a softened U-shaped roll of bite wax placed on the lower teeth and imprinted with the desired forward position, is a valuable practice and is recommended for all functional appliances. Fränkel now recommends that the construction bite not move the mandible farther forward than 2.5 to 3 mm. The vertical opening should be only large enough to allow the crossover wires through the interocclusal space without contacting the teeth. For most nighttime-wear activators, however, the construction bite requires a larger horizontal and more vertical posturing. Schmuth (1995) notes that most pa-

tients easily tolerate 4 to 6 mm of advancement and opening, which allows an end-to-end incisal relationship to be established for most Class II malocclusions. Fränkel originally subscribed to this amount of posturing, but clinical and experimental research showed that step-by-step activation produced a better and more continuous tissue reaction, particularly in the condyle, than did the "great leap forward" for full-time wear. Patients also were more likely to accept this amount, which frees the airway for enhancement of normal nasal breathing (Figure 12-16).

If an end-to-end relationship, or no more than 6 mm forward posturing, is used, the incisal contact determines the vertical opening. A clearance of at least 2.5 to 3.5 mm in the buccal segments is necessary to allow the crossover wires to pass through in the Fränkel appliance (or any occlusal appliance), so the incisal vertical relationship usually results in discluding these teeth. A tongue blade is sometimes placed between the teeth during taking of the construction bite to establish sufficient vertical clearance for the crossover wires. For many functional appliance clinicians a good rule of thumb is that the greater the horizontal movement, the less the vertical opening should be. For both the bionator and the Fränkel appliances, however, vertical opening is kept to a minimum.

Histologic research by Petrovic confirms the clinical impression that correcting the sagittal discrepancy in two or three stages may be more effective for both tissue response and patient adjustment to the forward posturing. Staged construction bites allow the practitioner to observe optimal prechondroblastic activity in the condyle. Chapters 2 and 5 to 7 cover the construction-bite technique and the important research at the tissue, cell, and molecular level.

For the Fränkel appliance, if 6 mm of sagittal movement is needed to correct the anteroposterior relationship, a construction bite of 3 mm forward posturing permits easy adaptation by the patient and reduces the likelihood of dislodgment during both day and night, muscle strain or fatigue, and unwanted proclination of lower incisors. The design and construction of the FR permit staged advancement of the

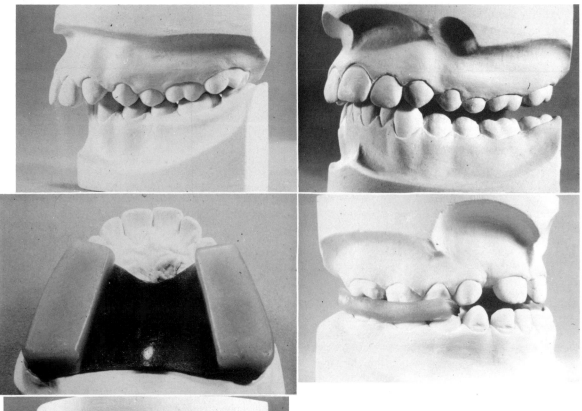

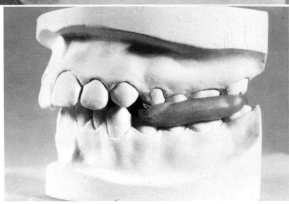

**Figure 12-14.** In the Fränkel technique the construction bite is not opened any more than needed to allow the crossover wires to pass through the interdental space. This measure is necessary for effective lip-seal exercises. The amount of forward positioning is usually about 3 mm, or half the width of a cusp. In mild Class II malocclusions this can correct the sagittal discrepancy in one step. Fränkel uses an adapted baseplate to which wax is added and softened for the construction bite. By leaving the anterior region open, he visualizes the midlines for proper registration in all three dimensions.

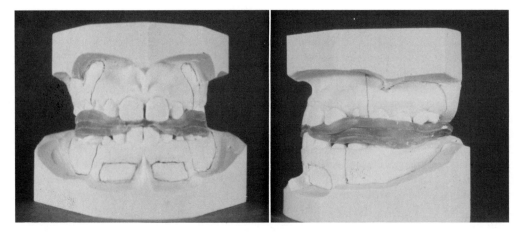

**Figure 12-15.** The horseshoe-shaped wafer is made up of three layers of softened beeswax. It is cut away on the incisal to permit determination of the correct vertical, sagittal, and midline registration. Lip pads and buccal shields are already outlined on the stone models.

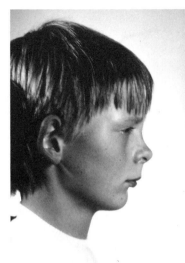
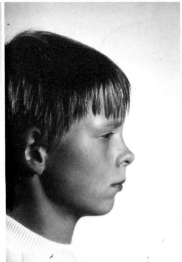
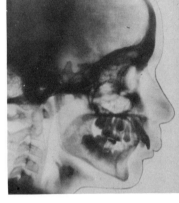
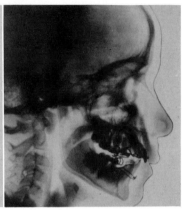

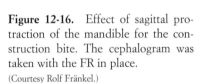

**Figure 12-16.** Effect of sagittal protraction of the mandible for the construction bite. The cephalogram was taken with the FR in place.
(Courtesy Rolf Fränkel.)

mandible after a favorable response to treatment from the original construction bite has been noted, usually after 6 months of appliance wear. The patient readily adjusts to the new advancement of the lip pads and lingual acrylic flange because the appliance is already comfortable in other aspects.

Even though the step-by-step forward-posturing procedure is used for the FR, the vertical opening still cannot be increased much beyond an end-to-end bite without endangering lip closure and lip-seal exercises or losing control of tongue activity and increasing the danger that the appliance will bob up and down. Some clinicians consider this a limitation of the Fränkel appliance—in contrast to the other functional appliances in which the height of the bite can be modified to take advantage of the different directions of growth (the H versus the V or Harvold-Woodside type–activators). Previous chapters by Rakosi cover this topic in depth.

The construction bite can be either a softened roll of beeswax or a semisoft horseshoe wafer made up of three thicknesses of yellow wax. (See Chapter 9 for details and illustrations.) For both the trial or practice bite and the final construction bite the wax is only partially softened in warm water. If the wax is too hot, the outside portion becomes mushy while the inside remains too hard to obtain the correct occlusal relationship. The wax should be cut away at the midline to permit checking of midline relationships. An improper

midline registration may lead to the patient's inability to adapt, with treatment failure the ultimate outcome. If the dental midlines do not coincide in habitual occlusion, the skeletal midlines must be determined and then used for taking the construction bite. *Midline discrepancies are usually caused by tooth drift and should not be corrected in the bite by manipulation during forward posturing.* Such discrepancies, if correctable, may be handled later with fixed appliances. After the practice bite has been obtained (and the patient commended for cooperating), the final bite is taken. It should be removed carefully, chilled in cold water, and placed on the models to confirm the fit. The chilled wax is then pressed on the upper arch (Figures 12-15 and 12-17). The patient is instructed to posture the lower jaw gently forward until it fits into the bite. The teeth and bite are checked for correct midline registration and full seating, and both the vertical and the horizontal openings are reevaluated to verify proper registration (see Chapter 9).

After confirmation of the construction bite the heavy elastic separators are replaced in the maxillary canine and first molar embrasures. The patient is instructed to come to the office immediately if the separators are lost. Adequate space *must* be present when the appliance is delivered 2 or 3 weeks later. This is essential if the appliance is to fit properly and lock on the maxillary arch.

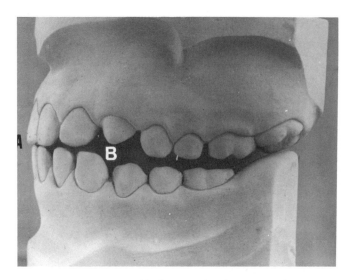

**Figure 12-17.** In a mild Class II malocclusion an end-to-end incisal relationship (*A*) should be registered in the construction bite (*B*). If the crossover wires do not have enough room, however, the bite must be opened slightly. The less the vertical opening, the more easily the patient can perform effective lip-seal exercises.

*Working model pour-up and trimming.* The newly taken impressions are poured immediately in yellow stone, with an adequate base to permit proper carving of the models and mounting on the articulator. The model must extend away from the alveolar process at least 5 mm to allow subsequent application of wax relief. The practitioner must be careful not to cut the tuberosity areas too closely when trimming the stone to the level of the vestibular sulcus (Figure 12-18).

After the working models have been separated from the impressions, they are carefully trimmed for the lip pads and buccal shields. Fränkel believes this is necessary because, even with the best trays and impressions, the depths of the sulci are not adequately reproduced to permit full extension of the acrylic for periosteal pull and maximal benefit from the lip-seal exercises. The 1 to 2 mm carving can be done by either the orthodontist or the technician. Ideally the operator will do it before sending the models to the laboratory. Furthermore, if the carving can be done in the patient's presence, the anatomic conditions of the particular areas can be inspected while carving for the buccal and anterior sulci. Meticulous care during carving produces the tissue tension necessary to stimulate appositional bone development in the basal areas without ulcerating the mucosa by overextension. If the buccal shields do not extend far enough into the sulci, the cheek will invaginate into the space and either dislodge the shield or fold inside it, negating its activity. Having to polish the peripheral portions somewhat because of overextension after the first visit is preferable to undershooting the mark on the buccal shield and lip pad extension.

LIP PADS. Because the impression-taking procedure may distort the tissue and actually diminish sulcular depth, the stone of the mandibular model is carefully carved back about 5 mm from the greatest curvature of the alveolar base with a

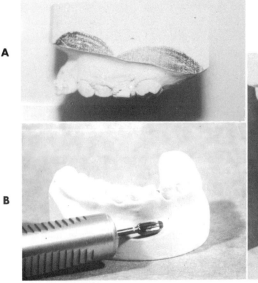

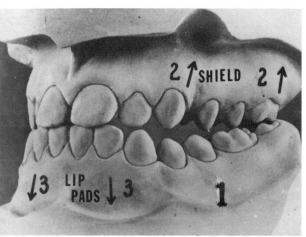

**Figure 12-18.** Correct model trimming is necessary before appliance fabrication. The desired amount of stone to be cut away can be outlined in pencil, **A,** and then cut away with a round or oblong acrylic bur, **B.** Final detailing is done with a plaster knife, **C.** No trimming is needed for the buccal shields on the mandible (*1*), but extension is required for the maxillary buccal shield periphery (*2*) and the mandibular lip pads (*3*). Care must be taken not to disturb muscle attachments.
(Courtesy Max Hall and Dick Allessee.)

pear-shaped carbide bur and office knife. Again, this procedure ensures optimal extension, puts the sulcus connective tissue under slight tension, and prevents the lip mucosa from working in between the pads and the labial mucosal tissue of the alveolar process. In Figure 12-19, *A* and *C,* the solid line marks the real depth of the sulcus, whereas the dotted line delineates the corrected peripheral limits, allowing for possible distortion by the impression-taking technique. The correct trimming is shown in Figure 12-19, *B* and *D.* A profile view of the working model should show the alveolar surface to be nearly vertical after the carving. The lower relief should be at least 12 mm below the gingival margin, according to Fränkel, to permit the wire framework for the lip pads to lie 7 mm below the incisor gingival margin. This distance allows properly formed rhomboid acrylic lip pads to be made over the wire skeleton. The technician may do some further fine carving, but this should be minimal because no record of the original extent of the sulci exists after the impression. Ideally, either the operator or the laboratory technician, not both, has the trimming responsibility. Any overextension of acrylic can be polished from the pads at appliance placement.

BUCCAL SHIELDS. The maxillary stone model also must be trimmed, after first removing the excess from the base. In the trimming for the buccal shields the sulcular depth must be 10 to 12 mm above the gingival margin of the posterior teeth. The muscle attachments and the tuberosity area deserve particular attention. The region next to the muscle attachment over the deciduous first molar and the superior limit of the lateral incisor depression, just mesial to the canine, must be well defined. This definition allows optimal extension of the buccal shields for all possible appositional bone growth (see Figure 12-18). *Trimming of the lower buccal vestibular sulcus is not required for the shields.*

SEATING GROOVES. If adequate space has not been created by the special heavy elastic separators, seating grooves must be cut in the permanent first molar–deciduous second molar and deciduous canine–first molar embrasures. These must be parallel to permit lateral expansion. Prior separation usually makes seating grooves unnecessary, but a 1.5 mm wide groove can be made with a sharp blade or saw on the cast.

Grooves that are too deep are better than those too shallow, because the seating wires should be deep enough to anchor the inserted FR firmly on the maxillary dentition (see Figures 12-5, 12-9, and 12-12). The seating grooves cut on the model must be duplicated in the patient's mouth when the appliance is placed. Therefore if the heavy separators have not created enough room, the mesial marginal ridges of the deciduous first molars must be notched as well as the distal marginal ridges of the deciduous second molars. Care must be exercised not to injure the permanent first molars.

FINAL TRIMMING. Before the working models are sent to the technician, the wax construction bite should be replaced and the backs of the models trimmed so they are flush, much like the original study casts (Figure 12-20). This allows the technician to check the bite when the casts are received and the operator to double check it when the finished appliance is returned.

**Laboratory prescription and procedures.** Because few clinicians fabricate their own Fränkel appliances and specific instructions are required by the laboratory for proper appliance fabrication, prescription pads (Figure 12-21) have been developed. Different laboratories require different information, but the prescription blank shown provides the important information needed by the technician to make the appliance as desired. If the notching described has not already been done by the operator, the laboratory should be given precise instructions on the prescription blank.

The laboratory must be informed on the prescription blank of any midline deviation or other abnormalities. The appointment time for appliance placement must be clearly marked. Furthermore, the operator should not hesitate to call and discuss fabrication personally or leave instructions for the technician to call, because the precision demanded for FR construction requires complete clarity of the clinician's needs and desires.

**Working model mounting.** After carefully unpacking and checking the casts and construction bite, the laboratory personnel assemble the parts to verify that nothing has gone

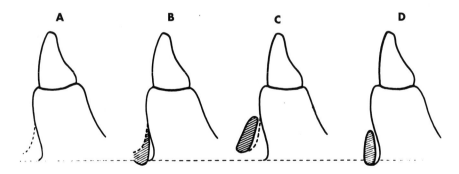

**Figure 12-19.** Correct and incorrect trimming and lip pad position are shown in this drawing. **A** and **C,** Inadequate carving and incorrect positioning of the lip pad. **B** and **D,** Proper carving and parallel pad orientation. Tissue damage may result from improper model carving and pad fabrication.

(Courtesy Rolf Fränkel.)

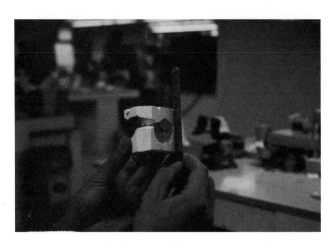

**Figure 12-20.** The backs of the working models must be properly trimmed with the casts mounted in the construction bite, either before sending to the technician or by the technician before mounting the models on the fixator. Backs should be parallel and in the same plane.

(Courtesy Max Hall and Dick Allessee.)

Doctor _____

Address _____

_____ Zip _____

Patient's Name _____

Original Malocclusion—Class _____ Division ____

Date shipped by Doctor _____

Appliance Placement Date _____

### WAX RELIEF FOR EXPANSION

The standard relief on the FR1, FR2, and FR4 is 3mm on the upper and ½mm on the lower. The standard relief on the FR3 is 3mm on the upper and 0 on the lower.

☐ Standard Relief   ☐ Alternate Relief — use diagram

### MODEL PREPARATION

Please trim the backs of the models parallel, with the wax construction bite in place. This will help insure accuracy in mounting the casts.
☐ Do not alter models in any way.
☐ Trim vestibules to best height and symmetry.
☐ Flatten lower sulcus to ____ mm depth.

### DISCING TEETH

Deciduous — Notching of the model interproximal to the c's and d's and the distal of the e's on the upper.
☐ Yes   ☐ No

Permanent — Notching of the model interproximal to the upper 3 and 4, 5 and 6, with equal amounts removed on each (this should duplicate the space created by the separators placed by doctor).
☐ Yes   ☐ No

### SPECIAL INSTRUCTIONS

_____

_____

_____

_____

---

PLEASE CONSTRUCT THE FOLLOWING TYPE OF FRANKEL APPLIANCE ON THE ENCLOSED MODELS:

☐ FR I          ☐ FR III
☐ FR II         ☐ FR IV

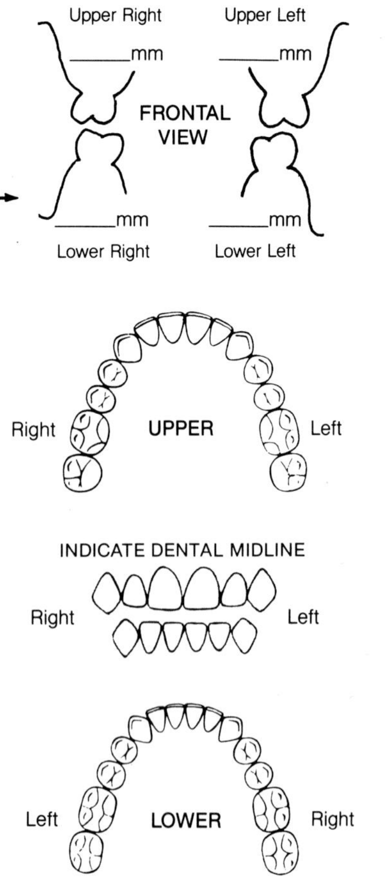

Upper Right          Upper Left
_____ mm          _____ mm

FRONTAL VIEW

_____ mm          _____ mm
Lower Right          Lower Left

Right     UPPER     Left

INDICATE DENTAL MIDLINE

Right                    Left

Left     LOWER     Right

**Figure 12-21.** Typical prescription pad used by orthodontic laboratories for instructions for FR fabrication. Proper attention to detail at this point can prevent problems later.

(Courtesy Max Hall and Dick Allessee.)

wrong during shipping. The first step is to mount the models on a straight-line fixator or articulator, with both fully inserted in the wax bite. After the casts have been mounted with plaster, the wax bite is removed. A minimum of 2.5 mm interocclusal space must be present for the crossover wires. A number of different kinds of fixators are available, but the one most commonly recommended is made by Dentaurum (072-000) (Figure 12-22).

**Wax relief.** Because the buccal shields must stand away from the teeth and tissues if the desired expansion is to be achieved, the prescription should include information for thickness of wax relief in the various areas. Outlining the lip pads and buccal shields with pencil on the mounted work models before waxing them up is a good procedure (Figure 12-23). Then the buccal surfaces are covered with layers of wax (Figures 12-24 and 12-25). The thickness is determined

individually by the amount of desired expansion needed, but it should not exceed 4 or 5 mm in the tooth area or 2.5 to 3 mm in the maxillary alveolar region. Only 0.5 mm thickness is needed at the mandibular shield periphery. Pink baseplate wax of a known thickness can be applied in layers to obtain the correct thickness of wax, or 3 mm thick red boxing wax can be used in the thickest portions, and baseplate wax then added to fill in the rest of the penciled outlines in the prescribed thicknesses. Fränkel uses a pointed explorer-like instrument with millimetric markings on the tip to ensure the correct depth of the wax (see Figure 12-25). Sometimes the maxillary buccal contours are curved, or convex, and the wax relief must exceed 3 mm to allow proper insertion and withdrawal of the appliance over an undercut (particularly in the maxillary canine area). The wax covering is especially important in the region of the deciduous maxillary first molars because of arch narrowing in most Class II, division 1 malocclu-

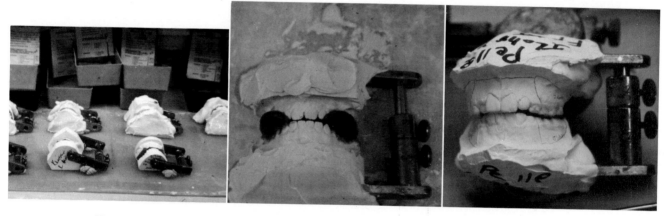

**Figure 12-22.** When the models reach the laboratory, they are assembled on fixators, after determination that the backs of the casts are trimmed correctly with the construction bite in place. After mounting, the Dentaurum 072-000 fixator permits easy separation and replacement of casts in the correct relationship without the wax bite in place.
(Courtesy Max Hall and Dick Allessee.)

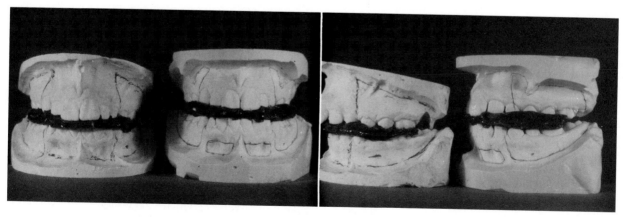

**Figure 12-23.** After the models are properly trimmed (as in Figure 12-18), buccal shields and lip pads are outlined on the casts in pencil before application of the wax relief and acrylic.
(Courtesy Max Hall and Dick Allessee.)

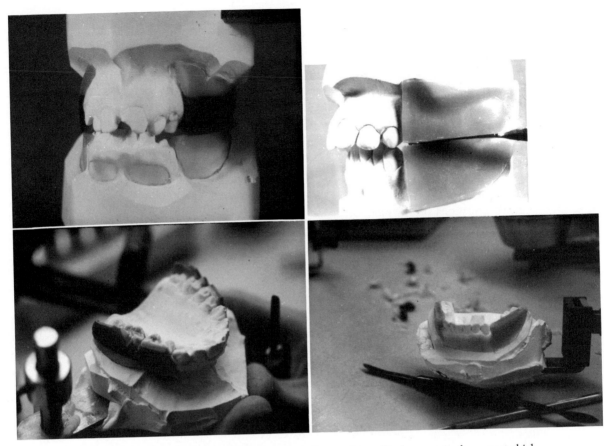

**Figure 12-24.** Wax relief is applied to the maxillary and mandibular casts in the correct thickness. Only 0.5 mm is needed on the mandibular cast, but 2.5 to 3 mm is required in the maxillary alveolar region. Not more than 4 mm relief should be used in the tooth area. Red boxing wax (3 mm) can be used for the thicker portions. Only a thin layer of wax is needed under the lip pads. Each cast may be waxed separately, and then the wax is joined when the models are placed together on the fixator.
(Courtesy Max Hall and Dick Allessee.)

sions. However, if the space between the shields and tissue over the alveolar bone at the depth of the vestibule is too great, preventing invagination of the cheek into this area, which negates the desired periosteal pull effect, is almost impossible.

Lower arch waxing requires only a very thin layer over the apical base (0.5 mm), thinning out to a rounded knife edge in the lower sulcus, where transverse changes are usually not desired. An overly thick wax layer makes the appliance too bulky, and the patient has a harder time adapting to it. The relief wax thickness is much greater in the dentition area, however, where as much as 4 or 5 mm is possible depending on the need for arch expansion. The usual amount needed is 3 mm. Upper and lower casts are waxed separately and then joined at the occlusal plane so that the outer surface has a gently flowing concave curve. Usually a thin layer of pink baseplate wax is placed under the lip pads to reduce the danger of abrasion of gingival tissue by the lip pads and the possible dehiscence of the canine or incisor gingival margins if the patient bobs the appliance up and down in the mouth during daytime wear. This iatrogenic effect is particularly

problematic for appliances not properly locked on the maxillary arch by notching.

**Wire forming.** The wires are formed and placed as shown in Figures 12-26 to 12-30 after the waxing has been completed. The palatal bow and occlusal rests are heavier (0.040 and 0.51 inch, respectively), because they are stabilizing and connecting wires. The tooth-moving wires, which are seldom indicated with the FR appliance, are a smaller gauge (0.028 inch). To prevent abrasion and irritation, the stabilizing and connecting wires should not contact the tissue. Wires situated in the vestibule that are not covered by acrylic should be 1.5 to 2 mm from the alveolar mucosa. On the lingual aspect the wires should be 1 to 2 mm from the mucosa and palate. Wire bending should follow the natural tissue contours to avoid impingement and irritation of the soft tissues.

*Lower lingual support wire.* This heavy, 0.051-inch stainless steel wire can be either three components soldered together or one continuous wire (Figure 12-26). Bending the crossover wires and horizontal reinforcing wires separately

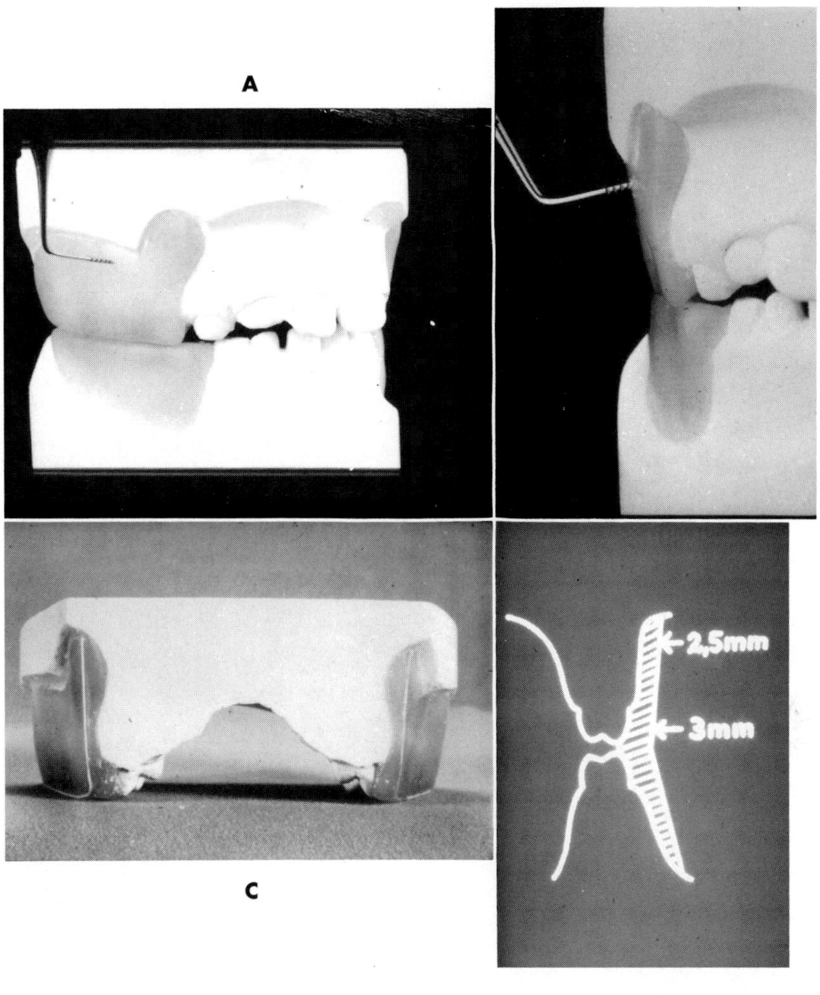

**Figure 12-25. A** and **B,** One technique Fränkel uses to ensure the correct thickness of wax is to make millimetric markings on an explorer and use this to measure the thicknesses applied. **C,** Wax-application thickness from the posterior before being finished down to a smooth surface. **D,** Minimal thickness recommended.

and then soldering them together or picking up the free ends in the cold-cure acrylic pad when it is fabricated is easier. The horizontal reinforcing wire element follows the contours of the lingual apical base at approximately 1 or 2 mm from the muscosa and 3 to 4 mm below the lingual gingival margin of the incisors to permit adding acrylic for the pad. The crossover wires pass between the occlusal surfaces at the embrasure between the deciduous first and second molars (or first and second premolars); avoiding contact with the upper and lower teeth is essential. The ends are then bent at about 90 degrees to insert into the buccal shields. The ends must be parallel to each other and the occlusal plane to allow for advancement of the anterior section later, if needed. This procedure is discussed in the latter part of this chapter. The wire must slide through the shield in the advancement procedure and must be perfectly straight. To prevent breakage, all wire bends in the Fränkel appliance (or any functional appliance) must be gradual. A right-angle bend can fatigue the wire and result in fracture during wear.

Wire parts embedded in the acrylic should not contact the wax (Figure 12-27), nor should they stand away more than 1 mm from the wax surface (Figure 12-30). This precaution prevents the buccal shields from becoming too thick and bulky.

*Lower lingual springs.* The 0.8-mm (0.028-inch) recurved spring wires are contoured to the lingual surfaces of the lower incisors right above the cingula, with the free ends about 3 mm below the incisal margins (Figure 12-26). The primary objective for these elements is to prevent extrusion of the lower incisors, but care must be taken not to activate them. This tips the lower incisors labially, an all too common problem with functional appliances. Fränkel stresses that these wires should usually be passive. If they are to be used for some special tooth-moving task, which is rare, a smaller-gauge wire (0.5 or 0.6 mm) is probably better suited to apply spring pressure. Tooth movements should be done before or after Fränkel therapy with fixed appliances.

*Lower labial wires.* These 0.9-mm (0.036-inch) wires serve as the skeleton for the lower lip pads (Figure 12-27). Fränkel prefers three wires for this unit instead of one, which is more prone to breakage. The lateral wires emerge from the buccal shields in a slightly inferior direction and follow the contour of the muscosa around to the lateral incisor embrasure at a distance of about 1 mm from the tissue so that they may be covered lingually and labially with the acrylic of the lip pads. The wire framework should be at least 7 mm below the

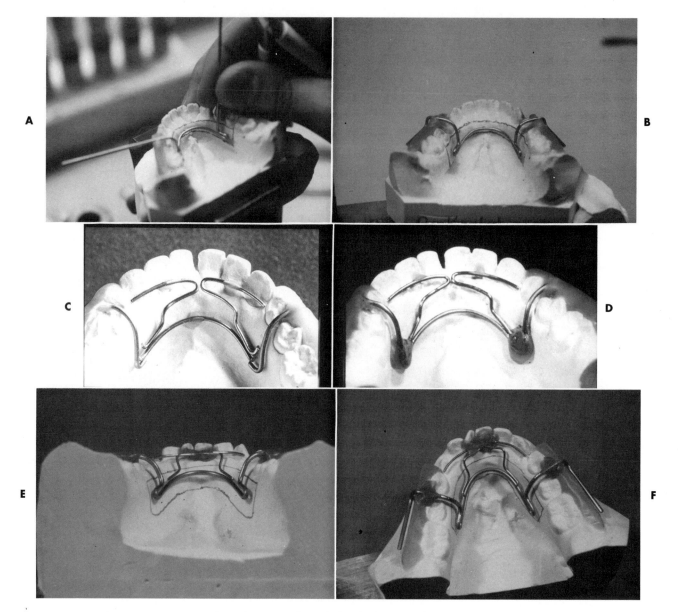

**Figure 12-26.** Lower lingual wires are formed after the lower model on the fixator has been separated. **A** and **B,** In forming the lingual pad skeleton wire that crosses over between the upper and lower deciduous molars or premolars, care must be taken that the hanger wire does not touch upper or lower occlusal surfaces. **C** and **D,** The passive lingual springs are then formed and affixed to the cast with sticky wax, with the hanger wire skeleton. **E** and **F,** The buccal ends are bent parallel to the buccal surface and stand away 1 mm from the relief wax so they can be encased in the acrylic shield.

(Courtesy Max Hall and Dick Allessee.)

gingival margin. The middle wire, or third component, is bent in the shape of an inverted **V** to prevent impingement on the labial muscle attachment.

*Palatal bow.* The 1-mm (0.040-inch, 18-gauge) thick palatal bow has a slightly posterior curve as shown in Figures 12-3 and 12-4. The curve provides an extra length of wire to facilitate adjustment for slight lateral expansion. This is sometimes necessary if the alveolodental area develops transversely

and begins to contact the buccal shields. The wire should cross the maxillary occlusal surfaces in the grooves that have been cut just mesial to the maxillary first molars to enhance the seating on the maxillary arch (Figure 12-28). The wire makes a loop in the buccal shield and emerges to lie between the maxillary first molar buccal cusps, ending in the fossa as an occlusal rest. The molar rests remain passive, unless the wire in the interproximal space moves up too high and impinges on the gingival tissue between the first molar and de-

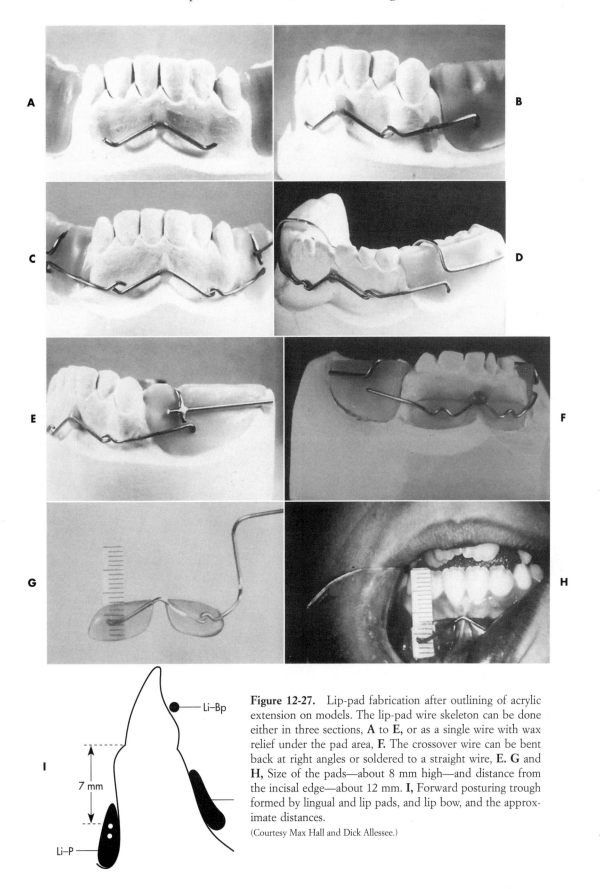

**Figure 12-27.** Lip-pad fabrication after outlining of acrylic extension on models. The lip-pad wire skeleton can be done either in three sections, **A** to **E,** or as a single wire with wax relief under the pad area, **F.** The crossover wire can be bent back at right angles or soldered to a straight wire, **E. G** and **H,** Size of the pads—about 8 mm high—and distance from the incisal edge—about 12 mm. **I,** Forward posturing trough formed by lingual and lip pads, and lip bow, and the approximate distances.

(Courtesy Max Hall and Dick Allessee.)

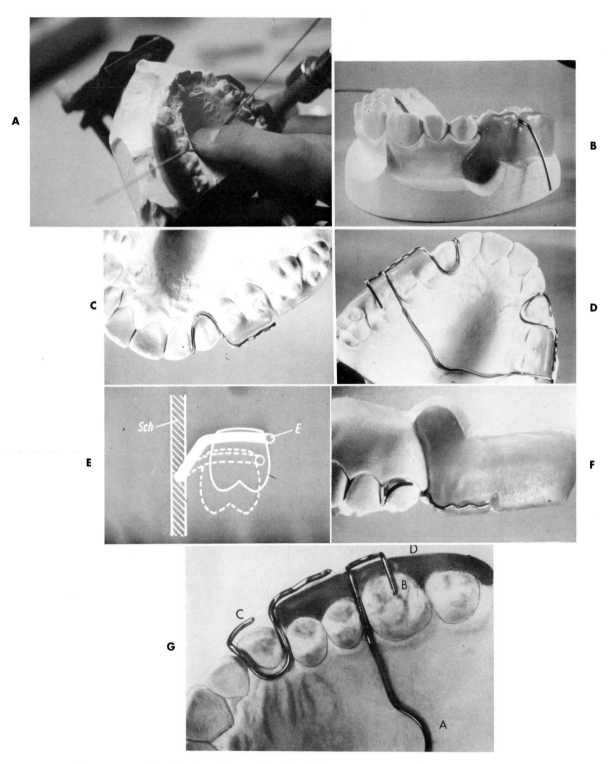

**Figure 12-28.** Maxillary lingual wires. **A** and **B,** The heavy palatal wire is formed partly by thumb and finger pressure and partly with a no. 139 pliers for the center loop. The bird beak pliers also works well for the canine clasps (Figure 12-29). **C** and **D,** The palatal bow crosses over in the embrasure between the permanent first molar and deciduous second molar or second premolar in the groove provided and then is bent around to form an occlusal rest. In the permanent dentition the maxillary rest is on the permanent first molar. If the deciduous second molar is present, the occlusal rest is bent forward to lie on this tooth. **E** and **F,** The canine clasp also passes through the embrasure provided by separation or slicing at the canine–first premolar region. As it passes through, it is bent occlusally; thus it may be adjusted down so as not to interfere with eruption of these teeth. In **G** the palatal aspect includes (*A*) palatal bow, (*B*) occlusal rest, (*C*) canine clasp, and (*D*) wax relief.

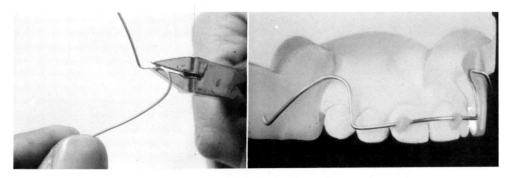

**Figure 12-29.** Fabrication of the passive maxillary bow is relatively simple with a bird beak no. 139 pliers. The bow is affixed to the model with sticky wax and must stand away enough for acrylic to incorporate the wire ends in the shield completely.

ciduous second molar. In this case the rests are bent slightly occlusally to reduce tissue contact (see Figures 12-5, 12-9, and 12-28). The rests should be parallel to the occlusal plane so the molars are free to expand laterally. If the FR Ib is used in the deciduous or mixed dentition and the permanent first molars have not erupted sufficiently, the occlusal rests can be bent mesially instead of distally, with the ends lying in the central fossae of the deciduous second molars (see Figures 12-15 to 12-19).

*Maxillary labial bow.* The 0.9-mm (0.036-inch, 19-gauge) maxillary labial bow shape and position are illustrated in Figures 12-2 and 12-29. The bow originates in the buccal shields and lies in the middle of the labial surfaces of the incisors. The wire leaves the acrylic with a slight bend toward the sulcus and then curves down in the natural depression between the canine and lateral incisors to form the canine loops. The canine loops form larger and more gentle curves, with the apex of each loop crossing the middle third of the canine root about 2 mm away from the mucosal surface. This important configuration permits canine eruption and expansion without contacting the labial wire. The loops should be wide enough to allow constriction later, if needed, to close maxillary incisor spaces. However, the labial bow is normally not used for tooth movement, which can be done before or after Fränkel appliance orthopedic growth guidance with fixed appliances. The wire is straight and not adapted to the individual tooth malpositions in the anterior segment. *Tipping of the maxillary incisors lingually with pinching of the labial bow loops,* as is done so often with a Hawley retainer, *is not a treatment objective with the Fränkel appliance.* Research by the author has shown that lingually tipped maxillary incisors can actually prevent full accomplishment of the mandibular growth pattern and thus reduce the benefit of forward posturing of the lower jaw. In addition, lingual tipping can cause the FR to become unseated from the maxillary interproximal grooves, letting the appliance drop and lose its maximal effectiveness. In the FR II a lingual wire behind the upper incisors prevents lingualizing of the maxillary anterior segment. This wire may be used to tip the central incisors labially in a Class II, division 2 malocclusion.

*Canine loops.* The canine loops (0.9 mm, 0.036 inch, 19 gauge) are embedded in the buccal shield at the occlusal plane level. They turn sharply toward the gingival margin of the deciduous maxillary first molars and fit in the embrasures between the deciduous first molars and canines, helping the palatal bow extensions at the first molar embrasures to anchor the FR on the maxillary arch. If the wires are formed properly, they can be bent occlusally to prevent interference with the erupting first premolars and canines. The loops wrap around the lingual surfaces of the canines and emerge labially at the canine–lateral incisor embrasures, curving distally over the canine cusps (Figure 12-28). The free ends can be bent occlusally if required.

**Fabrication of acrylic portions of the FR.** After the wires are bent and properly adapted to the models as just outlined, they are secured with sticky wax (Figure 12-30). The articulator should be closed again to ensure that the hangers or crossover wires do not touch either the upper or the lower tooth surfaces. Because of stress at this point, some clinicians recommend double hangers through the interdental space on each side to reduce breakage.

The lip pads, buccal shields, and lingual pads are usually fabricated in cold-cure acrylic. Laboratories use various techniques, but one (McNamara & Huge) completes the acrylic fabrication for the lower lingual pad and the labial lip pads first and then forms the maxillary wires and does the acrylic construction. Other laboratories bend the wires for the whole appliance and then do the acrylic work at the same time. Forming the lingual pressure pad with the two-step process is easier, but the buccal and lip pads can be done easily either way (see Figures 12-33 to 12-36).

Before the acrylic work for the buccal shields is done, the upper and lower wax portions are joined and the interdental space sealed to make a smooth lingual surface and prevent the acrylic from seeping through. The shields and pads are formed with alternate applications of monomer and polymer (the "salt-and-pepper" technique). Some laboratories prefer to mix the entire mass and mold the acrylic, claiming that the surface is more dense and the consistency better. With either technique the name and phone number of the patient can be

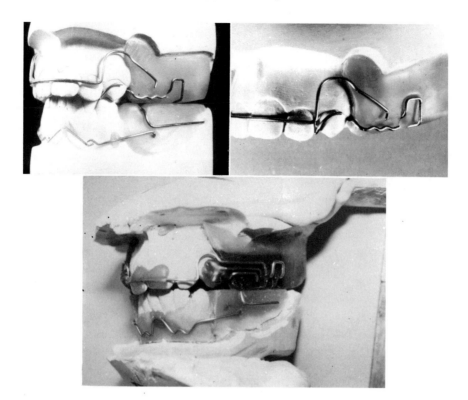

**Figure 12-30.**   Wire ends to be incorporated in the buccal shields. Each wire is held by sticky wax so it is not disturbed by the application of acrylic.

typed on a small piece of onionskin paper and incorporated in the buccal shields during the buildup phase. As the acrylic polymerizes, it can be molded to form the approximate desired shape. The total thickness of the shields and pads should not exceed 2.5 mm. If the polymerized appliance is then placed in a pressure cooker for 15 to 20 minutes at 25 to 30 pounds of pressure, the consistency and density improve (see Figure 12-37). The articulator should be placed in icewater to harden the wax and thereby facilitate separation of the appliance from the models after they are removed from the pressure cooker. Wires are gently freed from the models before separating the appliance from the work models to prevent distortion. Rough polishing and shaping can be done with a sandpaper arbor chuck or cherry-stone–type bur (see Figure 12-38). Because of the inherent complexity of the FR appliance and difficulty in polishing some of the lingual surfaces, practitioners should be careful not to nick the wires or catch the appliance on a rag wheel in the polishing process. Distortion is likely in such cases, or the wires break soon after the patient starts wearing the appliance. For some reason, Fränkel appliances require repair more frequently than other functional appliances—with even the heaviest wires breaking at the exit point from the shields. The patient loses important wearing time and may become less compliant if the appliance must be sent back to the laboratory. An important step is to round off and polish all margins, particularly where they put sulcus tissue under tension.

The lip pads look somewhat like a parallelogram (see Figure 12-2), but individual anatomy permits variation to prevent unnecessary impingement and irritation, especially at the frenum borders. The superior periphery of the lip pads should be at least 5 mm from the gingival margin. Figures 12-19 and 12-27 illustrate the proper position and inclination of the pads. This attention to detail is essential in eliminating the mentalis muscle hyperactivity and abnormal functional lip trap that enhance the overjet.

Before the FR is inserted in the patient's mouth, it should be replaced on the models and checked carefully for tolerances, adaptation, and wire conformity. The anterosuperior margin of the vestibular shield should extend past the canine–deciduous first molar embrasure to the middle of the canine. Some clinicians actually carry this into the depression over the lateral incisors (see Figure 12-35). The posterior periphery of the shield should extend distally beyond the last erupted tooth.

**FR Ic.**   Fränkel recommends the FR Ic for the more severe Class II, division 1 malocclusions in patients with overjets of more than 7 mm and sagittal dysplasia that exceeds an end-to-end cuspal relationship. As others have observed, posturing the mandible forward into a Class I relationship and eliminating the excessive overjet in one step for the Fränkel appliance are neither feasible nor necessary. Experience has shown that tissue response is less favorable, and patient compliance is much poorer. Thus the mandibular protraction is done in two, or occasionally three, steps.

A simple maneuver can accomplish the advancement procedures and dispense with the need for a new appliance. The

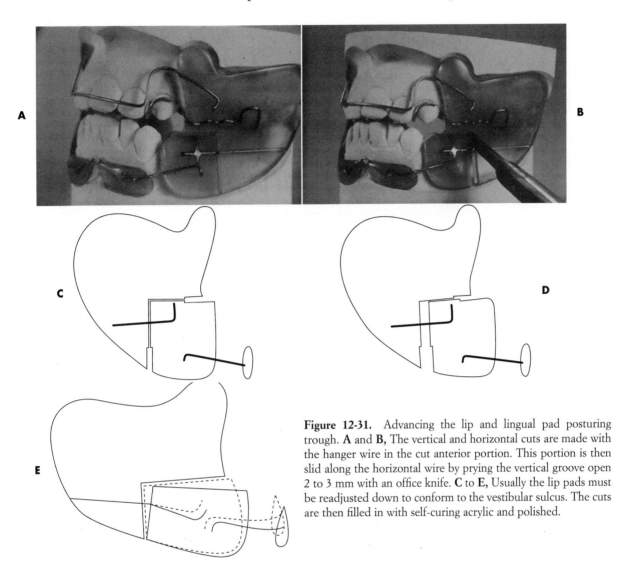

**Figure 12-31.** Advancing the lip and lingual pad posturing trough. **A** and **B,** The vertical and horizontal cuts are made with the hanger wire in the cut anterior portion. This portion is then slid along the horizontal wire by prying the vertical groove open 2 to 3 mm with an office knife. **C** to **E,** Usually the lip pads must be readjusted down to conform to the vestibular sulcus. The cuts are then filled in with self-curing acrylic and polished.

buccal shields (Figure 12-31) are split horizontally and vertically into two parts. The anteroinferior portion contains the wires for the lingual acrylic pressure pad and lower lip pads. The heavy through-the-bite hanger wire that connects the lingual pad and buccal shields permits advancement of the mandibular trough (formed by the lip pads on the labial side and the lingual pad on the inside) to allow for this maneuver. The ends of the hanger wires are incorporated in the buccal shield and are horizontal. This position allows the movement of the free portion in an anterior direction—after the acrylic cut has been made—by pulling the anterior section forward, with the wire slipping forward within the posterior part of the shield to accommodate the forward movement of the lingual pressure pad and labial lip pads. As Figure 12-31 shows, the vertical split is pried open with an office knife to the desired position by a 2- to 3-mm advancement, filled in with cold-cure acrylic, and polished. A new tactile engram is thus constructed for mandibular position, with both lip and lower lingual pads giving new exteroceptive and proprioceptive signals. Occasionally adjustments must then be made in the lip pads, bending the wires downward slightly. Parallelism with the contiguous tissue must be checked to prevent abrasion on placement and removal or during use. Also, because of the farther mandibular advancement, the posteroinferior buccal shield periphery may irritate the sulcus and require trimming.

In actual practice the FR Ic is seldom used now, because the FR Ib and FR II can be modified the same way, with the horizontal and vertical cuts for the advancement made when needed rather than ahead of time. The same connecting wire is pulled forward in the posterior part of the shield, opening the vertical slots to the desired 2- or 3-mm advancement of the lingual and labial pads. The slots are then filled in with cold-cure acrylic. An early variation of the FR Ic incorporated jackscrews in the slots of the buccal shields, permitting bilateral advancement as desired. This modification has been resurrected and is available on prescription. Fränkel, however, considers the thickening of the buccal shield to accommodate the jackscrews a disadvantage (Figure 12-32).

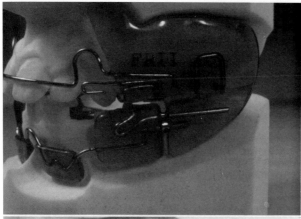

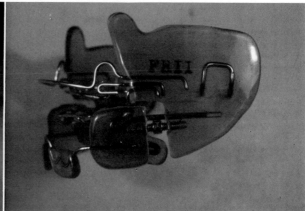

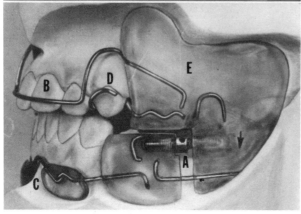

**Figure 12-32.** Advancing the shields with a jackscrew. This can be done gradually in two or three steps, as desired, or at one time (after 3 or 4 months) as shown in Figure 12-31. Jackscrew (*A*), labial wire (*B*), lip pads (*C*), canine clasp (*D*), buccal shield (*E*). Arrow on the shield shows the direction to turn the jackscrew to open it.

*Pre-Fränkel appliance fixed or removable mechanotherapy.* Before a description of the FR II is undertaken, a few words on pre-Fränkel appliance mechanotherapy are in order. *The Fränkel appliance is a deficiency appliance and an exercise device.* It was designed primarily to eliminate abnormal perioral muscle function and the deleterious effects on the dentition and optimal growth increments. It is *not* a tooth-moving appliance. Appurtenances can be added, as with any other functional appliance, but such modifications are usually not very efficient. More important, they jeopardize the effectiveness of the Fränkel appliance and increase the likelihood of its being unseated from the maxillary arch, which produces undesirable lower incisor procumbency and possible labiogingival stripping in the lower arch.

However, minor expansion of the upper arch is frequently desirable to correct rotations, change axial inclinations, and close spaces before placing the FR. Such movements actually enhance the success of the Fränkel appliance. Therefore careful diagnosis is essential. The clinician should not hesitate to use a simple active plate or direct-bonded attachments to achieve one or more of the aforementioned objectives in advance (see Chapter 18). Such limited corrective procedures also are possible afterward. The Fränkel appliance does not exclude use of other forms of therapy; in fact, it often demands them for optimal efficiency. This type of therapy is beyond the scope of the present chapter. Nevertheless, 3 to 6 months of tooth movement before treatment with the Fränkel appliance can improve the patient's final result.

## FR II

Although Fränkel has used the FR II mostly for Class II, division 2 malocclusions, more and more of his disciples are using it for Class II, division 1 patients (Figure 12-33). According to estimates, 80% to 90% of all Fränkel appliances now being made in the United States are the FR II type. Some clinicians report that the FR I canine loop can interfere with eruption of the permanent canines, which the FR II canine loop is less likely to do. Fränkel also has used active plates to align the maxillary anterior teeth before placing the FR II. However, other clinicians' experiences with fixed appliances before FR II placement for such cases have been more rewarding, as already noted. Final detailing also may be necessary after the eruption of canines and premolars. This is particularly true of the maxillary canines, which often are not corrected completely with Fränkel appliance therapy alone. Thus a period of fixed mechanotherapy after treatment with the Fränkel appliance is frequently needed for optimal results.

In any event, routine alignment of maxillary anterior teeth in Class II, division 2 malocclusions is suggested before FR II placement. One third to one half of all Class II patients require such fixed mechanotherapy for the maxillary anterior segment.

*FR II construction.* The FR II is modified by adding a stainless steel lingual bow (0.8 mm, 0.032 inch, 20 gauge) behind the maxillary incisors. This addition serves to maintain the pre–functional appliance alignment achieved and stabi-

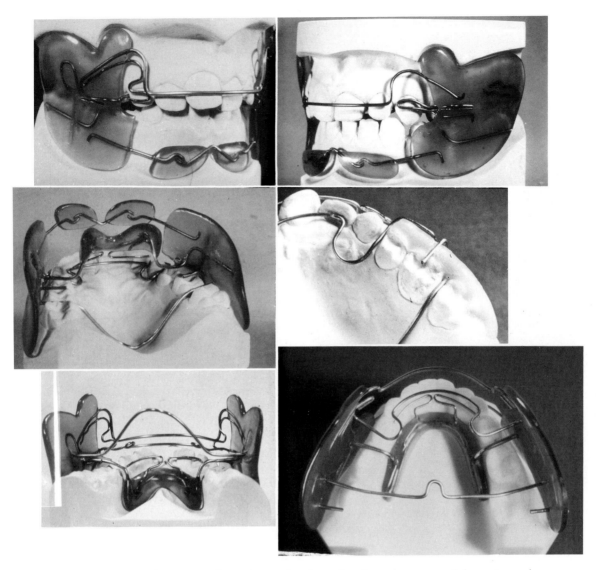

**Figure 12-33.** The FR II appliance has canine clasps that do not wrap around the canine and thus are less likely to interfere with eruption. The clasps continue through the distal canine embrasure and form a stabilizing lingual palatal bow. Formerly called a *protrusion bow* because of its use in Class II, division 2 malocclusions, it is now made of heavier wire and is passive, helping to anchor the appliance on the maxilla. The shields, lip pads, palatal bow, and lower lingual pad and wires are the same as for the FR I. The maxillary molar rest is bent mesially to lie in the occlusal fossa of the deciduous second molar.

lizes the appliance by helping to lock it on the maxillary arch, a prime requisite of FR therapy (Figures 12-5 and 12-33). An added factor, relative depression of the maxillary anterior teeth, also has been suggested. Fränkel originally called this modification a *protrusion bow;* but it no longer functions in this manner, with fixed or removable appliance pre-Fränkel mechanotherapy.

Because pre-FR therapy has achieved individual tooth alignment, a resilient lingual bow is unnecessary. A heavier stabilizing wire is thus recommended for improved structural support (0.030 to 0.036 inch). This wire assists the crossover wires in the embrasures between the permanent maxillary first molars and deciduous second molars and between the maxil-

lary canines and deciduous first molars, as described previously. After seeing cases by various clinicians or reading articles showing improper use of his appliance in the literature, Fränkel has stated that one of the major reasons for failure of FR therapy is the lack of a positive maxillary stabilization of the appliance. This is not a typical, loose-fit activator. The deleterious consequences of an unseated and free-floating appliance are seen in the proclining of lower incisors, mucosal irritation, and actual dehiscences in the lower canine and incisor areas, with wearing away of gingival mucosa.

The maxillary lingual bow of the FR II originates in the vestibular shield and passes to the lingual through the canine–deciduous first molar embrasure, which has been pre-

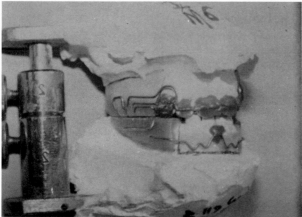

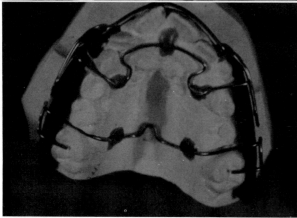

**Figure 12-34.** Waxing for the FR II is similar to that for the FR I; the lingual and labial wires are affixed with sticky wax before the application of acrylic. The lower lip-pad wire is a single piece in this particular appliance but can be made in three pieces if preferred.

viously notched. The wire forms loops that approximate the palatal mucosa and recurve vertically to contact the incisors at the canine–lateral incisor embrasure (Figure 12-33). A 90-degree bend allows the wire to follow the lingual contours of the four incisors, right above the cingula. The main objective of the FR II is to improve the mandibular sagittal relationship. Because little reciprocal retrusive maxillary response occurs in most cases, the additional lingual stabilizing wire has the desirable effect of preventing lingual tipping of the maxillary incisors (Figure 12-34). As pointed out earlier, lingually tipped maxillary incisors could prevent optimal mandibular forward posturing. So-called lingual tipping with the round wire labial bow of removable appliances is in reality a partial labial root tipping, because the incisors rotate about a centrum somewhere between the root apex and the gingival margin. Labial root tipping is seldom desirable for most Class II malocclusions. Preorthodontic and postorthodontic therapy with fixed appliances can prevent such undesirable sequelae, but the lingual bow also reduces this tendency. The lingual bow of the FR II passes through the notch created in the deciduous first molar–canine embrasure to penetrate the buccal shields. Like the canine loops of the FR I, the lingual bow of the FR II helps seat the appliance on the maxilla.

The FR II canine loops are modified. They originate in the buccal shields but contact the canines on the buccal surface only as a recurved loop (Figure 12-33). These 0.8-mm (0.032-inch, 20-gauge) loops actually serve as extensions of the buccal shields in the canine area, which is narrowed most by the abnormal perioral muscle function associated with the malocclusion. Placing these wires 2 to 3 mm away from the deciduous canines eliminates the restrictive muscle function, permitting the needed width development. The buccal shields may be extended forward into the canine fossa for the same reason (Figure 12-35).

As with the FR I, the therapeutic effect of the FR II is three dimensional. Selective eruption is encouraged to provide ver-

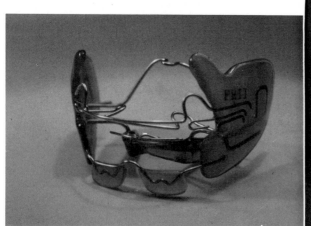

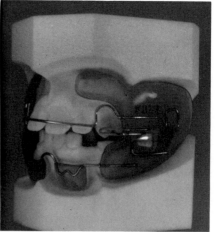

**Figure 12-35.** **A,** The appliance is polished after trimming and is ready for insertion. **B,** The FR II has been modified according to Diers, with the buccal shields projecting into the maxillary canine and lateral incisor fossae to screen off any deleterious or restricting effects on basal bone growth.

tical dentoalveolar adjustment. The need for bite opening is greater in Class II, division 2 malocclusions; therefore the FR II can and must be used to enhance selective eruption of the lower buccal segments. Maxillary expansion is often not needed in Class II, division 2 patients, who have broad dental arches. In such cases, minimal carving of the work model in the vestibular area occurs. The buccal shields need not stand away from the alveolar mucosa in the vestibule.

Because strong mentalis muscle activity usually occurs in Class II, division 2 malocclusions, lip pads are well rounded and polished to prevent mucosal irritation. In some cases of deep-bite Class I or Class II, division 2 malocclusions, with deep overbite and infraclusion of lower posterior segments, in which lip length and contact are ample, the vertical dimension can be opened to a greater degree without endangering lip seal. Particularly in an anteriorly rotating growth pattern, this tends to open the bite and direct mandibular growth in a more vertical direction, reducing the tendency to grow into a deeper bite during and after active treatment (Figure 12-36). Varying the vertical dimension of the construction bite to affect growth direction is discussed in Chapter 7.

The processing of the FR II is the same as for the FR I. The wire elements are affixed to the model with sticky wax after waxing and wire forming (Figure 12-37). The acrylic may be added either by using the "salt-and-pepper" technique or by mixing first to a moldable consistency and then applying with the fingers. Some experts claim that the acrylic is denser with the latter method, but most laboratories prefer the direct al-

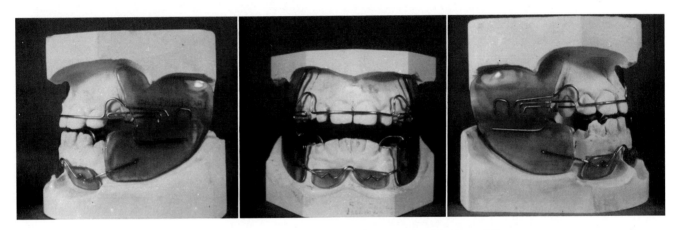

**Figure 12-36.** The FR II, with its wider-open vertical construction bite, is used if greater posterior eruption is needed and lip length is adequate and will not be affected (as far as lip-seal exercises are concerned) by the vertical increase. The wider opening is increasingly likely to produce a more vertical growth direction for anterosuperiorly rotating patterns, which tend to grow into deep overbites (e.g., in Class II, division 2 malocclusions). Note the interocclusal position of the hanger wires and space between the shields and the maxillary alveolar process.

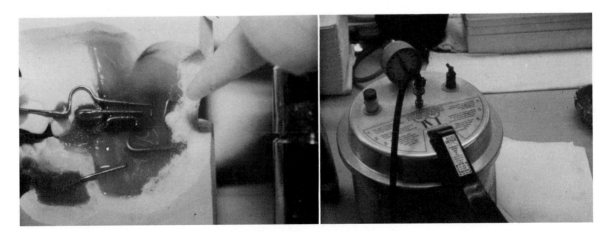

**Figure 12-37.** The "salt-and-pepper" technique of adding acrylic powder and monomer is most frequently used, but these materials can be mixed ahead of time, kneaded and rolled into a pliable mass, and applied by finger pressure with a light coat of petrolatum on the fingers to prevent sticking. In either case the curing appliance is then put into a pressure cooker under 20 pounds of air.

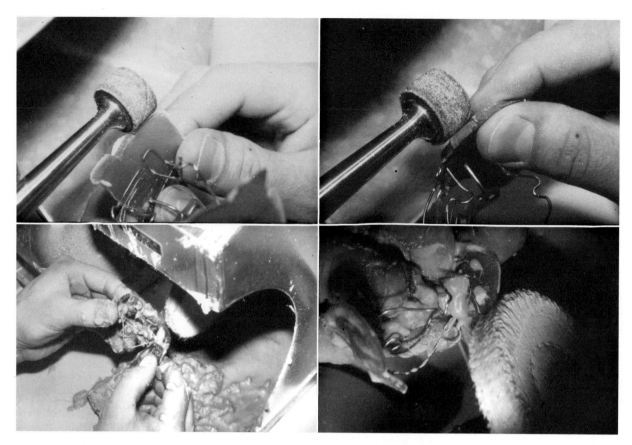

**Figure 12-38.** The polishing technique is similar to that used for Hawley retainers. However, the skeleton framework makes it easier to catch and distort the appliance. Greater care is required with both the sandpaper arbor and the rag wheel and pumice.

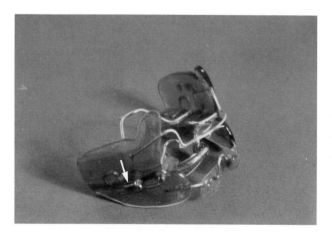

**Figure 12-39.** Some users of the Fränkel appliance have introduced modifications recently. Because little function occurs during sleep, use of extraoral force is possible for Class II malocclusions with maxillary protractions. The appliance is anchored on the maxilla, and light oblique or vertical pull force can be tolerated without dislodgment. Note the horizontal buccal tube embedded in the buccal shield (*arrow*).

ternate monomer-powder method illustrated. In any event the appliance is then placed in a pressure cooker, as with acrylic retainer fabrication, to provide a denser finished product. Polishing the appliance requires great care so as not to distort the wire elements (Figure 12-38).

New users should not attempt modifications, but some experienced clinicians have tried to incorporate extraoral force at night. Buccal tubes can be placed in the buccal

shields approximately at the deciduous second molar area (Figure 12-39). Before going to bed, the patient can place a face-bow with light force to enhance the maxillary retraction potential where needed. McNamara has shown minimal "headgear effect," or retrusion of the maxillary complex, with his conventional FR-treated cases. Case selection and patient cooperation are critical, however. Monitoring also is vital to prevent unfavorable sequelae, such as dehiscence of the lower

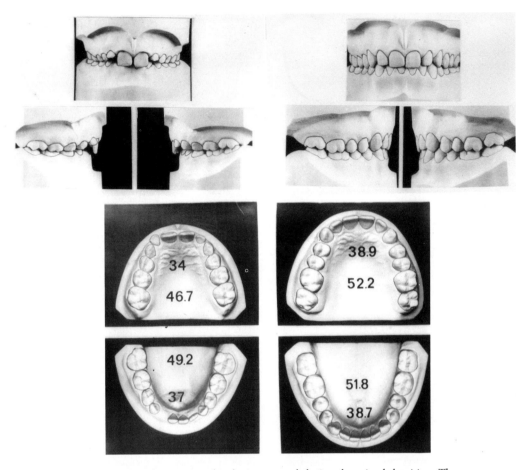

**Figure 12-40.** Class II, division 1 malocclusion treated during the mixed dentition. The excessive overbite and overjet have been eliminated, and the expansion achieved has corrected the arch-length deficiency. Again, a large and stable maxillary intercanine increase of almost 5 mm occurs.

incisors. Normally during sleeping this effect is unlikely, because the mandible tends to drop open. Nevertheless, the FR must be firmly anchored on the maxillary arch by the palatal bow at the molar and the lingual palatal incisor wire at the canine, or the results will be disastrous; however, if the extraoral force does not dislodge the appliance (by virtue of a vertical pull paralleling the Y-axis), greater maxillary retraction is possible with the combined appliances. (Combinations of functional and extraoral force appliances are discussed in more detail in Chapter 18.)

Examples of successful FR I and FR II treatment are illustrated in Figures 12-40 to 12-42.

## FR III

Because successful treatment of early correctional Class III malocclusion is more likely with combination protraction-retraction extraoral force, the FR III, or any functional appliance, is not usually the appliance of choice. However, it can be used for mild early mixed dentition, or even deciduous dentition, cases.

The concepts described for the FR I and FR II also apply to the FR III, which is still a deficiency appliance. A deficiency

in the maxillary arch instead of the mandible is usually the problem (Figure 12-43).

The lip pads are situated in the labial vestibular sulcus of the upper incisor segment, instead of the lower (Figures 12-43 and 12-44). The pads stand away from the mucosa and underlying alveolar bone in the same manner as with the FR II. The supporting metal framework is made up of 0.040-inch stainless wire. The purposes of the lip pads are threefold: (1) to eliminate the restrictive pressure of the upper lip on the underdeveloped maxilla; (2) to exert tension on the tissue and periosteal attachments in the depth of the maxillary sulcus for stimulation of bone growth; and (3) to transmit upper-lip force to the mandible via the lower labial arch for a retrusive stimulus. Admittedly, such force is quite minimal and probably has little effect other than to give a negative feedback signal to false anterior posturing (Figure 12-44). This is particularly true for a morphogenetic skeletal problem.

The labial bow rests against the mandibular teeth and not the maxillary incisors, which are free to move forward. Unlike the maxillary bow, however, the labial bow makes positive contact with the lower incisors by the 0.09-mm (0.036-inch) structural wire (Figure 12-44). Most experts recommend cutting a very shallow groove across the labial of the lower in-

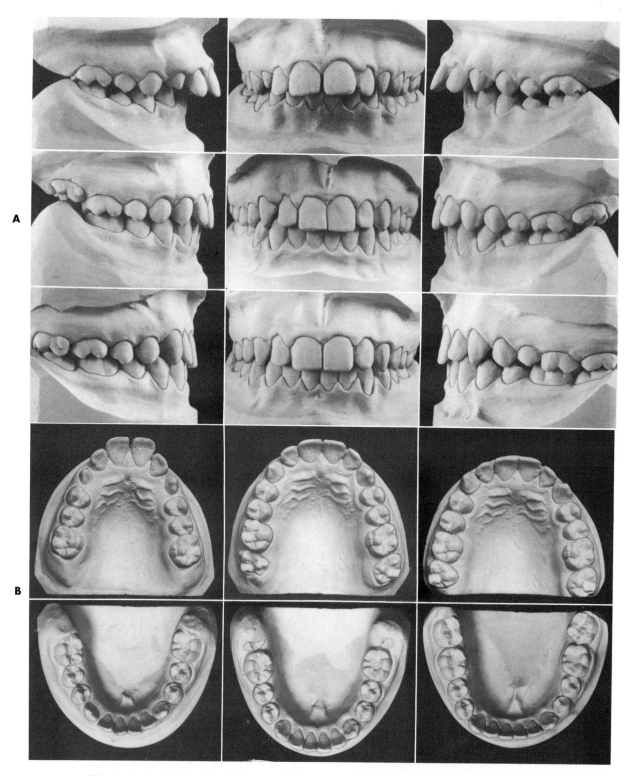

**Figure 12-41.** **A,** Class II, division 1 malocclusion treated after eruption of the lower second molars with a Fränkel FR. The middle row of casts shows improvement during therapy, and the lower row the final stable result achieved at 16 years of age. **B,** Expansion achieved and retraction of maxillary incisors. Lower incisor irregularity has been corrected, but no proclination of these teeth occurred.

(Courtesy Rolf Fränkel.)

cisors to ensure that a slight tension exists in this wire when the appliance is seated in the patient's mouth. The labial bow should cross the lower incisors at the lowest possible level, without impinging on the interproximal soft tissue, to keep lingual tipping of the lower incisors to a minimum.

The protrusion bow of the FR III is similar to that of the FR II, passing behind the upper incisors to stimulate slight to moderate forward movement of these teeth (Figures 12-43 and 12-44). The configuration is much the same as that used in the FR II, with the horizontal component of the wire contacting the teeth just above the cingula of the maxillary incisors. Occasionally the protrusion bow is divided at the midline to give more finger spring action to individual teeth (see Figure 12-43).

The palatal bow, a small posteriorly directed loop at the midline, approximates the palatal mucosa in the same manner as with the FR I and II (Figure 12-43). The difference is that the ends of the bow pass distal instead of mesial to the permanent first molar. The lateral extensions then pass into the buccal shields. The palatal bow is thus capable of delivering a slight anterior stimulus to the maxillary dentition by reforming this wire to contact the distal surfaces of the terminal molars on the tuberosities. The palatal bow is not primarily a tooth-moving wire but a stabilizing component replacing the acrylic palatal cover of the conventional activator.

The FR III is *not* locked on the maxilla by the crosswires from the protrusion bow and palatal bow. However, the close adherence of the buccal shields and lower labial wire to the

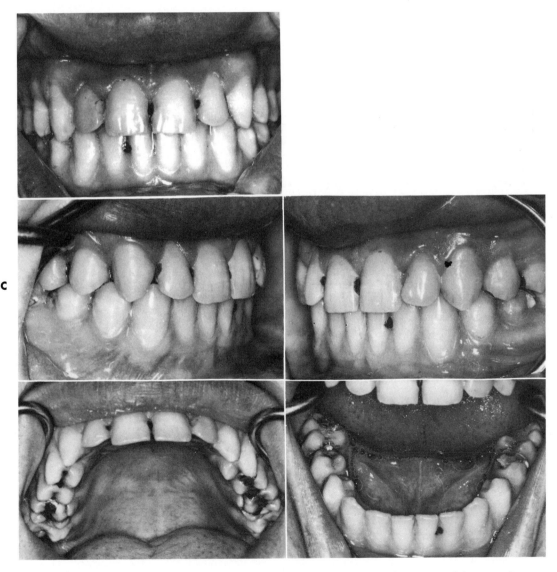

C

**Figure 12-41, cont'd.   C,** Many years out of treatment (adult). Despite the severity of the original overbite and overjet, the correction has proved stable and function is normal.
(Courtesy Rolf Fränkel.)

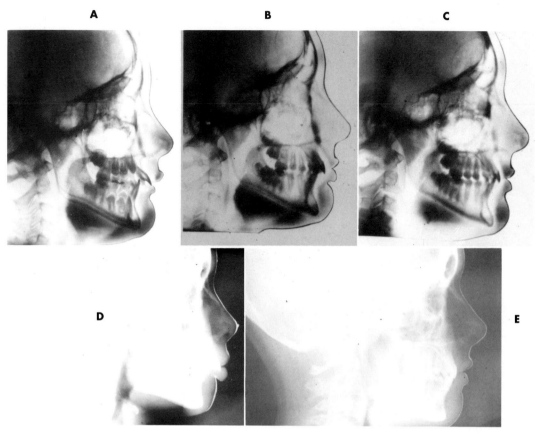

**Figure 12-42.** Major sagittal change accomplished in the FR treatment of a Class II, division 1 mixed dentition problem. **A,** Pretreatment, **B,** at the end of treatment, and **C,** 4 years later. The apical base relationship is normal. **D** and **E,** Both soft and hard tissue changes, achieved by FR therapy and lip-seal exercises.

(Courtesy Rolf Fränkel.)

mandibular basal bone and lower incisors gives a firm grip on the mandibular dentoalveolar structures.

The occlusal rests are on the mandibular first molar instead of the maxillary molar. In line with the concept of differential guidance of eruption, the mandibular molars are *prevented* from erupting upward and forward, whereas the maxillary buccal segment is free to erupt down and forward, reducing the Class III relationship. The rests thus enhance the mandibular anchorage of the FR III (Figure 12-45).

As with the FR I and II, the *buccal shields* stand away from the maxillary posterior dentoalveolar structures approximately 3 mm, but they are in contact with the mandibular teeth and mandibular apical base (Figure 12-46). This positioning recognizes that an inherent three-dimensional deficiency in the maxilla in most Class III malocclusions, which have buccal and anterior crossbite problems. Any constricting or deforming effect of the buccinator mechanism and orbicularis oris is screened from the maxillary arch and supporting bone. The approximation of the buccal shields to the mandibular arch, however, has a constricting effect on the mandibular dentition. The adapted labial wire increases this effect. The shields and lip pads theoretically exert outward pull or tension on the maxillary periosteum at the height of the vestibule.

*Construction bite.* Fränkel recognizes the probable maxillary deficiency and anteroposterior discrepancy in Class III malocclusions and the fact that a combined mandibular excess and accommodative forward posturing of the lower jaw may occur. The construction bite procedure involves clinically retruding the mandible as much as possible, with the condyle occupying the most posterior position in the fossa. The vertical dimension is opened only enough to allow the maxillary incisors to move labially past the mandibular incisors for crossbite correction. The bite opening is kept to a minimum to allow lip closure with minimal strain (see Figure 12-45). Muscle training and lip-seal exercises are as important for Class III as for Class II. Lip-seal exercises can improve the typically redundant and everted lower lips of patients with mandibular prognathism. The most retruded mandibular position varies among patients and also depends on whether the habitual Class III occlusion is a true basal malrelationship or an accommodative anterior mandibular displacement caused by incisor interference. The majority of Class III malocclusions are probably a combination of both sagittal basal discrepancy and adaptive tooth guidance.

To obtain the maximal posterior condylar position, the clinician gently taps on the patient's mandible with the flexed knuckles of the dominant hand while the patient opens the

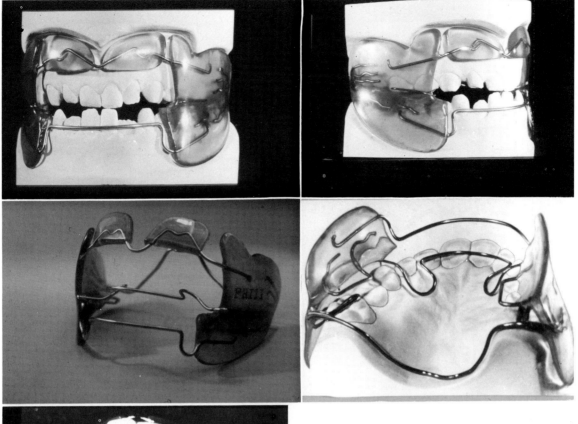

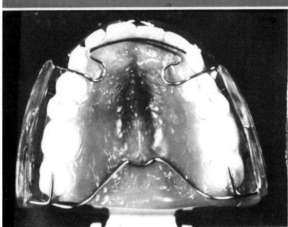

**Figure 12-43.** FR III for treatment of Class III malocclusions. The construction bite is in the most retruded mandibular position. The lip pads are in the maxillary arch, whereas the labial bow is resting against the mandibular teeth. The protrusion bow is against the upper incisors and can be activated to stimulate forward movement of the maxillary incisors, if desired. The palatal bar passes distal to the last molar but is not usually in contact with the tooth. The occlusal rest is on the mandibular molar.

bite approximately 1 cm. The clinician continues tapping gently and then asks the patient to close slowly and guides the final closure with posterior pressure applied by the thumb against the symphysis and the forefinger under the chin. Before taking the wax registration, the clinician must make sure the patient maintains this position for 1 or 2 minutes so the proprioceptive learning process and feedback to the muscles and tendons will be strong enough to overcome the natural tendency to protrude the mandible when closing into the construction bite wax wafer. The posterior guidance is essential during the actual bite-taking procedure. This position is easier for the patient to hold while the wax sets than that required by the Class II forward posturing, because it is the registration of a reproducible terminal position and the

wax can be softer. The wax is removed, chilled under cold water, and replaced and the bite registration is checked again, as with the FR I and II, before the patient is dismissed by the practitioner.

Deep-bite problems require a wider opening of the vertical dimension for the construction bite. This is done so the appliance can be fabricated to stimulate posterior eruption of the maxillary teeth. (Acrylic extensions and occlusal rests may be placed over the mandibular molars [Figure 12-46].) If the need for vertical development is minimal, the occlusal rests are sufficient to keep the lower molars from erupting, whereas the maxillary molars are free to move down and forward to correct the sagittal discrepancy. Separating elastics and notching are not necessary for the FR III because the appliance is

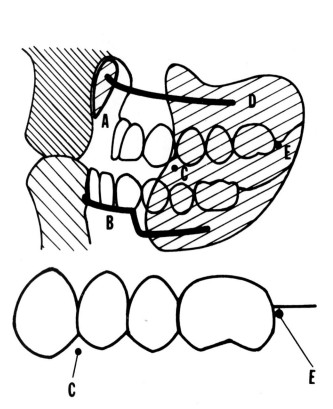

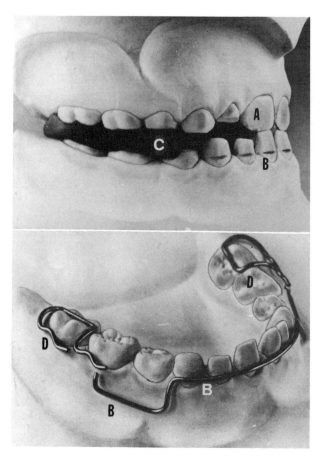

**Figure 12-44.** The lip pads (*A*) are in the maxillary labial vestibule for the FR III. The labial bow (*B*) is in contact with the six mandibular anterior teeth, exerting a very slight pressure on them. The protrusion bow (*C*) is in contact with the lingual surfaces of the upper incisors, passing interocclusally at the distal of the canines. The palatal bow (*E*) passes behind the last maxillary molar to enter the shield. It can then recurve and exit to form an occlusal rest over the lower molar, or a separate rest can be made. In most instances it does not touch the distal surface of the maxillary molar.

**Figure 12-45.** The construction bite for the FR III is taken in the most retruded mandibular position, opening the vertical dimension only as much as is needed to establish an end-to-end bite in the incisors (*A*). The lower labial wire position (*B*) is marked on the mandibular cast, and a slight groove is notched in the teeth at this line. The wax bite (*C*) must be thick enough to allow the protrusion bow, palatal bow, and occlusal rest wires (*D*) to pass through.

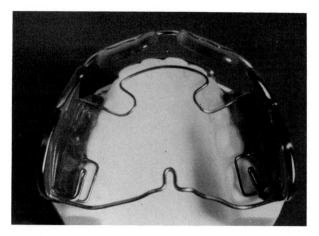

**Figure 12-46.** FR III in place on the lower model. It can be modified to allow an acrylic cover over the mandibular buccal segment, providing more stability because no locking wires are present at the embrasures. This also prevents eruption of the mandibular teeth while freeing selected maxillary teeth to erupt down and forward. The palatal bow, protrusion bow, and lip pads fit the maxillary arch.

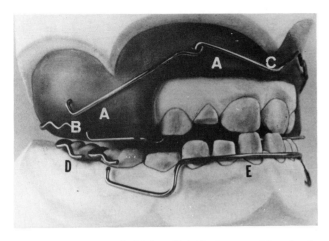

**Figure 12-47.** Wax relief (*A*) and labial wire assemblage for the FR III. The lip-pad assemblage (*C*) consists of three wires—two side wires parallel to each other that permit uniform advancement of the lip pads later and a central V-shaped wire bent to conform to the frenum attachment. The ends of the palatal bow and protrusion bow wires (*B*) stand about 1 mm away from the wax relief. The lower occlusal rest wire (*D*) and labial wire (*E*) will be incorporated in the mandibular portion of the buccal shield. No wax relief is placed on the mandibular arch for the FR III.

stabilized on the mandible by the buccal shields, labial wire, occlusal rests and, possibly, the acrylic cover.

*Working model pour-up and trimming.* The procedure for pouring and trimming the FR III is essentially the same as that for the FR I and II. The impressions are poured immediately in yellow stone, with an adequate base provided to permit proper carving of the maxillary model. The tuberosity must be faithfully reproduced for the palatal bow extension into the vestibular shield. The excess stone must be trimmed away (as noted previously).

The maxillary cast is trimmed for the lip pads. Trimming is extensive, after careful inspection of the patient's anatomic structures and palpation of the area in question. The pliable soft tissue of the upper lip usually accepts about a 5-mm deepening of the sulcus. Proper trimming positions the lower margin of the lip pads at a distance of some 7 to 8 mm from the upper incisor gingival border (see Figure 12-44). The pads are more teardrop shaped because of the midline muscle attachment and labial frenum.

The trimming of the model for the FR III buccal shields is the same as for the FR I and II and also is limited to the maxillary cast. Great care must be exercised to prevent creep of soft tissue under the shields at the height of the maxillary sulcus. Proper carving and appropriate wax relief prevent this undesirable occurrence. No trimming should be done on the mandibular model, although the operator must delineate the muscle attachments to prevent impingement and irritation from the proximity of the acrylic to the mucosa.

**Laboratory prescription and fabrication procedure.** The wax bite is reinserted, and the posterior surfaces of the upper

and lower casts are trimmed flush. The bite is then mounted on the fixator, as described previously, before the prescription is written and the models are sent to the laboratory. The laboratory can also mount the models, if requested, but doing so beforehand reduces the risk of distortion in mailing.

*Wax relief.* The maxillary expansion needs are the same for the FR III as for the other FR variations (with the exception of some Class II, division 2 problems in which the maxillary arch is broad enough and requires no more expansion). After the areas are outlined in pencil, the buccal and labial aspects of the maxillary teeth and alveolar process are again covered with wax. The thickness of the layer under the shields and pads is 3 mm. Boxing wax that is 3 mm thick works well. No wax is applied to the mandibular arch or teeth (Figure 12-47).

**Wire forming.** Both the mandibular labial bow and the palatal bow are formed from relatively heavy 1-mm (0.40-inch, 18-gauge) stainless steel wire. Because of the demands for flexibility for possible tooth movement, the maxillary protrusion bow requires 0.06 or 0.07 mm wire. Some operators make this wire heavier, however, because they plan to accomplish tooth movement therapy with the pre-Fränkel appliance. This is probably preferable in the long run because it reduces breakage of the FR III. All other wires are 0.9 mm (0.036 inch, 19 gauge).

For the lower labial bow (see Figures 12-43 and 12-45) a shallow groove is carved on the plaster casts across the six lower anterior teeth, just above the interdental papillae, to ensure a close fit. Cutting the groove and keeping the wire as low on the crown as possible reduce the tendency for lingual tipping of lower incisors, which could result from a wire position closer to the incisal margin. A 90-degree bend downward at the distal of the lower canine is then made, followed by another horizontal bend approximately 5 mm below the gingival margin. The horizontal leg of the labial bow embedded in the acrylic vestibular shield is parallel to the occlusal surface.

The occlusal rest originates in the vestibular shield and is adapted to lie snugly in the occlusal fissure of the last mandibular molar. The free ends should be far enough away from the mucosa to be incorporated in the acrylic when it is added on the model (Figure 12-45). Both ends of the 0.09-mm wire terminate in the shield.

The palatal bow also begins in the buccal shields and has a shape similar to that in the FR I and II but with the midpalatal loop curving posteriorly. It is kept about 0.5 mm away from the palatal mucosa. The wire runs distal to the last molar tooth, as described earlier, giving the molars freedom to erupt and move mesially. The wire can be adapted to the distal of the molar, below the distal convexity if possible.

The protrusion bow exits from the buccal shields, crossing the interocclusal space at the canine–deciduous first molar embrasure but not contacting the opposing teeth. After it is looped on the palatal mucosa, it comes forward to contact the lingual surfaces of the incisors just above the cingula, 2 or 3 mm below the incisal margin. If eruption is needed for the particular Class III malocclusion, in contradistinction to the Class II, division 2 type of problem (in which a depressive force is required), the protrusion bow must not contact the cingula because this would impede incisor eruption. The protrusion bow is always passive at the time of initial appliance placement.

The lip pad wiring of the FR III is formed much as that of the FR I and II but on the maxillary arch. Because the maxillary labial frenum attachment is heavier, the central wire V must avoid impingement on it. As with the FR I, these wires must be kept away from the relief wax to permit acrylic to cover them completely on the tissue side, even after polishing (see Figures 12-43 and 12-44).

**Fabrication of acrylic parts of the FR III.** The technique for fabricating acrylic parts of the FR III is essentially the same as for the FR I and II. The acrylic that contacts the gingival margin of the teeth in the lower dental arch must be ground away to prevent irritation, and the maxillary lip pads must parallel the slope of the alveolar process to prevent tissue damage and actual dehiscence. If properly designed, the tear-shaped lip pads do not cause damage as the appliance moves up and down during wear. The patient will probably find it easier to work the FR III up and down with the tongue and when opening the mouth, because the FR III is not locked in the interproximal spaces with crossover wires, even though gravity may help hold the appliance in place on the mandible.

Fränkel considers the maximal superior extension of the lip pads extremely important. He believes it pulls on the "septo-premaxillary" ligament (as described by Latham, Johnston, and Delaire, 1970) and the periosteum, enhancing bone deposition and freeing the pressure-sensitive membranous bone from adverse lip pressures. A dramatic example of an iatrogenic orbicularis oris effect is seen in patients with repaired cleft lips in whom severe maxillary retrusion can be attributed to the tight and unyielding scarified lip.

The FR III may be modified somewhat during the course of treatment. Because maxillary sagittal development is a major goal, any appreciable improvement may lead to mucosal contact with the maxillary lip pads. This contact can occur in as little as 3 to 4 months after appliance placement. If it happens, the acrylic is cut away from the anchoring tags of the lip pad skeletal wires, which are at right angles to the parallel lip-pad wires that emerge from the shields (Figure 12-48). The straight wires are grasped with an office pliers and pulled out of the shields to advance the upper lip pads and reestablish the proper distance. Endothermic acrylic can then be added to fill the holes cut in the shields. The appliance is repolished to prevent irritation. Minor adjustments of the lip pads are usually required to establish a parallel lip pad–mucosa relationship again.

With treatment progress the upper and lower incisors should approach an end-to-end bite. The maxillary protrusion bow may then be activated to stimulate forward tipping of the maxillary incisors. The clinician should check that the protrusion bow does not press on the upper incisor cingula at this time, because such action prevents eruption. The slight labial movement of the upper incisors by the protrusion bow prevents jiggling of the incisor teeth by accelerating the jumping

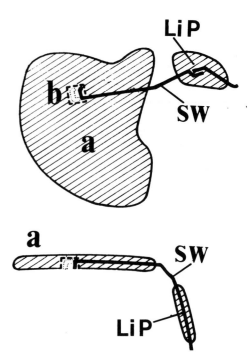

**Figure 12-48.** FR III lip-pad advancement is done by making a cut in the shield (*a*) and pulling the skeletal wire (*SW*) forward and upward. The cut section of the shield is then filled in with acrylic at (*b*) and polished.

of the bite. When the maxillary incisors are well over their mandibular counterparts, the protrusion bow can be removed to prevent any possible interference with maxillary incisor eruption. The occlusal rests on the mandibular molars should be left intact, however, so the posterior open bite that is usually produced by the sagittal correction closes by virtue of the down and forward eruption of unimpeded maxillary teeth.

Examples of successful FR III treatment are illustrated in Figures 12-49 and 12-50.

## FR IV

The etiology of the open-bite malocclusion is not as well delineated as that of Class II, division 1 problems. Clinicians must determine the degree to which the malocclusion is caused by morphogenetic pattern, direction of jaw growth, and abnormal perioral muscle function. They must also ask whether tongue posture and function are primary, perhaps a retained infantile deglutitional pattern, or adaptive to the morphology. Another consideration might be the role of finger sucking. With a potential multiplicity of contributing factors and considerable individual variation, therapeutic demands vary.

Fränkel designed a deficiency appliance and a muscle-training appliance. If the problem involves something else, the FR is not enough, except in carefully selected cases. One school of thought holds that lip seal exercises are easier to do, with obvious results, if a lip trap is present, as in Class II, division 1 malocclusions. Training the tongue posture and func-

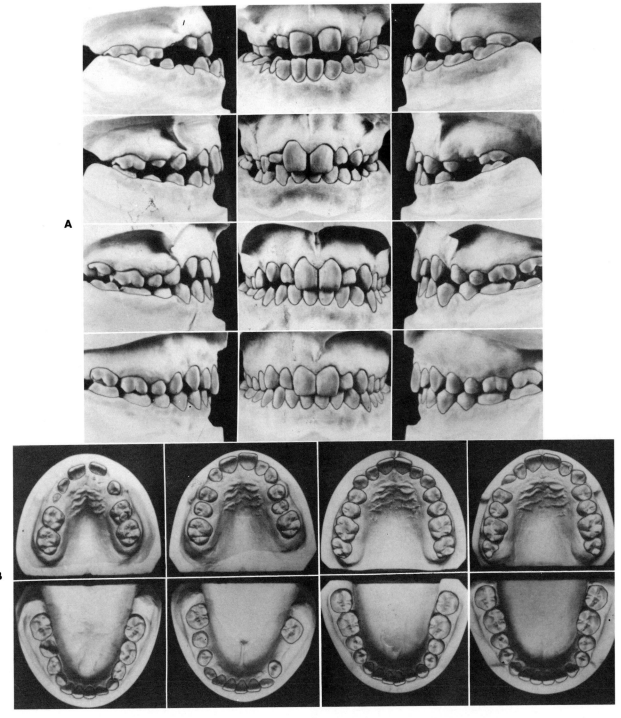

**Figure 12-49.** **A,** Starting treatment of Class III malocclusions with the FR III is desirable before the pubertal growth spurt. Preferably, treatment should begin as early as patient compliance can be assured. This may be in the deciduous dentition in some patients, although transitional dentition treatment has shown quite satisfactory results with the exchange of teeth. **B,** The mandibular arch has shown little change other than an uprighting of posterior segments and a rounding-out of the arch. The maxillary arch form and dimensional changes, however, are quite significant and stable out of treatment.

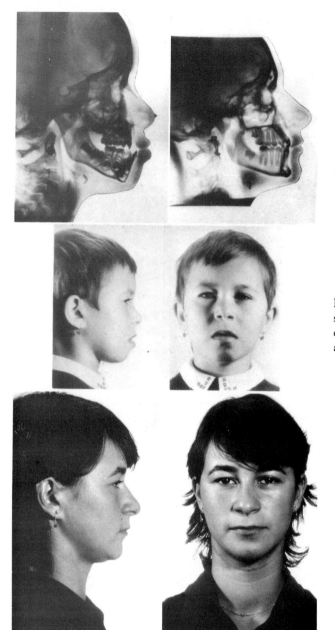

**Figure 12-50.** Class III malocclusion, with FR III treatment started in the deciduous dentition. The profile change is a major one, with significant improvement of lip posture. No chincap therapy was used.

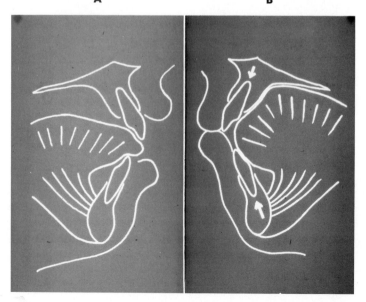

**Figure 12-51.** Anterior open-bite problems usually show protracted tongue posture, **A,** with incompetence of the lips. The tongue-tooth contact replaces the lip seal during deglutition to create a negative atmospheric pressure. This accentuates the tongue thrusting and enhances the anterior open bite. With the FR IV in place and with lip-seal exercises, **B,** lip contact takes over, reducing tongue protrusion and causing the tongue to move back into its normally raised position, in proximity to the palate, during deglutition. Incisors can then erupt normally to close the bite while the tongue reestablishes an interocclusal clearance between the posterior teeth. This allows the mandible to close up and forward into a more favorable growth direction, reducing the mandibular plane angle.

(Courtesy Rolf Fränkel.)

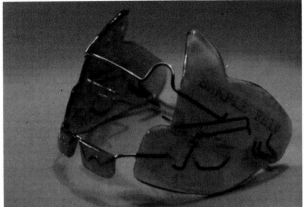

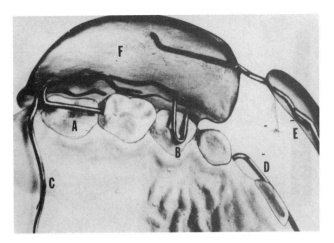

**Figure 12-53.** FR IV appliance on the maxillary cast. The rests for the permanent first molar (*A*) and deciduous first molar (*B*) usually contact both maxillary and mandibular occlusal surfaces. The palatal bow (*C*) passes to the distal of the last molar tooth. The maxillary labial arch (*D*), mandibular lip pads (*E*), and buccal shield (*F*) also can be identified.

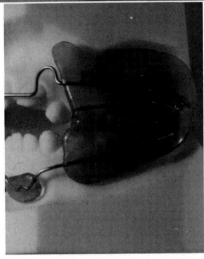

**Figure 12-52.** FR IV appliance. It has no maxillary lingual protrusion bow or canine clasp. The maxillary labial arch is usually passive at first, although it can be activated to retract the maxillary anterior teeth. Molar and premolar occlusal rests help stabilize the appliance. Because little or no interocclusal clearance exists, the rests contact both maxillary and molar posterior segments, preventing eruption. A thin layer of interocclusal acrylic is sometimes used for this purpose also, increasing appliance stability and enhancing a depressing force on the buccal teeth.

tion, however, is a different matter. A generation of orthodontists (and speech therapists) failed with their "tongue-thrusting" myofunctional therapy in most cases. Thus this modification of the basic FR appliance used by Fränkel in the correction of open bites depends primarily on careful case analysis and specific case selection (Figure 12-51). The philosophy of controlling tongue action from the vestibule instead of using a screening device within the arch is still not accepted, despite an article by Rolf and Christine Fränkel illustrating dramatic results. If the cases are chosen properly and patients cooperate completely, the lip-seal exercises are even more important than with the other FR types—if that is possible. Fränkel's report shows that the FR IV is truly a functional appliance, with evidence of significant basal bone

change. Above all the article shows that aberrant muscle activity can create open-bite problems and redirect growth in a more vertical direction. Because the FR IV reverses the unfavorable growth guidance, it must be used during an active growth period. Again, the mixed dentition is ideal for its influence, with a longer period of wear usually needed, into the permanent dentition. Diagnosis and case selection, however, along with patient compliance, are critical factors.

The FR IV has the same vestibular configuration as the FR I and FR II, but it has no canine loops or protrusion bow (Figure 12-52). Four occlusal rests on the maxillary permanent first molars and deciduous first molars prevent tipping of the appliance (Figure 12-53). The rests discourage eruption of posterior teeth—a vital requisite for anterior open-bite conditions. The palatal bow resembles that of the FR III and is always placed behind the last molar. The occlusal rests often require adaptation to the individual patient. They must not, however, prevent shifting of the appliance in a posterior (or dorsal) direction. Hence the appliance is not locked on either arch by interproximal wires. Occasionally a thin acrylic wafer is interposed between the upper and lower buccal segments, but the wafer cannot be too thick; otherwise lip closure becomes more difficult. Without the exercises the appliance is doomed to failure. A number of operators use the FR IV with vertical extraoral force–chincap therapy, which also helps close down the bite by virtue of a positive depressing action on the buccal segments. At least one modification has incorporated lingual crib spurs to discourage anterior tongue posture and compensatory tongue function, in a manner originally suggested by Kraus. A detailed discussion of this appliance and its manipulation is beyond the limits of this book. Figure 12-54 shows a successful treatment result.

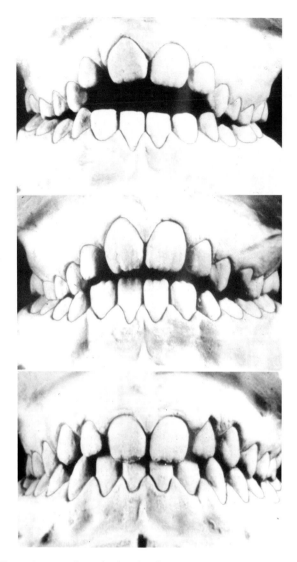

**Figure 12-54.** Open-bite malocclusion treated with only an FR IV appliance and the prescribed lip-seal exercises. Correction is a combination of retardation of posterior segment eruption with unimpeded incisor eruption, under the influence of the established normal lip and tongue function.

## CLINICAL MANAGEMENT OF THE FRÄNKEL APPLIANCE

The most well-made appliance will fail unless the operator follows a clinical discipline. This is particularly important for the Fränkel FR, which has more precise demands for fabrication and more exacting tolerances. This need for precision deters many clinicians, who are not willing to spend the time necessary in those critical first 6 to 8 weeks.

At the placement appointment the maxillary arch is checked to ensure that the special heavy spacing separators are still in place. If space is still not sufficient or the clinician has decided to notch the distal of the deciduous second molar and the mesial of the deciduous first molar for seating the crossover wires in the maxilla, a diamond cylinder bur is rec-

ommended to make the seating grooves. Stabilizing the appliance on the maxilla at the first visit is absolutely essential. Otherwise the patient cannot adapt to the fully extended shields and lip pads, and soreness develops. Under the best conditions this adjustment process takes time, effort, and constant encouragement. Knowledgeable clinicians provide parents and patients with good descriptive literature on the Fränkel appliance, which they can read while waiting for appliance placement and take home for future reference. The information also can be given at the time of impression taking so that it can be fully assimilated before appliance placement. Videotapes and slide sequences also are available to give a better idea of patient responsibilities and ways to handle the appliance in the critical first days. Watching one of these 7-minute tapes can make a potentially antagonistic patient into a cooperative one.

All margins are checked for smoothness before the appliance is inserted. The appliance is then seated on the maxilla to verify its stability on the dentition and the fit of the shields and labial and palatal wires. This procedure is repeated for the mandibular arch. The crossover wires must not contact the mandibular teeth, and the lingual wires arising from the acrylic pressure pad, behind the lower incisors, must be passive. The patient then bites into the appliance, and the tissue is checked in the pad and shield area. No blanching of tissue should appear, and the peripheral portions should contact sulcular tissue. Sufficient distance between the shields and the maxillary alveolar mucosa and teeth is crucial.

Tissue impingement is the most frequently encountered problem with initial appliance placement, and the areas of greatest concern are the buccal frenula and inferior margins of the lip pads. The lip pads must be in a vertical position so their lingual surfaces or margins do not contact the gingival tissue on insertion and removal. If the lower margins are tipped forward, the upper margins rub against the alveolar and gingival mucosa when the mouth is opened. Cutting a groove around the wires and rotating the pads to the correct vertical position can correct improper pad orientation. Alternately, the support wire can be freed in the buccal shields and moved backward or forward to ensure proper distance from the contiguous soft tissue. Then the slot in the acrylic is filled with self-cure acrylic and polished. Slight modification can be made with pliers, but care must be taken not to distort the shields in the process.

The anterosuperior periphery of the buccal shields over the maxillary canines is the next most likely area of irritation. Peripheral margins can be reduced and polished the same way as for overextension of the lip pads and shields. If possible, as with a new denture, awaiting actual tissue reaction is better than trying to anticipate it and cutting away acrylic. If no blanching of tissue occurs around the periphery of the shields and pads, the patient may safely start the break-in period at home, assuming that the appliance is fabricated properly and the construction bite is correct. Tissue redness around the periphery of shields and pads that are properly extended is a normal consequence of proper fit and good patient cooperation. The clinician must be careful not to cut away too much acrylic during the first visits. The patient should be shown the

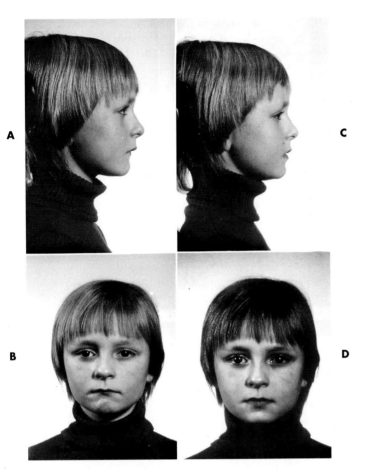

**Figure 12-55.** Without the FR II appliance, **A** and **B**, and with it inserted, **C** and **D**. Improvement is dramatic. Such pictures can help motivate beginning patients.

dramatic profile change and informed that irritation is possible for the first 2 weeks (Figure 12-55). Even the experienced clinician should allow ample time for initial placement of the FR, setting aside a half hour for instruction during the first appointment. If the lip-seal exercise regimen was not started at the time of taking the impressions and construction bite, this can begin with the appliance placement. Except during meals or when engaging in sports, the patient should hold a small piece of paper lightly between the lips.

After patients have grown accustomed to wearing the Fränkel appliance and can speak intelligibly, they should wear it all the time, except during meals. In the beginning, however, it should be worn for only short periods to allow the soft tissues and muscles to adjust to the "foreign body." Generally, during the first couple of weeks, the FR I and II are worn during the day only for 2 to 4 hours. During the first checkup or "control" appointment, the soft tissues are examined carefully and the necessary peripheral adjustments and polishing done. Again, the operator should always err in the direction of taking away too little rather than too much material. Of course, the appliance must not impinge on the muscle attachments, because these areas do not adapt to overextensions. However, the clinician should never trim the acrylic before verifying that

the appliance is truly overextended. An astringent mouthwash, warm saline rinses, benzocaine, or Orabase can help control the abrasion and inflammation.

During the interval between the second and third office visits, or a period of about 3 weeks, daytime wear extends to 4 to 6 hours and speaking exercises should begin. Speaking normally when wearing an FR is one of the most difficult challenges. Speech improvement can be accelerated by having the patient practice reading into a home tape recorder and listening to the sequence. Some clinicians prefer to wait until this time to initiate the lip-seal exercises, making sure first that the appliance fits well and is comfortable.

During the third appointment, after it has been determined that stabilization is good and tissues are not irritated, exercises may be prescribed in addition to the lip-seal regimen. These oral exercises are essentially isometric contractions of the perioral musculature, literally grasping the Fränkel appliance in the vestibule. A speech check should be made as the patient counts from one to ten.

At every appointment the clinician should use positive reinforcement to maintain a high level of patient compliance. The FR does not do the job by itself, and even the most cooperative 8- to 10-year-old gets discouraged. Showing pictures of the patient with and without the appliance in place and pictures and plaster models of the facial and dental changes achieved in other patients, along with having other Fränkel patients present at the same time for peer support, can be helpful (see Figure 12-55). Early appointments are particularly critical. The gingival mucosa and margins must be inspected for possible abrasions that might indicate manipulation of the appliance by the tongue in a free-floating status. Full-time daily wear is usually prescribed at the end of the third visit.

The average patient needs about 2 months before the FR I or II appliance is worn all night. Not every operator agrees with this rule, but Fränkel's experience indicates that nighttime wear should not be rushed. If the patient has difficulty adapting to the constructed forward-mandibular posture (even when it is only 3 mm) and is still uncomfortable, the jaw will drop open and back during sleep. Abrasions on the lower lingual mucosa are likely. Consequently an anterior-tipping stimulus to the lower incisors is possible as the lingual pressure pad rides on the lower incisors and rests on them for long periods. Patients adjust more easily to the FR III, however, and the appliance can usually be worn all the time after the first 2 weeks. This appliance also can cause ulceration and abrasion, which the clinician should monitor. Benzocaine or Orabase ointment soothe irritation and thereby enhance patient cooperation.

At first, treatment progress and appliance fit should be checked at 4-week intervals. The mucosa of the vestibule and gingivae should be examined at every visit, and (for the FR I and FR II) stabilization of the appliance on the maxillary arch verified. As with the bionator, minimal changes are necessary during treatment after the patient has grown accustomed to wearing the appliance; in fact, even less must be done, because the FR usually requires no interocclusal acrylic. The visit usually serves to stimulate motivation, show progress,

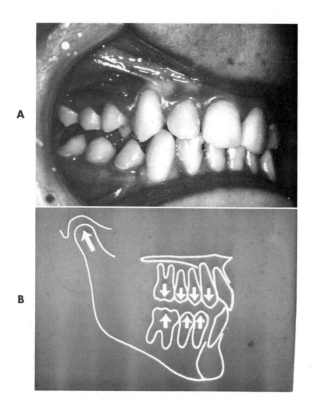

**Figure 12-56.** The FR I and FR II usually achieve sagittal correction more rapidly than eruption of posterior teeth. The result is often an incisal contact, with the posterior teeth being out of occlusion, **A.** The open bite that exists is caused by condylar growth that propels the mandible down and forward, **B.** Holding the corrected sagittal relationship with the FR until eruption has been obtained is a normal part of treatment.

and project future treatment time. Although they must be seated interproximally, the canine and molar crossover wires should be routinely checked for possible impingement on the interdental papillae as the deciduous teeth are exfoliated and the canines and premolars erupt. If tissue irritation is present, the FR I canine loops can be bent occlusally and the molar rests gingivally to relieve the pressure. The canine loops can be modified slightly to guide a buccally erupting canine into proper position. However, interference with normal canine eruption is possible; thus many clinicians prefer the FR II to the FR I. Also, any gingival margin abrasion or mucosal irritation must be eliminated, as must any labial tipping of the lower incisors or soreness of the lingual gingival tissue, which could indicate a destabilized, free-floating appliance.

As previously noted, planning for a short pre-Fränkel period of fixed appliance guidance for incisor alignment, space closure, or rotational correction is advantageous in some cases. Hence activation of the labial bow is seldom necessary. Minor residual spacing can be closed, however, if done gradually and with care not to retract the incisors too much in Class II, division 1 malocclusions. Too much pressure can cause the arch wire to slide gingivally and dislodge the appliance. The FR is not a tooth-moving appliance. The lingual protrusion bow (as Fränkel has called it) actually does little in

the way of protruding anything, except in Class II, division 2 patients in whom the maxillary central incisors may be tipped labially; moreover, this can be done much more quickly and accurately by pre–functional appliance guidance before the FR is placed. Rather, the lingual bow on the FR II helps maintain maxillary stabilization and also can prevent excessive lingual tipping of the maxillary incisors.

Sagittal, vertical, and transverse improvement should be apparent after 3 months of full-time wear. Frequently a lateral open bite develops (Figure 12-56). This is a sign of patient cooperation, because eruption of the lower posterior teeth is usually slower than the change in transverse and sagittal directions. With proper patient compliance, 6 months is usually adequate to correct an original cusp-to-cusp Class II malocclusion in the molar region. (The appropriateness of case selection and the presence of a normal increment of mandibular growth are assumed.)

More severe cases may require 9 to 12 months to correct a full distal relationship. These patients probably require a staged two- or three-step mandibular protraction approach to advance the lingual acrylic pressure pad and lip pads as previously described. With advancement of the anterior posturing trough of the appliance, a reciprocal distalizing thrust occurs on the body of the appliance. Thus the posteroinferior margins of the shields must occasionally be relieved during the staged mandibular advancement. Scheduling progress records at 6-month intervals is a good practice. Assessment of growth increments and direction and any treatment-induced changes requires a lateral cephalogram.

FR III adjustments are minimal and have been discussed in connection with appliance fabrication. Because of the relative ease of handling and the ease with which most patients adjust to the appliance, Fränkel recommends that inexperienced clinicians prescribe this appliance first in a mild Class III problem before using the FR I or II.

Although sitting on the appliance can distort it, making readaptation to its original shape almost impossible, breakage is usually minimal and confined to the buccal shields or crossover wires. If a fragment of the buccal shield is broken off (and this is usually the anterosuperior projection into the canine fossa), immediate repair can be done with cyanoacrylate adhesive. The original working models and mounting for the articulator must be saved so repairs or replacements can be made if the appliance is broken or lost.

## Treatment Timing

The best therapeutic effect of the Fränkel appliance and other functional appliances (e.g., Bio-Modulator of Fleischer, twin block of Clark), as far as expansion and resolution of arch-length deficiency are concerned, is achieved during the late mixed and transitional dentition period, when both hard and soft tissues are undergoing their greatest adaptational change, with as many as 52 teeth being present in their bony shell. Studies of growth and development and extensive research by Petrovic, Stutzmann, Moyers, McNamara, Graber, and others have shown that maxillary and mandibular growth is essential for sagittal and vertical skeletal change. The alternative is an accommodative or dual bite or major dental compensation, which is not likely to be stable. Use of functional appliances in nongrowing children or improperly chosen cases has already produced too many poor results.

The choice of the optimal time for Class II treatment initiation depends on the patient's rate of development. It varies somewhat, but a good indication of readiness is eruption of the four upper and lower incisors, which can happen as early as 7½ years but is more likely at 8½ to 9 years of age. For arch-deficiency problems with manifest maxillary narrowness that demand expansion to establish normal arch form, placing the FR at the beginning of this stage is better to take advantage of all possible dentoalveolar adjustment. For problems of sagittal and vertical concern, the appliance can be placed more toward the middle of the mixed dentition period, with the aim of carrying on into the transitional period as far as possible. Placing the FR in the late mixed or early transitional dentition, when the root resorption is already advanced for the deciduous teeth, is not recommended. Appliance stability and seating on the maxilla are critical, but this is more difficult with loose or missing deciduous teeth. Usually the clinician does not have the choice of when to start treatment. The patient comes in when parents or referring dentists think appropriate—and too often this is too late. If too late, awaiting the eruption of the maxillary and mandibular premolars and canines to provide the proper appliance stabilization is preferable. Such prepubertal timing is often more favorable from the standpoint of growth increment and direction for sagittal and vertical changes, particularly in male patients. The twin block appliance of Clark may be a better choice at that time.

Treatment for Class III and open-bite cases should usually start sooner than for Class II problems. This means immediately after eruption of the permanent first molars, even though chincap therapy may have been employed earlier as a pre-FR phase. The FR appliance effect in Class III problems is not so much a sagittal basal bone adjustment as it is in Class II cases. The construction bite for mandibular retrusion is minimal and seldom exceeds 1 or 2 mm. However, as a deficiency appliance and an exercise device the FR III stimulates anterior maxillary development, relieves abnormal perioral muscle pressures on the upper anterior teeth, and establishes normal lip tone and muscle function. FR III treatment in the deciduous dentition is usually not recommended, because patients at

this age are likely to lose or break the appliance. The patient undergoing FR treatment must be responsible enough to handle full-time wear, care of the appliance, and associated exercises. Another reason for waiting until the lower incisors have erupted is that lateral maxillary-arch growth is usually greater at this time and the potential for change per unit time is greater.

Most orthodontists regard Fränkel appliance therapy (and any pre-Fränkel fixed appliance preparation) as a first-phase attack on the malocclusion. Estimating treatment time is difficult, but figuring 15 to 24 months of guidance is advised so the patient is in the permanent dentition stage and future treatment decisions can be made. In the average case active treatment is completed after this period and the appliance may then be worn as a retainer, or a Hawley biteplate appliance may be used for the interval between the treatment phase and the permanent dentition time. Fränkel believes that if treatment is started during the permanent dentition, a retention phase of 2 to 3 years is needed. A long retention period is indicated especially in Class II, division 2, Class III, and open-bite problems.

Using Fränkel appliances in the treatment of patients with crowding in the permanent dentition is seldom indicated. However, in deep-bite sagittal problems, significant improvement can be achieved in one phase of treatment. Use of the Fränkel appliance then requires a depth of experience, recognition of appliance limitations, and knowledge of the time to institute other forms of mechanotherapy. Because the Fränkel appliance is not easy to construct or handle, the inexperienced clinician should begin with simpler malocclusions in patients who are likely to cooperate and not attempt to treat severe skeletal problems in the beginning. End-to-end molar relationships or flush terminal plane cases with an excessive overjet, a deeper-than-normal overbite, lingually inclined lower incisors, and pernicious lip trap and hyperactive mentalis habits are excellent choices for the neophyte. As indicated earlier, the FR III is the best appliance to begin with for mild Class III problems (Figures 12-49, *A* and *B*). Use of a chincap, which helps hold the appliance in place at night and exerts a retrusive force on the mandible, is permitted *with* the FR III. This fact underscores the degree to which many of these problems are combined maxillary deficiencies and mandibular overgrowths.

# Chapter 13

# The Twin Block Technique

William J. Clark

## ORTHODONTICS AND DENTOFACIAL ORTHOPEDICS

Orthodontics is specifically concerned with correcting irregularities of the teeth, but the term *orthodontics* does not adequately describe the treatment of skeletal disharmony and the wider esthetic aims of a specialty as concerned with facial balance and harmony as it is with balanced functional occlusion. Dental malocclusion is frequently secondary to abnormal skeletal development. The approach in treating such malocclusions changes from an orthodontic one with the primary emphasis on dental correction to an orthopedic one with the goal of correcting the underlying skeletal abnormality. This difference in approach recognizes the existence of two schools of thought in evaluating the aims of orthodontic treatment. An essential distinction in terminology exists between orthodontics and dentofacial orthopedics.

The term *dentofacial orthopedics* conveys to the patient that treatment can significantly alter and improve facial appearance in addition to correcting irregularity of the teeth. The adoption of this wider descriptive term has extended the horizons of the specialty and helped the public appreciate the various benefits of dentofacial therapy. The significance of this change in terminology was recognized in 1985 within the specialty of orthodontics when the *American Journal of Orthodontics* was renamed the *American Journal of Orthodontics and Dentofacial Orthopedics* by its editor, T.M. Graber. Subsequently the American Association of Orthodontics authorized a name change for the specialty, which was later approved by the Council on Education of the American Dental Association.

## THE FORM AND FUNCTION PHILOSOPHY

Functional orthopedics evolved mainly in Europe, whereas fixed appliance technique evolved mostly in America. At the beginning of the century the form and function philosophy was common to both Angle and Robin, the founders of modern fixed and functional appliance techniques. Further evolution occurred in various areas as the fixed technique continued to develop in America and functional technique evolved in Europe. Socioeconomic factors also played a significant part in the evolution of technique before and after the two world wars. The distance between the two areas of develop-

ment was responsible for a division in not only technique but also philosophy regarding the ability to correct malocclusion by controlling the functional environment of the developing dentition.

Since the development of the anterior biteplane by Kingsley and its modification by Case, functional therapy has been based on the form and function philosophy, the fundamental principle that function modifies anatomy. However, after a century of development in functional techniques, this simple principle is not yet universally accepted within the orthodontic community. This disagreement persists despite the increasing background of validated information supporting the case for the modification of skeletal form by functional therapy.

## THE EFFECTS OF FORCE ON BONE

Unlike other connective tissue, bone responds to a mild degree of pressure and tension by changing in form. The internal and external structure of bone is continuously modified by a process of bony remodeling to meet the changing requirements of function in development. The close correlation between form and function is well illustrated in dentofacial development from childhood to adulthood. In the newborn the glenoid fossa is virtually flat. At this stage the gum pads are at the same level as the condyle and articulation is well suited to the function of suckling, with no bony restriction to freedom of movement of the condyle in the glenoid fossa. The sigmoid outline of the glenoid fossa develops progressively in response to growth in the height of the maxilla and mandible and concomitant dental development as the occlusal plane moves down relative to the glenoid fossa. Changes in function from the infantile suckling pattern to mature deglutition and swallowing are important in this osseous morphologic adaptation.

During the development of the occlusion, incisal guidance and cuspal interdigitation progressively influence the movement of the mandible as deciduous and permanent teeth erupt. Occlusal forces transmitted through the teeth influence not only the teeth and dentoalveolar bone but also the supporting basal bone and the development of the temporomandibular articulation. Resorption of existing bone and deposition of new bone may take place on the surface of the bone, under the periosteum, or in the case of cancellous bone, on the surfaces of the trabeculae. In this respect, bone is more plastic than any other connective tissue.

The internal and external structure of bone is modified by functional demands to withstand the physical demands made on it with the greatest degree of economy of structure. This behavior is expressed by Wolff's law of transformation of bone. The architecture of bone is such that it can resist the forces brought to bear on it with the use of a minimal amount of tissue.

The challenge of functional therapy is to maximize the genetic potential of growth and guide the growing face and developing dentition toward a pattern of optimal development. In the dentition the force of occlusion of the teeth is the most natural functional mechanism that can be used to influence the structure of the supporting bone. This natural process of bony remodeling forms the basis of functional correction with the twin block technique.

The fundamental concepts of functional therapy have changed very little since the development of the monobloc by Robin (1902). Over the years, however, functional appliance design has been progressively modified for daytime and nighttime wear. Recent improvements in the design of functional appliances have led to more consistent results in functional orthopedic treatment. A significant advance is the introduction of appliances for full-time wear, including during eating, to maximize functional forces in the developing dentition.

## AIMS OF FUNCTIONAL THERAPY

In normal development a functional equilibrium is established under neurologic control in response to repetitive tactile stimuli. Occlusal forces transmitted through the dentition provide constant proprioceptive stimuli to influence the growth rate and trabecular structure of the supporting bone.

Malocclusion is frequently associated with discrepancies in arch relationships caused by underlying skeletal and soft-tissue factors that result in unfavorable cuspal guidance and poor occlusal function. The proprioceptive sensory feedback mechanism controls muscular activity and provides a functional stimulus or deterrent to the full expression of maxillary and mandibular bone growth. The unfavorable cuspal contacts of distal occlusion are obstructions to normal forward mandibular translation in function and as such do not encourage the mandible to achieve its optimal genetic growth potential.

If the mandible occludes in a distal relationship to the maxilla, the occlusal forces acting on the mandibular teeth in normal function have a distal component of force unfavorable to forward mandibular development. In such a malocclusion the inclined planes formed by the cusps of the upper and lower teeth in occlusion represent a servo mechanism that locks the mandible in a posteriorly occluding functional position (see Chapter 2).

Functional appliance therapy aims to improve the functional relationship of dentofacial structures by eliminating unfavorable developmental factors and improving the muscle environment enveloping the developing occlusion. Through alteration of the position of the teeth and supporting tissues,

a new functional behavior pattern or engram is established that can support a new position of equilibrium.

## THE INFLUENCE OF RESEARCH ON CLINICAL ORTHODONTICS

### Orthodontic Tooth Movement

The basic tenets of orthodontic tooth movement were validated by histologic examination in animal experiments. These experiments defined the sequence of histologic change in the periodontal membrane and alveolar bone in response to the application of orthodontic forces (Oppenheim, 1911; Reitan, 1951; Sandstedt, 1904, 1905; Schwarz, 1932). Indeed, philosophy and technique are influenced by research findings, and this interdependent relationship enables the determination of scientific bases for clinical orthodontic practice.

### Orthopedic Growth Response

A similar background of research underpins present concepts of functional orthopedic mechanisms in the correction of malocclusion. Comparative studies of growth and development in animal experiments lead to a better understanding of the growth response observed in clinical practice. With satisfactory resolution of the mechanism of orthodontic correction, the thrust of animal research over the past 25 years has concentrated more on the response to orthopedic forces applied by functional mandibular protrusion. A series of growth studies used fixed inclined planes to record growth changes by functional mandibular protrusion in monkeys and rodents. Studies in America and Europe have been remarkably consistent in their findings.

The response at the cellular level confirms the potential for bony remodeling of both the condyle and the glenoid fossa in experimental animals compared with untreated controls. The Michigan growth studies (McNamara et al, 1975) clearly demonstrate thickening of the condylar cartilage in the posterior and superior area compared with that observed in control animals, who experienced no such thickening. These results replicate the work of Petrovic et al reported in Chapter 2. Paulsen (1996) substantiates these conclusions with serial laminagraphic studies.

A histologic study in Toronto identified the deposition of new bone in the region of the postglenoid spine as evidence of bony remodeling in the glenoid fossa (Woodside, Metaxas, Altuna, 1987). The study led to the following conclusion:

In all the experimental animals, including, most importantly, the mature adult, a large amount of bone had formed in the glenoid fossa, especially along the anterior border of the post-glenoid spine. The glenoid fossa appeared to be remodeling anteriorly.

The current challenge in clinical research is to demonstrate that these same changes occur in a clinical setting in response to functional orthopedic technique with sufficient magnitude to achieve significant change in the pattern of dentofacial growth and development.

## EVOLUTION OF FUNCTIONAL APPLIANCES

As pointed out in Chapter 6, in the evolution of functional therapy, many variations in appliance design occurred after the original development of the monobloc at the turn of the century. Early appliances were bulky and cumbersome for the patient and only suitable for nighttime wear. Subsequent modification of design reduced the bulk of these appliances as clinicians sought to increase daytime wear by reducing palatal acrylic and replacing some acrylic with wire components. The labiolingual appliances of Bimler (1949) and the vestibular appliances of Fränkel (1967) exemplified this approach. These modifications improved patient acceptance of the appliances for daytime wear in many cases and therefore improved the consistency of response to treatment. The addition of wires increased the flexibility of the appliances but also made them more vulnerable to fracture and distortion and difficult to repair. The Balters bionator, a one-piece activator of reduced bulk, was adapted for daytime wear and became popular as a simpler alternative.

However, all these functional appliances shared the disadvantage of being made in one piece to fit the teeth in both jaws. The upper and lower components were joined together, and the patient could not eat, speak, or perform other normal oral functions with the appliances in the mouth. In addition, some variations were not esthetic and proved uncomfortable to wear. Full-time wear of the appliance was almost impossible.

Removing the appliance during meals inevitably interrupts the corrective process. When the appliance is removed, the patient usually functions with the mandible retruded and the benefits of unloading the condyle and encouraging protrusive mandibular function are lost as potential stimuli to mandibular growth.

Twin blocks free the patient from these restrictions. The patient can function normally in twin blocks and is able to eat and speak without restriction of normal movements of the tongue, lips, and mandible. This freedom enables the appliances to be worn full time.

## THE TWIN BLOCK TECHNIQUE

Twin blocks are simple bite-blocks that effectively modify the occlusal inclined plane; these devices use upper and lower bite-blocks that engage on occlusal inclined planes (Figure 13-1). Twin block appliances achieve rapid functional correction of malocclusion by transmitting favorable occlusal forces to the occlusal inclined planes covering the posterior teeth.

### The Occlusal Inclined Plane

The occlusal inclined plane is the fundamental functional mechanism of the natural dentition. In normal development, cuspal inclined planes play important roles in determining the relationship of the teeth as they erupt into occlusion. Occlusal forces transmitted through the dentition provide constant proprioceptive stimuli to influence the growth rate and adaptation of the trabecular structure of the supporting bone.

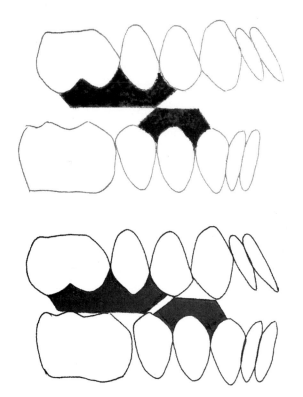

**Figure 13-1.** Twin blocks are simple bite-blocks with occlusal inclined planes.

Fixed occlusal inclined planes have been used to alter the distribution of occlusal forces in animal experiments investigating the effects of functional mandibular displacement on mandibular growth and adaptive changes in the temporomandibular joint (TMJ) (McNamara, 1980; Petrovic, 1978). (See Chapter 2.) The proprioceptive sensory feedback mechanism controls muscular activity and provides a functional stimulus or deterrent to the full expression of mandibular growth. If a distal occlusion develops, the occlusion of the teeth represents a servo mechanism that locks the mandible in a distally occluding functional position.

### Twin Blocks

Twin blocks are designed for full-time wear; they correct the maxillomandibular relationship through functional mandibular displacement. Twin blocks achieve rapid functional correction of malocclusion by modifying the occlusal inclined plane, guiding the mandible forward into correct occlusion. The forces of occlusion are used to correct the malocclusion (Figure 13-2).

Upper and lower bite-blocks interlock at a 70-degree angle; they are designed for full-time wear to take advantage of all functional forces applied to the dentition, including the forces of mastication. Wearing bite-blocks is similar in feel to wearing dentures, and patients can eat comfortably with the appliances in place. With twin blocks, full functional correction of occlusal relationships can be achieved in most cases without the addition of any orthopedic or traction forces.

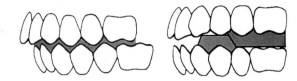

**Figure 13-2.** Twin blocks modify the occlusal inclined plane to guide the mandible forward into correct occlusion.

The twin block technique has two stages:

1. *Active phase:* Twin blocks use posterior inclined planes to adjust the vertical dimension and correct the malocclusion by functional mandibular protrusion.
2. *Support phase:* An anterior inclined plane is used to retain the corrected incisor relationship until the buccal segment occlusion is fully established.

## DEVELOPMENT OF TWIN BLOCKS

The twin block appliance (Clark, 1982, 1988, 1995) was developed in 1977 as a two-piece appliance resembling a Schwarz double plate and a split activator. In comparison with other functional appliances, a number of advantages result from using separate upper and lower appliances with occlusal bite-blocks. The functional mechanism is very similar to that of the natural dentition. Occlusal inclined planes give greater freedom of movement in anterior and lateral excursion and cause less interference with normal function. Appearance is noticeably improved when twin blocks are fitted, and the absence of lip, cheek, and tongue pads allows normal function. The goal in developing the twin block approach to treatment was to produce a technique to maximize the growth response to functional mandibular protrusion through the use of an appliance system the patient would find simple, comfortable, and esthetically acceptable.

The forces of mastication are the most active functional forces applied through the muscles of the masticatory apparatus. Mastication involves the whole face and even part of the cranium. Powerful functional forces are applied by active chewing movements in the mastication of food. Twin blocks are worn 24 hours a day. The patient eats with the appliances in the mouth, and the full forces of occlusion are harnessed as corrective forces for dental and facial development in the twin block technique to maximize the functional response to treatment.

Twin blocks are constructed in a protrusive bite that effectively modifies the occlusal inclined plane by means of acrylic inclined planes on occlusal bite-blocks. The occlusal inclined plane acts as a guiding mechanism, displacing the mandible down and forward. With the appliances in the mouth the patient cannot occlude comfortably in the former distal position, and the mandible is encouraged to adopt a protrusive bite with the inclined planes in occlusion. The unfavorable cuspal contacts of distal occlusion are replaced by favorable proprioceptive contacts of the inclined planes of the twin blocks, correcting the malocclusion and freeing the mandible from its locked distal functional position.

Twin blocks are designed for full-time wear to take advantage of all functional forces applied to the dentition, including the forces of mastication. The bite-blocks interlock at a 70-degree angle, usually covering the upper and lower teeth in the buccal segments. By causing a functional mandibular displacement, the interlocking occlusal bite-blocks alter the distribution of occlusal forces acting on the dentition to correct malocclusion during the development of the dentition.

Muscle behavior is immediately influenced through the placement of inclined planes between the teeth. The muscles of mastication must adapt to the altered balance of occlusal forces by guiding the mandible into protrusive function. This guidance results in rapid soft-tissue adaptation to achieve a new position of equilibrium in muscle behavior. Rapid improvement in facial appearance occurs during the first few weeks and months of treatment.

Animal experiments have confirmed that the muscles are primary factors in growth. The sensory receptors in the masticatory muscles, teeth, and surrounding tissues stimulate a functional response in the underlying bone to support the altered balance of functional forces acting to correct the maxillomandibular relationship. Bony changes are gradual and take several months to become established. Favorably directed occlusal forces transmitted through the dentition provide constant proprioceptive stimuli to influence the growth rate and architecture of the trabecular structure of the supporting bone.

The occlusal inclined plane has been used to demonstrate significant growth changes in animal experiments. Direct comparison with clinical results is now possible through the use of identical appliance mechanisms clinically and experimentally.

## BITE REGISTRATION

In Class II, division 1 malocclusion a protrusive bite is registered to reduce the overjet and distal occlusion by 5 to 10 mm on initial activation of twin blocks depending on the freedom of movement in protrusive function. This degree of activation allows an overjet as large as 10 mm to be corrected without further activation of the twin blocks.

In growing children with overjets as large as 10 mm, the bite may be activated edge to edge on the incisors with a 2-mm interincisal clearance if the patient can posture forward comfortably to maintain full occlusion on the appliances. In the vertical dimension, 2 mm of interincisal clearance is equal to approximately 5 or 6 mm of clearance in the first premolar region. This usually leaves 2 mm of clearance distally in the molar region and ensures that space is available for vertical development of posterior teeth to reduce the overbite.

This method of activation allows an overjet as large as 10 mm to be corrected on the first activation without further activation of the twin blocks. Larger overjets invariably require partial correction, followed by reactivation after initial correction.

The amount of initial activation for an individual patient is related to the ease with which the patient postures forward into a protrusive bite; in choosing the amount of activation, the clinician should consider the effect of forward posture on the profile. If the patient postures forward easily, an edge-to-edge occlusion is commonly activated. This occlusion is reproduced most easily by the patient and is equivalent to biting edge to edge on the incisors.

In considering guidelines for activation of functional appliances, Roccabado (personal communication, 1992) observes that the position of maximal protrusion is not a physiologic position. He concludes from examination of the function of the mandibular joint that the range of physiologic movement of the mandible is no more than 70% of the total

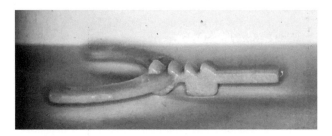

**Figure 13-3.** The Exactobite bite registration gauge.

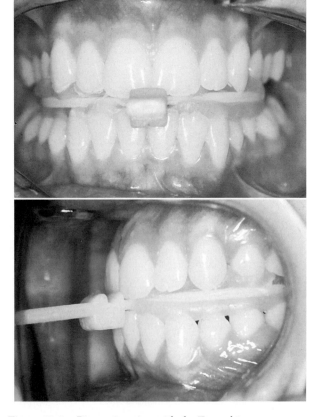

**Figure 13-4.** Bite registration with the Exactobite.

(From Clark WJ: *Twin block functional therapy: applications in dentofacial orthopedics,* London, 1995, Mosby-Wolfe.)

protrusive path. Thus the maximal activation of a functional appliance should not exceed 70% of the total protrusive path of the mandible.

Patients who may have difficulty in maintaining an edge-to-edge position in protrusion must be identified. Freedom of movement in forward posture is assessed by measuring the total protrusive path of the mandible. The overjet is measured in the fully retruded position and then in the position of maximal protrusion. The difference between these two measurements is the total protrusive path. Measuring the protrusive path helps identify patients who have a limited range of protrusive movement and would therefore be unable to maintain contact on the inclined planes if activation exceeds the physiologic range of movement. The George bite gauge is a convenient instrument to register a protrusive bite because it has a sliding jig attached to a millimeter scale; it is designed to measure the protrusive path of the mandible and can be subsequently adjusted to record a protrusive bite of no more than 70% of the total protrusive path.

Patients with horizontal growth patterns normally maintain an edge-to-edge incisor relationship more easily, provided the overjet is not excessive, whereas patients with vertical growth patterns may not tolerate the same degree of sagittal activation. A smaller initial activation is then necessary, and mandibular advancement must proceed more gradually by increments of activation.

Even in patients with horizontal growth patterns, a physiologic limit to the amount of protrusion that can be tolerated in initial mandibular advancement is evident. Overjets greater than 10 mm require stepwise reactivation by the addition of cold-cure acrylic to the anterior incline of the upper twin block during the course of treatment. However, even in treating patients with larger overjets, only one reactivation is normally required to correct most malocclusions.

The amount of vertical activation also is important and is determined by two factors. First, adequate vertical clearance must be available between the cusps of the upper and lower first premolars or deciduous molars to accommodate blocks of sufficient thickness to activate the appliance. The blocks are normally 5 to 6 mm thick between the first premolars. Second, the vertical activation must open the bite beyond the freeway space to ensure that the patient cannot drop the mandible into rest position and negate the proprioceptive functional response of the inclined planes. For the same reason, opening the bite beyond the freeway space may be an important factor in ensuring that the appliance is active when the patient is asleep.

## Bite Registration for Twin Blocks

The bite is registered for twin blocks in the same protrusive position used for other functional appliances. The Exactobite bite registration device is recommended for accurate control in registering a protrusive bite (Figure 13-3). This gauge allows the clinician to choose variable amounts of sagittal activation by selecting the appropriate groove to engage the upper incisors in registering the protrusive bite. The blue Exactobite gauge registers a 2-mm vertical clearance of the upper and lower incisors. Activation aims to achieve reduction of overjet, correction of distal occlusion, and midline correction (Figure 13-4).

When registering the bite, the clinician should give the patient a mirror. The patient should be shown the way to bite correctly into the Exactobite before the clinician applies wax to register the bite. The patient should be instructed to occlude with the midlines coincident, and the Exactobite should be positioned with the upper incisors occluding in the appropriate groove to reduce the overjet when the mandible closes into the incisal guidance groove. A relatively firm wax is used to register the occlusion. This wax is dimensionally stable and allows the occlusion to be correctly registered on models in the laboratory.

The activation of functional appliances normally exceeds the adaptive potential of periodontal and dentoalveolar tissues in altering the existing equilibrium of forces acting within the craniofacial structures and stimulating adaptive skeletal change in response to altered muscle activity. If the amount of activation significantly exceeds the mandibular growth potential, dentoalveolar compensation may occur to allow the stomatognathic system to adapt to a position of functional occlusal balance. Essentially, the rate of activation is related to the anticipated rate of sagittal growth. As with any functional appliance, care must be taken not to procline the lower incisors. Procumbent lower incisors in the initial malocclusion may militate against choice of a functional appliance or require a decision on possible extraction and combined fixed and removable appliance therapy.

## CONTROL OF THE VERTICAL DIMENSION

Occlusal bite-blocks provide an occlusal table that can be adjusted differentially to control the vertical dimension. Deep or reduced overbite is usually related to disproportion in upper and lower facial height. This diagnosis is determined by clinical examination of the patient in full-face and profile views to assess facial balance. The findings of clinical examination should be confirmed by cephalometric analysis. Cephalometric radiographs should be taken with the patient positioned in natural head posture.

Typically a patient with a brachyfacial growth pattern has a more horizontal growth pattern in the mandible, where deep overbite is associated with reduced lower facial height. A patient with a dolichofacial growth pattern on the other hand frequently has a reduced overbite related to a proportional increase in lower facial height. Management of overbite should take into account the facial proportions and improve facial balance by controlling the vertical dimension.

## VERTICAL ACTIVATION—TREATMENT OF DEEP OVERBITE

Vertical control in treatment of deep overbite associated with a brachyfacial growth pattern aims to increase lower facial height by correcting the incisors to an edge-to-edge relationship while adjusting the height of the upper bite-block in the molar region to encourage molar eruption. The goal is to

increase the vertical dimension and improve the profile by increasing lower facial height.

Deep overbite is reduced by overcorrecting to an edge-to-edge incisor relationship with an interincisal clearance of 2 mm in the protrusive bite. In recording the construction bite, the clinician normally leaves 5 mm of clearance in the first premolar region, which is equivalent to 2 mm of clearance distally in the molar region. Overbite reduction is achieved by trimming the occlusal cover on the upper twin block occlusodistally to encourage eruption of the lower molars. The inclined plane must remain intact, however, to maintain the activation to propel the mandible down and forward.

The occlusion is cleared over the lower molars by 1 to 2 mm only. This clearance is sufficient to allow eruption of lower molars but not large enough to allow the tongue to pass between the teeth, which would prevent eruption. In all functional techniques, vertical development in the buccal segments is commonly slower than sagittal correction. Vertical correction should therefore be made as early as possible in treatment to allow vertical development to proceed concurrently with sagittal correction.

The occlusal surface of the upper bite-block is progressively trimmed at each visit to maintain sufficient clearance over the lower molars to allow eruption. The clinician assesses clearance by passing an explorer between the teeth to ensure that the lower molars are not in contact with the upper block. Adequate interlocking wedges must be maintained to preserve the sagittal correction of arch relationships. The leading edge of the inclined plane of the upper bite-block is maintained intact throughout the twin block phase of treatment to preserve the active mechanism for functional correction (Figure 13-5).

At the end of the active phase the incisors and molars should be in correct occlusion. At this stage an open bite is still present in the premolar region because of the presence of the bite-blocks. The final adjustment is to trim the lower block slightly to reduce the open bite in the premolar region.

Eruption of lower molars occurs more quickly if separating elastics are placed in the interdental contacts with adjacent teeth at the start of treatment. Active eruption of lower molars may be encouraged by applying vertical elastics from the upper appliance to hooks on the lower molars. This is especially useful in older patients in whom eruption by natural forces tends to be slower.

## VERTICAL ACTIVATION—TREATMENT OF REDUCED OVERBITE

Patients with dolichofacial growth patterns have vertical growth patterns with increased lower facial height associated with reduced overbite and anterior open bite. This clinical situation requires careful management because the vertical growth pattern is often unfavorable for conventional functional correction.

All posterior teeth must be in occlusal contact with the opposing bite-blocks to prevent overeruption, which increases the anterior open bite and accentuates the vertical growth tendency. If second molars erupt distal to the appliance, eruption

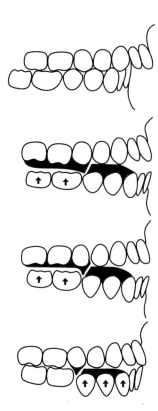

**Figure 13-5.** Sequence of trimming the blocks to reduce the overbite.

(Courtesy North Star Orthodontics, Park Rapids, Minnesota.)

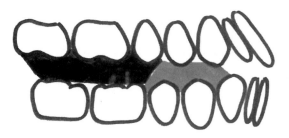

**Figure 13-6.** Occlusal cover is maintained over the posterior teeth to prevent eruption in treatment of anterior open bite.

should be controlled by placing occlusal rests or extending the upper twin block distally over the upper second molars to contact the lower second molars. Failure to observe this procedure complicates treatment considerably (Figure 13-6). Additional directional forces also may be used to help control vertical growth through the application of intrusive orthopedic forces to the upper posterior teeth.

## ORTHOPEDIC TRACTION

Where necessary, retractive and intrusive forces may be applied by the addition of headgear tubes to the upper first molars. These tubes apply retraction forces to the maxilla to reduce maxillary protrusion. This treatment can be combined with intermaxillary traction using a modified concorde face-

bow to advance the mandible by orthopedic traction in addition to functional correction by twin blocks.

## APPLIANCE DESIGN AND CONSTRUCTION

From the patient's perspective the two most important factors in appliance design are comfort and esthetics. The objective is to design appliances that are both comfortable and esthetic to improve patient compliance during treatment.

Twin blocks were originally conceived as simple removable appliances with interlocking occlusal bite-blocks designed to position the mandible forward to achieve functional correction of Class II, division 1 malocclusions. These basic principles still apply, but since the twin block technique was developed in 1977 many variations in appliance design have occurred; these variations have extended the scope of the technique to treat all classes of malocclusion. Appliance design has been improved and simplified to make twin blocks more acceptable to the patient without reducing efficiency (Figure 13-7).

Twin block appliances are tooth and tissue borne. To limit individual tooth movements, the appliances are designed to link the teeth as anchor units. In the lower arch, peripheral clasping and occlusal cover exert three-dimensional control on anchor teeth and limit tipping and displacement of individual teeth. In the lower arch, anchorage is increased by extending clasps around the labial and buccal segments. Where indicated, additional clasps may be placed on lower incisors; however, in practice, ball-ended clasps mesial to the lower canines have been found equally effective in controlling the lower labial segment.

### Evolution of Appliance Design

The earliest twin blocks were designed with the following basic components (Figure 13-8):

- Midline screws to expand the upper arch
- Occlusal bite-blocks
- Adams clasps on upper molars and premolars
- Adams clasps on lower premolars
- Interdental clasps on lower incisors
- Labial bows to retract the upper incisors
- Springs to move individual teeth and improve the arch form as required
- Provision for extraoral traction in treatment of maxillary protrusion

In essence, twin blocks attach a large handle to groups of teeth in both arches to minimize individual tooth movements and maximize the functional orthopedic response to treatment.

### Development of the Delta Clasp

If orthopedic forces are to be applied to removable appliances, the method of fixation is most important. The delta clasp was designed by Clark in 1985 to enhance the fixation of

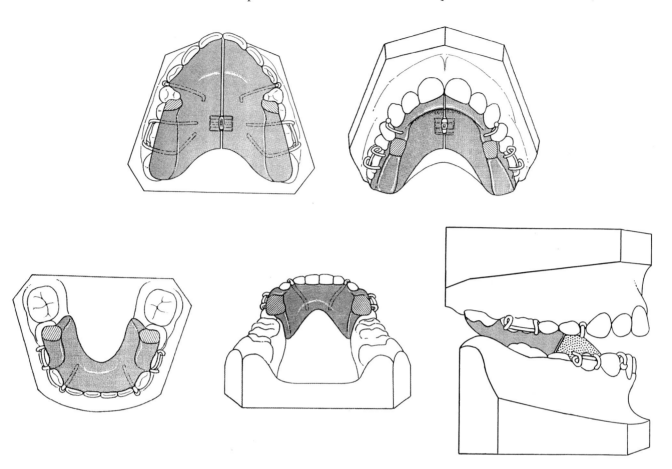

**Figure 13-7.**   Standard twin blocks.

(From Clark WJ: *Twin block functional therapy: applications in dentofacial orthopedics,* London, 1995, Mosby-Wolfe.)
(Courtesy W. Brudon and J.A. McNamara, Jr., University of Michigan.)

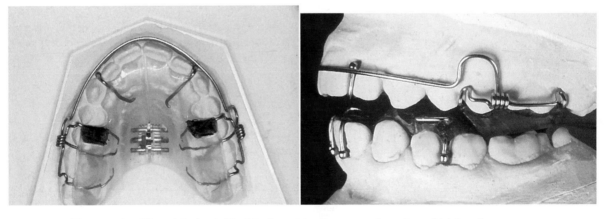

**Figure 13-8.**   The original twin block had provision for extraoral traction, which is no longer considered necessary.

twin blocks. It is similar in principle to the modified arrowhead clasp (Adams, 1949) but incorporates new features to improve retention, minimize adjustment, and reduce metal fatigue, thereby reducing breakage.

The Adams clasp is designed to fit individual teeth and incorporates interdental tags and mesial and distal retentive loops that are directed gingivally into undercuts and joined by a buccal bridge. The shape and position of the arrowheads allow the clasp to open slightly with repeated insertion and removal. The Adams clasp therefore requires routine adjustment at each visit to improve retention. Repeated adjustment increases the risk of metal fatigue.

The delta clasp retains the basic shape of the Adams clasp with its interdental tags, retentive loops, and buccal bridge. The essential difference is in the retentive loops, which are shaped in a closed triangle, unlike the open, V-shaped loop in the Adams clasp (Figure 13-9). Two methods of retention can be used with the delta clasp depending on the shape of the tooth. The apex of the triangle can be directed into the mesial or distal interdental area, or the base of the triangle can be adapted against the surface of the tooth to form a line contact.

The retentive loops were originally triangular (from which the name *delta clasp* is derived). Subsequent modification produced circular loops that are easier to construct; both types of loops have similar retentive properties. The circular loops may be adjusted to pass into the interdental space in cases in which the teeth are not favorably shaped at the mesiobuccal and distobuccal contours. Under these circumstances the best retention is obtained in the interdental areas between adjacent teeth.

The advantage of the triangular or circular loops is that the clasp does not open with repeated insertion and removal and therefore maintains better retention and requires less adjustment. The clasp gives excellent retention on lower premolars and can be used on most posterior teeth.

A comparison of the failure rate of both types of clasp has been performed by statistical analysis on two groups of 69 and 72 patients treated consecutively in Clark's practice between 1979 and 1993 (Clark, Stirrups, 1995). Results of this analysis indicated that the incidence of breakage of delta clasps was significantly reduced compared with that for appliances retained with the modified arrowhead clasp. The percentage of breakages was 10% for the modified arrowhead clasp (Adams clasp) and 1% for the delta clasp.

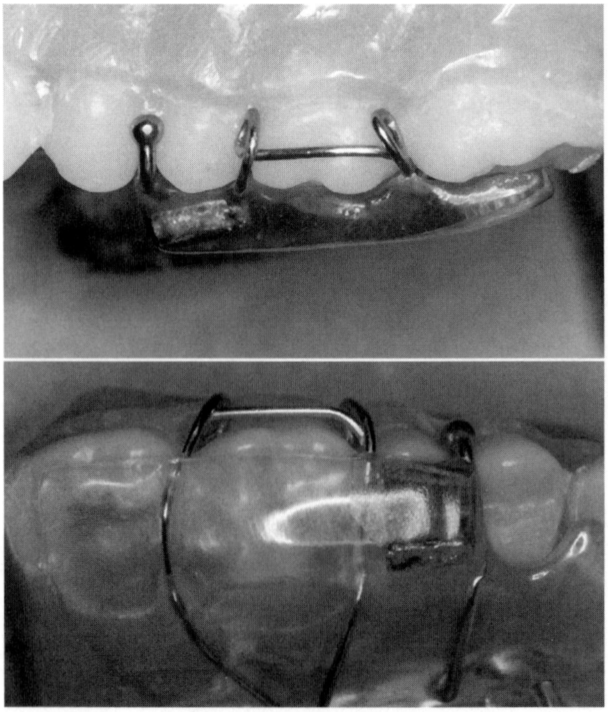

**Construction of the delta clasp.** The delta clasp is constructed from 0.70- or 0.75-mm stainless steel wire. Appropriate pliers to construct the delta clasp include the Adams universal pliers, which are snub nosed with square beaks, or "bird beak" pliers (RMO no. 139), which are snub nosed with one square and one round beak. The length of the beaks is an important feature of pliers for clasp construction; the distance between the tip and joint of the pliers must be short to achieve adequate strength and leverage to bend wire of sufficient diameter for clasp construction.

Two possible methods of construction may be used for the delta clasp according to the area of planned retention. The retentive loop may be angled to follow the curvature of the tooth into mesial and distal undercuts. This design is appropriate if the tooth is favorably shaped with good mesial and distal undercuts. However, if the individual teeth are not favorably shaped, the best undercuts lie interdentally below the contact points of adjoining teeth. The retentive loop of the clasp may then be directed interdentally; it is constructed at right angles to the bridge of the clasp and passes into the interdental undercut to gain retention from adjacent teeth. Before constructing the clasp, the clinician should examine the model to determine whether the tooth is only partially erupted. If sufficient supragingival undercut is not present, the gingival contour on the plaster model should be trimmed to expose the mesial and distal undercuts on the tooth, which are slightly subgingival. The method of preparation of the model is similar to the construction of the modified arrowhead clasp (Adams, 1970).*

## The Circular Arrowhead

The form of the clasp may be simplified by using circular arrowheads. These are bent using the round beak of the bird beak pliers (no. 139) (Figure 13-10). Circular arrowheads

---

*For detailed information on forming the delta clasp, see *Twin Block Functional Therapy* by William J. Clark, published by Mosby-Wolfe.

**Figure 13-9.** The delta clasp.

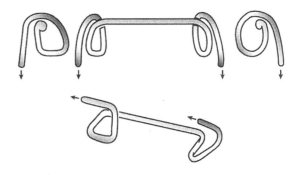

**Figure 13-10.** Delta clasp arrowheads.
(Courtesy J.A. McNamara, Jr., and W. Brudon, University of Michigan.)

need not be unduly small; they should be of sufficient size to engage the interdental or mesial and distal undercuts and still maintain at least 1 mm of clearance between the bridge of the clasp and the buccal surface of the tooth.

In the permanent dentition, delta clasps are routinely placed on upper first molars and lower first premolars. The shape of the clasp is modified on premolars to make the apex of the triangular arrowhead more acute to conform to the more slender shape of the tooth. The delta clasp also may be used on deciduous molars.

## Labial Bow

Removable appliances for the treatment of Class II, division 1 malocclusion have routinely incorporated labial bows, and in the early stages of development the upper twin block followed this pattern to improve appliance retention. If the labial bow engaged the upper incisors during functional correction, researchers observed that the overjet was reduced by retraction of the upper incisors, resulting in overcorrection of the incisor angulation. The labial bow therefore had to be adjusted at each office visit to prevent contact with the upper incisors.

If a labial bow is included in the appliance design and is activated prematurely to retract upper incisors, it acts as a barrier and limits functional correction by mandibular advancement. Retracting upper incisors prematurely reduces the scope for functional correction by mandibular advancement. A labial bow is therefore not required in most cases unless it is necessary to position severely proclined incisors upright. Even then, it must not be activated until the buccal segment relationship is fully corrected to a Class I relationship and functional correction is complete. In many cases the absence of a labial bow improves esthetics without reducing the effectiveness of the appliance.

A good lip seal often develops during twin block treatment without the necessity of any lip exercises. Improvement in lip posture and behavior can be attributed to functional adaptation to full-time appliance wear. The patient must form a good anterior seal when the appliance is worn during eating and drinking. The lips act in a similar manner to a labial bow, and lip pressure is effective in positioning upper incisors upright, thus making a labial bow redundant.

## Twin Block Construction

A good set of impressions and an accurate construction bite are necessary for accurate appliance construction. The appliance prescription should include detailed data required for the correction of the individual malocclusion rather than a vague and imprecise request for twin blocks. Variations in design should be specified. The construction bite registers the activation to be built into the appliance; it is recorded in a suitable modeling wax that retains its dimensional stability after it is removed from the mouth. Any excess wax extending over the buccal surfaces of the teeth should be removed to allow the models to seat correctly into the construction bite. In the laboratory the models are mounted on an articulator that registers the construction bite before the occlusal bite-blocks are constructed. A plasterless articulator may be used with adjustable screws to position the models in the correct relationship.

**The baseplate.** The baseplate and occlusal bite-blocks may be constructed from heat- or cold-cure acrylic. The main advantage of heat-cure acrylic is its additional strength, which is particularly important in later stages of treatment after the blocks have been trimmed to allow eruption in treatment of deep overbite cases. Fashioning the appliances in wax first allows the blocks to be formed with greater precision.

Cold-cure acrylic has the advantage of speed and convenience but sacrifices strength and accuracy. A top-quality cold-cure acrylic should be used to avoid problems with breakage, especially as the blocks are progressively trimmed during treatment. The inclined planes can lose their definition as a result of wear if soft acrylic is used.

The disadvantages of cold-cure acrylic can be overcome through the use of preformed blocks made from a good-quality heat-cured acrylic. These blocks are currently being manufactured in the correct size and shape for addition to cold-cure appliances. This addition makes constructing the occlusal bite-blocks easier and improves the accuracy of the inclined planes by providing a consistent angle for occlusion of the blocks (Figure 13-11).

**Occlusal inclined planes.** The position and angulation of the occlusal inclined planes are crucial to efficiency in correcting arch relationships. In most cases the inclined planes are angled at 70 degrees to the occlusal plane, and this angulation is usually effective in guiding the mandible into occlusion in a forward position. The position of the inclined plane is determined by the lower block and is important in the treatment of deep overbite. The inclined plane must be clear of mesial surface contact with the lower molar, which must be free to erupt unobstructed to reduce excessive overbite. The inclined plane on the lower bite-block is angled from the mesial surface of the second premolar or deciduous molar at 70 degrees to the occlusal plane. The lower block does not extend distally to the marginal ridge on the lower second premolar or deciduous molar to allow the leading edge of the inclined plane on the upper appliance to be positioned mesial to the lower first molar and thus not obstruct eruption. Buccolingually, the lower block covers the occlusal surfaces of the lower premolars or deciduous molars to occlude with the inclined plane on the upper twin block (see Figure 13-5).

The flat occlusal bite-block passes forward over the first premolar to become thinner buccolingually in the lower canine region. The full thickness of the blocks does not have to be maintained in the canine region. Reducing bulk in this area is important because speech is improved by allowing the tongue freedom of movement in the phonetic area. Because the canine region can be the most vulnerable part of the appliance, the lingual flange of the lower appliance in the midline should be sufficiently thick to provide adequate strength to avoid breakage.

The upper inclined plane is angled from the mesial surface

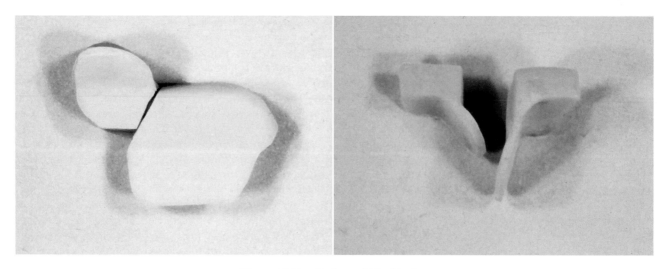

**Figure 13-11.**   Preformed bite-blocks.

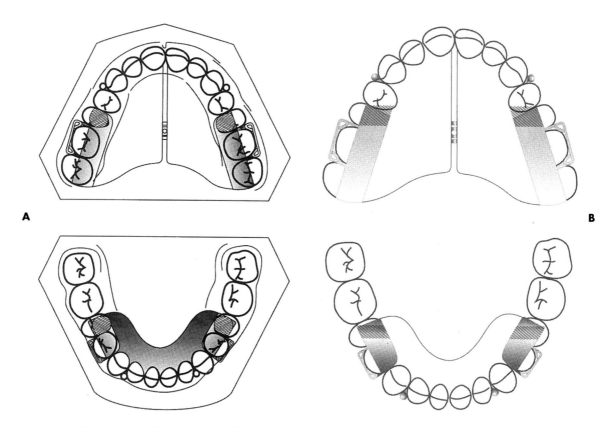

**Figure 13-12.**   The alignment of blocks relative to the line of the arch. **A,** Occlusal blocks aligned at right angles to the teeth in the buccal segments. **B,** Occlusal blocks aligned at right angles to the midline of the arch.

(Courtesy Johns Dental Laboratory, Terre Haute, Indiana.)

of the upper second premolar to the mesial surface of the upper first molar. The flat occlusal portion then passes distally over the remaining upper posterior teeth in a wedge shape, reducing in thickness as it extends distally.

Because the upper arch is wider than the lower, only the lingual cusps of the upper posterior teeth need to be covered rather than the full occlusal surface. This limited coverage makes the clasps more flexible and allows access to the interdental wires of the clasps for adjustment. In constructing the blocks, the clinician must make a decision concerning the alignment of the blocks in relation to the line of the arch. Two alternatives are effective in practice (Figure 13-12).

The blocks may be aligned in each quadrant at right angles to the line of the arch in the same pattern as the teeth are aligned. Alternatively, the lower blocks may be aligned at right angles to the midline, bisecting the arch. The upper blocks are constructed to match this angulation. In this second method the blocks maintain the same alignment relative to each other even if the midline screws are turned to widen the arch form (Figure 13-12, *B*).

*Angulation of the inclined planes.* The normal angulation of the inclined planes at 70 degrees to the occlusal plane has proved suitable in the majority of cases, although the angulation may be reduced to 45 degrees if the patient fails to posture forward consistently and thus occlude the blocks correctly. The angulation of 70 degrees was chosen after different angulations were tested for the inclined planes—from 90 to 45 degrees.

On the earliest twin block appliances the bite-blocks articulated at a 90-degree angle, forcing the patient to make a conscious effort to occlude in a forward position. Some patients could not consistently maintain a forward posture and tended to drop out of occlusion, which allowed the mandible to retrude to its original distal occlusion position. In the early stages of treatment, such patients were observed to be not posturing forward correctly, and as a result, posterior open bites developed as the bite-blocks occluded on their flat occlusal surfaces. In addition to developing posterior open bites, these patients did not make normal progress in sagittal correction. This complication arose in 30% of the earliest twin block cases. This problem was resolved by developing the occlusal inclined plane, based on the interdigitating cusps of the natural teeth and the functional mechanism of the natural dentition. The first modification set the angulation of the bite-blocks at 45 degrees to the occlusal plane to guide the mandible forward. This modification was immediately successful, and progress improved in patients who had previously been unable to maintain their forward mandibular postures (see Figure 13-1).

An equal down and forward force component is applied to the lower dentition by inclined planes angled at 45 degrees to the occlusal plane. The resulting occlusal force on the inclined planes applies an equal down and forward stimulus to growth. Taking this into account, clinicians chose the steeper angle of 70 degrees to the occlusal plane to apply a more horizontal component of force, reasoning that such force may encourage more horizontal mandibular growth. If the patient has difficulty in posturing forward, the activation may be reduced by trimming the inclined planes to reduce the amount of mandibular protrusion, thus enabling the patient to maintain a forward posture.

## APPLIANCE DESIGN

### Standard Twin Blocks

Standard twin blocks are suitable for treatment of uncrowded Class II, division 1 malocclusions with good arch

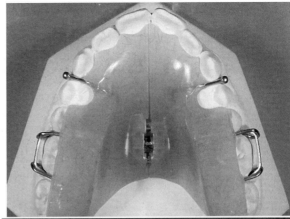
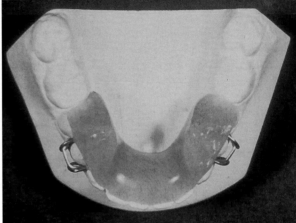

**Figure 13-13.** Standard twin blocks.

forms and overjets large enough to allow unrestricted forward translation of the mandible for full correction of distal occlusion (see Figure 13-12, *A*). Patients with Class II, division 1 malocclusions typically have narrow upper arches, with the lower arches in distal occlusion. During treatment a midline screw is routinely included in the upper appliance for compensatory expansion in the upper arch to accommodate the lower arch as the mandible translates forward. The standard design of twin blocks therefore has provision for midline expansion. The inclined planes are positioned mesial to the upper and lower first molars, with the upper block covering the upper molars and second premolars or deciduous molars. The lower blocks should not extend fully to the distal of the second premolar or deciduous molar. Therefore the inclined plane is positioned slightly forward of the lower first molar. Clearance is necessary to allow the lower molar to erupt to increase the vertical dimension in the treatment of excessive overbite.

The upper appliance has delta clasps on the upper first molars; additional ball clasps may be placed interdentally, distal to the canines, or between the premolars or deciduous molars. The lower appliance is a simple bite-block with delta clasps on the first premolars and ball clasps mesial to the canines (Figure 13-13).

## Variations in Appliance Design

**Arch development.** Twin blocks have the advantage of versatility of design in comparison with conventional one-piece functional appliances that apply an equal amount of expansion to both dental arches. Separate upper and lower twin block appliances allow independent control of arch development. Upper and lower midline screws may be used for unequal expansion in both arches. If the lower arch is expanded transversely, additional expansion is often required in the upper arch to compensate. The arches may be expanded at differential rates over time to achieve unequal expansion (Figure 13-14).

Appliance design may be modified by the addition of screws, springs, and bows to move individual teeth. Arch development can proceed in both arches by a combination of transverse and sagittal components to meet the requirements of the individual patient. Provision for combined transverse and sagittal expansion may be made by adding a three-way screw or using a three-screw sagittal design with a midline screw in addition to the two sagittal screws in the palatal acrylic.

## INTERCEPTIVE TREATMENT

### Twin Blocks in Mixed Dentition

The primary indication for twin blocks in early mixed dentition is in Class II, division 1 malocclusion in which prominent upper incisors rest outside the lower lip and are vulnerable to fracture because they are not protected by the lips. Twin blocks can fulfill three objectives at this stage of development:

1. They can reduce overjet and correct distal occlusion.
2. They can control overbite if the overbite is deep or anterior open bite is present.
3. They can improve arch form by transverse or sagittal development.

These objectives are achieved using a similar approach to treatment as is used in the permanent dentition, with modifications in appliance design to meet the requirements of the mixed-dentition stage of development.

The deciduous molars and canines may not provide adequate undercuts for fixation, but this problem is easily overcome. In mixed dentition the appliance design is modified by using **C**-shaped clasps that may be directly bonded to deciduous teeth with composite to temporarily fix the appliances in the mouth for 10 days to initiate full-time appliance wear. After a few days the clasps can be freed and the composite left in place to improve undercuts for fixation. In the initial stage the twin blocks may even be cemented or bonded directly to the teeth in addition to the application of composite to secure the clasps. This fixation enables the patient to adjust to wearing the appliance full time during the critical first few days. At this stage of development the procedure of temporary fixation of twin blocks to the teeth carries minimal risk, especially if first permanent molars are fissure sealed (Figure 13-15).

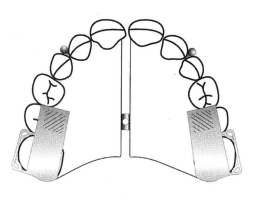

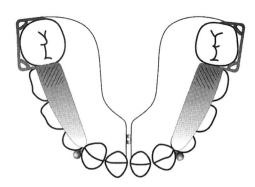

**Figure 13-14.** Twin block Schwarz appliances for independent expansion in both arches and correction of arch relationships in mixed dentition.

(From Clark WJ: *Twin block functional therapy: application in dentofacial orthopedics,* London, 1995, Mosby-Wolfe.)

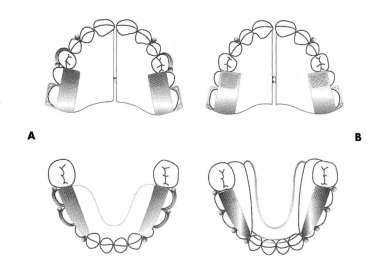

A                                                                     B

**Figure 13-15.** Variations in design for mixed dentition. **A,** **C**-shaped clasps can be bonded to deciduous teeth for temporary fixation. **B,** Upper Schwarz and lower Jackson twin blocks.

(From Clark WJ: *Twin block functional therapy: applications in dentofacial orthopedics,* London, 1995, Mosby-Wolfe.)

## Stages of Treatment

**Stage 1: active phase—twin blocks.** During the active phase of treatment, twin blocks are worn full time. The objective is to correct arch relationships in the anteroposteror, vertical, and transverse dimensions. Normally, overjet and overbite are corrected within 6 months, and the lower molars have erupted into occlusion within 9 months. The average wear time for twin blocks is 6 to 9 months.

**Stage 2: support phase—anterior inclined plane.** The objective of the second stage of treatment is to retain the corrected incisor relationship until buccal segment occlusion is fully established. To achieve this objective, an upper removable appliance is fitted with an anterior inclined plane to engage the lower incisors and canines (Figure 13-16). This appliance is worn full time initially to allow the buccal segment occlusion to settle; it is then used as a retainer.

The lower twin block appliance is left out at this stage, and the removal of posterior bite-blocks allows the posterior teeth to erupt. Full-time appliance wear is necessary to allow time for internal bony remodeling to support the corrected occlusion as the buccal segments settle fully into optimal interdigitation.

The upper and lower buccal teeth are usually in occlusion within 4 to 6 months. Full-time appliance wear is continued during the support phase for another 3 to 6 months to allow functional reorientation of the trabecular system before any reduction of appliance wear occurs during the retention period (Harvold, 1973) (Figure 13-17).

The support phase may be considered as important as the active phase. Stability is excellent after twin block treatment; this can be attributed partly to the support phase, during which a functional retainer is used to stabilize the corrected incisor relationship while the buccal teeth settle fully into occlusion.

## FITTING TWIN BLOCKS

### Instructions to the Patient

Patient motivation is an important factor in removable appliance therapy, and a protocol should be established for patient instruction when appliances are fitted. An ideal way to introduce a patient to twin blocks is to demonstrate appliances on models to explain the action of the inclined planes in correcting the bite. Simply by biting the blocks together cor-

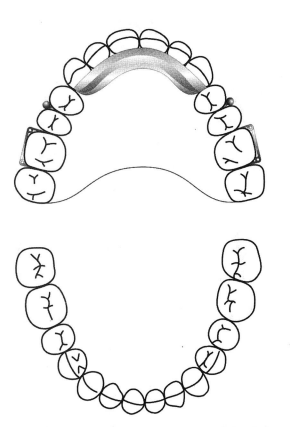

**Figure 13-16.** Support appliance with anterior inclined plane to engage lingual to lower incisors and canines.

(From Clark WJ: *Twin block functional therapy: applications in dentofacial orthopedics,* London, 1995, Mosby-Wolfe.)

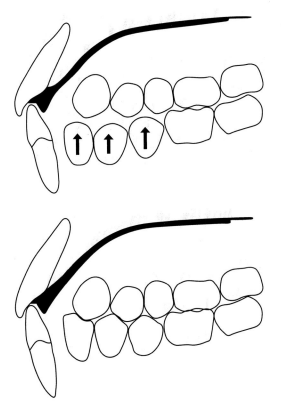

**Figure 13-17.** Anterior inclined plane supports corrected occlusion; lower premolars are free to erupt.

(From Clark WJ: *Twin block functional therapy: applications in dentofacial orthopedics,* London, 1995, Mosby-Wolfe.)

rectly, the patient encourages the lower jaw to adapt and grow to correct the malocclusion. The appliance system is simple and easily understood, even by young patients.

When the appliances are placed in the mouth, a noticeable improvement in facial appearance occurs immediately. This is an excellent motivating factor to encourage the patient to wear the appliance, especially if the clinician explains that this change will be permanent within a few months if the twin blocks are worn full time. The patient is instructed on the ways to insert and remove the appliances and operate the screw. The screw is turned for the first time after the appliance has been worn for 1 week.

Twin blocks achieve correction by the forces of occlusion, and therefore the patient must learn to eat with the appliances in place, removing them only for cleaning after every meal to avoid food stagnation under the appliances. Depending on the patient and the expected response, the appliances may be removed for eating for the first few days until they have settled in comfortably, but they must then be worn during meals because the forces of occlusion are used to correct the malocclusion, and these forces are most active when the patient is eating.

## CLINICAL MANAGEMENT

### Stage 1: Active Phase

**First visit—on fitting twin block appliances.** The overjet is measured before treatment with the teeth in occlusion and the mandible fully retruded; this measurement is recorded for future reference. The lingual flange of the appliance must be relieved slightly lingual to the lower incisors to avoid gingival irritation as the appliance is driven in by the occlusion during the first few days. The clasps are adjusted to hold the appliances securely in position without impinging on the gingival margin. If a labial bow is present, it should be out of contact with the upper incisors. The clinician should check that the patient bites comfortably in a protrusive bite. Selected cases benefit by bonding appliances for the first 10 to 14 days.

**Second visit—after 10 days.** The patient should be wearing the appliances comfortably and eating with them in position after 10 days. The initial discomfort of a new appliance should have resolved, and the patient should be biting comfortably in the protrusive bite. If the patient is failing to posture forward consistently, the clinician should consider reducing activation by trimming the inclined planes slightly.

Patient compliance is important in removable appliance therapy, and encouragement should be offered for success in becoming accustomed to the appliance quickly; reassurance should be provided on any difficulties. The patient should turn the screw under supervision, and at this stage, only minimal adjustment is made to the appliance if necessary. Improved muscle balance becomes evident quickly in the face because the appliance is worn full time. This improvement should be noted for the patient and parents as an encouraging sign of early progress.

**Overbite correction.** In cases of deep overbite the upper block should be slightly trimmed occlusodistally to leave the lower molars 1 mm clear of the occlusion to allow eruption and reduce the overbite by increasing lower facial height. In cases of reduced overbite, no trimming should be done on the blocks. All posterior teeth must remain in contact with the blocks to prevent eruption of posterior teeth.

**Third visit—after 4 weeks.** At each visit, progress is reviewed by measuring the overjet. At the same time the occlusion is checked for correction of the buccal segment relationships. Positive progress should now be noted in facial muscle balance; this should be confirmed by a reduction in overjet measured intraorally with the mandible fully retracted. Minor adjustment is necessary only to keep the labial bow out of contact with the upper incisors and ensure that the lower molars are not in contact with the upper block in cases of deep overbite. The clinician should check that the screw is operating correctly and adjust the clasps if necessary.

**Fourth visit—after 6 weeks.** A similar pattern of adjustment and checking of occlusion and overjet should occur after 6 weeks. The clinician should trim the blocks in the recommended sequence to reduce deep overbite.

Subsequent adjustment visits normally occur at 6-week intervals, and a steady correction of distal occlusion and reduction of overjet should occur, with concurrent eruption of lower molars to reduce the overbite.

**Progress in treatment.** Twin block appliances are simple, and treatment is normally uncomplicated. The upper arch must not be overexpanded into crossbite; it should be checked at each visit, and the clinician should stop the operation of the screw if necessary. An overjet as large as 10 mm can be corrected without reactivating the bite blocks if the rate and direction of mandibular growth are favorable.

Full correction of sagittal arch relationships can be achieved in as little as 2 to 6 months, thus producing a normal incisor relationship. At this stage the overjet is fully corrected, and the buccal segments are still out of occlusion because of the presence of the bite-blocks. In treatment of deep overbite, functional techniques consistently achieve sagittal correction of arch relationships before compensatory vertical development in the buccal segments is complete.

Clark holds that clinical management is simplified by introducing a single large activation when the appliances are fitted, provided the growth pattern is favorable for functional correction. On statistical analysis of the results of 76 consecutively treated patients, Clark (1994) found this regimen results in significant growth modification in comparison with untreated controls. Progressive mandibular advancement may be beneficial, however, in cases in which the growth pattern is less favorable.

If the patient's growth rate is slow or the growth direction is vertical rather than horizontal, the mandible should be advanced gradually over a longer period to allow compensatory mandibular growth to occur. Activation to increase mandibular protrusion can be provided by the addition of cold-cure acrylic to the inclined plane of the upper bite-blocks. In treatment of vertical growth, contact of the bite-blocks must be maintained on all posterior teeth to guard against eruption of posterior teeth, with resultant increases in anterior face height.

**Management of overbite.** As indicated previously, deep overbite is reduced by overcorrecting the incisors to an edge-to-edge relationship before reducing the height of the bite-blocks. Vertical development of the lower molars is encouraged from the beginning of the active phase of treatment by progressive trimming of the upper bite-block occlusodistally to allow the lower molars to erupt. At the end of the active phase the incisors and molars should be in correct occlusion.

At this stage an open bite is still present in the premolar region because of the presence of the bite-blocks. As a final adjustment at the end of the twin block stage the upper surface of the lower block is trimmed to allow the open bite in the premolar region to reduce before progressing to the support phase. Adequate interlocking wedges must be preserved to maintain anteroposterior correction of arch relationships. This method of reducing overbite through controlled eruption of posterior teeth supported by occlusal bite-blocks results in favorable changes in facial balance by increasing lower facial height.

If the overbite is reduced before treatment, overeruption of posterior teeth, which further reduces the overbite, should be prevented. All erupted teeth must then be in occlusal contact with the bite-blocks. If second molars erupt during the active phase, occlusal cover or occlusal rests must be extended to prevent overeruption of these teeth.

In treatment of cases of reduced overbite or open bite, clasps are placed on the posterior teeth and the appliances are left clear of the anterior teeth to encourage eruption of the incisors. In addition, a vertical-pull headgear may be used to apply intrusive force to the upper molars to reduce the vertical component of growth. Repelling magnets may be incorporated in the posterior bite-blocks to enhance depression of these teeth.

## Stage 2: Support Phase

The aim of the second stage of treatment is to retain the corrected incisor relationship until buccal segment occlusion is fully established by using an upper removable appliance with a steep anterior inclined guide plane. The lower appliance is left out at this stage, and the posterior bite-blocks are removed to allow the posterior teeth to erupt into occlusion. The anterior inclined plane extends distally to engage the lower canines. The lower incisors and canines should occlude on the base point of the upper incisors and canines, and the inclined plane should be positioned to fit directly lingual to the lower anterior teeth without interfering with occlusion.

The anterior inclined plane must be designed carefully to be unobtrusive but still retain the incisor relationship effectively. It should not interfere with speech, which might encourage the patient to remove the appliance. The patient should understand the importance of wearing this appliance full time to avoid the possibility of relapse at this critical stage of treatment. The upper and lower buccal teeth are usually in occlusion within 4 to 6 months, and the support phase is continued for a further 3 to 6 months to allow functional reorientation of the trabecular system before the position is retained.

## RETENTION

A normal period of retention follows treatment after occlusion is fully established. During the retention period, appliance wear can be gradually reduced to nighttime wear.

## CLINICAL RESPONSE TO TREATMENT

The clinical response observed after fitting twin blocks is analogous to changes observed and reported in animal experiments using fixed inclined planes. The rapid clinical response is similar to adaptive responses described by McNamara (1980) in animal experiments that studied functional protrusion with fixed inclined planes. (See Chapter 2 for Petrovic's studies concerning clinical response to treatment.)

McNamara's findings (1980) may be summarized as follows:

The placement of appliances results in an immediate change in the neuromuscular proprioceptive response. Provided all phasic and tonic muscle activity is affected, the resulting muscular changes are very rapid, and can be measured in terms of minutes, hours and days. Structural alterations are more gradual and are measured in months, whereby the dento-skeletal structures adapt to restore a functional equilibrium to support the altered position of muscle balance.

In comparison, within a few days of the fitting of twin block appliances, the position of muscle balance is altered so greatly that the patient experiences pain when retracting the mandible. This has been described as the *pterygoid response* (McNamara, 1980; Petrovic,), or the formation of a "tension zone" distal to the condyle (Harvold and Woodside). Such a response is rarely observed with functional appliances that are not worn full time.

Harvold (1973) and Petrovic et al described the histologic changes that occur after the fitting of fixed inclined planes during animal experiments. As noted, the area distal to the condyle is described as a tension zone. No vaccuum is created behind the condyle. Rather the response is one of tissue proliferation to fill in the area behind the condyle. Connective tissue and blood vessels apparently proliferate in the retrodiscal attachment within minutes or hours of fitting a full-time functional mechanism activated to advance the mandible. Johnston (1976) attributes this reaction to unloading the condyle (see Chapter 2).

The clinical signs in twin block treatment are consistent with previously discussed research findings and are evident after the first few days of treatment. The patient experiences discomfort in the condylar region when the appliance is removed (e.g., when brushing the teeth). On removal of the appliance the mandible is retracted and the condyle compresses

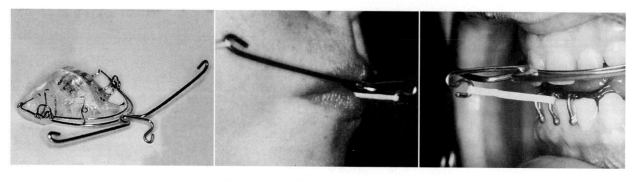

**Figure 13-18.**  The concorde face-bow.

connective tissue and blood vessels that have proliferated in the tension zone behind the condyle.

## Correction of Anterior Open Bite

In treating patients with vertical growth patterns in which anterior open bite is associated with increased lower facial height, the clinician must maintain contact of the posterior teeth on the occlusal bite-blocks to prevent eruption of lower molars. The blocks are not trimmed in the treatment of anterior open bite, and occlusal contact is effective in limiting molar eruption.

## Orthopedic Traction

If necessary, retractive and intrusive forces may be applied by the addition of headgear tubes to the upper first molars. In the original description of the twin block traction technique, high-pull extraoral traction force was applied to a modified face-bow worn at night to intrude the upper molars; this technique was effective in closing the anterior open bite. A distal component of force may be used to apply a retraction force to the maxilla to reduce maxillary protrusion. This force can be combined with intermaxillary traction to a modified concorde face-bow to advance the mandible by orthopedic traction along with functional correction by twin blocks.

## The Concorde Face-Bow

A conventional face-bow can be adapted by soldering a labial hook to provide for combined extraoral and intermaxillary traction (Figure 13-18). If traction is to be applied to a removable appliance, the outer bow of the face-bow should be adjusted to lie slightly above the inner bow. This position applies a slight upward component of force that helps retain the upper appliance. With the concorde face-bow the upward component of force is balanced by a horizontal elastic attached to the recurved labial hook. Traction is applied either as a straight pull to a cervical headcap or headgear, with provision for variable directional control.

The direction of extraoral force is especially important in treatment of patients with vertical growth patterns. A vertical component of orthopedic force is applied to the upper poste-

rior teeth to limit vertical development of the upper teeth and palate. The concorde face-bow is a unique method of delivering intrusive force to upper molars and protrusive force to the mandible and lower dentition. In treatment of reduced overbite the use of extraoral traction has been superceded in most cases by a simpler method using vertical intraoral elastics to achieve molar intrusion.

## Vertical Intraoral Elastics

One of the most interesting modifications of twin block treatment in recent years is the use of vertical elastics to reduce anterior open bite. The elastics are applied bilaterally and pass from the upper to the lower arch in the premolar region. They may be attached to either the twin block appliances or brackets on opposing teeth. They intrude the posterior teeth, especially the upper molars, by encouraging the patient to bite into the appliances consistently and therefore apply intrusive forces to the opposing molars. This effect is useful in the treatment of patients with vertical growth patterns who have weak musculature and do not close consistently on the appliance. This therapeutic approach was developed in the practice of Mills in Vancouver; she also is carrying out a study on the treatment of consecutive twin block patients. The addition of repelling rare earth magnets may assist in the endeavor to reduce anterior open bite.

## Temporary Fixation of Twin Blocks

Patient compliance is crucial in functional therapy, and any means of improving patient compliance contributes to the success of treatment. The clinician must do everything possible to be sure that the patient wears the appliance 24 hours a day, even if the appliance is removable. The two-piece design enables twin blocks to be fixed in the mouth temporarily for as long as 10 days to ensure that the patient wears the appliance 24 hours a day. This temporary bonding allows the orthodontist the same degree of control experienced with fixed appliances during the period when the patient is adapting to the new appliance. After 10 days of full-time wear the patient is more comfortable with the appliance in the mouth than without it. This technique is being used widely today with success.

## Reactivation of Twin Blocks

Response to treatment is related to the rate and direction of mandibular growth during treatment. The initial activation of the appliance should take into account the patient's growth pattern. An overjet of as much as 10 mm can be corrected without reactivating the bite-blocks for a brachyfacial patient with a horizontal growth pattern and favorable mandibular growth.

The initial activation should be reduced if the growth pattern is less favorable: for example, in treatment of patients with vertical growth patterns. Also, in treatment of larger overjets or in situations in which the protrusive path of the mandible is restricted, the inclined planes should be reactivated gradually in progressive increments during treatment.

Larger overjets of more than 10 mm cannot be corrected by a single activation of the inclined planes because the amount of activation required is beyond the normal physiologic range of movement of the mandible. The initial construction bite is taken to achieve a partial correction of the overjet, and the appliance is reactivated during the course of treatment.

Reactivation to increase the forward posture is achieved by the addition of cold-cure acrylic to extend the anterior incline of the upper twin block mesially. Cold-cure acrylic may be added at the chairside as the clinician inserts the appliance to record a new protrusive bite before the acrylic is fully set. Even in cases of excessive overjet a single reactivation of the twin blocks is normally sufficient to correct most malocclusions.

Especially in the treatment of deep overbite, no acrylic should be added to the distal incline of the lower twin block. Extending the occlusal acrylic of the lower block distally prevents eruption of the lower first molar. The lower first molars must be free to erupt to allow the overbite to be reduced through increases in the vertical dimension.

As already stated, the patient's growth rate should be taken into account in determining the amount of activation and timing the reactivation of the bite-blocks. If the growth rate is slow or the growth direction is vertical rather than horizontal, the mandible should probably be advanced gradually over a longer period to allow compensatory mandibular growth.

## Progressive Activation of Twin Blocks

Progressive activation of the inclined planes should be performed as follows:

- If the overjet is greater than 10 mm, the mandible should usually be stepped forward in two stages. The first activation is in the range of 7 to 10 mm. The second activation brings the incisors to an edge-to-edge occlusion.
- If full correction of arch relationships is not achieved after the initial activation, an additional activation is necessary.
- If the direction of growth is vertical rather than horizontal, the mandible may be advanced gradually to allow adequate time for compensatory mandibular growth.

- Phased activation is recommended in adult treatment, when the muscles and ligaments are less responsive to a sudden, large displacement of the mandible. Obviously dental compensation is a factor here.
- In the treatment of TMJ dysfunction the clinician must be careful not to introduce activation beyond the level of tolerance of injured tissue. The clinician should be conservative and advance the mandible slowly to a comfortable position that allows the patient to rest and function without discomfort.

## Integration of Twin Blocks with Fixed Appliances

Several indications exist for the integration of twin blocks with fixed appliances. A combined fixed and functional approach is necessary for correction of more complex malocclusions in which skeletal and dental factors require a combination of orthopedic and orthodontic techniques. Depending on the timing of treatment and the features of the individual case, alternative approaches may be considered to resolve multifactorial problems.

First, a preliminary stage of treatment with fixed appliances may be indicated before the fitting of twin blocks if upper and lower arch form does not match and the arches need to be leveled or aligned before functional correction. This technique may be useful if crowding is moderate or severe and cannot be resolved by twin blocks alone. Depending on the severity of the problem, lingual appliances may be fitted for interceptive treatment and arch development or full, bonded, fixed appliances may be used if required.

Second, because no anterior wires are used in twin blocks, brackets may be fitted in the labial segments during twin block treatment, and a segmented arch may be included. This allows the clinician to correct alignment while reducing overjet, correcting distal occlusion, reducing overbite, and correcting the transverse dimension. All these objectives can be achieved simultaneously during the twin block phase of treatment.

A third possibility is that a full lower fixed appliance may be fitted during the support phase. Alternatively, a lower lingual appliance may be fitted at this stage to allow the premolars to erupt while retaining the correct arch form.

Finally, twin blocks may be combined with bonded fixed appliances by two different approaches. Simple, removable twin blocks may be constructed to fit over a fixed appliance, and ball clasps may be used for retention. Another option is to construct fixed twin blocks designed for full-time wear and integration with fixed appliances. Clark has recently designed suitable components to achieve this objective. Prototype appliances are currently being used in clinical tests. This new approach to construction may extend the integration of twin blocks with fixed appliances.

### CASE STUDY

An 8-year-old boy began treatment in mixed dentition with a severe Class II, division 1 malocclusion and an overjet of

15 mm. The buccal segment relationship was a full-unit distal occlusion, and the overbite was excessive, with the lower incisors occluding in the soft tissue of the palate 5 mm lingual to the upper incisors (Figure 13-19). The lips were incompetent at rest, with a short upper lip. The lower lip was trapped lingual to the upper incisors. In profile the maxilla appeared well related to the cranial base and the mandible was retrusive.

Functional orthopedic correction was achieved with twin blocks after 14 months of treatment. At this stage the twin blocks were discontinued and replaced with an anterior inclined plane to support the corrected occlusion (Figure 13-20). The anterior inclined plane was worn full time for

6 months, after which it was worn at night as a retainer during the transition to permanent dentition (Figure 13-21). At this stage, slight spacing was present distal to the upper canines, and the overbite was slightly increased to 4 mm. The buccal segments were in Class I relationship, and the overjet was stable at 3.5 mm. Facial changes were rapid in the early stages of treatment and were sustained after treatment. A short period of treatment with fixed appliances was required to detail the occlusion (Figure 13-22).

Active treatment followed by retention and observation lasted for 3 years and 2 months before fixed appliances were fitted. During this time, mandibular length increased by 18 mm from hinge axis to gnathion. Mandibular corpus

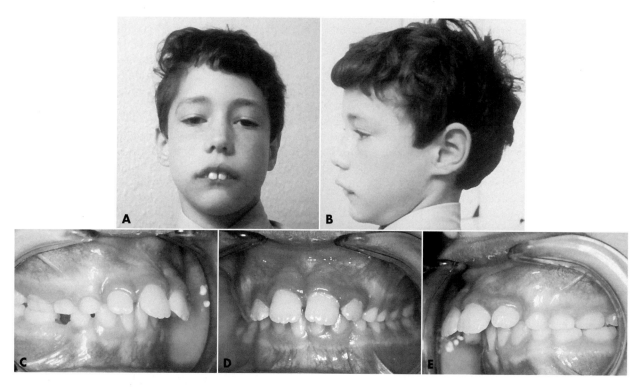

**Figure 13-19.** An 8-year-old boy before functional treatment. **A** and **B,** Extraoral views. **C** through **E,** Intraoral views.

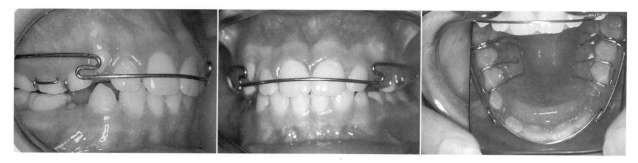

**Figure 13-20.** Same patient as in Figure 13-19 after 14 months of treatment. Support phase using palatal anterior guide plane.

length increased by 12.4 mm from 68.0 to 80.4 mm, and ramus height increased by 8.6 mm from 36.8 to 45.4 mm. Measurement along the facial axis using nasion-basion as the registration plane recorded 22 mm of growth during this period (equivalent to 8 mm per year). This compares with an average normal growth increment along the facial axis of 3 mm per year. Facial changes are dramatic.

Angular changes in this case study were not significant, underlining the fallacy of evaluating the response to functional therapy by angular cephalometric criteria alone. Linear analysis is more revealing and gives a clearer indication of the growth increments that occur relative to the norm, thus providing a more useful benchmark for comparing the orthodontic and orthopedic response in treatment.

Examination of growth increments in individual and consecutively treated cases treated with the twin block technique supports the view that functional orthopedic therapy can influence mandibular growth and produce highly significant growth change in treatment (Clark, 1995b). Figures 13-23 and 13-24 illustrate the changes in appearance possible with functional treatment.

Before planning surgical correction of facial imbalance caused by skeletal factors, the clinician should consider the alternative of functional orthopedics. If the problem is within treatable limits, twin blocks can achieve nonsurgical orthopedic correction, a treatment that is much more acceptable to the patient than the combined surgical and orthodontic approach used by some practitioners.

## TREATMENT OF CLASS II, DIVISION 2 MALOCCLUSION

Patients with Class II, division 2 malocclusions usually have mild Class II skeletal relationships with horizontal growth patterns and well-formed chins. In this type of malocclusion, minimal mandibular advancement is required to correct the anteroposterior relationship. Harvold and Woodside have shown that correction of a Class II molar relationship is possible through the placement of an occlusal table between the teeth and the selective trimming of acrylic to encourage eruption of lower molars. The lower molars can erupt along a mesial eruptive path to correct the molar relationship.

The original twin block appliances were modified from the standard design by the addition of springs lingual to the upper incisors to advance retroclined upper incisors. This addition allowed the mandible to be translated down and forward to correct the distal occlusion. At the same time the occlusal bite-blocks were trimmed to encourage eruption of the posterior teeth to reduce the overbite (Figure 13-25).

An edge-to-edge construction bite is registered to correct the distal occlusion in Class II, division 2 malocclusion. Control of the vertical dimension is achieved by adjusting the thickness of the posterior occlusal inclined planes.

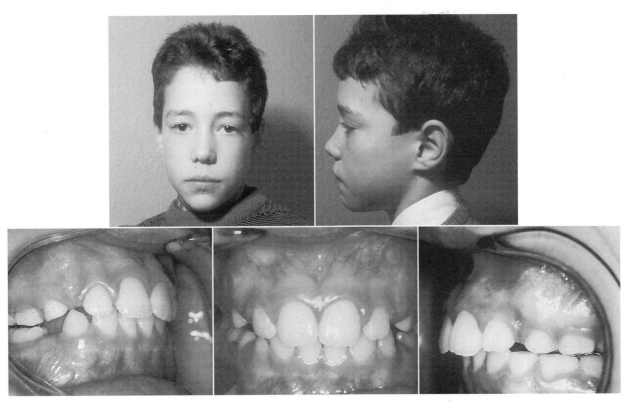

**Figure 13-21.** Same patient as in Figure 13-19 after 14 months of treatment. Facial and intraoral change after treatment.

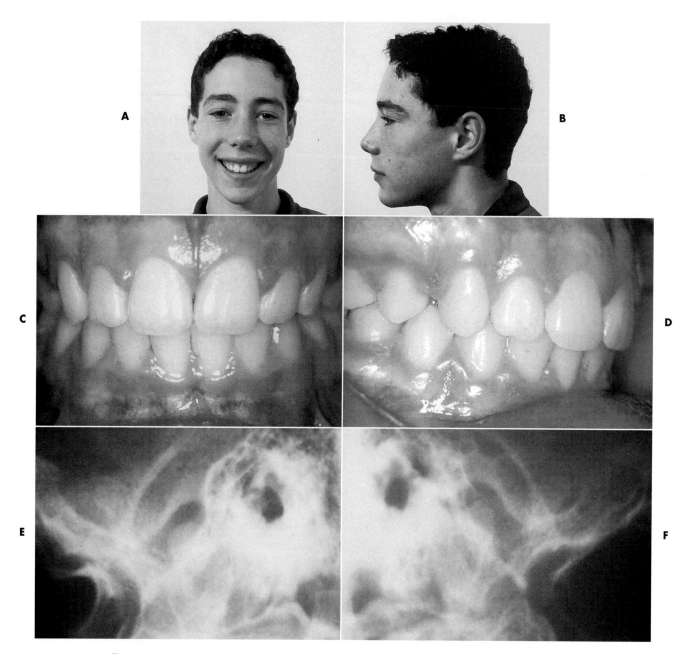

**Figure 13-22.** Same patient as in Figure 13-19. **A** through **D,** Final views after a short period of multiattachment fixed appliances. **E** through **F,** Tomograms show that condyles are properly seated.

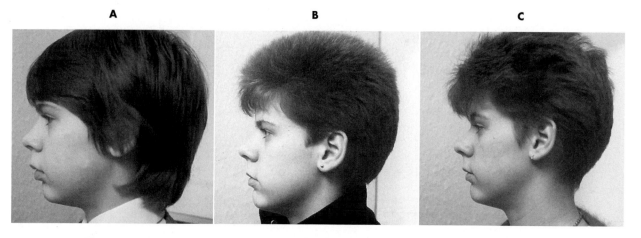

**Figure 13-23.** A 12-year-old patient. **A,** Beginning treatment. **B,** After treatment. **C,** After retention.

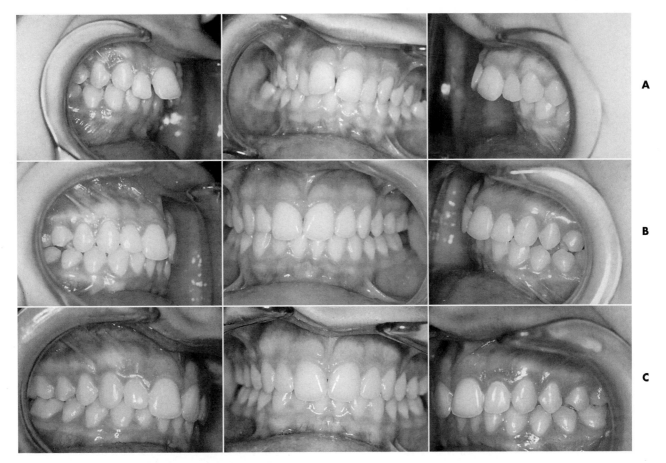

**Figure 13-24.** Some patients as in Figure 13-23. Changes in appearance with functional therapy. **A,** Before treatment. **B,** After 21 months of treatment. **C,** After retention at 15 years of age.

The leading edge of the inclined plane must be maintained intact because this is the functional mechanism instrumental in correcting the malocclusion. At the same time the incisor relationship is corrected by the labial tipping of the upper incisor crowns, which frees the mandible from any possible distally locked position.

## The Sagittal Twin Block Appliance

The Class II, division 2 malocclusion responds well to treatment with the twin block sagittal appliance (Figure 13-26). The sagittal twin block is suitable for treatment of both Class II, division 2 malocclusions and Class II, division 1 malocclusions with retroclined incisors. It also is effective in treatment of facial and dental asymmetries.

As the name implies the sagittal twin block is designed primarily for anteroposterior arch development. Two sagittal screws are positioned in the palate to advance the upper anterior teeth, similar to the mechanism of action of the Schwarz plate. Some oblique development also is possible by offsetting the angulation of the screws to achieve an additional component of buccal expansion. Normally the palatal screws are angled to drive the upper posterior segments distally and buccally along the line of the arch. This movement is necessary to

ensure that the arch expands in the molar region as the screws are opened. If the screws are set parallel in the palate, the molars are driven into crossbite.

In placing screws in the palatal acrylic, the clinician must ensure that they are set in the horizontal plane. The screws should not have a downward inclination anteriorly, which would cause the appliance to ride down the anterior teeth, reducing its effectiveness. The anteroposterior positioning of the screws and location of the cuts determine whether the appliance acts mainly to move upper anterior teeth labially or to distalize upper posterior teeth. The interdental clasps also affect the reciprocal action of opening the palatal screws.

The position of the anterior cut determines the number of anterior teeth included in the anterior segment. If only the central incisors are retroclined, these may be the only teeth moved labially; alternatively, the lateral incisors also may be advanced by placing the cut distal to the lateral incisors. The incisors are then opposed against the posterior teeth to advance the labial segment.

Space can be created for buccally or palatally malposed canines by advancing all four upper incisors. If the cut is positioned distal to the canines or first premolars, it increases the distalization of posterior teeth in proportion to the number of teeth included as anchorage in the anterior segment.

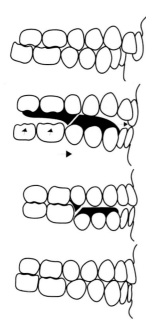

**Figure 13-25.** Management of Class II, division 2 malocclusion by advancing the mandible and proclining the upper incisors with springs or sagittal screws. Eruption of lower molars corrects the vertical dimension.

(From Clark WJ: *Twin block functional therapy: applications in dentofacial orthopedics,* London, 1995, Mosby-Wolfe.)

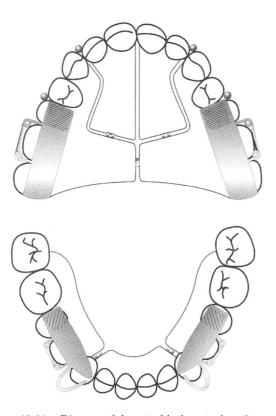

**Figure 13-26.** Diagram of the twin block sagittal appliance for anteroposterior development in Class II, division 2 malocclusion.

(From Clark WJ: *Twin block functional therapy: applications in dentofacial orthopedics,* London, 1995, Mosby-Wolfe.)

The sagittal design also is useful for unilateral correction through unequal operation of the sagittal screws according to the amount of activation required on each side. In cases of asymmetric arch development, the screw on one side may be activated more than the other to compensate if more space is required unilaterally. This technique is particularly effective in correction of facial or dental asymmetry and control of unilateral Class II malocclusion.

The lower twin block sagittal appliance applies similar principles in the lower arch. Curved screws are placed in the lower canine region to advance the lower anterior segment. Alternatively, to open premolar spaces, straight screws are placed in the region of the second premolar.

The sagittal screws are normally activated twice a week in growing children: one quarter turn of each screw at midweek and at the weekend. Less activation may be required for older patients whose tooth movements are slower. Often the clinician must trim away the acrylic over the soft tissue of the palate to avoid compression of tissue caused by operation of the screw. The acrylic must not be trimmed away where it contacts the lingual of the upper incisors; trimming should be limited to the area of the soft tissue.

Sagittal twin blocks may be combined with brackets on the upper anterior teeth with a sectional arch wire to correct individual tooth alignment (Figure 13-27). This combination of fixed and functional appliance treatment is effective in correcting arch relationships and alignment simultaneously during the twin block phase of treatment. An easy transition may then be made to a full, fixed orthodontic appliance phase to detail the occlusion and complete the treatment.

## Reverse Twin Blocks

Correction of Class III malocclusion is achieved by reversing the occlusal inclined planes to apply a forward component of force to the upper arch and a downward and backward force to the mandible in the lower molar region. The inclined planes are set at 70 degrees to the occlusal plane, with biteblocks covering the lower molars and upper deciduous molars or premolars and sagittal screws advancing the upper incisors (Figure 13-28).

In a Class III malocclusion the maxilla is frequently contracted laterally and anteroposteriorly. Three-way expansion is usually required in the upper arch to develop the maxilla anteroposteriorly and transversely. As in correction of Class II malocclusion, the clinician must match the width of the upper arch to the lower arch as the maxilla advances and the mandible is restricted in forward development. Therefore the upper arch must be expanded and the maxilla must be advanced relative to the mandible.

The bite is propped open in this type of malocclusion, and the only contact is on the inclined planes to increase the activation. The patient bites down into the appliance to drive the maxilla forward. This action may be combined with the application of Class III intermaxillary elastics or a reverse-pull face mask for forward orthopedic traction to maximize maxillary advancement.

## Monitoring the Condylar Position During Treatment

**Method.** High-quality joint x-ray films are recorded in a standardized procedure using an Orthophos Plus diagnostic x-ray unit. The films are recorded to show the following:

1. The position of the condyle in the glenoid fossa before treatment with the teeth in contact
2. The downward and forward position of the condyle in the fossa when the twin block appliance is inserted
3. The position of the condyle after the overjet has been reduced
4. The position of the condyle in the fossa on completion of treatment

A number of patients have been examined to establish a benchmark for location of the condyle in the fossa. At this stage, no quantitative results can be reported from research studies, but clearly repositioning of the condyle occurs during treatment, and the condyle relocates toward its former position in the fossa at a surprisingly early stage.

An example of this type of change is illustrated in the records of a 13-year-old boy with an overjet of 15 mm. The patient had been advised to have surgical correction but had sought a second opinion and decided on twin block orthodontic treatment.

The joint x-ray films clearly indicate the repositioning of the condyles in the glenoid fossa during treatment. Radiographs were taken before treatment with the teeth in occlusion. This film was repeated with the twin blocks inserted. The position of the condyles was measured relative to the nearest point on the bony outline of the external auditory meatus:

1. The distance from the condylar outline to the auditory canal before treatment was 3 mm on the right side and 4 mm on the left side.
2. When the appliance was inserted, the distance increased to 17 mm on the right and 15 mm on the left.
3. After 9 months of treatment the overjet was fully corrected and the distance reduced to 4 mm on both sides.

Lateral skull cephalograms show the change after 16 months of treatment with twin blocks. Models also show the improved occlusion.

Although studies of condylar position are still preliminary, they may help clarify the remodeling and repositioning changes that occur in the condyle-to-fossa relationship during twin block treatment. Again, Paulsen's laminagraphic studies (1996) substantiate these observations.

Examination of changes within the TMJ confirms that the condyles are initially displaced down and forward on the articular eminence when the appliance is fitted. As treatment progresses, the condyles are gradually repositioned in the glenoid fossa, which appears to be a typical response (Figures 13-29 and 13-30).

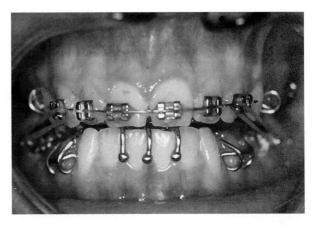

**Figure 13-27.** Twin blocks combined with anterior brackets and sectional arch wires to align the anterior teeth.

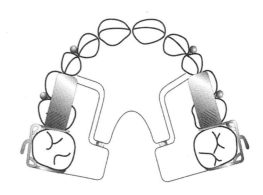

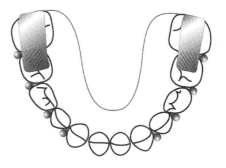

**Figure 13-28.** Reverse twin blocks for Class III treatment. Upper twin block sagittal appliance with screws to advance upper incisors and hooks for Class III traction.

(From Clark WJ: *Twin block functional therapy: applications in dentofacial orthopedics,* London, 1995, Mosby-Wolfe.)

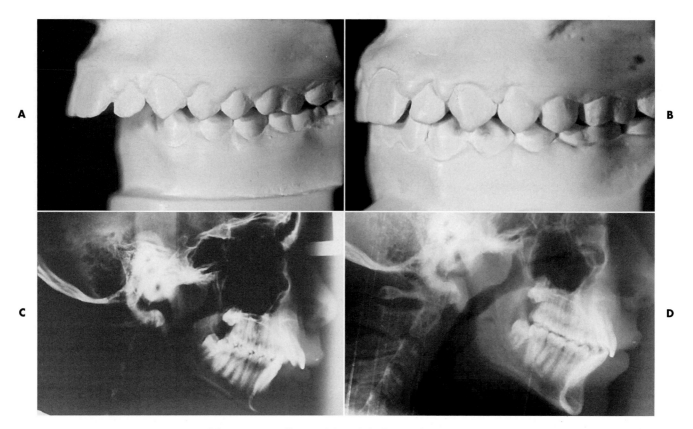

**Figure 13-29.** Models, joint x-ray films, and lateral skull x-ray films. **A,** Occlusion before treatment. **B,** Occlusion after 18 months of treatment. **C,** Cephalogram before treatment. **D,** Results after 18 months of treatment.

(Courtesy G. Kluzak, Calgary, Alberta, Canada.)

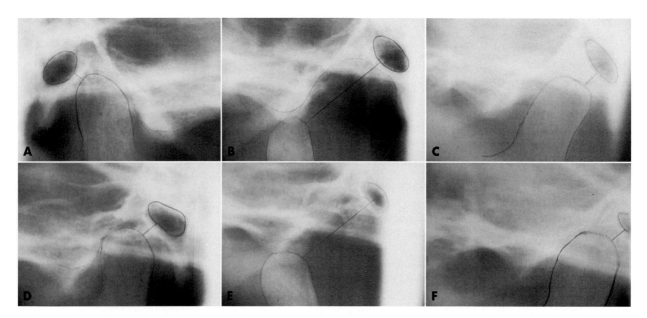

**Figure 13-30.** **A,** Left TMJ before treatment in occlusion. **B,** Left TMJ after fitting of twin blocks. **C,** TMJ after 9 months of treatment, with overjet fully reduced. **D** through **F,** Same views on right side.

(Courtesy G. Kluzak, Calgary, Alberta, Canada.)

## MAGNETIC TWIN BLOCKS

The use of magnets in occlusal inclined planes as functional appliance mechanisms is a new development. Magnetic force is under investigation as an activating mechanism in orthodontic and orthopedic treatment. Animal experiments in mandibular advancement (Vardimon et al, 1990) indicate an enhanced mandibular growth response to magnetic functional appliances compared with nonmagnetic appliances of similar design (see Chapter 14). Similar experiments using a magnetic appliance with an adjustable screw for maxillary advancement showed midfacial protraction with horizontal maxillary displacement and anterosuperior premaxillary rotation (Vardimon et al, 1990; see Chapter 14).

Clinical investigations are now proceeding to develop new appliance systems to harness magnetic forces. The twin block technique lends itself to the addition of magnets to occlusal inclined planes. Reports by Darendeliler and Joho (1991, 1993, 1995) describing the magnetic activator device (MAD) II appliance for treatment of Class II, division 1 malocclusion illustrate the possibilities for the addition of magnets to twin blocks, as reported by Clark to the E.O.C. in 1990. The mechanism of correction in magnetic twin blocks is the application of occlusal forces to the occlusal inclined planes. The clinician should consider the normal frequency of tooth contacts when planning treatment.

Normal interjaw tooth contacts have been measured between 8 minutes (Sheppard, Markus, 1962) and 20 minutes (Lear, Flanagan, Moorrees, 1965) in a 24-hour period but only 1 to 2 minutes during nighttime wear (Powell, 1965). Lear et al found 8.2 deglutition-free periods per night, each 20 minutes long. In addition, the clinical rest position, with 1- to 2-mm interocclusal clearance, does not coincide with the electromyographic relaxed position, with a larger, 5- to 12-mm interocclusal clearance.

Witt and Komposh reported a physiologic limitation in the effects of activators during sleep. An activator with no sagittal displacement and a 4- to 6-mm posterior bite clearance delivered less cranial force (70 to 150 g) than horizontal force (145 to 270 g); an activator with a 3.5-mm sagittal displacement and the same clearance delivered an increased dorsal force (315 to 395 g) but caused almost no change in cranial force (120 to 175 g). These findings indicate that patients might wear their appliances in completely unproductive positions. Increasing the construction bite beyond the habitual postural position (i.e., increasing the vertical clearance) does not improve the mandibular protrusive response.

Given the normal frequency of interjaw tooth contacts, a similar unproductive pattern may develop during twin block treatment. As the patient adapts to the presence of occlusal inclined planes and the muscles establish a new postural position of equilibrium, the blocks may only contact intermittently. With respect to the normal physiologic resting posture, the patient will likely develop an adaptive protrusive resting position with space between the opposing bite-blocks. Comparison of the frequency of occlusal contact between magnetic and nonmagnetic appliances of similar design is an area meriting further research. Such research could test the hypothesis that occlusal contact is enhanced by the use of magnets in the attracting mode.

## Attracting or Repelling Magnets

The first consideration in the use of magnets in inclined planes is whether the opposing poles should attract or repel. Logical reasons support the use of both systems. The advantages of both methods may be summarized as follows, with examples of clinical application.

**Attracting magnets.** Increased activation may be built into the initial construction bite for the appliances using attracting magnets. The attracting magnetic force pulls the appliances together and encourages the patient to occlude actively and consistently in a forward position. The attracting magnets increase the frequency of occlusal contact on the inclined planes. Indeed, patients have observed that on waking, the blocks are in contact, probably as a result of the attracting magnets. This contact may increase the effectiveness of the appliances at night. Care must be taken to limit attractive force magnitude. If the force is too strong, the appliances may be displaced or become a monobloc, thus losing the advantage of twin block flexibility.

Rare earth magnets generate a high magnetic force from small magnets that can be inserted in the inclined planes of the twin block appliance. Clark has used two materials—samarium cobalt and neodymium boron—to test the clinical response to magnetic twin blocks. Neodymium boron applies a higher magnetic force from smaller magnets but is more likely to corrode if not adequately protected from abrasion.

Attracting magnets were tested clinically in five different situations:

1. *Class II, division 1 malocclusion with a large overjet*—The addition of magnets results in more rapid correction of distal occlusion than would normally be expected with nonmagnetic appliances. After 1 month of treatment one patient's overjet reduced from 10 to 6 mm, and after 2 months of treatment a further reduction to 2 mm was observed.
2. *Mild residual Class II buccal segment relationship*—A mild residual Class II buccal segment relationship is difficult to resolve with nonmagnetic twin blocks. This malrelationship is usually a unilateral problem, and magnetic inclined planes can be used to accelerate correction of the buccal segment relationship to a "super Class I" relationship. This correction can be quickly achieved, thus allowing treatment to be completed satisfactorily (Figure 13-31).
3. *Mild Class II, division 1 malocclusion*—Some patients fail to posture forward consistently with conventional twin blocks and as a result make slow progress. The addition of attracting magnets noticeably improves occlusal contact of the bite-blocks, and progress improves as a result. Patients with this type of malocclusion do not respond to conventional functional therapy because they fail to make the muscular effort required to acti-

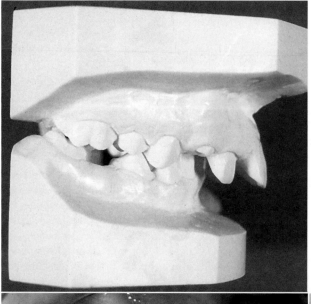

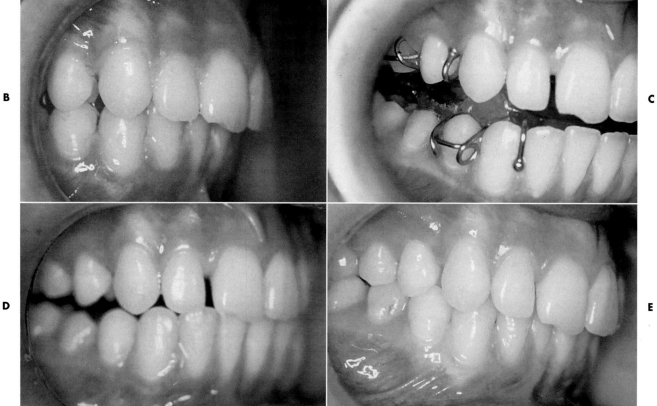

**Figure 13-31.  A,** Appearance before twin block therapy. **B,** Appearance after twin block therapy with incomplete correction. **C,** New magnetic twin blocks. **D,** Overcorrected appearance. **E,** Appearance after occlusion settles.

vate the appliance. Attracting magnets benefit these patients by increasing favorable occlusal contacts.

4. *Adults with severe Class II, division 2 malocclusions and persistent headaches associated with occlusal interference*—Magnets can be used in sagittal twin blocks to correct distal occlusion. This technique is usually combined with vertical elastics to elevate the lower molars to reduce the overbite. A finishing stage with fixed appliances is normally followed by restoration of the upper anterior teeth to complete treatment. Magnets assist in posterior eruption.

5. *Marked skeletal Class III malocclusion*—The patient studied in this clinical example had a severe hereditary type Class III skeletal pattern with a persistent unilateral crossbite. The patient was advised to consider surgical correction but did not agree. A 9-month period of treatment with rapid maxillary expansion and Class III intermaxillary traction was undertaken (Figure 13-32). No improvement was noted in the lingual occlusion or lateral crossbite; the patient failed to respond to conventional mechanics because of unforeseen adverse skeletal factors.

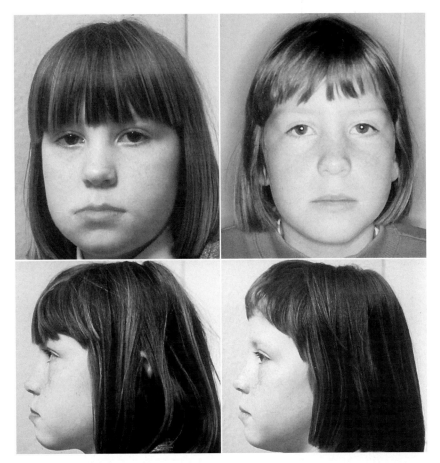

**Figure 13-32.** Facial improvement in Class III malocclusion after treatment with magnetic twin blocks for 2 months.

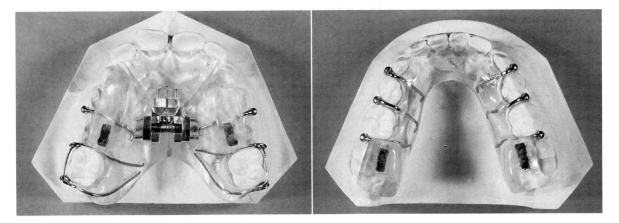

**Figure 13-33.** Class III twin block construction with appliances on models.

Because both the patient and her parents were anxious to continue with an orthopedic approach, a further attempt at treatment was made using Class III magnetic twin blocks to control the unfavorable growth (Figure 13-33). Orthopedic forces were applied to correct mandibular displacement and advance the maxilla; an additional sagittal expansion component also was applied. This technique was quickly effective in improving the mandibular displacement, and the initial response to Class III correction was excellent (Figure 13-34). A reverse-pull face mask was fitted to combine functional correction

with forward traction to the maxilla. This combination of mechanics continued for 16 months. However, the improvement proved temporary, and the condition later relapsed when as anticipated the Class III growth pattern reasserted itself. This approach may nevertheless prove effective in other cases in which the skeletal pattern is within treatable limits.

*Correction of facial asymmetry.* Facial asymmetry provides an obvious indication for the use of magnets to counteract asymmetric muscle action. Mandibular displacement can

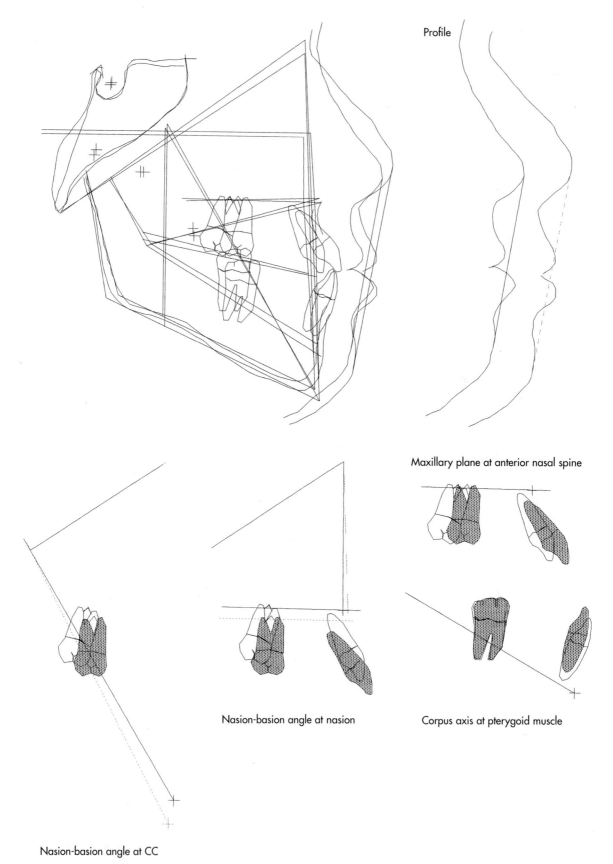

Profile

Maxillary plane at anterior nasal spine

Nasion-basion angle at nasion

Corpus axis at pterygoid muscle

Nasion-basion angle at CC

**Figure 13-34.** Cephalometric tracings show position before and after reduction of overjet with superimpositions. Shaded areas indicate posttreatment results.

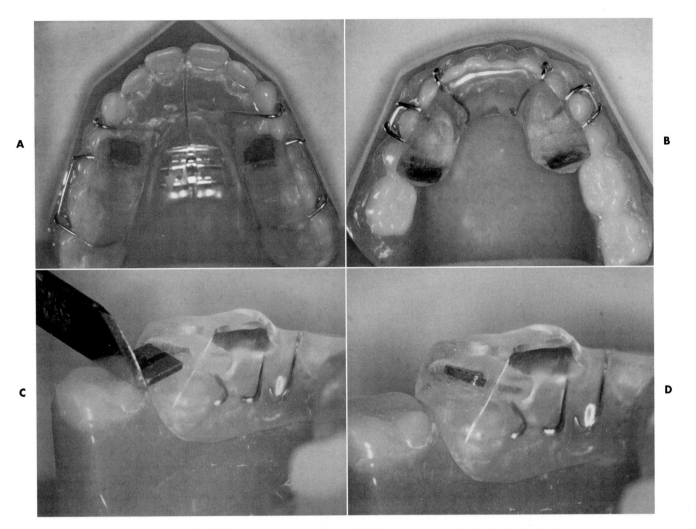

**Figure 13-35.** **A** and **B,** Magnets mounted on an incline to correspond with the inclined plane. **C** and **D,** Application of the magnet into a horizontal slot in the inclined plane.

quickly be corrected using attracting magnets in the occlusal inclined planes on the working side to correct unilateral mandibular displacement in growth. The inactive side may be an upper bite-block only, or inclined planes may be activated to a lesser degree to encourage midline correction. Magnets may be included either unilaterally or bilaterally. Early interception of facial asymmetry with magnetic inclined planes should theoretically improve the rate of correction achieved by conventional functional appliances by providing an excellent training mechanism to improve facial balance.

**Repelling magnets.** Repelling magnets may be used in twin blocks with a lesser mechanical activation built into the occlusal inclined planes. The repelling magnetic force is intended to apply additional stimulus to forward posture as the patient closes into occlusion. A possible disadvantage of repelling magnets may be that the amount of activation needed is not clear, and proprioceptive contacts on the blocks are not enhanced by repelling forces.

Moss and Shaw (1990) reported at the European Orthodontic Congress on a controlled study of 12 patients treated with repelling magnets placed in the occlusal inclines of twin block appliances. The results indicated a 100% increase in the rate of correction compared with a similar group of patients not treated with magnets. The repelling magnets were intended to induce additional forward mandibular posture without the need for reactivation of the blocks. Although speed of correction was improved, an improved skeletal response to orthopedic forces was not observed; significant changes were observed in incisor angulations.

Whether attracting or repelling magnets are used, reactivation of the blocks by addition of acrylic to the inclined planes deactivates the magnets. Screws may therefore need to be included in the appliance design for magnetic twin blocks to achieve continuous reactivation of magnetic force.

## Response to Magnetic Twin Blocks

A short period of investigation reveals that magnetic twin blocks may help resolve some of the problems in the management of difficult cases. Figure 13-35 shows placement of magnets for correction of Class II malocclusion.

Initial assessment of the use of magnets as activating mechanisms for improved response to functional therapy is excellent. Whether attracting or repelling magnets will be more effective must still be resolved; both are probably appropriate in different applications. Attracting magnets are indicated in cases in which the patient does not or cannot make the muscular effort to posture consistently to the corrected occlusion. (See Chapter 14 on the use of magnets in functional appliances.)

## ADVANTAGES OF TWIN BLOCKS COMPARED WITH OTHER FUNCTIONAL APPLIANCES

1. A major advantage of twin blocks compared with other functional appliances is that they are designed to be worn full time, even during most sports (except swimming). Full-time wear allows the patient to adapt completely to the appliance and provides continuous application of light physiologic forces to stimulate the maximal possible growth response to correct the skeletal relationship.

2. In comparison with other functional appliances, twin blocks cause less interference with normal function because the mandible is free to move normally in anterior and lateral excursion without being restricted by a bulky one-piece appliance. The functional mechanism of twin blocks is very similar to that of the natural dentition.

3. Appearance is noticeably improved when twin blocks are fitted. This is an excellent motivating factor. The absence of lip, cheek, and tongue pads allows the freedom of normal function and does not distort the patient's facial appearance during treatment.

4. Patients quickly learn to speak normally with twin blocks, just as patients do with dentures. In comparison with other functional appliances, twin blocks do not distort speech by restricting movement of the tongue, lips, or mandible.

5. Twin blocks can be designed with no visible anterior wires without losing efficiency in correction of arch relationships.

6. Because they are worn full time, twin blocks achieve more rapid correction of malocclusion. This benefits patients in all age groups.

7. Twin blocks allow independent control of upper and lower arch width.

8. Integration with conventional fixed appliances is simpler than with any other functional appliance.

9. One limitation of functional appliances in the past has been that they are removable by the patient. Clark has recently designed a new means of attachment for twin blocks to molar bands that achieves better stability and should extend the option for fixed twin blocks.

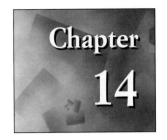

# Chapter 14

# The Magnetic Functional System

Alexander D. Vardimon

Dieter Drescher

Christoph Bourauel

Gottfried P.F. Schmuth

T.M. Graber

Introduction of a new treatment modality is prone to reservation and criticism. This reaction is related to the comfort of practitioners who for years have had full control over routinely used treatment techniques. Years of experience make the orthodontist an expert in certain techniques. Unfortunately, however, objectivity is lost with time. Treatment failures with the old technique are underestimated, whereas treatment successes are overestimated. For example, open-bite cases achieving stable treatment results are more likely to be recognized than those that develop posttreatment relapse. The same is true for functionally treated cases that develop "Sunday bite" or orthopedic failures in Class III correction with chincap or facial mask; these failures are often easily erased from memory. Moreover, clinicians tend to discredit side effects associated with current treatment procedures such as loss of attached gingiva adjunct with alignment of impacted teeth and apical root resorption linked to incisor torque and intrusion movements. Another hurdle in presenting a new technique is overcoming the convenience of practicing a technique that requires no further training. The difficulties in learning the fixed appliance technique for orthodontists trained with removable appliances and for experienced fixed appliance orthodontists to acquaint themselves with functional treatment are excellent examples of the problems faced in promulgating a new technique. The challenge in breaking through these problems is analogous to the difficulty of eradicating mouth-breathing and tongue-thrust habits in open-bite patients. These problems are especially troublesome for experienced clinicians because preconceptions and habits are more resistant with age. The initial phase for beginners in a new technique is highly demanding, especially because time is required until intuitive perception develops to a point where the clinician is able to insert the correct modification in the appliance if tooth movement deviates from original treatment strategy. Finally, approval or disapproval of the new technique must be based on the clinician's treatment results. This stage is a necessity and should rely on statistically proven analysis. Unfortunately, clinical inferences often are concluded from anecdotal episodes.

If orthodontics is to be held as part of the medical sciences, striving for advancement should be continuous. No hurdle should impede the goal of providing better patient care. That few advancements have occurred in the field of removable functional appliances (FAs) in the past 40 years with the exception of Fränkel appliances is perplexing; in contrast, fixed-appliance techniques have experienced major improvements in the past few decades. These improvements include changes in the chemical and physical properties of arch wires (nickel-titanium, beta-titanium, super elasticity), bracket design (straight-wire technique, lingual brackets) and material (ceramic), and bonding materials (etching technique, composites, glass ionomer). This chapter introduces a novel FA based on a unique mode of action—magnets—aimed at expanding the range of treatment productivity.

## MAGNETIC PROPERTIES

The rationale for introducing magnets to the arsenal of FAs is based on the necessity of decreasing the incidence of treatment failure associated with conventional appliances. The assumption that the functional magnetic system (FMS) can provide an answer to these failing cases is related to the unique characteristics of magnetic attractive force systems compared with conventional mechanotherapy. These characteristics include the following:

- High force-to-volume (F/V) ratio
- Maximal force at short distances

- Three-dimensional centripetal orientation of attractive magnetic force
- No interruption of magnetic force lines by intermittent media
- No friction in attractive force configuration
- No energy loss

## High Force-to-Volume (F/V) Ratio

The breakthrough in the use of permanent magnets in dentistry came with the introduction of new magnetic alloys. These rare earth magnets, which belong to the lanthanide elements such as the samarium cobalt alloys ($SmCo_5$, $Sm_2Co_{17}$), are 20 times stronger than the previous strongest permanent magnet, the aluminum-nickel-cobalt ($AlNiCo_5$). Thus for the same force magnitude a 20-times smaller magnetic unit can be applied with rare earth alloys (Figure 14-1). Because the oral cavity dictates the size of the appliance, this increase in F/V ratio (also known as the *miniaturizing effect*) makes the use of magnets in dentistry a beneficial modality. In physical terms the new magnetic alloys are characterized by a high coercive force (H) (i.e., a high magnetic field strength), which indicates their ability to encounter demagnetization forces; a high remanence (B), or magnetic induction, which indicates the extent of spontaneous magnetization; and a high energy product (B × H), which indicates the ability to attract or repulse (Becker, 1970).

A new magnetic alloy, neodymium-iron-boron ($Nd_2Fe_{14}B$), has been discovered in the past 15 years (Chin, 1980). This neodymium (Nd) compound is 3 times stronger than Sm-Co magnets (Robinson, 1984). However, the Nd magnet is 240 times more susceptible to corrosion in the salivary milieu than the Sm-Co magnets (Vardimon, Mueller, 1985) and possesses a lower Curie temperature (the temperature at which a permanent magnet irreversibly starts to lose its magnetic properties). These two limitations currently make Sm-Co alloys the magnetic compounds of choice in dentistry. Extensive studies have demonstrated that lanthanide magnets maintain good biocompatibility (Bondemark, 1994; Bondemark et al, 1994; Cerny, 1980a,b).

## Maximal Force at Short Distances

In contrast to conventional forces (e.g., coil springs, elastics, screws) that react according to Hooke's law (F ~ Ed) (where the force [F] is proportional to a constant such as the elastic modulus [E] times the distance [d]), magnetic force reacts according to Coulomb's law—that is, the force is proportional to the inverse square of the distance (F ~ 1/d²) (Tsutsui et al, 1979) (Figure 14-2). For example, in cases of impaction and final adjustment, in which little space is usually provided between the impacted tooth or slightly misaligned teeth and the dental arch, the magnetic force system offers a better-controlled system than conventional forces. This advantage has been used to design a new bracket with a magnetic base (Kawata et al, 1987) and develop magnetic eruption appliances (Sandler, 1991; Vardimon et al, 1991). Another consequence of this different force behavior facilitates intermaxillary me-

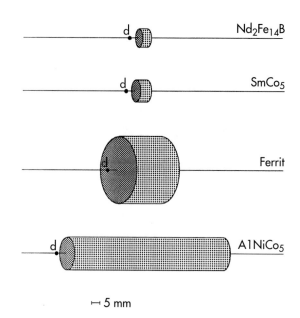

**Figure 14-1.** Increase in F/V ratio with improvement in magnetic alloys. To receive the same magnetic field of ferrite (the most common magnetic alloy) at 1 cm from the magnetic pole surface, the volume of $AlNiCo_5$ is reduced by 77%; $SmCo_5$, 4.4%; and $Nd_2Fe_{14}B$, 1.6%.

chanics. Conventional intermaxillary elastics are mostly efficient in the open mouth, whereas magnetic force reaches its peak during mouth closure. At maximal mouth opening the vertical force component of the elastics increases; a decrease in the horizontal force vector also occurs. Consequently, not only is the desired horizontal force inadequate for Class II correction, but the vertical force vector may also cause unfavorable steepening of the occlusal plane in high-angle cases. Clinicians considered this effect when introducing the first orthodontic magnetic appliances to substitute for Class II or III elastics in orthodontic treatment (Blechman, 1985; Blechman, Smiley, 1978).

## Three-Dimensional Centripetal Orientation of Attractive Magnetic Force

The three-dimensional orientation of attractive magnetic force implies that if two magnets are displaced from each other in more than one plane, they attract to a full overlap. If a first, mobile magnet is displaced in the x, y, and z dimensions in relation to a second, fixed magnet, the mobile magnet moves toward a full overlap with the fixed magnet. Thus if the stationary magnet is linked to a plate, and the mobile magnet is attached to an impacted tooth, and if the stationary magnet is in the final tooth position, it attracts the mobile magnet toward a full engagement. Centripetal attraction in all three spatial dimensions can be obtained from initial to complete traction phases (Vardimon et al, 1991). This feature also is implemented in magnetic FAs and is discussed later in this chapter (Vardimon et al, 1989, 1990).

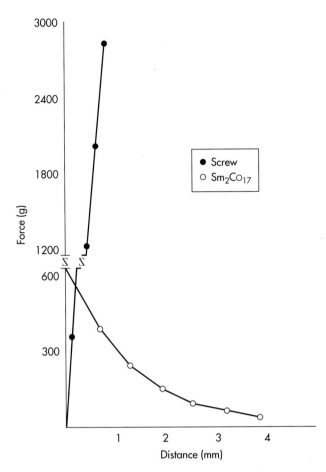

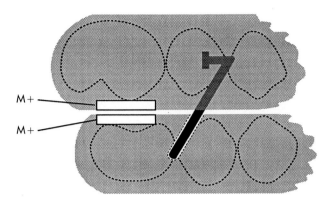

**Figure 14-3.** Müller prongs used to correct the mode of repelling magnets from detachment in arbitrary directions to a controlled, unidirectional vertical displacement.

**Figure 14-2.** Force to distance (F/D) diagram for expansion screw and magnets used for rapid maxillary expansion. The expansion force increases in a linear manner according to Hooke's law ($F \sim Ed$) with every one-fourth revolution of the screw and decreases hyperbolically according to Coulomb's law ($F \sim 1/d^2$) as the repelling magnets detach from one another.

## No Interruption of Magnetic Force Lines by Intermittent Media

Another unique feature of magnetic forces is that any media interposed between two magnets cannot bar the passage of magnetic force lines. If a magnet attached to an impacted tooth is embedded in the tissue, it is attracted by an intraoral magnet even if soft or hard tissues are interposed in the gap between the two magnets. This advantage has been applied in the design of the hygienic magnetic eruptor for the alignment of impacted teeth (Vardimon et al, 1991).

## No Friction in Attractive Force Configuration

As previously discussed, attracting magnets are useful in controlling the three spatial dimensions. This feature is called *centripetal orientation.* Because the slot–arch-wire technique does not have to be applied when an attractive force configuration is used, friction forces are excluded. This advantage has been implemented by Darendeliler and Joho (1992) in their

magnetic arch wires. In contrast, if repulsive forces are used, repulsion occurs in arbitrary and unpredictable directions. Therefore if repulsion is to occur in a given direction, guiding elements must be incorporated in the appliance. For example, when magnets are used to expand the upper dental arch, they are installed in a repulsive configuration, and guiding elements control repulsion along the transverse axis (Vardimon et al, 1987). Likewise, guiding elements must be incorporated in the Dellinger active vertical corrector, which intrudes posterior teeth with magnets in a repulsive configuration. These elements, known as *Müller prongs* (Figure 14-3), counteract deleterious mandibular lateral shift and the development of unilateral crossbite (Vardimon et al, 1994). However, the clinician should remember that these guiding elements introduce friction in the appliance. Occasional increases in the force threshold may be required to compensate for the energy loss from friction.

## No Energy Loss

Elastics are the classic examples of force systems that deteriorate over a short time; the viscoelastic properties of elastics are prone to relaxation. This change is accelerated in dental use because of fluid adsorption that occurs when elastics are exposed to the saliva milieu (Kuster et al, 1986). However, energy loss also can occur in metals. A reverse curve of Spee incorporated in a stainless steel arch wire frequently decays into an almost flat form if the arch wire is removed from the patient's mouth after 3 to 5 weeks. In this case the energy loss is caused by deactivation. Because most active elements operate around the yield strength, plastic deformations and even fatigue failure (repeated application of loads below the maximal stress) are often seen in springs of removable plates and at high-stress points along arch wires (e.g., loops and helices in high-tempered stainless steel, TMA, nickel-titanium wires). In contrast, the high coercive force suggests that this new generation of rare earth magnets can maintain energy capacity for years without any loss. However, as previously mentioned, the high-energy product of the magnet ($B \times H$) lasts only as long as the magnets are protected against corrosion (salivary assault) and the temperature does not exceed the Curie temperature (around 350° C for $SmCo_5$ and 200° C for $Nd_2Fe_{14}B$).

Before any discussion of the implementation of these characteristics in the FMS occurs, the etiology of treatment failure should be described because the new appliances are designed to affect the causative factors.

## ETIOLOGY OF TREATMENT FAILURE

Treatment failures caused by FAs are classified according to the following categories:

- Unfavorable skeletal growth pattern
- Default differential diagnosis
- Inadequate patient compliance
- Incompetent neuromuscular adaptation

*Unfavorable skeletal growth pattern* is a broad term encompassing several manifestations. The most common manifestations are time-related difficulties. The close relationship between growth and time is demonstrated by the decrease of skeletal growth potential beyond the age of approximately 14 years in boys and 12 years in girls, the period of peak pubertal growth (Björk, 1963; Björk, Helm, 1967; Hägg, Taranger, 1984; Lewis et al, 1982; Taranger, Hägg, 1980). Consequently, because functional correction is determined by growth, such correction requires time-dependent treatment (Pancherz, Hägg, 1985). Almost unanimous agreement exists that after growth cessation, no functional treatment can be commenced. However, no study has demonstrated that FAs are effective only at peak growth periods. Adverse growth magnitude and direction are other factors (Mamandras, Allen, 1990). The most common example is inadequate mandibular horizontal growth, which produces skeletal Class II malocclusion. In a more severe but less frequent dysfunction, aberration in the expected growth pattern takes place. For example, the horizontal growth pattern unexpectedly transforms into a vertical one. However, because growth generally maintains its pattern, the attribution of failure of FAs to an unfavorable growth pattern is a misleading dogma. On the contrary, in most functionally treated cases, some skeletal improvement of mandibular posture can be detected. Nevertheless, skeletal correction may be insufficient. This insufficient correction has led to debate regarding whether the skeletal change that occurs during treatment would have happened naturally without any treatment. Although supporting the notion that mandibular growth is partially determined by factors other than genetics is difficult (Petrovic et al, 1981), the fact that functional correction subsides after growth ceases supports the strong relationship between the two processes. An argument can be made that in cases in which conventional FAs fail to perform against the genetic pattern, FMSs also may produce no improvement or only dental improvement. However, a more plausible hypothesis is that FMSs act more effectively in propelling dormant genetic tendencies than conventional FAs. For instance, a locked mandibular growth pattern caused by a Class II, division 2 malocclusion that may have failed to respond to FA therapy may be revived by the FMS.

*Default differential diagnosis* refers to treatment failure as a result of false analysis of the given malocclusion. For example, certain Class II malocclusions result from maxillary or bimaxillary arch length deficiency and thus require headgear therapy or extraction treatment, using fixed mechanotherapy, and not treatment by FA. Another form of default differential diagnosis occurs in borderline cases. In such cases the preliminary diagnostic evaluation often suggests that both nonextraction and extraction treatment approaches may work appropriately with removable or fixed mechanotherapy. In these cases the clinician should judiciously apply a diagnostic therapy procedure in which an FA is applied for a limited time and then evaluated after at least 1 year to determine whether to continue the initial treatment strategy. At this stage, treatment failures frequently occur as the clinician postpones the application of new treatment approaches. The FMS may expand the number of borderline patients who, by the end of the diagnostic therapy period, successfully continue their functional nonextraction therapies.

*Inadequate patient compliance* is an often misused term. Frequently the orthodontist responds to lack of treatment progress by increasing the appliance wear time to as much as 24 hours a day. Such overwhelming requirements often result in patient noncompliance and lead the clinician to condemn the patient. Successfully treated patients normally have average wearing times of 10 to 12 hours per day (Remmelink, Tan, 1991; Vargervik, Harvold, 1985). Moreover, some investigators recommend nighttime wear only because growth is accelerated during this time (Petrovic, 1994); others require daytime wear to stimulate functional activity (Ahlgren 1978). These contradicting recommendations result from the fact that an FA can be worn by the patient nonproductively. The net effective time functional correction is performed during appliance wear contributes to treatment success, not the extent of time an FA is placed in the mouth. In addition, lack of patient compliance is most often affected by categories such as deficient growth pattern and incompetent muscle adaptation.

Incompetent neuromuscular adaptation is probably the most difficult hurdle a functional treatment must clear. The oral neuromusculature is the first complex affected by the spatial displacement of the mandible. Thus functional correction of dentoalveolar and skeletal structures only occurs after oral neuromuscular adaptation. This sequence of events is supported by Petrovic and Stutzmann (1972), McNamara (1973), Petrovic et al (1975), Oudet et al (1988), and Easton and Carlson (1990), who found that a change in the activity of the lateral pterygoid muscle (LPM) is a predetermined factor in triggering the functional correction cycle. However, reservations regarding the role of the LPM have been raised (Sessle et al, 1990). The adjustment of the oral musculature to the functional displacement of the mandible is accomplished by two groups of muscles. The first group of muscles (LPM, digastric, posterior bundles of the temporalis) undergoes adaptation that affects the anteroposterior (horizontal) jaw posture; the second group incorporates the muscles responsible for the superoinferior position of the mandible (masseter, anterior bundles of the temporalis, suprahyoid group of muscles, medial pterygoid).

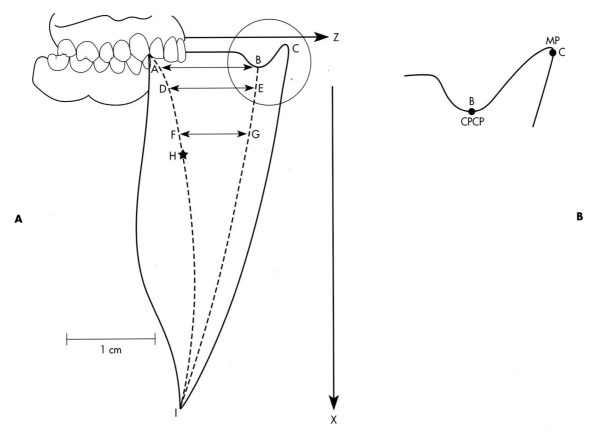

**Figure 14-4.** **A,** Posselt diagram demonstrating that the extent of the constructive mandibular advancement (*z axis*) decreases on mouth opening (*x axis*) from z = 11.2 mm (*A to B*) at minimal opening (x = 2 mm), to z = 9.6 mm (*D to E*) at the rest position (x = 3.0 mm), to z = 7.6 mm (*F to G*) at mouth opening with a Harvold-Woodside activator (x = 8.5 mm), and to z = 0 mm (*I*) at maximal bite opening (x = 38 mm). **B,** The constructive protrusive closure position (*CPCP*) is the most inferior point along the upper border of the Posselt diagram (*B*) when the upper and lower anterior teeth are posed in an edge-to-edge relationship.

In macaque monkeys a functional neuromuscular adaptation occurs if three criteria are met: first, positioning of the mandible at a protrusive displacement adjacent to the maximal protrusive point, second, accomplishment of the first requirement at maximal closure position (Figure 14-4), and third extension of the duration at which the first two criteria occur (Vardimon et al, 1989). The point at which the first two requirements are accomplished is referred to as the *constructive protrusive closure position* (CPCP) (Vardimon et al, 1989) (see Figure 14-4, *B*). The essential requirement of capturing the mandible at the CPCP for effective functional correction raises the question of how often the jaw rests at this position during appliance wear. No direct answer is available for this question. However, Gibbs et al (1981) have demonstrated that during each swallow a maximal contact position is achieved that lasts approximately 638 milliseconds. Kydd and Neff (1964) measured 1200 to 3000 swallows per day. In normal physiologic activity the maximal contact position occurs only 8 to 20 minutes a day (Lear et al, 1965; Sheppard, Markus, 1962), suggesting that even with complete patient compliance, the net duration in which a functional device is performing at the full optimal

CPCP is short. Moreover, Witt and Komposch (1971) found inadequate vertical support to maintain the mandible in a closed position during activator wear. This finding indicates that the elevation group of muscles is a major causative factor for the failure of functional treatment. In an attempt to counteract the tendency of the jaw to rest in an open position, Harvold and Woodside (Woodside, 1984) designed an FA that operates at or below the rest position. However, a close examination of the Posselt diagram of mandibular border movements (Posselt, 1952) reveals that mandibular protrusive movement decreases constantly from maximal value at no bite clearance to no value at maximal bite opening (see Figure 14-4, *A*). Thus the increase in bite clearance of the Harvold-Woodside activator limits mandibular advancement (Sander, Schmuth, 1979), and improved performance through increase in the duration at the CPCP does not occur. The unequivocal importance of mandibular advancement compared with bite opening is clearly demonstrated in the study of Moore et al (1989).

Patients wearing FAs in nonproductive ways by separating the jaws are frequently observed in the clinical setting. This acquired position of a dropped mandible can aggravate Class II malocclusion. At night, the longest time at which an FA operates, the maximal intercuspation contact decreases to 1 to 2 minutes (Lear et al, 1965; Powell, 1965), and the rest position is inferiorly located from an interocclusal clearance of 1 to 3 mm during the day to an electromyographic (EMG) relaxed position of 5 to 12 mm (Manns et al, 1981; Peterson et al, 1983; Rugh, Drago, 1981; Van Sickels et al, 1985). Thus Vardimon et al (1989) suggest that the unique characteristics of magnetic forces offer a solution to counterbalance the issue of incompetent neuromuscular adaptation.

## CONSTRUCTION AND CLASSIFICATION

The FMS incorporates some principles of the Schwarz appliance (*Vorschubdoppelplatten*) (Frass, 1992; Sander, 1988ab;

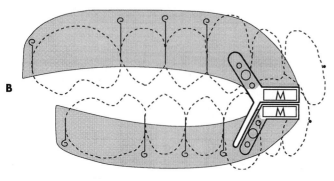

Schmuth, 1983; Schwarz, 1956). It consists of upper and lower removable plates that each contain a magnetic unit; both units are arranged in an attractive pole orientation (Figure 14-5) (see Chapter 13).

The upper magnetic unit comprises a stainless-steel magnetic housing with a single prong attached to it. The magnetic housing incorporates two cylindric rare earth magnets ($SmCo_5$) (Vardimon et al, 1994). If expansion of the maxillary arch is required, an expansion screw is linked to the magnetic housing and prong. The juncture between the magnetic housing, prong, and expansion screw is such that on activation of the expansion screw, the position of the magnetic housing and prong remains unchanged along the initial sagittal plane (Figure 14-6). An extension arm with a bend of 130 degrees connects the expansion screw with the magnetic unit (Figure 14-7), allowing a better fit of the magnetic unit with the anatomic outline of the anterior segment of the hard palate (see Figure 14-7, *B*). The prong is inclined at 70 degrees to the magnetic interface or occlusal plane (see Figure 14-7, *B*), to meet the requirements of mandibular movement along a slanted line (see Figure 14-7, *C*), as indicated by the hinge axis of the temporomandibular joint (Posselt, 1962). The prong

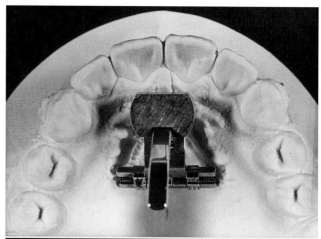

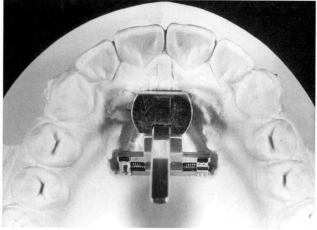

**Figure 14-5.    A,** An FMS appliance. **B,** A midsagittal view of the FMS appliance.

(Courtesy Dentaurum.)

**Figure 14-6.**    The upper magnetic screw in closed (**A**) and open (**B**) modes. Regardless of the amount of screw opening, the upper magnetic housing always remains along the same sagittal plane.

also has a small bend of 45 degrees at its occlusal end to enable a smooth initiation of guidance (see Figure 14-7, *B*).

The lower magnetic unit consists of a magnetic housing that encompasses two cylindric rare earth magnets ($SmCo_5$) corresponding to those in the upper magnetic housing. The lower magnetic housing has a posterior inclined wall that forms an oblique plane (Figure 14-8, *A*). Guidance of the mandible into the CPCP is provided by the sliding of the mandibular oblique plane along the maxillary prong on mouth closure (see Figure 14-8, *A*). This guidance mechanism is enhanced by a semifunnel groove in the oblique plane (Figure 14-8, *B*). In accordance with therapeutic requirements an expansion screw can be linked to the lower magnetic unit (Figure 14-9, *A* and *B*). In such a case, on activation of the lower expansion screw, the position of the magnetic housing remains invariable (Figure 14-9, *C* and *D*). Regardless of the amount of expansion in each arch the prong and magnetic housing of the upper appliance always correspond with the oblique plane's groove and the magnetic housing of the lower appliance along the same sagittal plane.

The anchoring units of the plates include Adams, triangle (arrowhead), and elastic clasps. The first two are well described in the literature (Adams, 1988; Schmuth, 1983; Witt, Gehrke, 1988). The elastic clasp (Figure 14-10) was designed to meet the specific requirements of magnetic forces (i.e., to counteract the elevation of both plates toward the occlusal plane produced by the attractive force). If the elastic clasp is being designed for a canine tooth, two hooks are soldered on the vertical extension of the U-shaped loop of the labial bow (see Figure 14-10, *A*). The hooks' heads point outward, away

from the loop. A two-unit elastic chain is then stretched between the hooks (see Figure 14-10, *B*). The anchor tooth is affixed with a bonded button, cleat, or Begg bracket. When the appliance is placed in the mouth, the stretched elastic chain is snapped beneath the undercut of the button attachment, eliminating the tendency of the plate to rock (see Figure 14-10, *C*). The hooks (or extensions) should align with the occlusal edge of the attachments (see Figure 14-10, *B*). In such a position the elastic chain provides adequate support to the FMS. A specially designed U-shaped loop with bending extensions to receive the elastic chain can be used instead of soldered hooks (see Figure 14-10, *D* and *E*). Both methods are acceptable, and orthodontists and orthodontic technicians should choose the one that works best. A longer elastic chain consisting of three or four rings between two hooks soldered to the inside of the mesial leg of the two U-shaped loops of the labial bow is recommended for the upper incisors. Alternatively, a right-angle U-shaped loop can be designed for the two upper central incisors (see Figure 14-10, *F*). Because the functional correction is applied in the mixed dentition, elastic clasps are used on both deciduous and permanent teeth. However, the application of elastic clasps on deciduous teeth is of limited value because increased mobility and sensitivity during the exfoliation of deciduous teeth hinder the patient in the use of the appliance. No cases have demonstrated extrusion of anchored teeth because of acrylic support on the lingual tooth aspect and force equilibrium at maximal closure. At maximal closure the extrusive force generated by the lower appliance is balanced by the counterforce produced by the upper appliance. This counterbalance also applies to the ex-

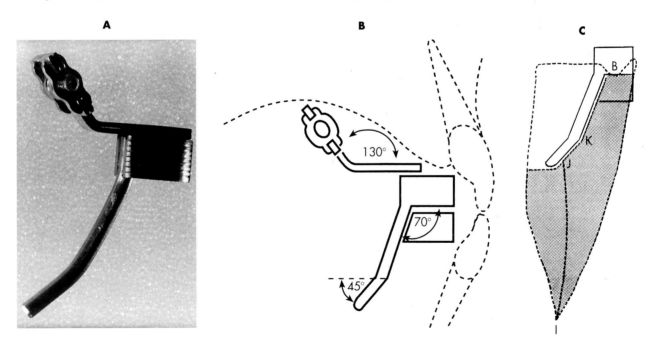

**Figure 14-7.   A,** Upper magnetic unit. **B,** The prong has a 70-degree inclination to the upper magnetic housing and a small bend of 45 degrees at its inferior edge. The extension arm linking the upper magnetic housing to the screw has a bend of 130 degrees. This bend is dictated by the contour of the palate. **C,** The lower jaw traverses a path of closure from maximal jaw opening (*I*) to the CPCP (*B*) comprised of the following segments: *I* (x = 40 mm) to *J* (x = 15 mm), no prong guidance; *J* to *K* (x = 2 mm), guidance along the 45-degree bend of the prong; and *K* to *B* (x = 10 mm), final guidance along the 70-degree bend of the prong.

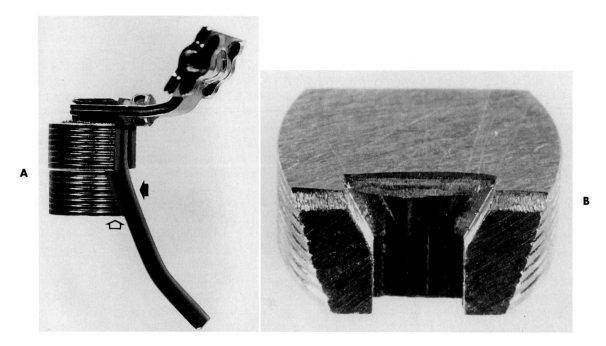

**Figure 14-8.** **A,** The lower magnetic housing has an inclined plane (*empty arrow*) coinciding with the inclination of the prong (*full arrow*). **B,** A semi–funnel-shaped groove provides mechanical support for guiding the prong into a centered position for treatment of functional and skeletal lower midline deviations.

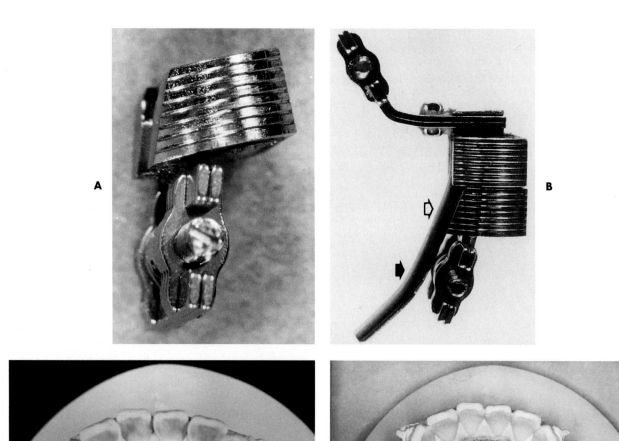

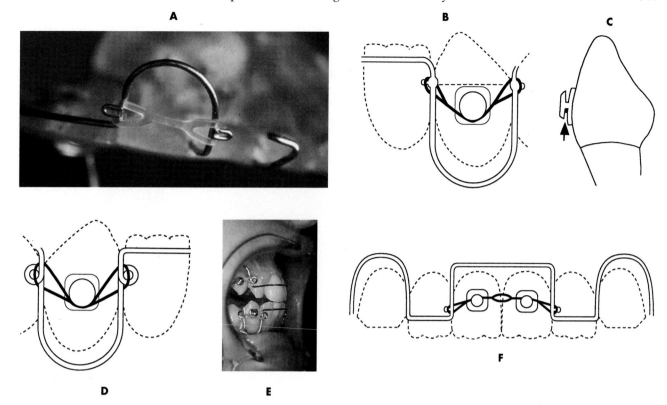

**Figure 14-10.** **A,** The elastic clasp is designed so that its soldered hooks can receive a medium to long elastic chain. **B,** The soldered hooks align with the incisal rim of the bonded attachment (*dotted line*). When stretched between the hooks, the elastic chain forms a slight crescent outline. **C,** Side view of the elastic span when snapped in the undercut of the bonded attachment (*arrow*). **D** and **E,** The hooks also can be formed during arch-wire bending as integrated parts of the U-shaped loop. **F,** In mixed dentition, before the upper canines have erupted, the upper central incisors can serve as the anchor teeth. In such cases, U-shaped loops with hooks embracing the two upper central incisors are applied.

trusive force generated by the upper appliance. The elastic chain should be changed every 4 to 6 months depending on the fatigue rate of the elastic material. A two-unit segment of elastic chain connected by an intermediate elastic span should be used.

For severe Class II malocclusions with augmented overjet (> 8 mm) the orthodontist should consider a stepwise advancement of the mandible. Such a regimen is recommended to hinder a neuromuscular stretch exceeding the adaptation threshold. Exacerbated tissue adjustment produced by a one-step mandibular advancement could lead to a counterreaction of the neuromuscular system and collapse of the functional correction (Fränkel, 1969; McNamara, 1982ab; Van Beek, 1982). In response, a sagittal protraction screw may be added to the upper magnetic unit, allowing a gradual advancement of the mandible as treatment progresses (Figure 14-11).

**Figure 14-9.** **A,** Lower magnetic housing with screw. **B,** The screw (*full arrow*) is aligned with the oblique plane (*empty arrow*). **C,** Closed positions of the screw. **D,** Open positions of the screw. In both closed and open positions the lower magnetic housing remains on the same sagittal plane with the upper magnetic housing.

Upper magnetic units can take three forms: magnetic units with no screws, magnetic units with expansion screws, and magnetic units with expansion and protraction screws. Lower magnetic units can be designed with or without expansion screws. Theoretically, the FMS can have a total of six combinations of design. However, almost all Class II malocclusions can be treated clinically by one of the following four types of FMS:

*Type 1*—An upper magnetic unit with an expansion screw combined with a lower magnetic unit with no expansion screw (Figure 14-12, *A*)

*Type 2*—An upper magnetic unit with an expansion screw combined with a lower magnetic unit with an expansion screw (Figure 14-12, *B*)

*Type 3*—An upper magnetic unit with expansion and protraction screws combined with a lower magnetic unit with no expansion screw (Figure 14-12, *C*)

*Type 4*—An upper magnetic unit with expansion and protraction screws combined with a lower magnetic unit with an expansion screw (Figure 14-12, *D*)

A type 1 FMS is applied clinically in Class II cases characterized by minute overjet with ideal and harmonized upper and lower arches or a slightly narrowed upper arch when models are placed in Class I relationship. A type 2 FMS is

A    B    C

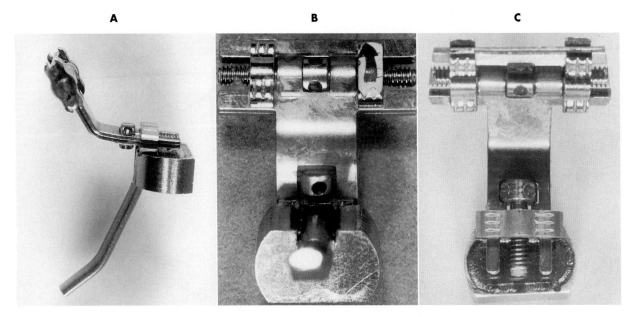

**Figure 14-11.** Upper magnetic housing with expansion and protrusion screws viewed from lateral (**A**), occlusal (**B**), and palatal (**C**) aspects. The protrusion screw is adjacent to the magnet.

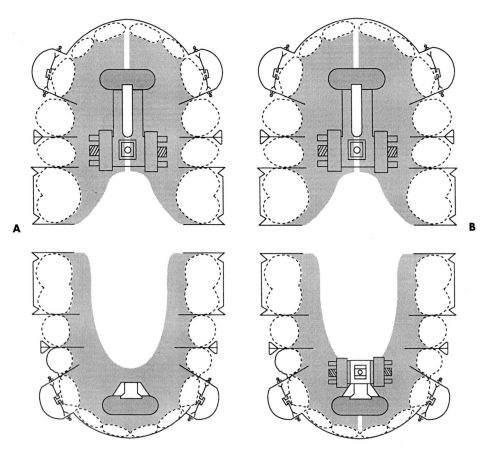

**Figure 14-12.** The four combinations of the FMS. **A,** Type 1 FMS applied in Class II, division 1 malocclusion with moderate to severe overjet, transversal deficiency of the upper arch, and ideal lower arch. **B,** Type 2 FMS applied in Class II, division 1 malocclusion with severe overjet and transversal deficiency of both arches.

used in Class II malocclusion distinguished by moderate to severe overjet and transversal deficiency of both arches. A type 3 FMS (Figure 14-13, *A*) is implemented in Class II malocclusion characterized by severe overjet in which a one-step mandibular advancement will not be tolerated by the neuromuscular system (Falk, Fränkel, 1989). This malocclusion is characterized by transversal deficiency of the upper arch and an ideal lower arch. A type 4 FMS is applied in Class II malocclusion with extremely severe overjet and transversal deficiency of both dental arches. A progressive mandibular advancement is required. Type 3 and 4 FMSs also are used in Class II, division 2 malocclusion (Figure 14-13, *B*).

## DESIGN CONSIDERATIONS

The bite registration is usually taken at an almost edge-to-edge incisal relationship (see Figure 14-16, *A*), or a "super" Class I molar relationship. In cases of severe overjet in which a type 3 or 4 FMS is indicated, the working bite can be registered at a half–Class II relationship and corrected during treatment to a Class I relationship using the upper protraction screw. The working models are then mounted in a fixator in accordance with the bite registration. The lower magnetic

unit is placed close to the lingual aspect of the lower incisors. When the upper and lower magnetic units match, the prong is aligned with the midsagittal line. However, if the patient exhibits a midline deviation, the orthodontist must consider whether midline correction should be designed in the appliance (as in functional or skeletal deviation) or excluded (as in dental deviation). In the former case the construction bite is taken at matched midlines; in the latter, no attempt is made to correct midline deviation during bite registration.

In designing the elastic clasp, the clinician must give special consideration to constructing the U-shaped loops of the labial bow wide enough that the vertical legs of the loops do not contact the bonded attachments. The elastic span, before insertion into the gingival undercut of the bonded attachment, should rest passively aligned with the occlusal edge of the bonded attachment (see Figure 14-10, *B*). The patient should be instructed to hook the elastic clasp on the bonded attachments using an expansion screw-key.

If a type 3 or 4 FMS is applied to correct a Class II, division 1 malocclusion, the upper magnetic screw should be placed away from the upper incisors, leaving a space with no acrylic for the later progressive advancement of the magnetic housing by the protraction screw (see Figure 14-13, *A*). Alternately, some acrylic may be left initially in this area between the ante-

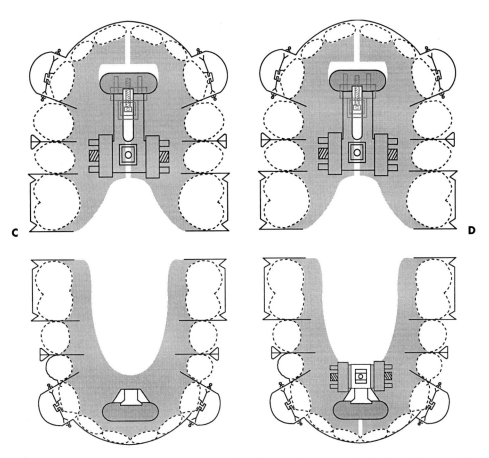

**Figure 14-12, cont'd.   C,** Type 3 FMS applied in Class II, division 1 malocclusion with extremely severe overjet, and in cases of Class II, division 2 malocclusion in which gradual mandibular advancements are required. **D,** Type 4 FMS applied in malocclusions similar to those requiring type 3 correction, with transversal deficiency of both arches.

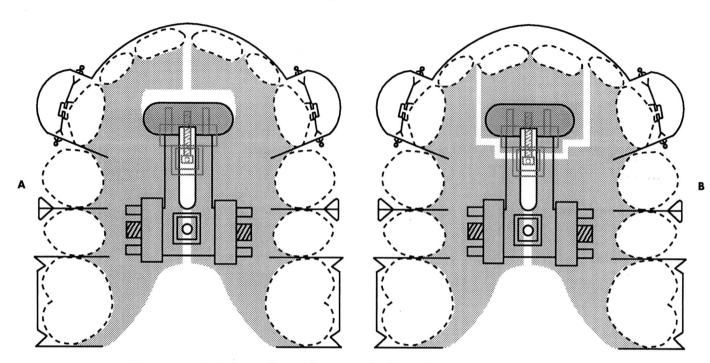

**Figure 14-13.** **A,** In severe Class II, division 1 malocclusion, if an upper magnetic housing with expansion and protrusion screws is applied, the acrylic anterior to the upper magnet is gradually removed as the protrusion screw is activated. **B,** In Class II, division 2 malocclusion the acrylic between the magnetic housing and central incisors remains attached to the magnetic housing but is separated from the rest of the plate. White lines indicate sectional cuts along the acrylic.

rior wall of the upper magnetic housing and the palatal aspect of the upper incisors; this acrylic will be gradually removed from its contact with the magnet each time the protraction screw is activated. This procedure advances the magnet without protruding the upper incisors. In contrast, in Class II, division 2 malocclusion in which mandibular advancement proceeds simultaneously with protraction of the upper central incisors, full acrylic coverage is maintained between the magnetic housing and upper central incisor teeth. However, this acrylic part is separated from the bulk acrylic of the upper plate; only the acrylic in contact with the upper central incisors is attached to the magnetic unit (see Figure 14-13, *B*). Additionally, the labial arch should be separated from these teeth by offset bends or by periodic activation of the canine's U-shaped loops.

## MODE OF ACTION

Two definitions are important in understanding the mode of action of the FMS (Vardimon et al, 1994). *Spatial magnetic force system* refers to the dissociation of the attractive magnetic force into its three vector components: the vertical force ($F_x$) acting along the craniocaudal axis (x), causing jaw closure; the lateral shearing force ($F_y$) acting along the transverse axis (y), producing medial mandibular shift from any lateral excursion; and the sagittal shearing force ($F_z$) acting along the posteroanterior axis, generating mandibular advancement in

protrusive excursions. *Centripetal spatial orientation* describes the attraction of a mobile mandibular magnet by a stationary maxillary magnet toward a full overlap of their magnetic interfaces at the CPCP (x, y, and z = 0 mm) from any point within a spatial domain of mandibular movements confined by the attractive force system.

A maximal vertical attractive force ($F_x$) of almost 3 newtons (N) acts between the upper and lower magnetic units at occlusion (Bourauel et al, 1995; Vardimon et al, 1994) (Figure 14-14, *A*). Such a force level enables normal physiologic oral activity during active periods (e.g., mastication, deglutition, speech) and constraint of the mandible in the CPCP during rest periods (e.g., sleep). The chosen maximal force level acts as a mitigating stimulus in guiding the jaw from rest to CPCP. Generally, active jaw activities differ from nocturnal activities with respect to the location of the rest position; this difference is caused by diverse muscle tonicity. During daily FMS wear, two control patterns exist. The first is at rest, during which no physiologic activity occurs and the jaw is posed in a rest position with an interocclusal clearance of about 2.3 mm (Posselt, 1962). During this phase, movement of the jaw along almost a straight line (vertical axis = x) from the rest position (x = 2.3 mm, $F_x$ = 1.5 N) to the CPCP (x = 0 mm, $F_x$ = 3 N) is performed by the magnets, whereas the effect of the guiding prong is secondary (Vardimon et al, 1994). The second daily control pattern occurs during activity of the oral musculature (i.e., speech, deglutition, yawning) in which only the prong governs mandibular advancement because the jaw's vertical borderline movements often exceed the range of magnetic activity (x > 6 mm) and muscle tonicity surpasses magnetic attractive forces. Because of this tonicity, even small gaps (x < 6 mm) such as those between the rest position and the CPCP provide no restriction to open and closure movements. For example, Proffit and Field (1982) found in children that an occlusal force of 1.7 ± 3.02 kilogram force (kgf) developed during swallowing; this force is about six times greater than the maximal attractive force. During chewing, these forces increase to 5.01 ± 4.24 kgf, 17 times greater than the magnetic attractive force. However, during the night, because of muscle relaxation, the mandible reposes at a rest position with an increased interocclusal clearance of about 5 to 12 mm. This rest position also is assigned as the EMG rest position (Manns et al, 1981; Peterson et al, 1983; Rugh, Drago, 1981; Van Sickels et al, 1985). During sleep, when the patient resumes sporadic swallowing approximately once a minute, the jaw traverses from the EMG rest position (x = 8.5 mm, $F_x$ = 0 N) toward the CPCP (x = 0 mm, $F_x$ = 3 N) (Kydd, Neff, 1964). A nocturnal control pattern is instituted along this path of closure. The initial guidance from x = 8.5 mm to x = 2.3 mm is regulated by the guiding prong, whereas the final constraining of the jaw into the CPCP from x = 2.3 mm to x = 0 mm is commenced by the magnets. Magnetic attraction may possibly affect nocturnal jaw guidance to the CPCP at an even earlier stage of mouth closure (i.e., at bite clearance greater than the rest position [x = 4 mm, $F_x$ = 0.9 N]) because of the decline in muscle tonicity.

With the exception of mastication the effect of the medial shearing force ($F_y$) is minor during free mandibular movements (Figure 14-14, B) because mandibular movements hardly deviate from the midsagittal plane (Gibbs et al, 1982). However, even if lateroexcursive movements are exerted (e.g., if the patient chews gum with the FMS in place), the lateral shift produced ( ± 4 mm) falls within the range of the $F_y$ (y = ± 8 mm), directing the jaw medially to the midsagittal plane and simultaneously to the CPCP. More important, this centripetal spatial orientation feature is an important factor in the management of functional and skeletal mandibular midline deviations. In such cases the bite registration for appliance construction should be taken at a centered position so that the magnets can correct the acquired malocclusion. Moreover, even in nondeviated Class II cases the initial onset of mandibular advancement generally causes an interarch transversal discrepancy because of maxillary transversal deficiency. As long as upper compensatory expansion has not been fully established, the patient tends to shift the lower jaw sideways or posteriorly to overcome the imbalance by maintaining a good unilateral intercuspation. This transitional unbalanced intercuspation often causes the "Sunday bite" (SB)

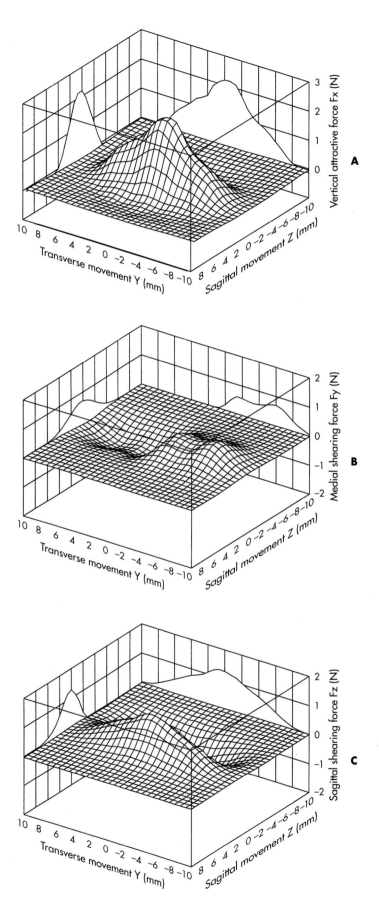

**Figure 14-14.** Spatial F/D diagrams of the FMS as horizontal movements of the lower jaw are performed (y = transversal, z = sagittal) at maximal closure of the mouth (x = 0 mm). **A,** $F_x$ = vertical force. **B,** $F_y$ = lateral force. **C,** $F_z$ = sagittal force.

phenomenon often blamed for FA failure (Storey, 1988). SBs have been divided into constructive SBs, short-term malocclusions occurring in early functional correction before the establishment of permanent mandibular repositioning, and destructive SBs, long-term conditions associated with breakdown of functional correction. Because $F_y$ (see Figure 14-14, B) is only about one third the magnitude of $F_x$, it is enforced mechanically by the guiding groove along the oblique plane of the lower magnetic housing and moved along the same sagittal plane as the corrected midline. Additional reinforcement is offered by the semi-funnel at the occlusal edge of the groove.

The use of a single prong instead of the two prongs of the conventional Schwarz appliance offers patient comfort and a mechanical advantage of self-governing upper-arch expansion (Schmuth, 1983; Schwarz, 1956). In conventional Schwarz appliances, frequently the two prongs of the upper appliance meet the lateral corner of the oblique plane of the lower appliance, impeding the completion of upper-arch expansion. A compensatory grinding of the lingual acrylic wall of the lower appliance to extend the lateral range of the oblique plane often results in a slim and fragile juncture between the posterior acrylic extensions and oblique plane, increasing the risk of fracture of the lower appliance in the canine–first premolar region.

The sagittal shearing force component, $F_z$ (Figure 14-14, C), is a major contributor to the centripetal spatial orientation feature of the FMS. The path of movement of the lower jaw, even in short distances such as from the rest position to the CPCP, does not follow a straight vertical x line. This jaw movement, which ensues along a 70-degree slope, implies that at rest position the lower magnet is displaced both apart (x = 2.3 mm) and posteriorly (z = −0.84 mm). Thus the lower magnet is attracted at the rest position toward the CPCP by a vertical force of $F_x$ = 1.55 N and a sagittal force of $F_z$ = 1.6 N. This equivalence in force magnitude demonstrates the significant contribution of the force vector $F_z$ to the centripetal spatial orientation effect. With further mouth closure as the magnets approach full overlap and the z dimension decreases, significant attraction to the CPCP is managed by $F_x$. However, although the $F_z$ magnitude increases continuously, it reaches levels of half the magnitude of $F_x$ (at z = 0 mm, $F_x$ = 3 N, $F_z$ = 1.7 N) (see Figure 14-14, A through C). The contribution of $F_z$ to locating the jaw in the CPCP occurs not only as protrusion occurs to the zero overjet point (z = 0 mm, CPCP = 0) but also if the jaw performs a further protrusion reaching a Class III relationship. The force vector $F_z$ then directs the jaw posteriorly to the correct CPCP position.

The FMS is designed for all three force components of the attractive magnetic force system, and the mechanical components (prong, oblique plane) act synergistically to guide and constrain the jaw in the CPCP. Regardless of the anteroposterior displacement or other movement the mandible undertakes, it always moves to the CPCP in the shortest three-dimensional way. This centripetal spatial orientation feature extends the duration the mandible is located in the most functionally efficacious corrective position and thus increases the

functional performance. Surprisingly, the net effective operating time of functional appliances has not been considered in previous studies (Carels, Van der Linden, 1987). The primary effect of the FMS is to increase the duration of maximal mouth closure at the CPCP beyond the limited interval of 8 to 20 minutes a day (Lear et al, 1965; Sheppard, Markus, 1962). That only 1 to 2 minutes of this interval occur at night emphasizes the need to augment this shortage of physiologic support to accomplish treatment requirements (Lear et al, 1965; Powell, 1965). This lack of support is of major concern because 70% of the wear time of conventional functional appliances or FMS occurs at night. The unique mode of action of the FMS implies an improved therapeutic performance in this regard.

## CASE STUDY

A 12½-year-old boy with protruded teeth was transferred to the Department of Orthodontics at Tel Aviv (Israel) University by the dentist. He had an unremarkable medical history. The extraoral clinical examination revealed a retrognathic soft tissue profile and an incomplete lip seal at rest position with an everted lower lip (Figure 14-15, A and B). The patient had a full Class II malocclusion of the right and left molars and canines (Figure 14-15, C through E), deep overbite, excessive overjet (9 mm), mild upper (−4 mm) and lower (−3 mm) crowding, a submerged and distally tipped lower right second premolar (Figure 14-15, F), excessive curve of Spee (Figure 14-16, A), and ovoid dental arches. The Bolton analysis showed a 1.4-mm mandibular excess for the 6 anterior teeth and a 3.1-mm mandibular excess for the total 12 teeth. Cephalometric analysis (Table 14-1 and Figure 14-15, G and H) disclosed a severe skeletal Class II malocclusion related to a retrognathic and short mandible.

Bite registration was taken at edge-to-edge incisal relationship (see Figure 14-16, A), and an FMS appliance was constructed with expansion screws in both the upper and lower appliances (Figure 14-16, B through F) and a retraction screw in the lower appliance between the right lower second premolar and the first molar (see Figure 14-16, E). Anchorage buttons were bonded to the buccal surfaces of all four canines (Figure 14-16, G through I). The patient was instructed to wear the FMS 14 hours a day and activate the expansion screws in both arches and the retraction screw in the lower appliance one-quarter turn once a week (see Figure 14-16, E). Thus sagittal and transversal corrections of the dental arches and single tooth and segmental movements such as correction of arch-length deficiency were achieved with the FMS. The patient adjusted quickly to the FMS. After 3 months of treatment the overjet decreased to 4 mm, the molars obtained a Class I relationship, and the canines reached an edge-to-edge relationship (Figure 14-17, A through C). At this stage the FMS was unable to force the mandible into the initial position, a posterior bite clearance still existed, the distalization of the lower first molar was discontinued, and the lower right second premolar reached full alignment. After noting the remarkable improvement in the

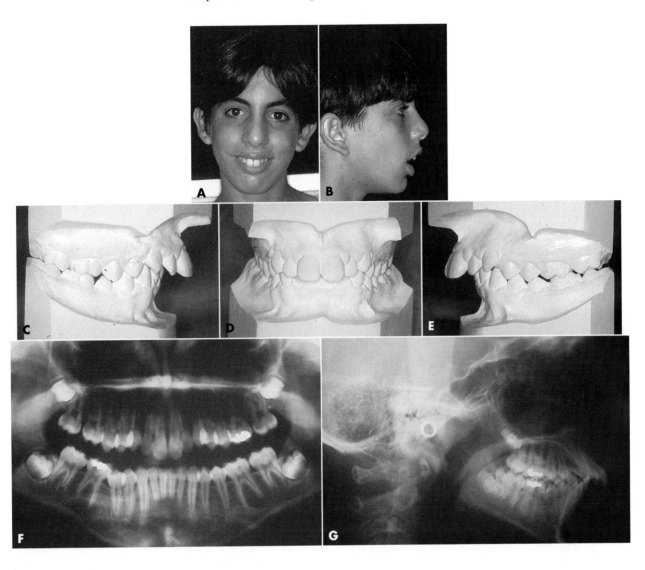

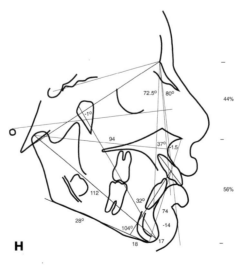

**Figure 14-15.** Initial records of a 12½-year-old boy referred for treatment. **A,** Facing forward. **B,** Profile view. **C** through **E,** Initial models. **F,** Panoramic radiograph. **G,** Lateral head radiograph. **H,** Cephalometric tracing.

(Courtesy Visit Chaijindaratana, Tel Aviv, Israel.)

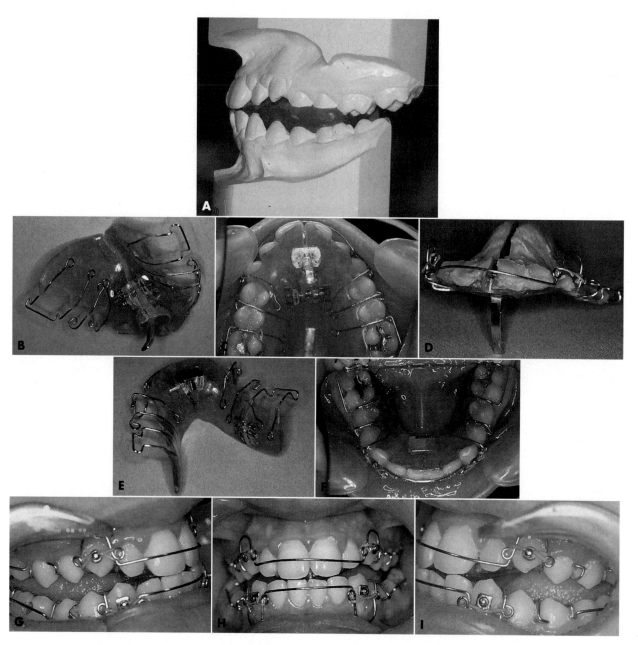

**Figure 14-16.   A,** Registration wax. **B,** Upper FMS appliance. **C,** Upper FMS appliance intraorally. **D,** Rebased upper FMS appliance. **E,** Lower FMS appliance with distalization screw. **F,** Lower FMS appliance intraorally. **G** through **I,** FMS at CPCP; note the extend of posterior bite clearance.

(Courtesy Visit Chaijindaratana, Tel Aviv, Israel.)

malocclusion, the patient put himself on a wearing schedule of 24 hours a day. He could speak without impairment and removed the appliance only during meals. After an additional 2 months of FMS treatment (Figure 14-17, *D* through *F*) the overjet decreased to 3 mm and a reduction in bite clearance was demonstrated; within a month the overjet subsided to 2 mm. At this stage the canines reached an almost full Class I relationship. After 7 months of treatment the upper appliance was rebased (see Figure 14-16, *D*) to obtain a bet-

ter fit between the acrylic and the palate, and because of the consequent control of the transverse expansion at this stage, an overcorrection of the molar relationship occurred (headgear effect) (Figure 14-17, *G* through *I*). In an additional 2 months, complete interdigitation of the posterior bite occurred, with the right side ahead of the left dentition (Figure 14-17, *J* through *L*).

The final records of FMS treatment (Figure 14-18) revealed that all goals of FA correction were accomplished, and the

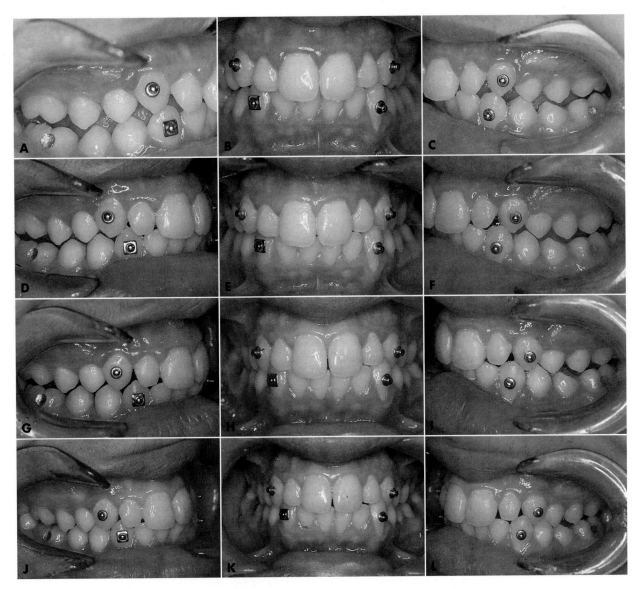

**Figure 14-17.** Progression in FMS treatment of patient from Figure 14-15. **A** through **C**, After 3 months of FMS treatment, Class I occlusion was established in the molar region, and an early reduction of bite clearance occurred (compare with Figure 14-16, *G* through *H*). **D** through **F**, After 5 months of FMS treatment an almost complete Class I occlusion was established in the canine region in conjunction with continuous reduction of bite clearance. **G** through **I**, After 7 months of FMS treatment a full Class I occlusion was accomplished in the canine region. **J** through **L**, After 9 months of FMS treatment super Class I occlusion developed in the molar region (headgear effect).

(Courtesy Visit Chaijindaratana, Tel Aviv, Israel.)

patient was ready for final adjustment with fixed-appliance mechanics, especially to correct the left maxillary canine (see Figure 14-18, *F*).

In general, six target areas are affected by functional correction:

1. Mesial movement of the lower dental arch
2. Distal movement of the upper dental arch
3. Mesially oriented eruption (extrusion) of the lower posterior dental segment
4. Distally oriented eruption (extrusion) of the upper posterior dental segment
5. Acceleration of the mandibular anterior growth component
6. Retardation of the maxillary anterior growth component

The superimposition of the before- and after-treatment cephalograms of the patient in the case study revealed that the overall facial change was characterized by a vertical

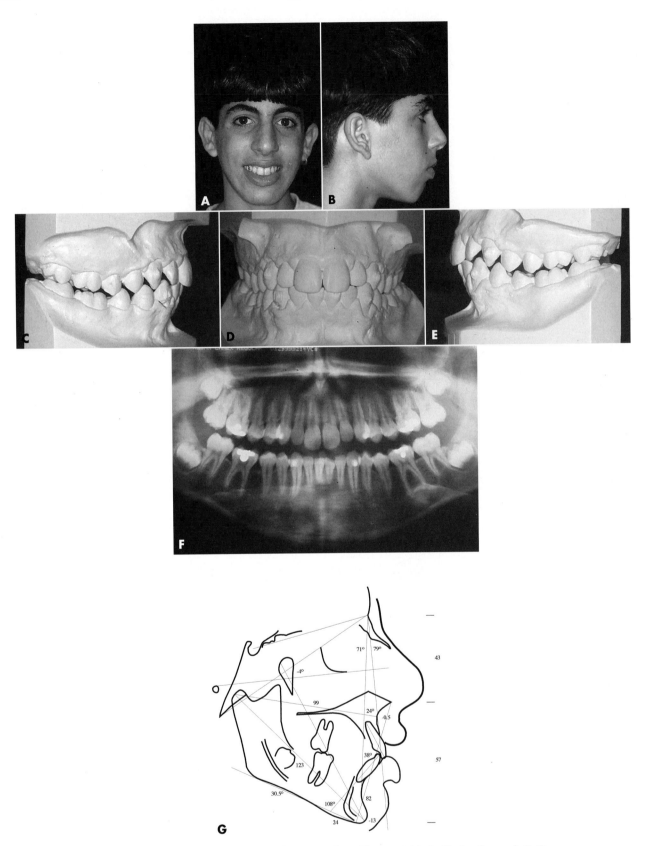

**Figure 14-18.** Final FMS records of the patient from Figure 14-15. **A,** Facing forward. **B,** Profile. **C** through **E,** Final FMS models. **F,** Panoramic radiograph. **G,** Cephalometric tracing.

(Courtesy Visit Chaijindaratana, Tel Aviv, Israel.)

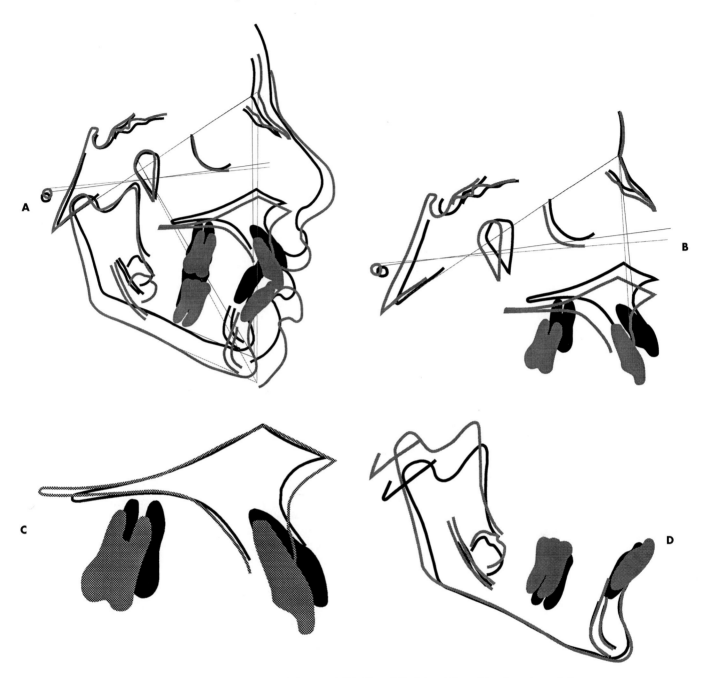

**Figure 14-19.** Superimposition of the initial (*black*) and final (*grey*) lateral head tracings of the patient from Figure 14-15 1 year after FMS treatment. **A,** Superimposition along reference line basion-nasion (Ba-N) at the most posterosuperior aspect of the pterygomaxillary fissure. **B,** Superimposition along reference line Ba-N at N. **C,** Superimposition along internal structures of the maxilla (i.e., nasal floor). **D,** Superimposition along internal structures of the mandible (i.e., mandibular canal, lingual border of the symphysis).

growth pattern (Figure 14-19, *A*). This vertical pattern was evident by a 3-degree increase in the mandibular plane to Frankfort horizontal angle and a 3-degree decrease in the facial axis (see Table 14-1). Maxillary dental change was characterized by retraction of the incisors (target area 2) combined with distalization and extrusion of the molars (target area 4) (Figure 14-19, *B* and *C*). This change is referred to as a *headgear effect* and is produced by the FMS (see Figure 14-17, *G* and *I*).

Ignoring facial growth, point A moved forward mainly because of retraction of the upper incisors (see Figure 14-19, *C*). However, the N point moved forward more than did the A point (see Figure 14-19, *A*), producing a reduction of −1 degree in the S-N-A angle and indicating maxillary growth retardation (target area 6) in relation to the upper face complex (see Figure 14-19, *B*). The most striking feature of the FMS treatment occurred skeletally in the lower jaw (see Figure 14-19, *D*). The

**TABLE 14-1. · CEPHALOMETRIC DATA OF CASE STUDY PATIENT**

| Parameter | Pretreatment Measurement | Posttreatment Measurement | Normal Value |
|---|---|---|---|
| Sella-nasion-subspinale (S-N-A) angle | 80 degrees | 79 degrees | 82 degrees |
| Sella-nasion-supramentale (S-N-B) angle | 72.5 degrees | 71 degrees | 80 degrees |
| Facial axis | 89 degrees | 86 degrees | 90 degrees |
| Condylion-subspinale Co-A | 94 mm | 99 mm | 95 mm |
| Condylion-gnathion Co-Gn | 112 mm | 123 mm | 122 to 125 mm |
| (Co-Gn) − (Co-A) | 18 mm | 24 mm | 28.5 mm |
| Anterior nasal spine (ANS) to menton (Me) | 74 mm | 82 mm | 67-69 mm |
| N⊥A | −1.5 mm | −0.5 mm | 0-1 mm |
| N⊥pogonion (Pg) | −14 mm | −13 mm | −2 to −4 mm |
| Incisor superior (1) to N-A | 37 degrees | 24 degrees | 22 degrees |
| 1 to N-B | 32 degrees | 38 degrees | 25 degrees |
| 1 to mandibular plane | 104 degrees | 108 degrees | 93 degrees |
| Mandibular plane to Frankfort horizontal | 28 degrees | 30.5 degrees | 22 degrees |
| UAFH/LAFH ratio | 44%:56% | 43%:57% | 45%:55% |

Co-Gn distance increased by 11 mm (target area 5). This increase was necessary to compensate for not only the maxillary horizontal growth (increase in Co-A = 5 mm) but also the vertical growth pattern (see Figure 14-19, *A*). In addition to skeletal correction, dental change occurred in the mandible in the form of a slight increase in the lower incisors' proclination (target area 1) (change in 1 to NB = 5 degrees, change in 1 to mandibular plane = 4 degrees) and in molar extrusion (target area 3) (see Figure 14-19, *D*).

Although the S-N-B angle did not change and the S-N-A angle even increased in the case study, an overall successful skeletal correction occurred because of complementary mandibular growth (i.e., a catching-up to the facial vertical growth pattern). In other words, if the mandibular increase (change in Co-Gn = 11 mm) had not been twice as large as the maxillary increase (change in Co-A = 5 mm), aggravation of the Class II malocclusion would have developed.

One reason for the continuous debate between proponents and opponents of functional treatment is the overweighted value given to target area 5 (i.e., the accelerating mandibular anterior growth component) in cephalometric analysis. Functional correction is a combined effect of all six target areas. The amount that each component contributes to the overall functional correction varies according to the patient. However, because functional correction is age related and cannot be applied after growth cessation, some improvement of target area 5 is a prerequisite for successful FA treatment. The contribution of target area 5 can be low (less than 25%) and that of the other five target areas predominant (greater than 75%), and the result may nevertheless be successful FA correction. However, if the contribution of target area 5 drops to zero, an unstable FA correction is established. The unique characteristics of the FMS provide increased efficacious functional duration, thus expanding the contribution of target area 5 and the five other target areas.

# Chapter 15

# Early Treatment— The Emancipation of Dentofacial Orthopedics

David C. Hamilton

*"$T$he crux of the variety of reports implying a direct or stimulating link between function and size is that tissue size is not an inheritable trait per se. Instead, the tissues and the organs which they comprise have a predetermined capacity to modify their sizes in response to the changing physiological conditions which impact these tissues and organs."*

Alphonse R. Burdi,
Professor of Anatomy, University of Michigan

## FACIAL AND SKELETAL ORTHOPEDICS

In 1985, largely through the efforts and influence of its editor, Dr. T. M. Graber, and with the approval of the trustees and House of Delegates of the American Association of Orthodontics (AAO), *The American Journal of Orthodontics* changed its title to *The American Journal of Orthodontics and Dentofacial Orthopedics*. This seemingly modest change, unnoticed by many, was wise and in many ways portended the future of the orthodontic specialty. Only in 1994 did the AAO officially change the name of the specialty known as *orthodontics* to *orthodontics and dentofacial orthopedics*. In the same year this change was approved by the American Dental Association, making the new name official. Changing the titles of orthodontic departments, documents of the Association, and names of related organizations such as the American Board of Orthodontics is a slow, ongoing process. Individual orthodontists are gradually changing their letterhead, stationery, business cards, and phone book listings to acknowledge the change.

Although more accepted in Europe, facial orthopedic practice in America remains relatively quiescent, receiving little positive recognition or enthusiastic acceptance. In several recent seminars, groups of orthodontists were asked whether they considered themselves "facial orthopedists." About 15% responded affirmatively. An extensive survey that provided a better assessment of current attitudes about and appreciation of the potential of dentofacial orthopedics was conducted and presented by Hamilton (1995) at a recent Angle Society meeting. (The survey is summarized in the Prologue.) In many communities, well-informed and progressive younger dentists and pediatric dentists who are aware of the research and literature, are frustrated in their attempts to refer their younger orthodontic patients for care that they perceive should be accomplished at an early age. In other communities, many dentists lacking appropriate training but interested in practicing orthodontics have taken advantage of the void and stepped in to provide treatment.

Although many medical and dental specialties are engaged in contentious disputes involving overlaps of practice and are challenging one another to be recognized as the appropriate discipline to provide a specific modality of care, no discipline is seriously challenging the orthodontic specialty in the area of facial orthopedics (with the exception of a small number of pediatric dentists). For years, orthodontists have considered themselves to be in the business of straightening teeth—the "put your plaster on the table" syndrome. Orthodontists are the best qualified practitioners to provide facial orthopedic therapy because of their education and experience. Failure by orthodontists to provide facial orthopedic care seriously inhibits their capacity to treat patients with severe facial dysplasias appropriately and efficiently. Observing patients' growth with the intent to perform orthognathic surgery later is not sound clinical practice. As third-party health care–benefit programs continue to deny benefits for orthognathic surgery, dentists will be forced to seek other, less invasive, less potentially iatrogenic alternatives.

More dental schools and graduate orthodontic programs need to cultivate the biologic background and research necessary to reinforce and expand scientific knowledge and understanding of facial orthopedics and early treatment precepts and techniques. Residents should be required to treat at least

319

two preschool children as a part of their clinical programs. Orthodontists must shift paradigms and accept the challenge of scientific and timely orthopedic treatment of younger patients with severe facial growth dysplasias. They must develop their skills and enthusiastically accept the role of facial orthopedist, expanding their scopes of practice to include this important health care responsibility. Failure to make this transition may seriously and adversely affect the future of the specialty.

## GENERAL CONSIDERATIONS

The practice of orthodontics is a complex dental medical specialty that is both an art and a science, albeit an inexact science. A large number of complex issues must be considered when evaluating an individual patient, especially when evaluating the wide variations of problems among patients. Evaluating all factors is vitally important; it affects the following practice elements:

1. The number and sophistication of diagnostic records necessary
2. The diagnosis
3. The treatment plan
4. The appliances and laboratory services necessary for treatment
5. Patient management
6. Business and financial arrangements
7. Whether treatment will be single or multiple phase
8. The length of treatment
9. The method and length of retention
10. The determination of a reasonable fee
11. The quality and stability of the final outcome

In addition to evaluating the patient's specific dentofacial problem, the orthodontist must carefully consider the following factors:

1. The patient's age and race
2. The patient's potential for additional growth
3. Possible etiologic factors
4. Possible palliative or preventive techniques
5. The patient's possible biologic, physiologic, and psychologic response to treatment
6. The patient's unique, personal reasons for seeking treatment and expectations of treatment
7. The patient's expected compliance and cooperation with responsibilities during treatment
8. The possible risks of the proposed treatment and risk management and informed consent issues
9. The business and economic details, including possible third-party benefits, that apply to the patient's circumstances

### Functional Matrix Theory

As promulgated by the eminent functional anatomist Moss (see Chapter 1), skeletal facial growth has a compensatory re-

sponse to the functional matrix, which consists of components such as muscles, nerves, glands, and teeth. Functional matrix growth is primary, and skeletal structure growth is secondary. This is particularly apparent in membranous bone areas (i.e., the craniofacial complex).

## Nature's Inclination to be Normative

During growth, the body attempts whenever possible under existing conditions to compensate for deficiencies by altering growth to improve or normalize functional relationships (see Chapters 1 and 2).

## Dominance of the Morphogenetic Pattern

Gans (1996) states the following regarding the morphogenetic pattern:

Several times . . . speakers have emphasized that particular aspects of the phenotype might or might not be inherited. I would like to suggest that the question is irrelevant in the present context. In fact, it is probably worse than irrelevant because the concept that something is [inherited] seems to imply fixity and resistance to modification. . . . It is unimportant whether a particular malocclusion or deformation of a jaw is produced by a faulty genetic program or by a temporary or long-lasting environmental disturbance of the developmental process. From the viewpoint of treatment, all that is necessary is that the condition exists and that it may be dealt with by prosthesis or medical manipulations. The only appropriate questions asked are whether the therapy works and whether it may have deleterious side effects.

## The Four Possible Stages of Orthodontic Treatment Timing

1. Preschool/primary dentition: typically 3 to 6 years of age
2. Preadolescent/mixed dentition: *early*—typically 7 to 9 years of age; *late*—typically 10 to 11 years of age
3. Adolescent/early permanent dentition: typically 12 to 15 years of age
4. Adult/permanent dentition: more than 16 years of age

Multiple-stage treatment has both advantages and disadvantages that must be carefully considered before the clinician decides whether to initiate early treatment. Unnecessary early treatment should be discouraged. If an early beginning of treatment is indicated, the clinician must completely inform both the parents or family and the referring dentist that a second and even third stage of treatment may be necessary; this information should be thoroughly documented as well. This process is routine in general orthopedics when treating skeletal deformities. Craniofacial growth guidance should not be less time dependent. This is especially important if traditional third-party benefits may be exhausted during an early stage of treatment.

Before treatment, the clinician must identify and rectify deleterious habits, medical problems, and environmental factors that may negatively influence treatment results if they persist during or after treatment. Early recognition, referral, and treatment of abnormal habits and airway problems and chronically enlarged tonsils or adenoids are particularly important. Enlarged tonsils and adenoids alter the functional matrix, resulting in misdirected growth. The earlier the correction, the greater the chance for a successful and stable result.

Skeletal growth modifications in early treatment are generally predictable and stable. Perhaps the greatest *disadvantage* of early treatment is the possibility that in spite of a well-conceived, properly diagnosed, well-planned, and successful early treatment, the patient's adverse growth or genetic pattern may reassert itself, requiring the patient to be treated later in a second stage. This circumstance does not necessarily indicate that the physician's original diagnosis and treatment plan were incorrect or that the patient relapsed.

Treatment outcomes have a close association with the individual orthodontist's ability and comfort with the prescribed treatment methods and the patient's attitude and compliance. Therefore after an appropriate period of time and after treating several patients, orthodontists must evaluate their personal success rates with various treatment disciplines for patients of different ages in the light of the expanding, biologically oriented therapy.

## EARLY PRESCHOOL TREATMENT

The fundamentals of biology, growth, and development supported by current research dictate that in the presence of recognizable and significantly severe facial dysplasias, orthodontists acquit themselves by judiciously practicing facial and skeletal orthopedics (see Chapters 1, 2, 3, and 4). The same fundamentals dictate that treatment of children with many of these facial dysplasias be initiated at the earliest appropriate opportunity. The earliest age in most instances would be 3½ or 4 years. Timing of treatment should be directly and differentially related to the individual child's emotional maturity level and parents' attitudes and expectations; age 4 or 5 is ideal.

**Advantages of preschool treatment.** The numerous advantages of preschool treatment include the following:

1. Cellular response to growth modification is optimal. Skeletal sutures are open and reposturing of skeletal components is enhanced.
2. Experience indicates that in using the treatment modalities recommended in this chapter, failure occurs so infrequently that in the vast majority of the patients, the advantages of early treatment far exceed the disadvantages.
3. Use of bonded appliances largely eliminates the need for strict patient and parent compliance.
4. Treatment times are greatly reduced.
5. After possible initial apprehension, patients are highly cooperative, easy to treat, and present few treatment problems.
6. Patients are usually highly compliant.
7. Because the patients are at home most of the time and under constant parent supervision, extraoral appliances such as face cribs, face-bows, extraoral anchorage, and chincaps present few problems. Clients may in fact wear these appliances for as many as 20 hours daily.
8. Although undesirable and improbable, decalcification of primary teeth results in no permanent damage if appliances and hygiene are properly handled.
9. Parents appreciate treatment of children at an early age, particularly if treatment involves bonded appliances.
10. Early correction of skeletal dysplasias to enhance optimal growth patterns is conducive to a natural appearance.
11. Early correction greatly reduces the risk of peer ridicule, which permanently damages self-esteem in highly sensitive and emotional patients.
12. Early correction, particularly in the transverse dimension, enhances chances of permanent results.
13. Early treatment may reduce the total treatment cost if it negates completely or greatly simplifies and shortens the time required for second-stage orthodontic or dentofacial orthopedic treatment.

**Disadvantages of multiple-phase or multiple-stage treatment.** In addition to the problem of unfavorable morphogenetic patterns discussed previously, other disadvantages from a pragmatic standpoint include the following:

1. Patients may burn out. Prolonged treatment, whether in stages or continuous, may seriously compromise the patient's and parents' patience and willingness to continue treatment. This is particularly evident in treatment regimens in which success depends on wearing elastic, removable functional appliances, or extraoral traction appliances. Burnout may manifest itself in the following behaviors: neglect of oral hygiene, failure to keep appointments, or even in discontinuing payment of monthly fees.
2. When first-stage treatment goals are moderately successful with fair to good results, the parent may either resist or reject the second stage of treatment for financial or other reasons. In this instance the orthodontist's reputation may be jeopardized if the patient, parents, and referring dentist later forget that the family elected not to complete treatment and are critical of the results, expense, and time spent in early treatment.
3. The establishment of realistic and fair fees, risk management, and public and professional relations associated with a second period of treatment all may be difficult. Patients and referring dentists may perceive staged treatment as being unnecessarily long or feel that treatment has been extended so patients will have to pay unnecessary or excessive additional fees.

Although these issues will not be discussed in depth in this chapter, they should be considered and properly addressed by the orthodontist before any recommendation to initiate treatment is made.

## TRIAGE

After identifying the four possible dental stages during which orthodontic treatment can be considered, the next essential decision concerning differential patient management is called *triage*. Triage is a word that originated in World War I to describe the priorities established for field hospitals during the initial examination of wounded soldiers. Casualties brought into the field hospitals during extremely busy periods were divided into three classes: (1) those whose injuries demanded and were amenable to immediate treatment; (2) those whose treatment could reasonably be postponed and carried out after transportation to a larger base hospital; and (3) those whose injuries were so severe that it was decided that they should not be treated for one of several reasons.

Triage of orthodontic patients—or the decision of whether to treat the patient—at any age or stage of growth and dental development involves several fundamental decisions: (1) whether the patient should receive orthodontic treatment; (2) whether treatment should be deferred until later; (3) whether the patient should not be treated at all or treated at an older age with combined orthodontics and orthognathic surgery. The younger the patient, the greater the number of options. Understandably, as the patient grows older the number of options decreases.

If the decision is made to treat a child during the primary dentition period, the clinician should at least contemplate the possible need for additional stages of treatment; on rare occasion, additional stages are needed at an older age. In the early mixed dentition period the chances that two stages of treatment will be required also are increased. In instances of severe skeletal dysplasia the older the patient, the greater the probability that achieving optimal results will require coordinated orthognathic surgery. As mentioned previously, when considering orthognathic surgery, determining the appropriate age for intervention is critical. In unique or difficult cases in which several legitimate options or treatment plans might be considered, the final decision may be to begin staged treatment early but delay irreversible decisions until early treatment outcomes can be evaluated.

## THE SYNERGISTIC SYSTEM AND ITS PRECEPTS: 2 + 2 = 5

More than 35 years of experience, successes, and failures have resulted in the development of what has been called the *synergistic system*. Any consideration of the system or acceptance of its components depends significantly on the orthodontist's views regarding the following precepts and the system's development and use.

### Conceptual Precepts

1. Proper facial and orthopedic treatment of a growing child at an early age with functional orthopedic appliances can modify and enhance facial growth. This results in improved facial esthetics and in many instances

a reduction in the need for or length of time of more comprehensive treatment later.

2. Use of orthopedic functional techniques demands the highest level of education, training, and experience and exceptional attention to detail. Education of general dentists is critical because many do not realize the potential of orthopedic therapy. Both dentists and orthodontists too often argue that Class III cases are morphogenetic and thus cannot benefit from early treatment. This is patently wrong, but case selection is critical and a thorough diagnostic study is essential. Hereditary patterns do not always guarantee that offspring will have the same configuration (see Figure 15-4). Alterations in growth of the skeletal pattern achieved by facial orthopedic treatment using functional orthopedic appliances are usually irreversible. Compromises are unacceptable unless absolutely dictated by unusual circumstances.

   Orthodontists who are genuinely proficient in the use of functional orthopedic appliances are often disconcerted to note other orthodontists who, having failed in their efforts to achieve successful treatment using functional concepts, state that the concepts are not viable and the appliances are not effective. These practitioners may have been improperly trained in appliance usage, led to believe the appliances were simple to use, may not have comprehended or paid adequate attention to the myriad of important options and details involved with the concepts and use of the appliances, and failed to gain the cooperation and/or wearing time necessary to produce satisfactory results.

   Even more disturbing are the use and misuse of these technique-sensitive and irreversible growth-modifying appliances and procedures by inadequately trained general dentists and pediatric dentists who have been convinced by questionably motivated entrepreneurs at weekend courses that they can triple their incomes by incorporating orthodontics into their practices. At this time (1997) the federal government and state boards have *not* adequately defended the best interests of the public with regard to advertising and the provision of orthodontic care by inadequately educated and trained practitioners.

3. Functional appliances are not generic. Each functional appliance has unique characteristics and treatment effects. The use of these appliances by different clinicians may produce very different results. Caution should be used when accepting research that attempts to generalize and draw conclusions based on either single appliance usage or the results of a single practitioner.

4. The younger the patient and the earlier the patient is treated, the more successful the results, the less time it takes to achieve goals, and the greater the stability of the results.

5. The maxilla and midfacial structures are predisposed to environmental and functional forces that contribute to deficiencies or deformities, particularly in the trans-

verse development of the maxilla and midfacial area. The attendant alteration of the functional matrix is the primary cause of a significant number of dentofacial problems. Failure to recognize and correct adequately the maxillary deficiency causes a high percentage of posttreatment failures (e.g., mandibular dental crowding, Class II relapse, transverse relapse).

6. As a result of maxillary constriction the mandible may be trapped and inhibited in its normal forward and lateral growth. Over time the form, posture, and size of the mandible are affected. Maxillary constriction and its attenuating effect on mandibular growth may be a primary cause of Class II skeletal deficiencies. Maxillary constriction also is the primary contributing cause of dental crowding in both the upper and lower arches. The earlier the maxillary problem is corrected, the greater the opportunity for the mandible and face to achieve their greatest normal growth potentials (see Chapter 17).

7. Orthopedic, sutural, and frequently differential (anteroposterior) expansion of the maxilla is necessary in a high percentage of patients with Class II skeletal patterns and maxillary constriction with attendant crowding of upper and lower teeth. Expansion also is indicated in Class III patients using face cribs for maxillary protraction. Orthopedic disarticulation of all maxillary sutures with other bones occurs when the midline suture is expanded. Disarticulation of these sutures greatly facilitates orthopedic manipulation and repositioning of the maxilla in all three dimensions.

8. In many patients the constriction, or transverse mutation, is greater in the intercanine dimension than it is in the intermolar dimension. A bonded palatal expansion appliance with occlusal coverage and two expansion screws that disarticulates the teeth is highly recommended and permits patient-specific, differential, anteroposterior expansion. Sufficient and stable *skeletal* expansion of the maxillary canine area is essential to avoid mandibular anterior dental relapse. Such expansion appears to be stable and greatly reduces the incidence of relapse in both the upper and lower anterior dental segments.

9. Both the success and stability of treatment are directly related to the clinician's ability to alter and maintain the changes in the functional matrix of the patient's developing, and eventually mature, face.

10. Dentoalveolar compensation, or the compromised alteration and compensatory repositioning of the dental and dentoalveolar structures in response to adverse skeletal growth problems, is nature's attempt to functionally accommodate facial and skeletal dysplasias.

11. Dentoalveolar decompensation is as essential to successful treatment with functional orthopedic reposturing of the jaws as it is to successful orthognathic surgical repositioning. Decompensation as early in treatment as possible facilitates optimal reposturing of the skeletal components, enhances function, and encourages continuing normal facial and skeletal development.

12. Disarticulation of the teeth and condyles 24 hours a day, including when eating, permits the patient's neuromuscular complex to position the mandible naturally and facilitates the normal function of the mandible relative to the maxilla. When the teeth are disarticulated, the condyles also are automatically disarticulated. Disarticulation of the teeth facilitates tooth movements. Anchorage preparation in the lower arch may occur at the same time. To varying degrees, sutural expansion of the maxilla also disarticulates the other bones articulating with the maxilla. Disarticulation permits repositioning in all three dimensions and greatly reduces the length of treatment time.

The wax registration bite used by a laboratory for making an appliance must be detailed and accurate and provide sufficient space for the acrylic between the upper and lower teeth. The bite must be carefully taken by the clinician; it determines the sagittal and vertical functional and orthopedic forces incorporated in the appliance.

13. Bonded appliances that are in place 24 hours a day (eliminating the need for patient cooperation) are important for achieving successful treatment with the functional therapeutic milieu. Patients readily adapt to the new appliances and parents greatly appreciate the fact that they are not responsible for making their children comply with appliance-wearing instructions.

14. Functional orthopedic appliances are not simple devices, and their proper use demands attention to clinical and laboratory procedure details. Appliances and progress must be carefully checked and if necessary, the appliances should be adjusted by the orthodontist at each appointment. The perception of optimal achievement is important to consistent and successful results. Impressions and registration bites must be retaken several times to achieve the desired result.

15. Comprehension of the appliance's design and use and excellent craftsmanship of the finished appliance are essential to the success of treatment.

16. During early treatment the synergistic use of state of the art edgewise or straight-wire techniques greatly enhances the results of early treatment. Comprehensive treatment may or may not be a goal of early phased treatment. Certainly, parents are happier when their children's teeth are straightened and they can see visible progress during the early phases of treatment. As many as 65% of comprehensively and properly treated phase I patients require little or no additional or phase II treatment.

17. The use of a 0.022-inch slot bracket is strongly recommended for orthodontists planning early mixed dentition treatment. The larger slot permits significant variability in wire types and sizes. In 2 × 4 appliances, larger arch wires can be used in the fragile intermolar tube–lateral bracket distance. This is particularly useful in the lower arch and greatly reduces the number of breakages and nonscheduled appointments.

18. The recognition that in any given patient, some natural rebound toward the original condition occurs necessitates programmed overtreatment. Natural settling and rebound should not be confused with relapse; they should be anticipated and accommodated by the treatment plan and treatment.

19. Specific differential retention of skeletal orthopedic corrections is essential to ensure stability of results. For example, a patient using a functional, activator-type retainer after Class II skeletal correction should be slowly weaned from the appliance with a reduction of the wearing time over a period of months to achieve the optimal result.

20. Proper treatment (including maxillary expansion) of a growing child at an early age using functional orthopedic appliances can greatly enhance facial esthetics, improve oral and physical health, reduce the possibility of periodontal complications, and in many instances eliminate the need for extraction of permanent teeth.

## Facial and Skeletal Treatment Modalities

The alteration of facial and skeletal configuration can be accomplished using three methods:

1. *Functional appliances* (e.g., screening appliances, conventional activators, bionators, and Fränkel appliances) are designed to change the patient's pattern of function, alter the jaw relationships, and reprogram the neuromusculature, thus altering the functional matrix of the face.

2. *Orthopedic appliances* are designed to transfer forces as directly as possible to the facial skeletal components. Forces generated may be much higher than those used for orthodontic tooth movement. The appliances effectively influence sutural changes and bone growth. If used at an early age, functional appliances favorably alter the continuing facial growth pattern.

3. *Orthognathic surgery,* in which the orthodontist cooperates with an oral and maxillofacial surgeon and the treatment plan involves the surgical repositioning of the jaws and skeletal components of the face, is another option.

The use of functional and orthopedic appliances is highly growth dependent, and patients are best treated with these appliances at the earliest possible age. In all but a few special instances, orthognathic surgery is most successful when the patient is mature; therefore it is usually deferred until growth is completed. Discussion in this chapter is directed toward treatment with orthopedic functional appliances in patients with primary and early mixed dentition.

## The Synergistic System: 2 + 2 = 5

More than 30 years of experience with functional appliance use, many failures and disappointments, and considerable frustration have contributed to the development of a system of appliances that with few exceptions competently resolves most dentofacial problems. Used with sound edgewise and straight-wire techniques, the system requires minimal patient or parent cooperation and produces excellent and stable results. Excessive office time, unscheduled appointments, length of treatment time, and costs associated with the provision of treatment have all been dramatically reduced. Few problems arise with patient and parent relations, and few conferences or parent complaints occur. The system encourages staff involvement and provides a generally positive office atmosphere.

**Appliances of the system.** Appliances of the system can be divided into those considered principally orthopedic, functional, tooth-moving or orthodontic, stabilizing or holding, and retentive. The comprehensive treatment of most patients, and certainly of those with skeletal and dental problems, dictates that these appliances be synergistically combined to meet treatment goals. Appliances of the *synergistic system,* with the exception of the molar distalizing appliance (MDA) that must be bonded, may all be used either as bonded (the preferred type) or removable appliances. In the following section, they are arranged from the most basic to the most complex.

*Palatal expansion appliance (PEA).* The palatal expansion appliance (PEA) is the basic *orthopedic* appliance of the system (see Figures 15-1, 15-2, 15-5, 15-6, and 15-7). It is primarily a maxillary expansion appliance, is almost always bonded, has full palatal acrylic coverage, and very frequently incorporates both an anterior and posterior expansion screw. If the second molars have erupted, they should *not* be included in the acrylic indexing because of the risk of decalcification. An 0.028-inch occlusal wire spur should be incorporated in the appliance to prevent overeruption of these teeth during disarticulation.

APPLIANCE OPTIONS. The following options may be incorporated into all of the orthopedic and functional appliances (except when otherwise noted):

- As discussed previously, use of two screws permits differential expansion; the greater opening is usually in the intercanine width, as opposed to the intermolar width.
- Use of 0.03-inch tubes simultaneously with labial arch wires (see Figure 15-7) provides a unique wire framework permitting attachment of soldered auxiliaries. The tubes are routinely soldered to the framework in a position equivalent to those of buccal tubes on either the primary second molars or permanent first molars, if these are in place. The tubes permit use of anterior brackets and labial arch wires, thus permitting alignment, intrusion or extrusion, opening or closing of spaces, and rotations of the anterior teeth simultaneously and synergistically with the stabilization of the sutural expansion (see Figure 15-7). In mixed dentition, this method is equivalent to using an upper 2 × 4 appliance (see Figure 15-5, *E* through *G*). In permanent dentition the arrangement results in a highly efficient use of time and

anchorage that can be used to complete upper anterior tooth alignments. Therefore when the bonded functional orthopedic appliance is removed, treatment of the upper dentition may be conveniently completed by bracketing and banding only the premolars and molars.

- IMPORTANT: The mesial-distal movement of the maxillary incisor teeth should *not* be inhibited in any way during the actual expansion of the appliance. Ideally, bracketing the incisors should be delayed for 1 month after the final turn of the expansion screws. Figures 15-1 and 15-2 show single-screw PEA appliances, and Figure 15-1, *D* shows the sutural opening of a patient in primary dentition.

- If *orthopedic* retraction of the maxilla or maximal reduction of severely procumbent maxillary anterior teeth is needed, a face-bow with either cervical or oblique forces may be adapted by adding 0.045-inch or 0.050-inch tubes to the wire framework of the appliance (see Figure 15-7, *C*). Because the appliance is bonded to the buccal quadrant teeth, this technique is highly capable of tipping the occlusal plane, depending on the amount of force used and the direction of pull and adjustment of the face-bow's outer arms. Ease of movement is enhanced by the expansion as the appliance disarticulates the maxilla from its neighboring bones.

- Hooks may be used in the canine area to accommodate the use of a face crib for maxillary protraction (see Figure 15-2, *J* and *K*). The direction of pull should be parallel to the occlusal plane, unless tipping the maxillary plane is a treatment goal.

- A biteplane may be incorporated into the acrylic appliance in deep-bite cases. This method, in addition to permitting the mandible to settle in its own position, permits eruption of the lower posterior teeth and results in an increase in the vertical dimension of the face when needed. The wax registration bite must be specially adapted to properly allow a predetermined amount of freeway space necessary for contact with the lower incisors. At the same time, sufficient space must be available to permit the eruption of the lower buccal teeth. In severe cases, vertical elastics to lower buccal sectional arches may facilitate the eruption of the lower teeth. Facial vertical correction obtained with these mechanics at an early age and properly retained over a sufficient period of time is highly stable.

- An occlusal buccal bite-block may be incorporated in the PEA if the treatment goal is to intrude or inhibit the eruption of posterior teeth and reduce the Frankfort–mandibular plane angle and the vertical facial dimension (see Figures 15-5, *E,* and 15-7, *A*). The wax registration bite should be taken at a predetermined increased vertical dimension that exceeds the freeway space by several millimeters. Ideally the appliance should at least be made on a hinged articulator in the laboratory. Bonded appliances worn for 6 months under these circumstances and at an early age can significantly reduce the vertical dimension of the face. In severe cases a vertical-pull chincap may facilitate the closure.

*Dual arch expansion appliance (DAE).* The DAE appliance was originally conceived with the intention of expanding both the maxilla through sutural opening and the mandible through alveolar expansion using a single maxillary expansion appliance (see Figures 15-8 and 15-9). The PEA appliance was modified by the addition of lower flanges very similar to those on a Harvold-type activator, which contact (with no relief) the buccal alveolar processes of the mandible. Design and fabrication of the appliance requires a carefully executed registration bite and detailed models of both the upper and lower teeth. The registration bite is very important and should be taken with the condyles in centric relation with about 2 to 3 mm of vertical space. In high-angle patients, this opening may be increased to accommodate occlusal acrylic coverage of the posterior teeth. The appliances must be fabricated using the "salt and pepper" technique. The lower impression must be deep and lingually accurate. The lingual flanges should be long and exceed the freeway space by 5 to 10 mm.

In addition to expanding the maxilla and mandible, the DAE appliance has been able to produce forward reposturing, growth, and remodeling of the lower jaw to accommodate its new position. The rationale for Class II skeletal correction is that as the maxillary suture expands because of the tapering of the lower jaw, the patient (who is unconsciously seeking additional comfort) automatically repositions the mandible forward. In all but the most severe Class II skeletal conditions, the molar relationship is totally corrected after 6 months of 24-hour wear.

Experience has proven that if a 7 mm screw is used in the appliance, the maxilla may expand by approximately 6.5 mm, while at the same time the mandible may expand by about 4.5 mm. Interestingly, these measurements are closely related to the Bolton ratio. Of additional interest are the two apparently different patient responses to appliance stimuli: (1) patients who resist forward posturing and demonstrate a significantly greater increase in the expansion of the lower arch, and (2) patients who readily posture the mandible forward and demonstrate greater Class II corrections and less mandibular expansion.

A significant advantage in using the DAE appliance is that the effects of the appliance are highly synergistic with other treatment goals. For example, the leveling, alignment, and anchorage preparation of the lower arch may be accomplished and is usually completed during the 6 months of DAE usage, particularly in full dentition treatment. When the DAE appliance is removed, the upper teeth may be immediately banded and bracketed, an arch wire may be placed, and modest-force Class II elastics may be used to reinforce the correction of the molar relationship (see Figure 15-8). In the early treatment of moderate Class II skeletal deficiencies the results of DAE appliance use are highly stable and may eliminate the need for additional functional or orthopedic treatment.

(NOTE: Because of its positive effect on mandibular growth, it is critical that the DAE appliance *not* be used in growing patients with any tendency toward Class III skeletal growth.)

If the teeth are crowded in these patients and a need for expansion of both arches is apparent, the treatment plan of choice may include a PEA in the maxilla and a well-designed Schwarz-type expansion appliance in the lower arch (see Chapter 17).

*Activator or expansion activator (ACT).* The ACT is highly effective for correcting Class II skeletal patterns when properly designed and either bonded or worn conscientiously by the patient for an appropriate period. If the ACT is removable, the time worn should be no less than 9 months and if bonded it should be 6 months. Either of these times should be followed by a period of functional retention (see Figure 15-6, *F* and *G*). All the options described for the PEA appliance also are options for the bonded activator. In Class II skeletal malocclusions requiring both maxillary expansion and mandibular advancement, the three following options are possible:

1. A bonded PEA may be used for about 2 months. When it is removed, impressions and a wax registration bite for a bonded activator are taken. The PEA is worn as a removable appliance until 1 to 2 weeks later, when the activator is bonded in place. The activator is then worn for about 6 months, at which time it is removed and a removable functional retainer is put in place.
2. An alternate method involves the use of an expansion activator (preferably bonded). Expansion is initiated at the first appointment after bonding; the screws are turned once every 3 days until the prescribed amount of expansion is achieved. The appliance is worn for 6 months and then replaced with a functional type of removable retainer.
3. A bonded maxillary Herbst-type appliance (see Chapters 16 and 17) may be substituted for the activator if indicated or preferred. Differences in use and effects must be considered. All the options available with the PEA also are options with the Herbst appliance. The Herbst appliance should be worn a maximum of 6 months; it should then be removed and impressions and a registration bite taken for a functional retainer.

*Bonded molar distalizing appliance (MDA).* The MDA, whether bilateral or unilateral, provides a simple, a predictable, an advantageous, and an effective alternate to extraoral traction if differential diagnosis indicates the need for distalization of maxillary molars. The appliance also may be used if the patient will not cooperate with using headgear, functional appliances, or Class II elastics and an alternate or compromise treatment approach is necessary. This appliance is mentioned only because it is part of the synergistic system treatment; it is not presented in this chapter.

Early treatment case reports (Figures 15-1 to 15-9) demonstrate the use of the PEA, ACT, DAE appliance, and combinations with fixed attachments.

*Text continued on p. 335*

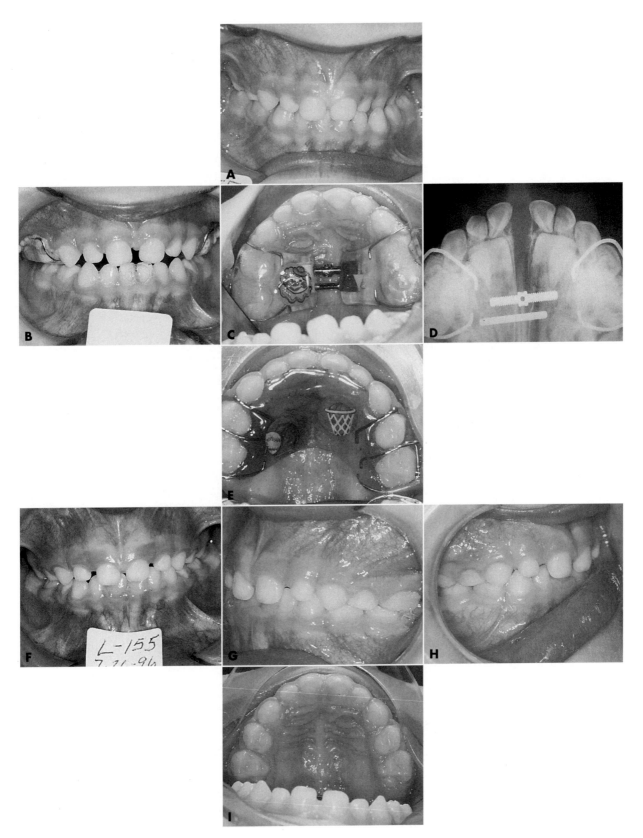

**Figure 15-1.** Bonded PEA. **A,** Patient is 4 years and 6 months old with a Class I occlusion with Class II skeletal and dental tendencies, maxillary constriction, and left unilateral crossbite and mandibular convenience swing to the left. **B** and **C,** Treatment with a bonded PEA. Note the disarticulation and amount of expansion achieved by a single expansion screw. **D,** Sutural opening is seen in occlusal radiograph. **E,** The holding appliance after removal of the PEA. **F** through **I,** Results 2 years and 7 months postretention. No further treatment required.

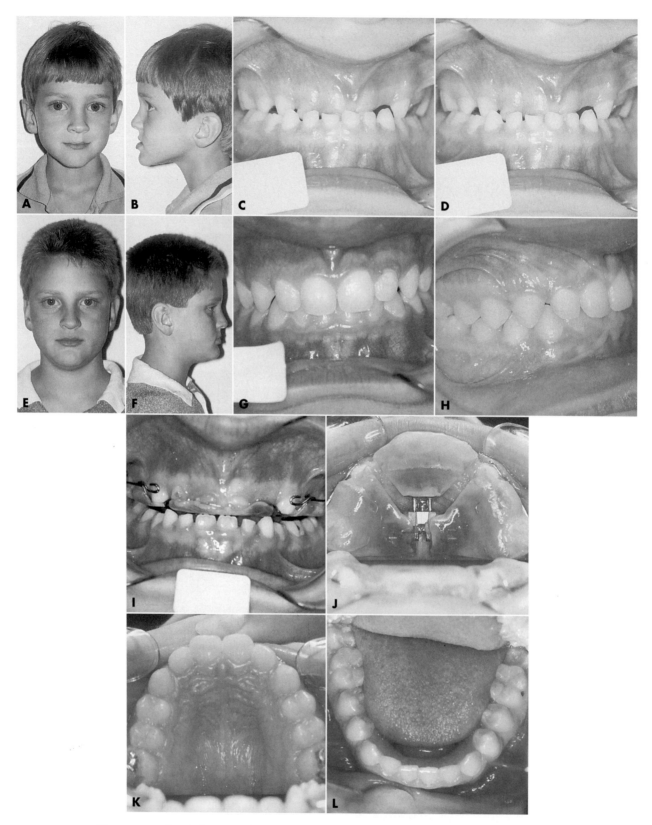

**Figure 15-2.** Bonded PEA. **A** through **D,** Patient was 5 years and 6 months old at start of treatment and had a severe Class III malocclusion with maxillary constriction, vertical overclosure, and upward and forward rotation of the mandible. **E** through **H,** Intraoral, facial, and profile views at 11 years and 1 month of age, 2 years and 3 months postretention. **I** and **J,** Three-way PEA in place. **K** and **L,** Posttreatment occlusal views.

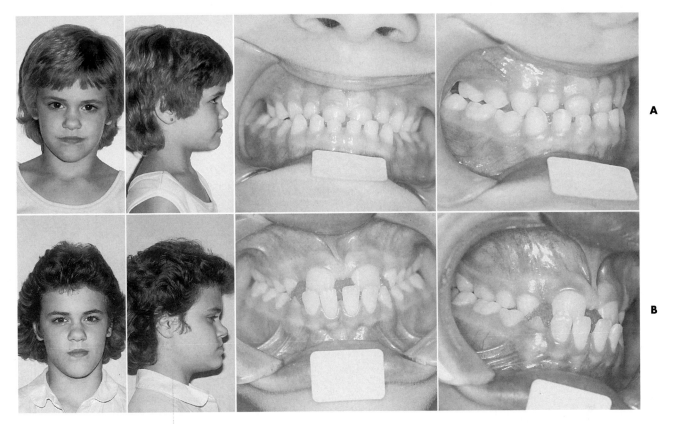

**Figure 15-3.** **A,** Patient with a Class III malocclusion at 6 years and 6 months of age. **B,** Same patient at 10 years and 3 months. Second-opinion orthodontist advised against orthopedic guidance because patient was too young. As a result, 4 years of adverse growth occurred unnecessarily.

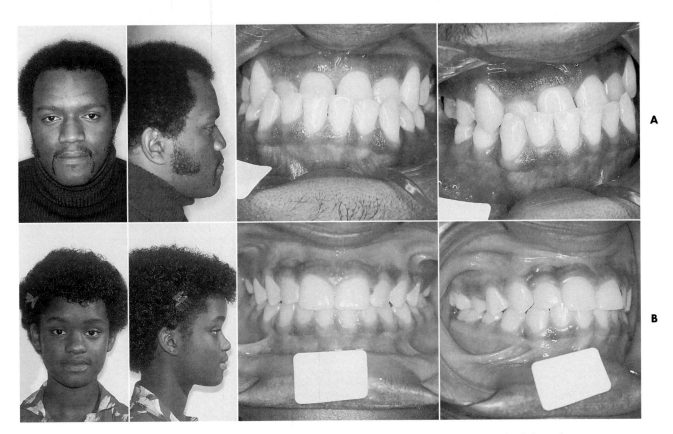

**Figure 15-4.** Prognathic parents do not always produce prognathic children. **A,** The father of this patient had a marked untreated prognathic pattern type of malocclusion. **B,** The daughter was treated at 5 years with a bonded PEA, protraction headgear, and limited retention. The finished photographs are taken at 12 years with no additional treatment.

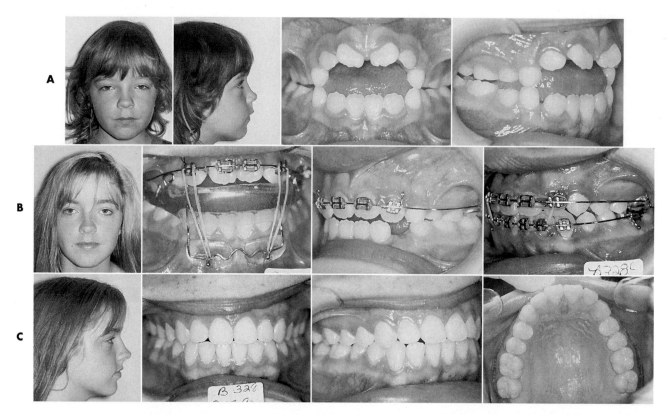

**Figure 15-5.** **A,** A patient with Class II, division 1 malocclusion with open bite and abnormal tongue function and posture. **B,** Treatment employing a bonded PEA, followed by a modified activator with fixed appliances and a lip bumper successfully closed the open bite. **C,** 8 years later and well out of treatment, the orthodontic correction is stable.

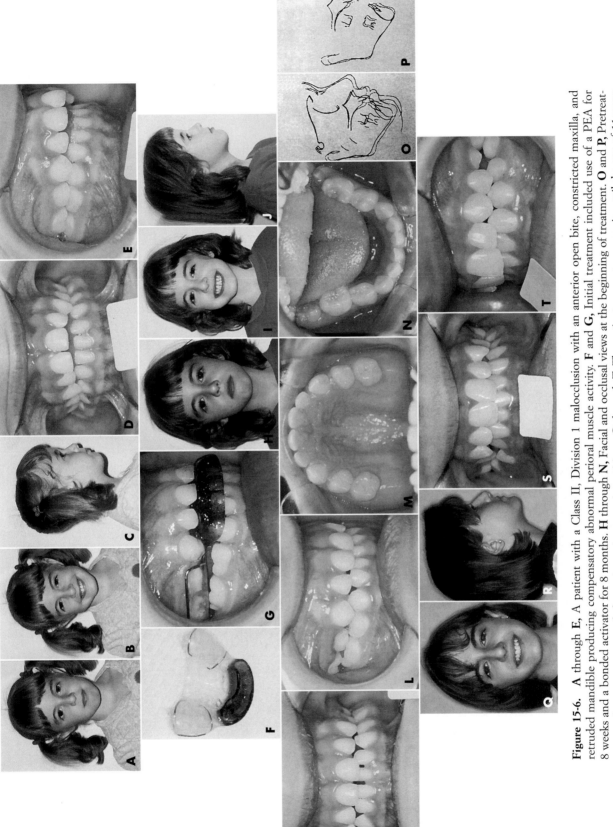

**Figure 15-6.**   A through E, A patient with a Class II, Division 1 malocclusion with an anterior open bite, constricted maxilla, and retruded mandible producing compensatory abnormal perioral muscle activity. F and G, Initial treatment included use of a PEA for 8 weeks and a bonded activator for 8 months. H through N, Facial and occlusal views at the beginning of treatment. O and P, Pretreatment and posttreatment cephalometric tracing superimpositions. Q through T, The patient was not seen again until the age of 11 years and 6 months. She will require modest fixed mechanotherapy, but the facial improvement remains. No extractions are planned.

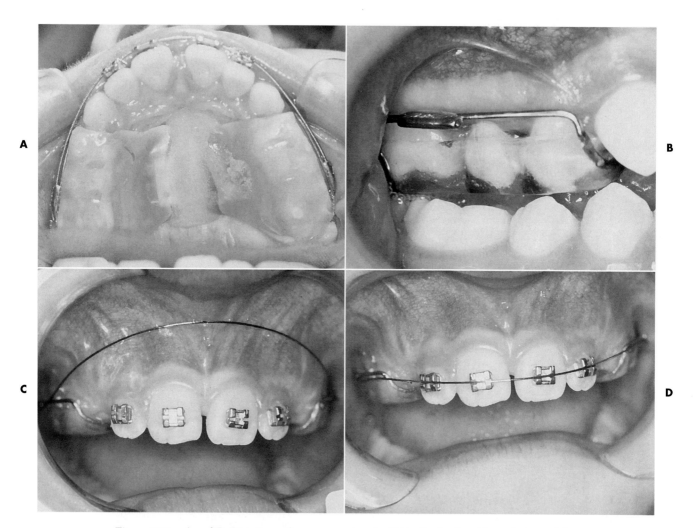

**Figure 15-7.**  **A** and **B,** Variations of treatment using the PEA. Occlusal and buccal views of the PEA after closure of midpalatal expansion area with acrylic. **B,** Buccal tubes on bonded PEA. **C** and **D,** PEA use with 2 × 4 fixed attachments and incisor intrusion arch before and after placement in anterior brackets.

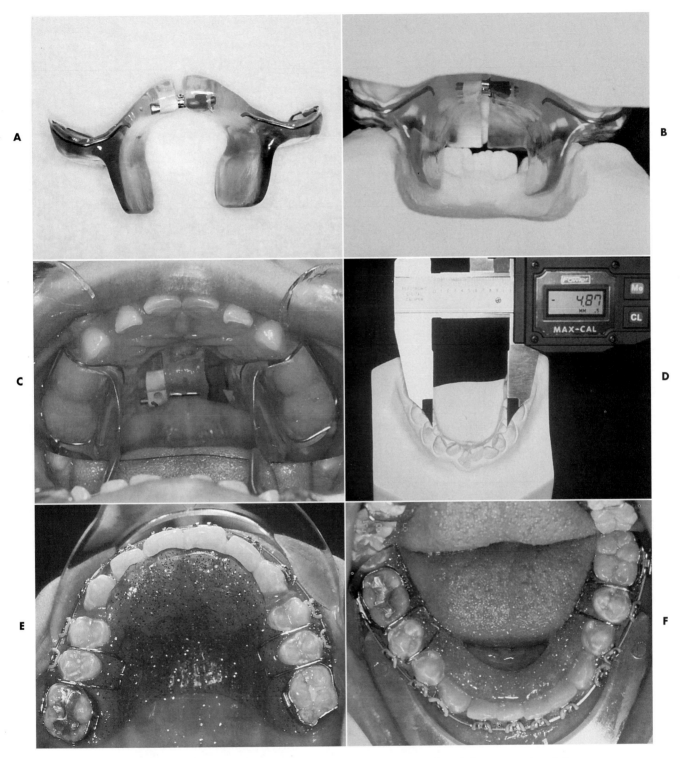

**Figure 15-8.** Treatment with DAE appliance. **A** and **B,** The length and close apposition of the mandibular flanges. **C,** DAE bonded in the mouth. Note the expansion screw. **D,** Plaster casts showing caliper measurements of 4.87 mm of expansion achieved in the lower arch. **E** and **F,** Maxillary and mandibular holding arches.

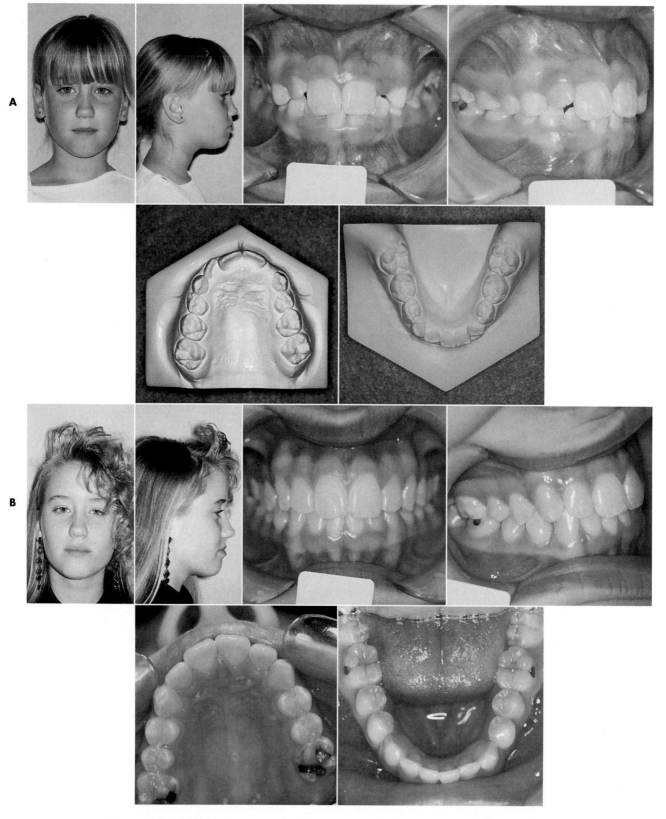

**Figure 15-9.    A,** This 8-year, 9-month-old girl was considered a borderline extraction case. Note blocked out lower canines. Clinical indications were for two-phase treatment, starting with a bonded DAE appliance. A lower, 2 × 4 fixed appliance also was used in the first phase. **B,** The patient returned at 14 years and 7 months with no second period of treatment. Some slenderizing of lower incisors occurred with use of a spring retainer. Treatment timing was vitally important in this case.

## STATE OF THE ART ORTHODONTICS: 2001

Facial orthopedics and functional treatment, particularly at early ages, are inexact and incompletely understood clinical sciences at this time. Orthodontists' improved abilities to scientifically, accurately, and differentially diagnose preschool children with dentofacial problems will eventually help establish more definitive criteria for early treatment. However, the biology of facial growth and development dictates that in the presence of a recognizable and significantly severe facial dysplasia, orthodontists acquit themselves as facial orthopedists. The same biology dictates that treatment of children with facial dysplasias be initiated at the earliest possible and convenient age. The earlier the child with a severe facial and skeletal dysplasia is treated, the sooner normal function and enhanced facial growth and development can ensue.

In the meantime, state of the art orthodontic treatment largely embraces the sound and perhaps more comfortable (from pragmatic practice management and orthodontist's peace of mind perspectives) posture of initiating treatment in patients in the late mixed dentition stage of development. With varying degrees of success, orthodontists preserve the "E" space, take advantage of the limited remaining potential for facial skeletal growth, choose their own appliances, and manage the patient's dentition through the final eruption of the permanent teeth. Although the synergistic system is an excellent treatment modality to use during these procedures, treatment timing must be carefully coordinated with the exchange of dentition and eruption of teeth; the appliance should fit the needs of the patient, not vice versa.

Orthodontists have taken modest strides toward recognizing their potentials as facial orthopedists; the potential is beyond imagination. Only when most graduate orthodontic departments become excited about not only the biologic, scientific, and research aspects of facial and skeletal orthopedics but also the clinical methodologies of early correction and require that residents treat preschool patients as a part of their clinical experiences will the art and science of facial orthopedics in the United States achieve its full potential.

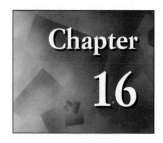

# Chapter 16

# The Modern Herbst Appliance

Hans Pancherz

At the International Dental Congress in Berlin in 1909, Herbst presented a fixed–bite jumping device called *Scharnier,* or joint (Figure 16-1). (Bite jumping is the production of a change in sagittal intermaxillary jaw relationship by anterior displacement of the mandible.) The Herbst appliance keeps the mandible continuously in a protruded position both when the jaws close and the teeth are not in occlusion. Because jaw and muscle function is changed, the appliance can be considered a fixed functional appliance.

In 1934, Herbst (1934) and Schwarz (1934) presented a series of articles on their experiences with the appliance. Herbst employed the appliance most usefully in the following instances: (1) in patients with Class II malocclusions and retrognathic mandibles, (2) in the facilitating of healing after mandibular ramus fractures, (3) in the capacity of an artificial joint after surgical resection of the condylar head, and (4) in patients with temporomandibular joint (TMJ) problems such as clicking and bruxism. After 1934, however, very little was published about the Herbst appliance, and the treatment method was more or less forgotten.

In 1977, Pancherz resurrected the Herbst appliance for use as an experimental tool in clinical research. In comparison with removable functional appliances such as the activator, bionator, and Fränkel appliance, the Herbst appliance has several advantages:

1. It is fixed to the teeth.
2. Patient compliance is not required for its correct function.
3. It works 24 hours a day.
4. Treatment time is short (approximately 6 to 8 months).

In the October 1979 issue of the *American Journal of Orthodontics,* Pancherz (1979) called attention to the possibilities for stimulation of mandibular growth by means of the Herbst appliance. In subsequent articles, he and various coworkers* evaluated the short- and long-term effects of the appliance on occlusion, the dentofacial complex, and the masticatory system.

Since 1979 the Herbst appliance has gained increasing attention, especially in Europe and the United States.* The Herbst appliance method has been found most useful in the management of severe Class II malocclusions.

## DESIGN

The Herbst appliance can be likened to an artificial joint working between the maxilla and mandible. A bilateral telescopic mechanism attached to orthodontic bands keeps the mandible in an anterior jumped position (see Figure 16-1). Each telescopic device consists of a tube, a plunger, two pivots, and two locking screws that prevent the telescoping parts from slipping past the pivots (Figure 16-2). The pivot for the tube is usually soldered to the maxillary first molar band, and the pivot for the plunger is affixed to the mandibular first premolar band. The length of the tube determines the amount of bite jumping. Usually the mandible is retained in an incisal end-to-end relationship.

A large interpivot distance prevents the plunger from slipping out of the tube when the mouth is opened wide. Therefore the upper pivot should be placed distally on the molar band, and the lower pivot should be placed mesially on the premolar band. The length of the plunger should be kept at a maximum to prevent it from disengaging from the tube. If the plunger is too long, however, it may protrude too far behind the tube and injure the buccal mucosa distal to the maxillary permanent first molar. If the plunger disengages from the tube on mouth opening, it may get stuck in the tube opening on subsequent mouth closure and damage the appliance (i.e., break or loosen the bands).

The anchorage system of the Herbst appliance deserves consideration. In the maxillary dental arch the first premolars

*Hägg, Pancherz (1988); Hansen, Ieamnuseiuk, Pancherz (1995); Hansen, Pancherz (1992); Hansen, Pancherz, Hägg (1991); Hansen, Pancherz, Petersson (1990); Pancherz (1981, 1982ab, 1985, 1991, 1994); Pancherz, Anehus-Pancherz (1980, 1982, 1993, 1994); Pancherz, Fackel (1990); Pancherz, Hägg (1985); Pancherz, Hansen (1986, 1988); Pancherz, Littmann (1988, 1989); Pancherz et al (1989); Pancherz, Stickel (1989); and Sarnäs et al (1982).

*Amoric (1995); Bakke, Paulsen (1989); Breads (1984); Champagne (1989); Hägg (1992); How (1982, 1983, 1984, 1987); Langford (1981, 1982); McNamara (1988); McNamara, How (1988); McNamara, How, Dischinger (1990); Pangrazio-Kulbersch, Berger (1993); Paulsen et al (1995); Rider (1988); Schiavoni (1988); Schiavoni, Grenga, Macri (1992); Sessle et al (1990); Sidhu, Kharabanda, Sidhu (1995); Wieslander (1993); Windmiller (1993); Woodside, Metaxas, Altuna (1987); and Zreik (1994).

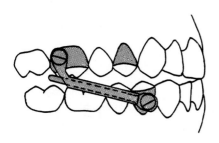

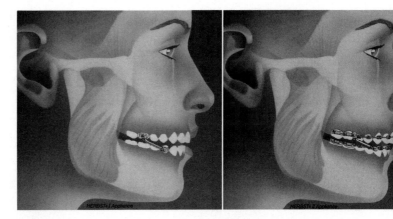

**Figure 16-1.** Working position of the Herbst appliance with the teeth in occlusion. (Middle and right illustrations courtesy Dentaurum, Newtown, Penn.)

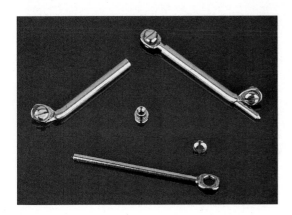

**Figure 16-2.** The disassembled telescopic mechanism of the Herbst appliance. This mechanism is available in pairs; it is of a standard length.

and permanent first molars are banded and interconnected on each side with a half-round (1.5 × 0.75 mm) or round (1 mm) lingual or buccal sectional arch wire. In the mandibular dental arch the first premolars are banded and connected with a half-round (1.5 × 0.75 mm) or round (1 mm) lingual sectional arch wire that touches the lingual surfaces of the front teeth. This form of anchorage is called *partial anchorage* (Figure 16-3, *A*). In some instances this type of anchorage is insufficient and therefore must be increased by the incorporation of additional dental units. In the maxillary dental arch a labial arch wire is attached to brackets on the first premolars, canines, and incisors. In the mandibular dental arch the lingual sectional arch wire is extended to the permanent first molars, which are also banded. This form of anchorage is called *total anchorage* (Figure 16-3, *B*).

In the current version of the Herbst appliance the bands are replaced by splints cast from a cobalt-chromium alloy and cemented to the teeth with a glass-ionomer cement. The upper and lower front teeth are incorporated into the anchorage through the addition of sectional arch wires (Figure 16-3, *C*). The cast-splint appliance ensures a precise fit on the teeth. It is strong and hygenic, saves chair time, and causes very few clinical problems.

## Modifications in Appliance Design

In patients with Class II malocclusions who have narrow maxillary arches, expansion can be performed using the Herbst appliance by soldering a quad-helix lingual arch wire (Figure 16-4, *A*) or a rapid palatal expansion device (Figure 16-4, *B*) to the upper premolar and molar bands or to the splint.

## CONSTRUCTION OF THE BANDED HERBST APPLIANCE

The bands should be formed individually of orthodontic band material that is at least 0.15 mm thick to prevent the problems of loose and broken bands. Prefabricated bands break under the strains placed on them during treatment.

### First Visit

Alginate impressions for plaster casts of the upper and lower dental arches are made and sent to the laboratory. Separating springs are placed mesially and distally to the teeth that are to be banded.

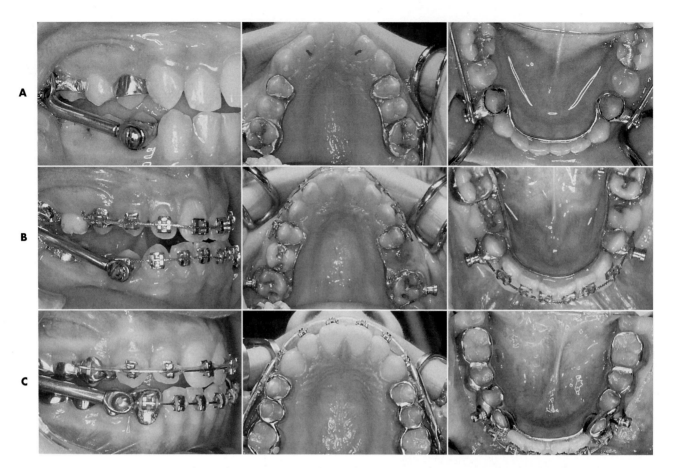

**Figure 16-3.** The anchorage system of the Herbst appliance. **A,** Partial anchorage (banded appliance). **B,** Total anchorage (banded appliance). **C,** Total anchorage (cast-splint appliance).

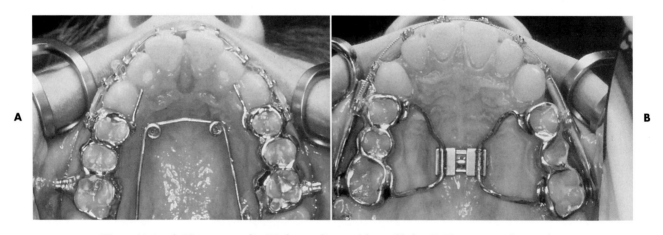

**Figure 16-4.** **A,** Upper cast-splint Herbst appliance with quad helix. **B,** Upper cast-splint Herbst appliance with rapid palatal expansion screw.

**Laboratory.** Bands are made at the laboratory from 0.15- to 0.18-mm thick orthodontic band material for the upper permanent first molars and upper and lower first premolars (Figure 16-5, *A*). The finished bands are sent back to the orthodontist.

## Second Visit

The bands are placed on the patient's teeth (Figure 16-5, *B*), and a construction bite is taken with the mandible advanced to the desired position (Figure 16-6). Alginate impressions are made while the bands are still on the teeth. The im-

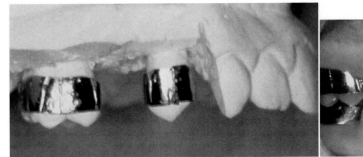
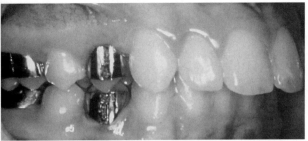

**Figure 16-5.** **A,** Bands made individually on maxillary plaster casts using orthodontic band material (5.0 mm × 0.15 mm). **B,** Appearance of the bands on the patient's teeth.

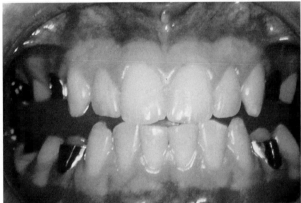
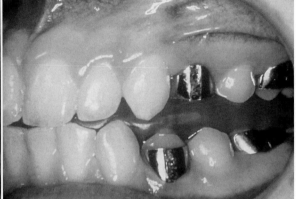

**Figure 16-6.** Different views of the construction bite. The mandible is advanced to an incisal end-to-end relation, and the teeth are in the correct midline position.

pressions, bands, and construction bite are sent back to the laboratory, and new separating springs are placed.

**Laboratory.** The bands are fixed in the impressions, and plaster models are poured. The banded models are oriented to each other in the construction bite and mounted in a fixator (Figure 16-7, *A*). The lingual arch wires and pivots for the telescoping mechanism are soldered to the bands. The use of a jig (Figure 16-7, *B*) facilitates orienting and soldering of the pivots to the bands. The tube and plunger are adjusted to fit the interpivot distance (Figure 16-7, *C*), and the pivot openings for the tube and plunger are widened (Figure 16-8, *A* and *B*) to provide a loose fit of the telescoping parts at their points of attachment, thus increasing the lateral movement capacity of the lower jaw (Figure 16-8, *C* and *D*). These mechanisms reduce the load on the anchorage teeth and bands during mandibular lateral excursion. The finished appliance (Figure 16-8, *E*) is then sent back to the orthodontist.

## Third Visit

At the third office visit the bands are cemented and the telescopic mechanism is attached to the pivots using a screw-

driver that firmly grips the locking screws (Figure 16-9). After placing the appliance, the clinician should assess the function of the telescoping mechanism as the patient opens the mouth. Interferences between the plunger and tube must be removed. The midline also should be noted; any necessary correction is accomplished by unilateral shortening of the appropriate tube or through the addition of advancement shims on the contralateral plunger (Figure 16-10, *A*). Finally, the lateral movement limit should be checked (Figure 16-10, *B* through *D*). The amount of lateral mandibular movement may be increased by the orthodontist by further widening of the maxillary and mandibular pivot openings (see Figure 16-8, *A* and *B*).

Before dismissal, the patient must be informed about the function of the Herbst mechanism and warned about the possibility of muscle discomfort and eating difficulties during the first week. After that time, however, adaptation to the appliance usually occurs and no further discomfort is felt. The patient is instructed by the practitioner to avoid hard and sticky food that may dislodge the appliance. If the telescoping elements come apart on wide opening of the mouth, the patient quickly learns to replace the lower plunger into the upper tube.

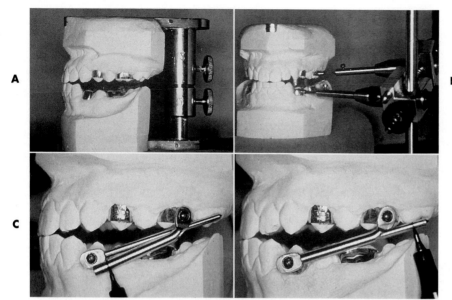

**Figure 16-7.** **A,** Dental casts in the construction bite in the fixator. **B,** Jig for the orientation of the telescoping pivots to the bands. The orientation jig is not currently available for purchase. **C,** Adjustment of the tube and plunger to fit the interpivot distance.

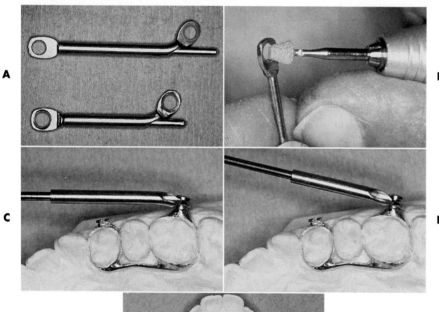

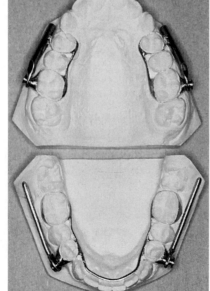

**Figure 16-8.** The telescoping tube before (**A**) and after (**B**) widening of the pivot openings. The lateral movement capacity of the tube before (**C**) and after (**D**) widening the pivot opening. **E,** The finished Herbst appliance. Note the brackets welded on the upper first premolar bands.

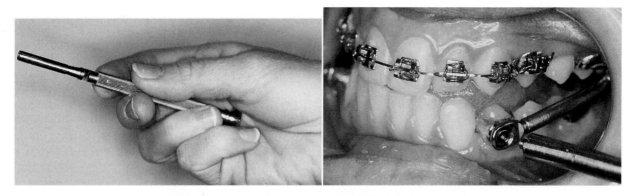

**Figure 16-9.** Screwdriver for firm gripping of the locking screws.

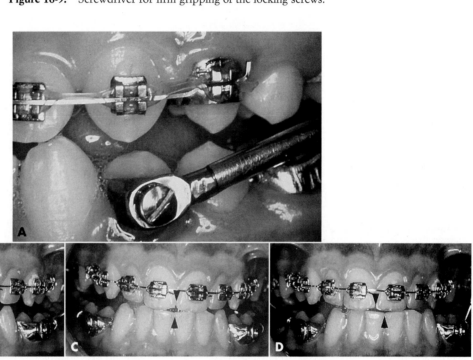

**Figure 16-10.** **A,** Mandibular advancement shim added to the plunger. Lateral mandibular movements with the Herbst appliance. **B,** To the right. **C,** In neutral position. **D,** To the left.

## CONSTRUCTION OF THE CAST-SPLINT HERBST APPLIANCE

In comparison with the banded Herbst appliance, the orthodontist's clinical work with the cast-splint appliance is much easier, and chair time is shortened. The laboratory work, on the other hand, is more time consuming, and the appliance is more expensive.

### First Visit

Alginate impressions for plaster casts of the upper and lower dentition are made, and a construction bite is taken. The impressions and the wax bite are sent to the laboratory.

**Laboratory.** Maxillary and mandibular splints are cast from cobalt-chromium alloy. The lower lingual arch wire and

the pivots for the plunger and tube are soldered to the splints. The lengths and pivot opening of the telescoping tube and plunger are adjusted. The same procedure is used as with the banded Herbst appliance (see Figures 16-7 and 16-8).

### Second Visit

The splints are cemented and the telescopic mechanism is adapted. Patient education is the same as with the banded Herbst appliance.

## EFFECTS ON THE DENTOFACIAL COMPLEX

The effects of the Herbst appliance on occlusion and maxillary and mandibular growth are discussed in this chapter.

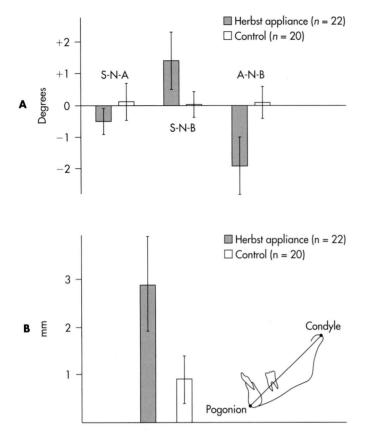

**Figure 16-11.** **A,** Changes (mean and standard deviation) in the sella-nasion-subspinale angle (*SNA*), the sella-nasion-supramentale angle (*SNB*), and the subspinale-nasion-supramentale angle (*ANB*) over 6 months. **B,** Increase (mean and standard deviation) in mandibular length over 6 months.

The results are based on analyses of dental casts, lateral head films (in full occlusion and with the mouth wide open), and TMJ radiographs from consecutively treated patients with Class II, division 1 malocclusions and deep bites. Untreated patients with Class II malocclusions served as controls.

## Treatment Effects

The Herbst appliance is the most powerful and effective modality in the treatment of Class II malocclusions. Normalization of occlusion is generally accomplished with 6 to 8 months of treatment. Overcorrected sagittal dental arch relationships and incomplete cuspal interdigitation at the end of treatment are to be expected before settling occurs. The improvement in the sagittal and vertical occlusal relationships during treatment is a result of both skeletal and dental changes (Pancherz, 1982ab).

**Sagittal changes.** The Herbst appliance restrains maxillary growth and stimulates mandibular growth (Hägg, Pancherz, 1988; Pancherz, 1979, 1982a; Pancherz, Hägg, 1985) (Figure 16-11, *A* and *B*). Sagittal condylar growth increases, whereas vertical condylar growth is relatively unaffected (Pancherz, Littmann, 1988, 1989) (Figure 16-12). Furthermore, bone re-

modeling processes in the lower mandibular border change the morphology of the mandible (Pancherz, Littmann, 1989). This change may be a result of an altered muscle function pattern during therapy (Pancherz, Anehus-Pancherz, 1980). The ultimate condylar position is unaffected by treatment (Pancherz, Stickel, 1989) (Figure 16-13). Some experimental and radiographic evidence indicates, however, that the articular fossa is repositioned anteriorly in the skull (Decrue, Wieslander, 1990; Pancherz, 1979, 1981) (see Chapter 4). These findings are in agreement with histologic studies performed in monkeys.*

Extensive dental changes occur in the maxilla and mandible during therapy (Pancherz, 1982a; Pancherz, Hansen, 1986). The mandibular teeth are moved anteriorly, the incisors are proclined, and the maxillary molars are moved posteriorly (Figures 16-14 and 16-15). The effect of the Herbst appliance on the maxillary molar teeth is essentially comparable with that of a high-pull headgear (Pancherz, Anehus-Pancherz, 1993). The teeth are both distalized and intruded. (A quantitative evaluation of sagittal skeletal and dental changes contributing to Class II molar correction and overjet correction is provided in Figures 16-16 and 16-17.)

In summary, the following changes contribute to Herbst appliance correction of Class II malocclusion:

1. Stimulation of mandibular growth
2. Inhibition of maxillary growth (a less important change)
3. Distal movement of the upper dentition
4. Mesial movement of the lower dentition (proclination of the incisors)

**Vertical changes.** In Class II malocclusions with deep bites, overbite may be reduced significantly by Herbst therapy (Pancherz, 1982b). Overbite reduction is primarily accomplished by intrusion of the lower incisors and enhanced eruption of the lower molars (Figure 16-18). Part of the registered changes in the vertical position of the mandibular incisors results from proclination of these teeth, however.

Because of the vertical dental changes, the maxillary and mandibular occlusal planes tip down (see Figure 16-18, *B*). Nevertheless, the appliance has a limited effect on maxillary and mandibular jaw position as expressed by the palatal plane angle (NL/NSL) and mandibular plane angle (ML/NSL) (see Figure 16-18, *C*).

## Early Posttreatment Effects

After the Herbst appliance is removed at the end of treatment, overcorrected sagittal dental arch relationships and incomplete cuspal interdigitation are generally seen. Because active treatment is short (6 to 8 months), the occlusion is unstable and adaptive occlusal changes tend to occur (Pancherz, 1981; Pancherz, Hansen, 1986) (Figure 16-19).

During the first year posttreatment the occlusion settles into a Class I relationship (Figure 16-20). The overjet and

*Baume, Derichsweiler (1961); Breitner (1930); Elgoyen et al (1972); McNamara (1973, 1976); Stöckli, Willert (1971); and Woodside, Metaxas, Altuna (1987).

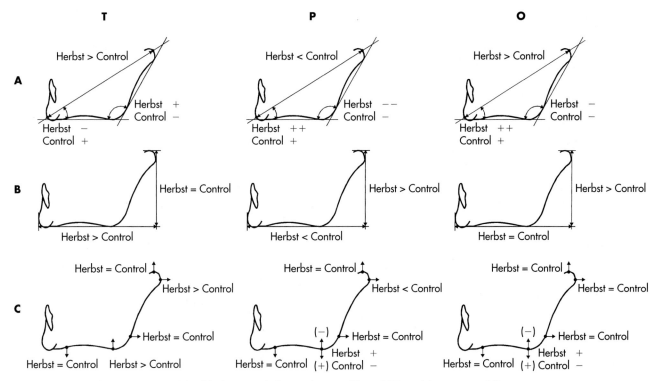

**Figure 16-12.** Mandibular morphologic changes (**A** and **B**) and bone remodeling processes (**C**) in 12 boys with Class II, division 1 malocclusions treated consecutively with the Herbst appliance. *T,* Treatment period of 6 months; *P,* posttreatment period of 7 years (to the end of growth); *O,* total observation period of 7½ years.

sagittal molar relationships recover about 30% of their previous dimensions. Approximately 90% of the posttreatment occlusal changes occur during the first 6 months after treatment and are mostly of dental origin (Pancherz, Hansen, 1986) (see Figure 16-20). The upper teeth (especially the molars) move anteriorly, the lower teeth move posteriorly, and the incisors become upright.

An unfavorable maxillomandibular growth relationship contributes to only a minor degree to early posttreatment occlusal changes. A catch-up in maxillary growth and a minor reduction in mandibular growth are apparent in subjects treated with the Herbst appliance in comparison with untreated controls (Pancherz, 1981; Pancherz, Hansen, 1986).

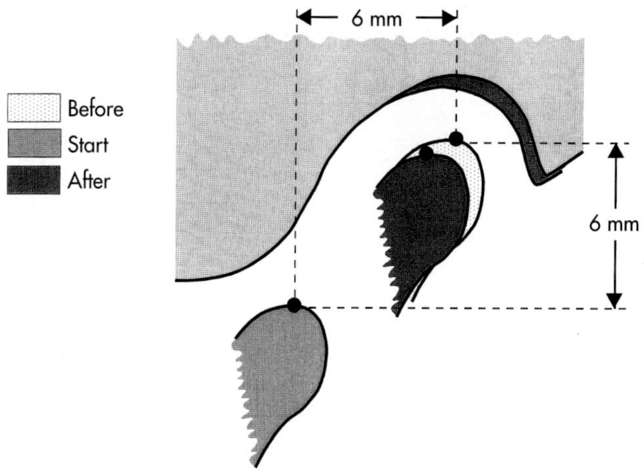

## Late Posttreatment Effects

When examining patients treated with the Herbst appliance 5 to 10 years after treatment, the clinician usually notes several effects. A Class I dental arch relationship is maintained by a stable cuspal interdigitation of the upper and lower teeth, whereas relapse tends to occur in cases with unstable occlusal conditions (Pancherz, 1981). In several Herbst studies* the importance of a good posttreatment occlusal intercuspation has been emphasized for the prevention of dental and skeletal relapse. Teeth locked in a stable Class I intercuspation are

*Text continued on p. 348*

**Figure 16-13.** Average changes in condylar position as observed in an analysis of 30 boys treated consecutively with the Herbst appliance. Measurements were taken before treatment, at the start of treatment (when the appliance was placed), and after treatment (when the appliance was removed).

*(Pancherz, 1982a, 1991, 1994; Pancherz, Hägg, 1985; Pancherz, Hansen, 1986; Wieslander, 1993).

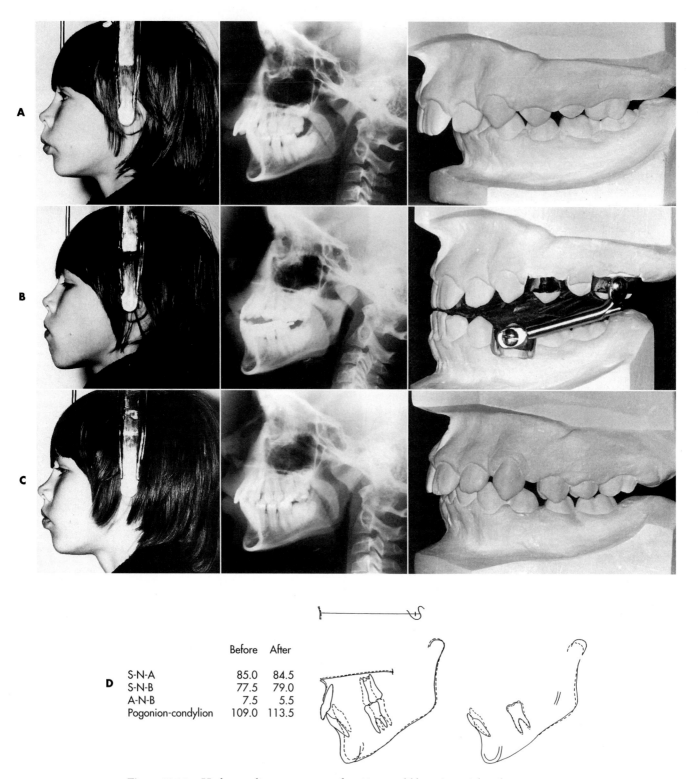

|   | Before | After |
|---|--------|-------|
| S-N-A | 85.0 | 84.5 |
| S-N-B | 77.5 | 79.0 |
| A-N-B | 7.5 | 5.5 |
| Pogonion-condylion | 109.0 | 113.5 |

**Figure 16-14.** Herbst appliance treatment of an 11-year-old boy. A partial anchorage system was used. **A,** Before treatment. **B,** At the start of treatment. **C,** After treatment and removal of the appliance. **D,** Superimposed cephalometric tracings from before *(dotted lines)* and after *(solid lines)* treatment.

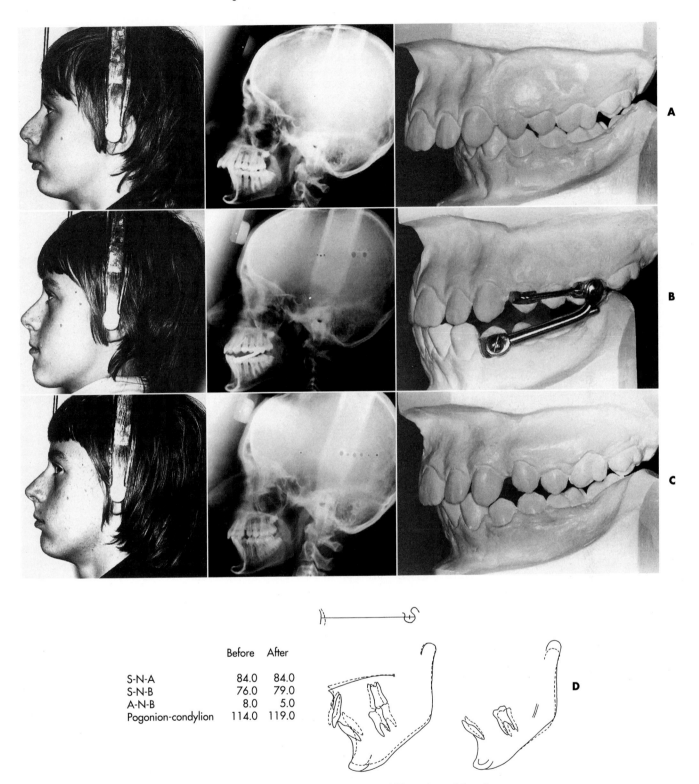

|  | Before | After |
|---|---|---|
| S-N-A | 84.0 | 84.0 |
| S-N-B | 76.0 | 79.0 |
| A-N-B | 8.0 | 5.0 |
| Pogonion-condylion | 114.0 | 119.0 |

**Figure 16-15.** Herbst appliance treatment of a 12-year-old boy. A partial anchorage system was used. **A,** Before treatment. **B,** At the start of treatment. **C,** After treatment and removal of the appliance. **D,** Superimposed cephalometric tracings from before *(dotted lines)* and after *(solid lines)* treatment.

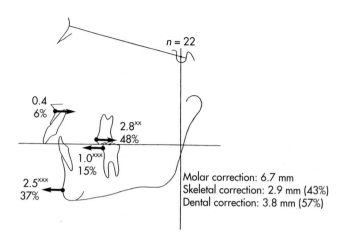

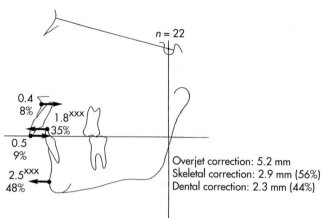

Molar correction: 6.7 mm
Skeletal correction: 2.9 mm (43%)
Dental correction: 3.8 mm (57%)

Overjet correction: 5.2 mm
Skeletal correction: 2.9 mm (56%)
Dental correction: 2.3 mm (44%)

**Figure 16-16.** Sagittal skeletal and dental changes in millimeters (mean values) and percentage of contribution to Class II molar correction during 6 months of Herbst appliance treatment. *xx,* Significant at 1% level; *xxx,* Significant at 0.1% level.

**Figure 16-17.** Sagittal skeletal and dental changes in millimeters (mean values) and percentage of contribution to overjet correction during 6 months of Herbst appliance treatment. *xxx,* Significant at 0.1% level.

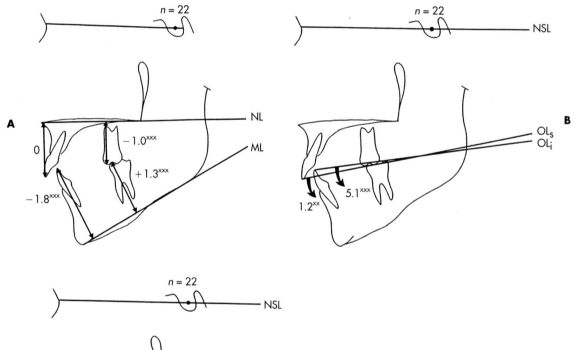

**Figure 16-18.** Vertical linear changes (in millimeters) and angular changes (in degrees) (mean values) during 6 months of Herbst appliance treatment. **A,** Tooth position changes. **B,** Occlusal plane changes. **C,** Jaw base changes. *xx,* Significant at 1% level; *xxx,* Significant at 0.1% level.

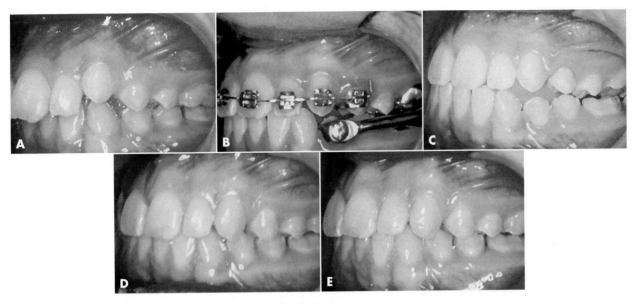

**Figure 16-19.** Herbst appliance treatment of a 12-year-old girl. **A,** Before treatment. **B,** During treatment. **C,** After 8 months of treatment (on the day the appliance was removed). Note the overcorrected sagittal dental arch relationships. **D,** Approximately 6 months posttreatment. The occlusion has settled. **E,** Approximately 12 months posttreatment.

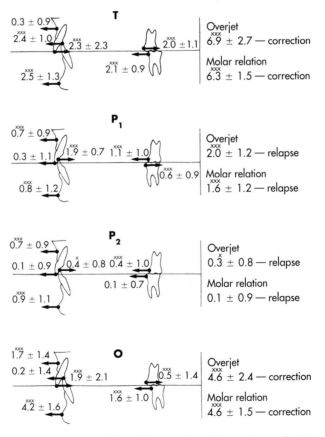

**Figure 16-20.** Sagittal, skeletal, and dental changes (in millimeters) contributing to alterations in overjet and molar relationships in 40 Class II, division 1 malocclusions treated with the Herbst appliance. Registrations (mean and standard deviation) during the treatment period (*T*) of 7 months, posttreatment period 1 (*P₁*) of 6 months, posttreatment period 2 (*P₂*) of 6 months and total observation period (*O*) of 19 months. *x,* Significant at 5% level; *xxx,* significant at 0.1% level.

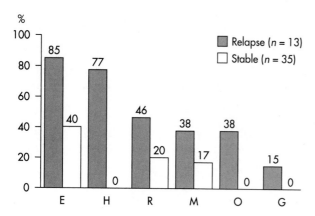

**Figure 16-21.** Long-term effects of Herbst appliance treatment on overjet. Analysis of patients 5 to 10 years posttreatment to assess frequency of relapse factors in 13 relapse and 35 stable cases. *E,* Early treatment; *H,* persisting habits; *R,* no posttreatment retention; *M,* mixed dentition treatment; *O,* unstable posttreatment occlusion; *G,* unfavorable posttreatment growth.

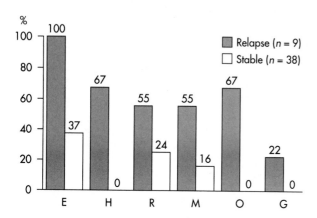

**Figure 16-22.** Long-term effects of Herbst treatment on sagittal molar relationships. Analysis of patients 5 to 10 years posttreatment to assess frequency of relapse factors in 9 relapse and 38 stable cases. *E,* Early treatment; *H,* persisting habits; *R,* no posttreatment retention; *M,* mixed dentition treatment; *O,* unstable posttreatment occlusion; *G,* unfavorable posttreatment growth.

more likely to transfer maxillary growth forces to the mandible (or vice versa) and thus possibly act as restricting or stimulating factors on mandibular growth. Thus a functionally stable occlusion after Herbst or any orthodontic therapy could be more important for lasting treatment results than the posttreatment growth pattern (Pancherz, Fackel, 1990).

When comparing Herbst patients with and without relapse in overjet and sagittal molar relationships and relating the relapse to selected relapse-promoting factors, Pancherz (1994) found that the most frequent combination of factors was early treatment, mixed dentition treatment, persistent lip or tongue dysfunction habits, and unstable posttreatment occlusion (Figures 16-21 and 16-22). Unfavorable posttreatment growth, however, is not a significant factor for occlusal relapse.

Although early treatment seems to be an important factor for relapse, it may not be responsible for the relapse. Because early treatment usually implies mixed dentition treatment, a solid Class I cuspal interdigitation is usually not attained. Thus the primary cause for the relapse is the unstable occlusion after therapy and not the maturity period in which the patients are treated.

In the same way, clinicians have to interpret the consequences of the atypical swallowing habits found in a large number of subjects who relapse (see Figures 16-21 and 16-22). Because of these habits, normal retention by the functionally occluding teeth is impaired; the teeth are less fre-

quently in occlusal contact than is the case in normal swallowing (Ballard, 1953; Rix, 1953).

A relapse example is presented in Figure 16-23. The subject is a girl whose Class II malocclusion was treated twice with the Herbst appliance, first in the mixed dentition and then in the permanent dentition.

In analyzing the long-term effects of Herbst treatment in relation to normal growth records of subjects exhibiting excellent occlusion (Bolton standards), researchers have noted that the appliance improves the sagittal jaw base skeletal relationship but does not normalize it (Broadbent, Broadbent, Golden, 1975; Hansen, Pancherz, 1992) (Figure 16-24). The sagittal dental arch relationship, on the other hand, is almost normalized (Hansen, Ieamnuseiuk, Pancherz, 1995). Thus the dental effects of the Herbst appliance used as part of a long-term treatment can compensate for an unfavorable jaw base relationship.

The high-pull headgear effect of the Herbst appliance on the upper molars (distalization and intrusion of the teeth) seems temporary. In cases of improper retention, recovering tooth movements occur posttreatment as the molars move mesially and extrude (Pancherz, Anehus-Pancherz, 1993) (Figures 16-25 and 16-26). Some changes, however, result from normal growth and development.

The long-term effect of Herbst appliance treatment on mandibular growth is difficult to judge. The increase in sagittal condylar growth and changes in mandibular morphology

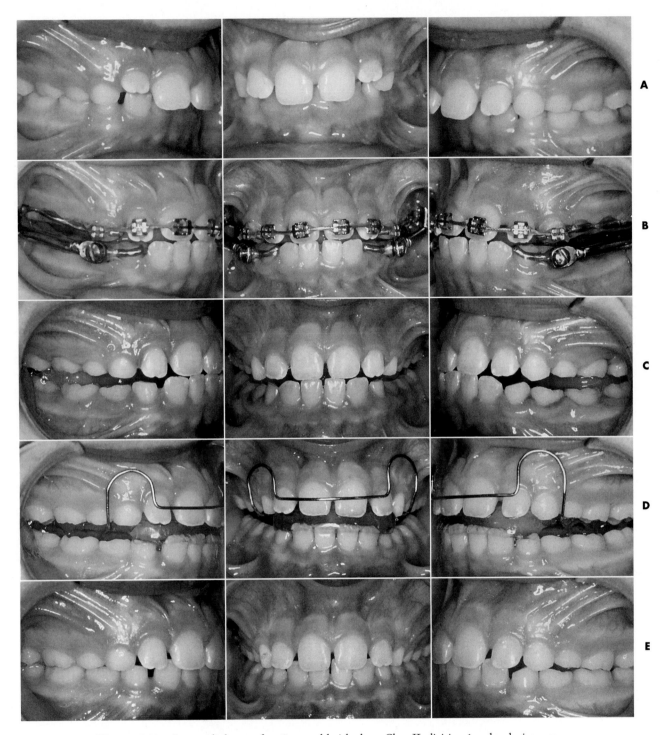

**Figure 16-23.** Intraoral photos of an 8-year-old girl whose Class II, division 1 malocclusion was treated twice with the Herbst appliance, once in the mixed dentition and once in the permanent dentition. **A,** Before treatment. **B,** During the first phase of Herbst treatment. **C,** After 6 months of treatment, when the appliance was removed. Note the overcorrected Class I dental arch relationship and the incomplete cuspal interdigitation. **D,** During retention with an activator for 9 months. **E,** After activator retention. Note the unstable occlusion.  *Continued.*

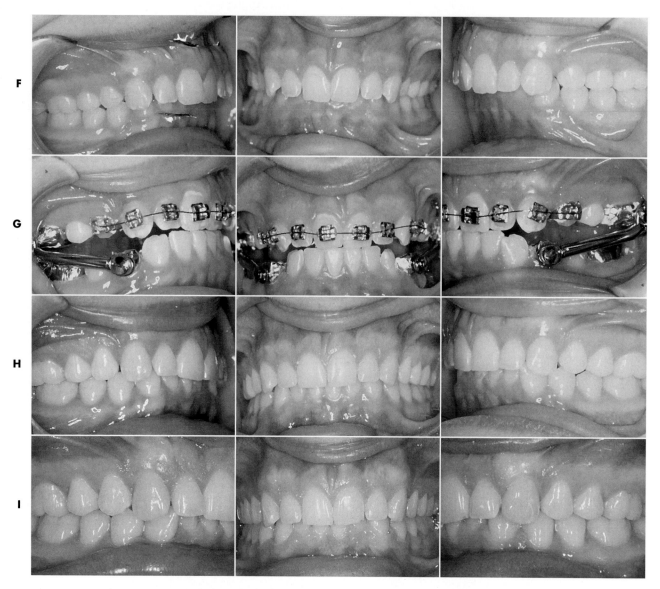

**Figure 16-23, cont'd.** **F,** Appearance 4 years after activator retention. A complete Class II relapse is present. **G,** Retreatment with the Herbst appliance for 7 months. **H,** Appearance 6 months after the second phase of Herbst treatment and activator retention. Note the good cuspal interdigitation. **I,** Appearance 5 years posttreatment at the age of 19 years. Note the stable long-term result.

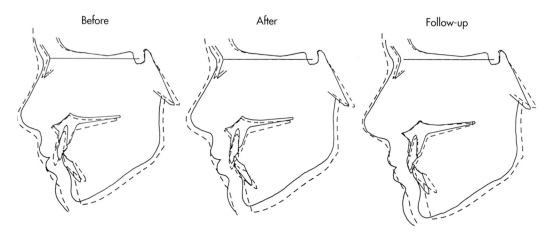

**Figure 16-24.** Composite tracings of 32 patients (16 girls and 16 boys) with Class II, division 1 malocclusions treated with the Herbst appliance (*dashed lines*), and composite tracings of 32 patients (16 girls and 16 boys) exhibiting excellent occlusion (Bolton standards) (*solid lines*). Registrations taken before treatment, 6 months after treatment, and 6¾ years after treatment.

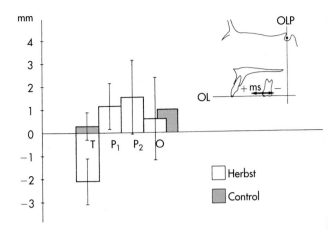

**Figure 16-25.** Sagittal maxillary molar position changes (mean and standard deviation) in 45 patients with Class II, division 1 malocclusions treated with the Herbst appliance. Registrations during four examination periods: treatment period of 7 months ($T$), posttreatment period 1 of 6 months ($P_1$), posttreatment period 2 of 5 to 10 years ($P_2$), and total observation period ($O$), comprising the periods T, $P_1$, and $P_2$.

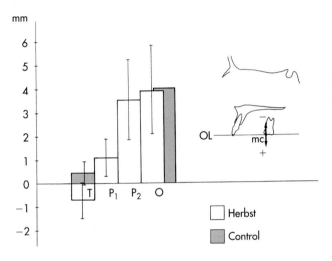

**Figure 16-26.** Vertical maxillary molar position changes (mean and standard deviation) in 45 patients with Class II, division 1 malocclusions treated with the Herbst appliance. Registrations during four examination periods: treatment period of 7 months ($T$), posttreatment period 1 of 6 months ($P_1$), posttreatment period 2 of 5 to 10 years ($P_2$), and total observation period ($O$), comprising the periods T, $P_1$, and $P_2$.

seen during treatment cannot be verified 7 years after therapy (Pancherz, Littmann, 1989) (see Figure 16-12). The Herbst appliance, as any other orthopedic appliance, has only a temporary impact on the existing skeletofacial growth pattern (Pancherz, Fackel, 1990). After the orthopedic intervention, maxillary and mandibular growth strives to catch up with its earlier pattern (Figure 16-27). Despite recovering growth changes after Herbst treatment, functional stability of the occlusion obviously counteracts occlusal relapses.

## EFFECTS ON THE FACIAL PROFILE

In one evaluation of the short- and long-term effects of the Herbst appliance on the soft-tissue profile, 49 patients with successfully treated Class II, division 1 malocclusions were surveyed (Pancherz, Anehus-Pancherz, 1994). The patients were treated for 7 months and followed for 5 to 10 years posttreatment. Lateral cephalometric radiographs from before treatment, start of treatment (when the appliance was placed), after treatment, 6 months posttreatment, and 5 to 10 years posttreatment were analyzed.

## Treatment Changes

Herbst appliance treatment generally results in a reduction of the hard- and soft-tissue profile convexity (Figure 16-28). The upper lip becomes retrusive, whereas the lower lip remains almost unchanged (Figure 16-29).

## Posttreatment Changes

As with other techniques, large individual variations exist in facial profile changes after Herbst therapy. On average, however, the following long-term posttreatment changes can be expected:

- Reduction in the soft-tissue profile (excluding the nose) convexity (see Figure 16-28) because of normal jaw growth changes (increases in mandibular prognathism)
- Increase in the soft-tissue profile (including the nose) convexity (see Figure 16-28) because of normal nose growth
- Retrusion of the upper and lower lips in relation to the esthetic line (see Figure 16-29) because of normal nose and chin growth

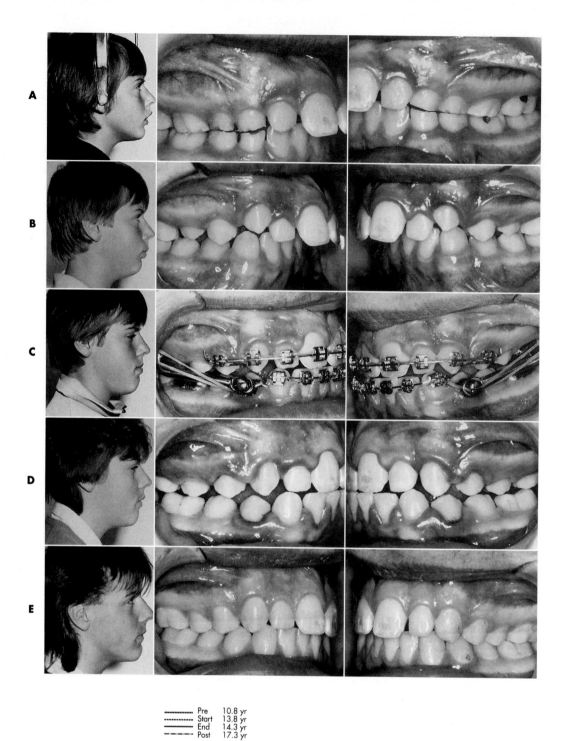

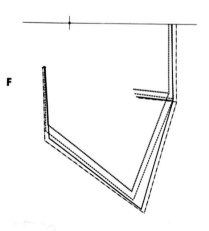

|  |  |  |
|---|---|---|
| ·················· | Pre | 10.8 yr |
| - - - - - - - - | Start | 13.8 yr |
| ——————— | End | 14.3 yr |
| —·—·—·— | Post | 17.3 yr |

**Figure 16-27.** Herbst appliance treatment of a 14-year-old boy. The pretreatment skeletofacial growth pattern changed during Herbst treatment and recovered after treatment. A stable cuspal interdigitation after Herbst therapy counteracted an occlusal relapse. **A,** Appearance 3 years pretreatment. **B,** At the start of Herbst treatment, before the appliance was placed. **C,** During Herbst treatment. Lower anchorage was increased with Class III elastics. **D,** At the end of 7 months of Herbst treatment and after appliance removal. **E,** Appearance 3 years posttreatment. **F,** Superimposed cephalometric polygons.

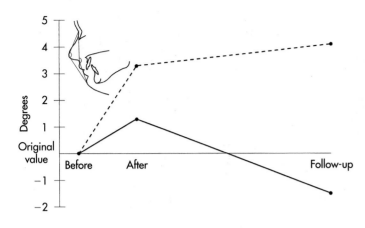

**Figure 16-28.** Mean changes in the soft-tissue facial profile angles, excluding *(dotted line)* and including *(solid line)* the nose, in 49 subjects treated with the Herbst appliance. Positive values imply profile convexity reduction. Negative values imply profile convexity increase. Measurements taken before treatment (the original value at 0), after 7 months of treatment (when the appliance was removed), and at follow-up 5 to 10 years posttreatment.

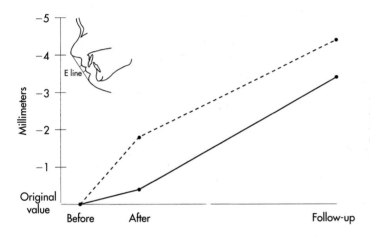

**Figure 16-29.** Mean changes in the position of the upper *(dotted line)* and lower *(solid line)* lips in relation to the esthetic line in 49 subjects treated with the Herbst appliance. Negative values imply lip retrusion. Measurements taken before treatment (the original value at 0), after 7 months of treatment (when the appliance was removed), and at follow-up 5 to 10 years posttreatment.

The facial profile photographs of four subjects whose Class II, division 1 malocclusions were successfully treated with the Herbst appliance are shown in Figure 16-30. Both short- and long-term improvement in facial appearance is apparent in all four cases.

The Herbst appliance improves the soft-tissue profile. The most favorable soft-tissue profile changes are seen in subjects with protrusive upper lips and retrusive chins and lower lips (see case 4 in Figure 16-30). Because of posttreatment growth changes, the long-term effects of therapy are, however, variable and unpredictable.

## EFFECTS ON THE MASTICATORY SYSTEM

Because the Herbst appliance continuously keeps the mandible in a protracted position, the harmonious interaction among the occluding teeth, masticatory muscles, and jaw joints is challenged.

### Masticatory Ability

Patients adapt to the appliance very quickly and accept it readily despite the fact that at the beginning of treatment, they have contact between the anterior teeth only. Chewing diffi-

culties are experienced only during the first 7 to 10 days of treatment. No subsequent problems are usually reported, although masticatory efficiency measurements indicate that the test material is poorly comminuted during the first 3 months of treatment (before antagonist contacts in the buccal segments have been established) (Pancherz, Anehus-Pancherz, 1982).

### Functional Disorders

Minor functional disturbances in the masticatory system (tenderness on palpation of the TMJ and masticatory muscles) are occasionally noted. These disturbances, however, are temporary and generally appear in the beginning of the treatment period (Pancherz, Anehus-Pancherz, 1982) (Figure 16-31). No adverse long-term effects of the Herbst appliance on the craniomandibular system have been found during examinations of patients at the end of their growth periods 7½ years posttreatment (Hansen, Pancherz, Petersson, 1990).

### Muscle Activity

Class II malocclusions produce deviations from the norm in electromyographic (EMG) patterns of the temporal and masseter muscles compared with normal occlusions (Pancherz,

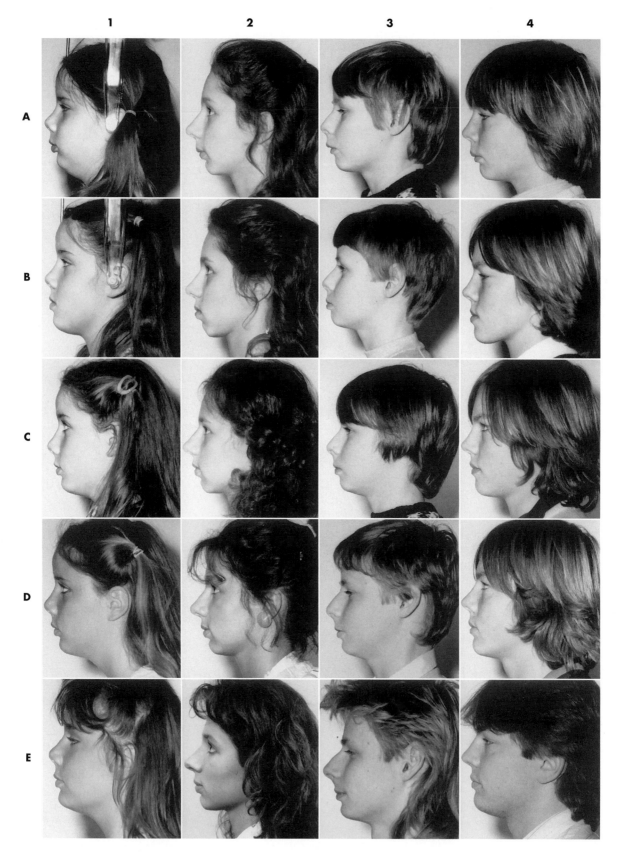

**Figure 16-30.** Facial profile photographs of two girls (cases 1 and 2) and two boys (cases 3 and 4) whose Class II, division 1 malocclusions were successfully treated with the Herbst appliance. **A,** Before treatment. **B,** At start of treatment (when the appliance was placed). **C,** After treatment (when the appliance was removed). **D,** Appearance 6 months posttreatment. **E,** Appearance 7 years posttreatment.

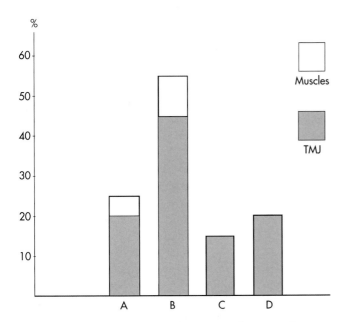

**Figure 16-31.** Frequency of tenderness on palpation in the masticatory muscles and TMJ. Registrations taken in 20 male subjects with Class II, division 1 malocclusions treated consecutively with the Herbst appliance. *A,* Before treatment. *B,* After 3 months of treatment. *C,* After 6 months of treatment (when the appliance was removed). *D,* Appearance 12 months posttreatment.

1980) (Figures 16-32 and 16-33). Treatment with the Herbst appliance normalizes the EMG pattern for these two muscles (Pancherz, Anehus-Pancherz, 1980) (Figure 16-34). Over time the muscle-contraction pattern in Herbst-treated patients becomes more like that seen in untreated adults with normal occlusion (Figures 16-35 and 16-36).

## Temporomandibular Joint

When analyzing lateral tomograms of the TMJ in consecutively treated Herbst patients at the end of their growth periods (7½ years posttreatment), researchers have noted a normal condyle-fossa relationship (Hansen, Pancherz, Petersson, 1990). No structural changes in the bony components of the condylar head and fossa can be found. Thus Herbst treatment apparently has no adverse effects on the TMJ over time. Research evidence indicates anterior positioning of the articular fossa, however (see Chapter 4).

## MANDIBULAR ANCHORAGE PROBLEMS

The telescopic mechanism of the Herbst appliance produces a posteriorly directed force on the upper dentition and an anteriorly directed force on the lower dentition. Resulting

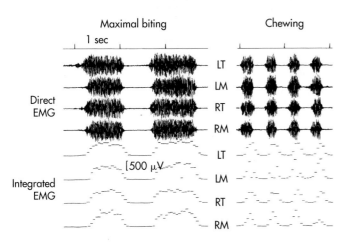

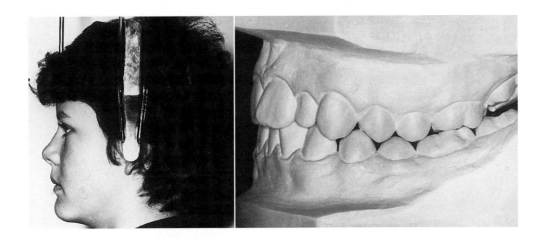

**Figure 16-32.** Electromyogram from a 12-year-old boy with a normal (Class I) occlusion. Note the harmonious EMG pattern. EMG registrations taken during maximal biting in intercuspal position and during chewing of peanuts. *LT,* Left temporal muscle; *LM,* left masseter muscle; *RT,* right temporal muscle; *RM,* right masseter muscle.

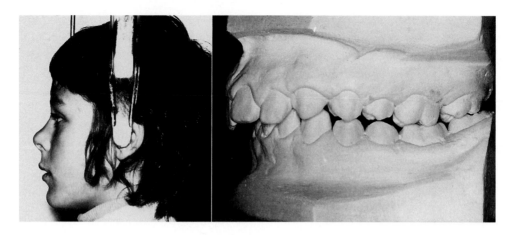

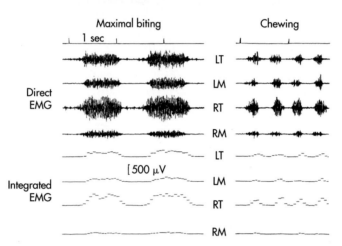

**Figure 16-33.** Electromyogram from a 12-year-old boy with a Class II, division 1 malocclusion. Note the disharmonious EMG pattern. EMG registrations taken during maximal biting in intercuspal position and during chewing of peanuts. *LT,* Left temporal muscle; *LM,* left masseter muscle; *RT,* right temporal muscle; *RM,* right masseter muscle.

tooth movements are consequences of anchorage loss. Clinically, anchorage loss in the maxilla (during the use of a partial anchorage system) appears as spaces developing between the canines and first premolars (see Figures 16-14 and 16-15). In the mandible, anchorage loss results in proclination of the anterior teeth (see Figures 16-14 and 16-15). In the correction of Class II malocclusion, posterior tooth movements in the maxilla are often desirable, whereas proclination of the lower incisors is generally undesirable.

Clinically, lower anchorage is difficult to master. In a comparison of five different nonextraction mandibular anchorage systems incorporating different numbers of teeth or using the lingual mucosa for anchorage (Figure 16-37), Pancherz and Hansen (1988) found that none of the systems prevented anterior movement of the lower dentition and proclination of the incisors (Figure 16-38). Although the lingual Pelot anchorage (acrylic lingual pad) seemed more effective than the tooth-borne anchorage, clinically it is less useful because it has a great tendency to cause ulceration of the lingual mucosa. Even in the updated cast-splint Herbst appliance (see Figure 16-3, *C*), proclination of the lower incisors is unavoidable.

The development of posttreatment lower incisor crowding

caused by relapsing incisor tooth movements seems not to be a clinical problem because not only the incisors but also the molars tend to move back to their former positions after Herbst therapy (see Figure 16-20). In one analysis of 65 patients treated with the Herbst appliance (Pancherz, Hansen, 1988), minor incisor crowding (less than 1 mm) developed 1 year posttreatment in 18% of the subjects; the available space was unchanged or increased in 82% of the subjects.

The possible development of mandibular incisor crowding over time is difficult to foresee and does not seem related to Herbst treatment itself. Figures 16-39 to 16-43 present mandibular dental arch changes in five patients with Class II, division 1 malocclusions treated with the Herbst appliance using different lower anchorage systems.

## INDICATIONS

The primary objective of the Herbst appliance is to stimulate mandibular growth; it is therefore especially useful for growing patients with skeletal Class II malocclusions (including division 1 and 2 malocclusions).

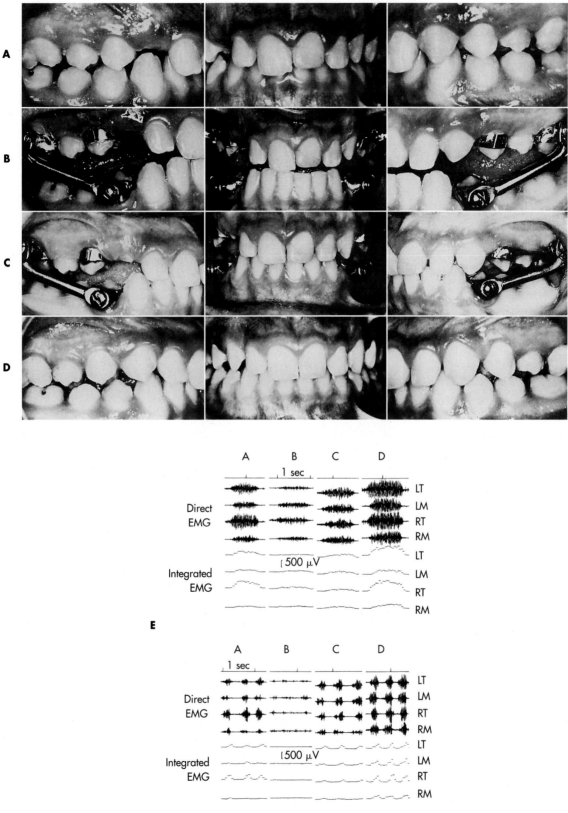

**Figure 16-34.** Intraoral photographs and EMGs from a 12-year-old boy with a Class II, division 1 malocclusion treated with the Herbst appliance. **A,** Before treatment. **B,** At the start of treatment (when the appliance was inserted). **C,** After 3 months of treatment. **D,** After 6 months of treatment (when the appliance was removed). **E,** EMG recordings during maximal biting in intercuspal position (*top*) and during chewing of peanuts (*bottom*). *LT,* Left temporal muscle; *LM,* left masseter muscle; *RT,* right temporal muscle; *RM,* right masseter muscle.

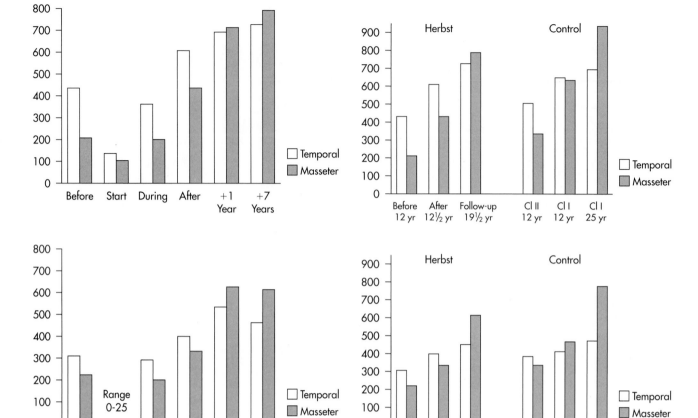

**Figure 16-35.** Maximal integrated EMG activity in μV from the temporal and masseter muscles during maximal biting in intercuspal position (*top*) and during chewing of peanuts (*bottom*). Registrations (mean values) were taken in 10 boys with Class II, division 1 malocclusions treated consecutively with the Herbst appliance. *Before,* Before treatment; *Start,* at start of treatment (when the appliance was inserted); *During,* after 3 months of treatment; *After,* after 6 months of treatment (when the appliance was removed); *+ 1 year,* 1 year posttreatment; *+ 7 years,* 7 years posttreatment.

**Figure 16-36.** Maximal integrated EMG activity in μV from the temporal and masseter muscles during maximal biting in intercuspal position (*top*) and during chewing of peanuts (*bottom*). Registrations (mean values) were taken in 10 boys with Class II, division 1 malocclusions treated consecutively with the Herbst appliance and in three groups of control subjects: 23 untreated boys with Class II, division 1 malocclusions; 23 boys with normal occlusions; and 21 young men with normal occlusions.

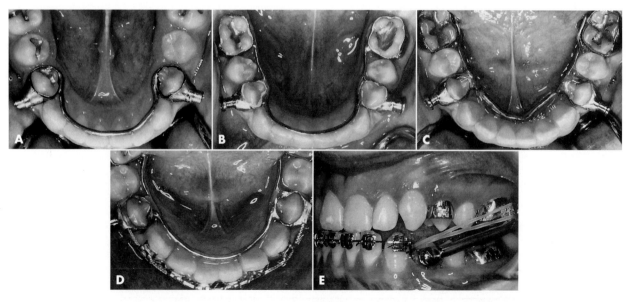

**Figure 16-37.** Intraoral photographs of five mandibular anchorage systems. **A,** Premolar anchorage. **B,** Premolar-molar anchorage. **C,** Acrylic and wire Pelot anchorage. **D,** Labial-lingual anchorage. **E,** Class III elastics.

This treatment method should be used with great caution in patients who have stopped growing. Skeletal alterations will be minimal, and treatment effects will be confined to the dentoalveolar area. Furthermore, risk for the development of a dual bite increases (Held, Spirgi, Cimasoni, 1963), with dysfunctional symptoms from the TMJ as a possible consequence (Egermark-Eriksson, Carlsson, Ingervall, 1979).

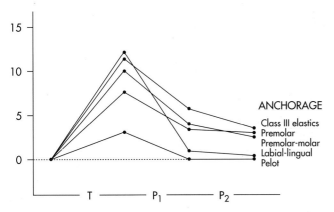

**Figure 16-38.** The average change (in degrees) in lower incisor tooth inclination in 65 patients with Class II, division 1 malocclusions treated with the Herbst appliance. Patients were divided into five anchorage groups: premolar anchorage ($n = 16$), premolar-molar anchorage ($n = 20$), Pelot anchorage ($n = 6$), labial-lingual anchorage ($n = 10$), and Class III elastics ($n = 13$). Registrations of changes were taken during the treatment period of 7 months (T), posttreatment period 1 of 6 months ($P_1$), and posttreatment period 2 of 6 months ($P_2$).

The same prerequisites for successful treatment apply for the Herbst appliance as for removable functional appliances such as the activator, bionator, and Fränkel appliance. The maxillary and mandibular dental arches should be well aligned and should interdigitate properly in the normal sagittal relation. The Herbst appliance can be used successfully in groups in which removable functional appliances fail.

## Postadolescent Patients

Patients who have passed the maximal pubertal growth but still have some growth potential may be too old for conventional removable functional appliances because treatment with these appliances extends for a relatively long period (2 to 4 years). Treatment with the Herbst appliance, on the other hand, can be completed within 6 to 8 months, thus allowing the use of the residual growth left in these older patients.

## Mouth Breathers

Nasal airway obstructions can make the proper use of removable functional appliances difficult or impossible. However, such obstructions do not interfere with the correct function of the Herbst appliance because of obligatory mandibular propulsion.

## Uncooperative Patients

The Herbst appliance is fixed to the teeth and works continuously without any assistance from the patient. These factors make it a useful modality for treating uncooperative patients.

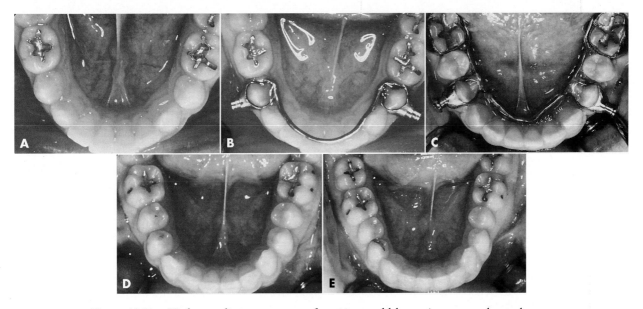

**Figure 16-39.** Herbst appliance treatment of an 11-year-old boy using a premolar anchorage system. No retention was performed after treatment. During the treatment period the mandibular incisors were proclined 5 degrees. During the posttreatment period of 1 year the incisor position recovered completely. **A,** Before treatment. **B,** Start of Herbst treatment. **C,** After 6 months of treatment (when the appliance was removed). **D,** Appearance 1 year posttreatment. **E,** Appearance 7 years posttreatment at the age of 19 years. No anterior crowding is present.

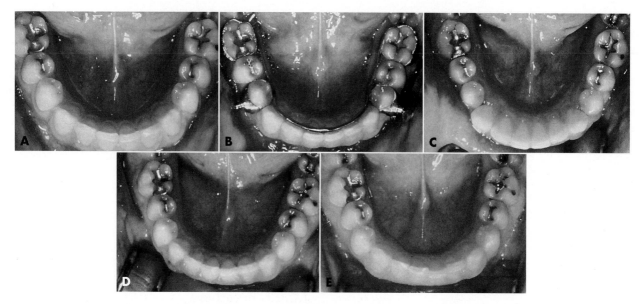

**Figure 16-40.** Herbst appliance treatment of a 16-year-old boy using a premolar-molar anchorage system. Retention with an activator after treatment was performed for 18 months. During the treatment period the mandibular incisors were proclined 23.5 degrees. During the posttreatment period of 1 year the incisors recovered by 17.5 degrees. **A,** Before treatment. **B,** Start of Herbst treatment. **C,** After 6 months of treatment (when the appliance was removed). **D,** Appearance 1 year posttreatment. **E,** Appearance 5 years posttreatment at the age of 21 years. Slight anterior crowding is present.

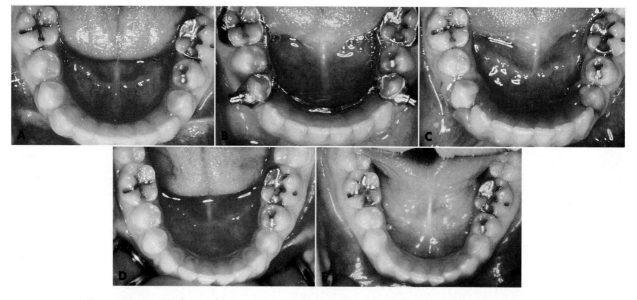

**Figure 16-41.** Herbst appliance treatment of an 11-year-old girl using a pelot anchorage system. Retention with an activator after treatment was performed for 18 months. During the treatment period the mandibular incisors were proclined 5.5 degrees. During the posttreatment period of 1 year the teeth recovered by 3.5 degrees. **A,** Before treatment. **B,** Start of Herbst treatment. **C,** After 5½ months of treatment (when the appliance was removed). **D,** Appearance 1 year posttreatment, **E,** Appearance 6 years posttreatment at the age of 18 years. Insignificant anterior crowding is present.

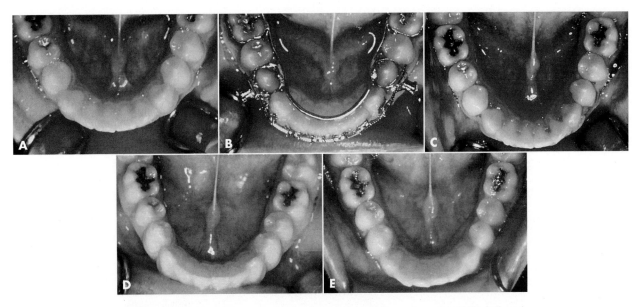

**Figure 16-42.** Herbst appliance treatment of a 14-year-old boy using a labial-lingual anchorage system. No retention was performed after treatment. During the treatment period the mandibular incisors were proclined 9 degrees. During the posttreatment period of 1 year the teeth recovered by 8.5 degrees. **A,** Before treatment. **B,** Start of Herbst treatment. **C,** After 6 months of treatment (when the appliance was removed). **D,** Appearance 1 year posttreatment. **E,** Appearance 5½ years posttreatment at the age of 20 years. Slight anterior crowding is present.

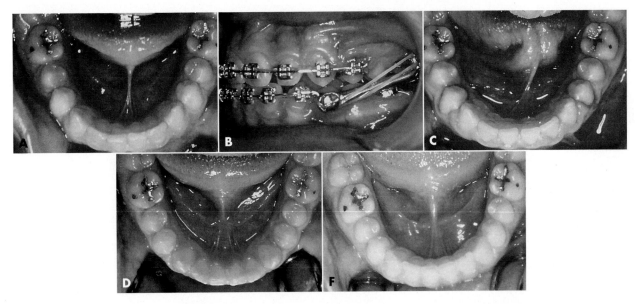

**Figure 16-43.** Herbst appliance treatment of a 13-year-old boy using a Class III elastic anchorage system. No retention was performed after treatment. During the treatment period the mandibular incisors were proclined 10.5 degrees. During the posttreatment period of 1 year the teeth recovered by 5.5 degrees. **A,** Before treatment. **B,** Start of Herbst treatment. **C,** After 7 months of treatment (when the appliance was removed). **D,** Appearance 1 year posttreatment. **E,** Appearance 5 years posttreatment at the age of 19 years. No anterior crowding is present.

## Patients Who do not Respond to Removable Functional Appliances

Removable mandibular protraction appliances are generally used only part of the day (12 to 14 hours). In certain patients the optimal threshold for adaptive growth changes in the condylar region is never reached because of this part-time appliance wear.

## MULTIPHASE TREATMENT APPROACH

As a rule, patients with Class II malocclusions cannot achieve a perfect end result with the Herbst appliance exclusively. Practitioners have found that many cases require a subsequent (or initial) dental alignment treatment phase using multibracket appliances.

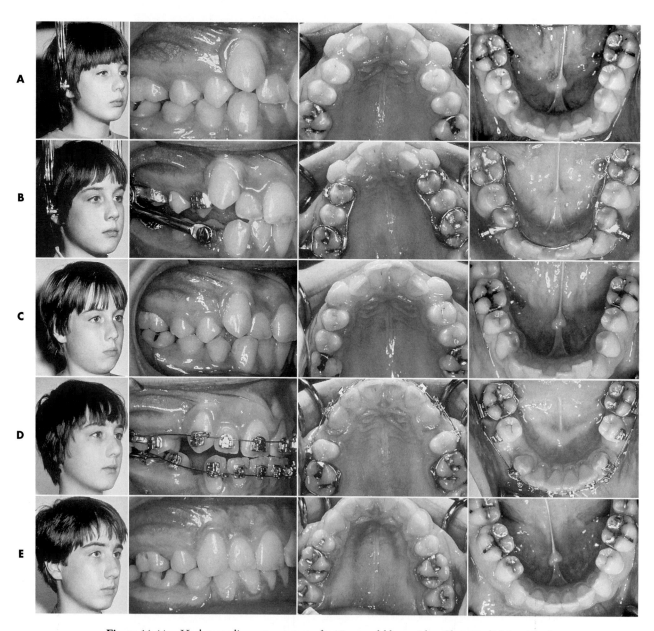

**Figure 16-44.**   Herbst appliance treatment of a 12-year-old boy with a Class II, division 1 malocclusion and severe maxillary and mandibular crowding. A two-step extraction treatment approach was used. **A,** Before Herbst treatment. **B,** Start of treatment (orthopedic treatment phase). **C,** After 6 months of Herbst treatment (when the appliance was removed). Note the corrected sagittal dental arch relationship and the normalized overjet and overbite. **D,** During multibracket appliance treatment with extractions of four first premolars (orthodontic treatment phase). **E,** After 12 months of treatment (when appliances were removed).

Treatment of a Class II, division 1 malocclusion usually occurs in two steps (Figure 16-44):

1. *Orthopedic phase*—The Class II malocclusion is corrected to a Class I occlusion using the Herbst appliance.
2. *Orthodontic phase*—Tooth irregularities and arch discrepancy problems are treated with a multibracket appliance (with or without extraction of teeth).

Treatment of a Class II, division 2 malocclusion may require a three-step treatment approach:

1. *Orthodontic phase*—Alignment of the anterior maxillary teeth is achieved by means of a multibracket orthodontic appliance.
2. *Orthopedic phase*—The Class II malocclusion is corrected to a Class I occlusion by means of the Herbst appliance.
3. *Orthodontic phase*—Tooth irregularities and arch discrepancy problems are treated with a multibracket appliance. Extractions should be avoided in the treatment

of Class II, division 2 malocclusion, if possible, as they are in fixed mechanotherapy.

## TIMING OF TREATMENT

On a short-term basis the most favorable time to treat patients with the Herbst appliance is at the peak of the pubertal growth spurt (Pancherz, Hägg, 1985) or at the skeletal developmental stages MP3 FG-G (Hägg, Pancherz, 1988; Hägg, Taranger, 1980). At this time the influence on mandibular condylar growth is greatest and the risk of undesirable dental effects on the mandible (e.g., proclination of the incisors) is small (Figures 16-45 through 16-47). However, clinicians must remember that large individual variations exist in skeletal and dental treatment responses (Pancherz, Hägg, 1985).

Over time, however, the growth period does not seem to have any significant influence on the final result (Hansen, Pancherz, Hägg, 1991) (Figure 16-48). Therefore late Herbst

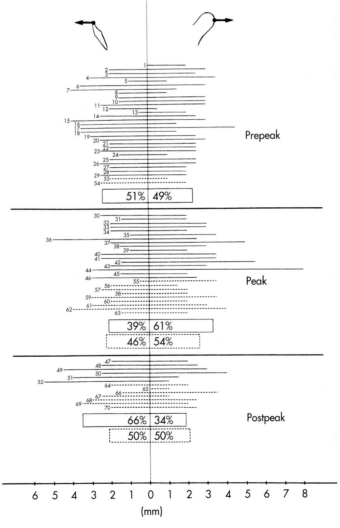

**Figure 16-45.** Mandibular condylar and incisor changes contributing to overjet correction in 52 boys (*solid lines*) and 18 girls (*dashed lines*) treated with Herbst appliances. Note the large individual variations in skeletal and dental responses.

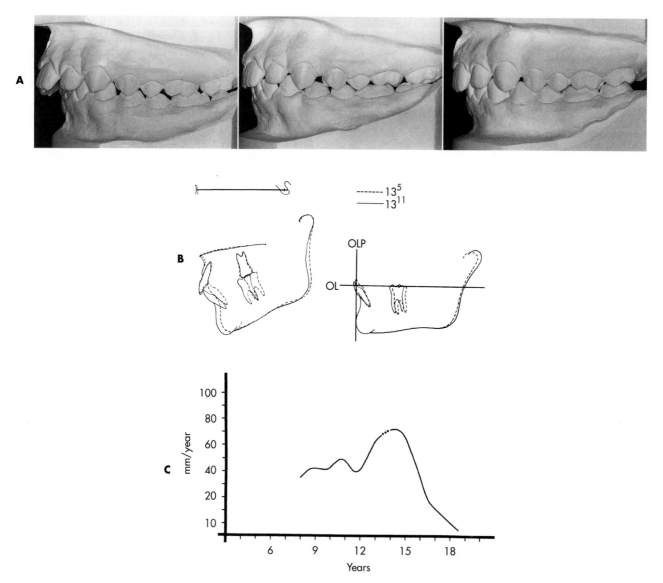

**Figure 16-46.** Herbst appliance treatment of a boy aged 13 years and 5 months in the peak growth period. **A,** Plaster casts from before treatment *(left),* after 6 months of treatment (when the appliance was removed) *(middle),* and 5 years posttreatment *(right).* **B,** Cephalometric tracings from before and after treatment superimposed on the nasion-sella line at sella. Mandibular tracings superimposed on the anterior and inferior mandibular bone contours. **C,** The velocity growth curve (in mm/year), with the treatment period given *(dots).*

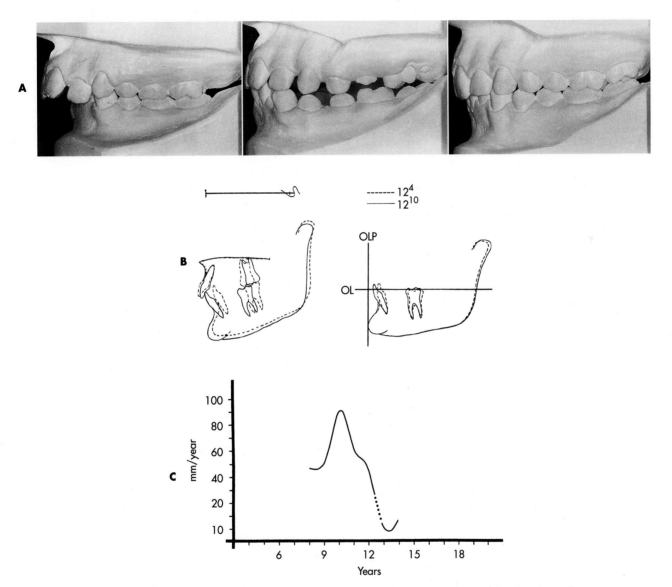

**Figure 16-47.** Herbst appliance treatment of a girl aged 12 years and 4 months after the peak growth period. **A,** Plaster casts from before treatment (*left*), after 6 months of treatment (*middle*), and 5 years posttreatment (*right*). **B,** Superimposed cephalometric tracings from before and after treatment superimposed on the nasion-sella line at sella. Mandibular tracings superimposed on the anterior and inferior mandibular bone contours. **C,** The velocity growth curve (in mm/year), with the treatment period given (*dots*).

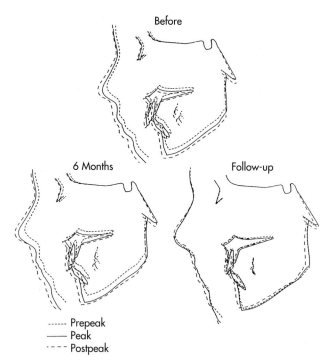

**Before**

**6 Months**

**Follow-up**

----- Prepeak
—— Peak
- - - - Postpeak

**Figure 16-48.** Composite tracings of 40 male patients with Class II, division 1 malocclusions treated with Herbst appliances. The distance between the hard- and soft-tissue profile is enlarged. Of the patients studied, 19 were treated before maximal pubertal growth (*Prepeak*), 15 at maximal growth (*Peak*), and 6 after maximal growth (*Postpeak*). Registrations were taken before treatment (*Before*), 6 months after treatment (when the occlusion had settled) (*Six months*), and at the end of the growth period 6½ years posttreatment (*Follow-up*).

appliance therapy in the permanent dentition and just after the peak of growth velocity is recommended to favor occlusal stability after treatment and reduce the time of posttreatment retention (Pancherz, 1994) (see Figures 16-21 and 16-22). In subjects with unfavorable posttreatment growth patterns (sagittal maxillary growth exceeding sagittal mandibular growth), stable Class I intercuspations certainly help counteract occlusal relapse (Pancherz, 1991). The interlocking teeth transfer maxillary growth forces to the mandible, and vice versa.

Early treatment in the deciduous or mixed dentition is not recommended because a stable cuspal interdigitation is difficult to achieve after Herbst appliance therapy and retention time thus has to be extended until all permanent teeth have erupted. If insufficient retention is applied, a dental relapse is likely to occur (Pancherz, Hansen, 1986) (see Figure 16-23). Furthermore, early treatment may be fruitless in the long run because severe Class II discrepancies seem to strive constantly

to reassert themselves (a phenomenon known as *predominance of the morphogenetic pattern*). Long-term studies of the results achieved in Herbst appliance treatment support this assumption (Hansen, Pancherz, 1992; Pancherz, Fackel, 1990).

## RETENTION AFTER HERBST TREATMENT

As has been shown (see Figures 16-16 and 16-17), the improvement in sagittal molar and incisor relationships accomplished during Herbst appliance therapy mainly results from an increase in mandibular growth, distal tooth movement in the maxilla, and mesial tooth movement in the mandible. Any posttreatment relapse initially results from maxillary and mandibular dental changes. A stable functional occlusion after treatment counteracts this relapse. However, treatment generally leads to overcorrected sagittal dental arch relationships with incomplete cuspal interdigitation. Thus a period of active retention is necessary until the occlusion has settled or a second treatment phase with a multibracket appliance must be instituted.

The Andresen activator is a suitable active retention device after Herbst appliance treatment. The appliance holds the teeth in the desired position while allowing interocclusal adjustments. Furthermore, the activator trains and accommodates the musculature to the new mandibular position. Musculature in harmony with the dentofacial structures is certainly of tremendous importance for stable treatment results. As demonstrated from the EMG analyses (Pancherz, 1980) (see Figure 16-34), the disharmonious muscle contraction pattern seen in patients with Class II malocclusion is normalized during Herbst appliance treatment (Pancherz, Anehus-Pancherz, 1980). The treatment time of 6 to 8 months is rather short, however, and the musculature probably needs more time for significant permanent adaptation.

## SUMMARY

The Herbst appliance is a fixed functional appliance that is most effective in the treatment of Class II malocclusions provided it is used as indicated. It should not be looked on as a substitute for removable functional appliances such as the activator, bionator, and Fränkel appliance. In the mixed dentition a removable functional appliance should be used to make Class II treatment most effective. If, however, the treatment response is slow and insufficient or patient compliance is poor, the clinician should wait until the permanent teeth have erupted and then use the Herbst appliance in the early postpeak growth period as part of a two- or three-step treatment approach as indicated.

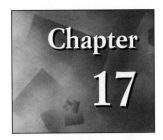

# Chapter 17

# The Modified Herbst Appliance (Jasper Jumper)*

J. J. Jasper

James A. McNamara, Jr.

Barry Mollenhauer

## Section I

## The Correction of Interarch Malocclusions Using a Fixed-Force Module

J.J. Jasper
James A. McNamara, Jr.

### BASIC PRINCIPLES

A number of fixed and removable appliance systems have been advocated for the correction of malocclusions characterized by sagittal discrepancies between the dental arches and their bony bases. The most frequently occurring sagittal malocclusion is the Class II type, for which a wide variety of treatment modalities has been developed.

This chapter describes the basic components of the Jasper jumper (JJ) mechanism, a mechanism that can be viewed as a modification of the Herbst bite-jumping mechanism (Herbst, 1910) (see Chapter 16). This interarch flexible-force module allows the patient greater freedom of mandibular movement than that possible with the original bite-jumping mechanism of Herbst.

### Extraoral and Intraoral Appliances

Appliances traditionally used to treat Class II malocclusion can be divided into two categories: extraoral and intraoral. Typical extraoral appliances include face-bows attached to tubes on the upper first molar bands and headgears attached directly to the arch wires or to auxiliaries connected to

*The illustrations for this chapter were provided by William L. Brudon. The authors also acknowledge the technical contributions of Lee W. Graber, William C. Machata, and Mart McClellan to this chapter.

the arch wires (Graber, 1955; Kloehn, 1953; Poulton, 1967; Watson, 1972).

The typical extraoral traction device used in the correction of Class II malocclusion applies forces to the maxillary dentition to retard forward movement or growth of the teeth and maxilla and push the maxillary teeth posteriorly. Equally important is the associated vertical vector of force produced by these appliances. A high-pull face-bow produces an intrusive force vector, whereas a cervical-pull face-bow tends to produce an extrusive force vector (Baumrind et al, 1983). The use of a cervical face-bow in a patient with a short lower facial dimension may be indicated, but this type of appliance often is contraindicated in patients with normal to long lower anterior facial heights because of the adverse vertical forces produced (Figure 17-1).

A wide variety of intraoral appliances also have been advocated for the treatment of Class II malocclusions. These appliances can be categorized into two groups: appliances that pull and appliances that push.

**Appliances producing pulling forces.** The most commonly used modality to produce pulling interarch force vectors is intermaxillary elastics. Class II elastics are perhaps the most commonly used means of changing dentoalveolar (and skeletal) relationships in Class II malocclusions. Not only do Class II elastics produce sagittal forces, they also create extrusive forces (Figure 17-2) at the points of attachment (usually the upper canines and lower first or second molars). Such extrusive forces typically are indicated only in patients in whom increases in lower anterior facial height are desired. McNamara (1981) has shown that only about 10% of pretreatment Class II mixed dentition patients have decreased lower facial heights, whereas 30% to 50% have excessive vertical development.

Another appliance system that produces a similar type of pulling force is the severable adjustable intermaxillary force (SAIF) spring developed by Armstrong in 1957 (Armstrong, 1993). In contrast to intermaxillary elastics that are removed and replaced by the patient, SAIF springs provide a fixed

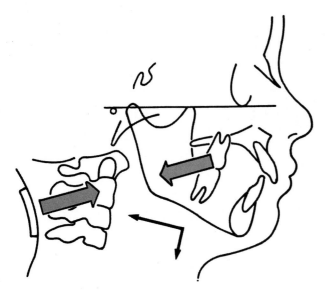

**Figure 17-1.** Forces produced by the cervical-pull face-bow. Note the extrusive force vector.

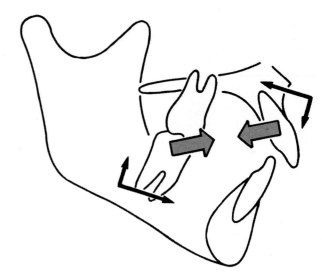

**Figure 17-2.** The vector of force produced by Class II intermaxillary elastics. Although the primary force is directed along the occlusal plane, extrusive forces also are produced.

pulling force. However, this mechanism has not been used widely because of difficulties encountered in appliance management, including breakage, hygiene, and comfort problems.

**Appliances producing pushing forces.** The second category of intraoral appliances used in the correction of Class II malocclusion includes appliances that deliver a pushing force vector, forcing the attachment points of the appliance away from one another. This resultant force contrasts with pulling devices such as intermaxillary elastics that bring their insertions closer to one another.

Not included in this discussion are the vast number of removable functional appliances that act as active pushing (protrusive) appliances; the use of these appliances typically results in a change in the postural level of muscle activity and in most instances results in a change in mandibular posture (Ascher, 1968; Balters, 1964; Fränkel, 1976; Fränkel and Fränkel, 1989).

One of the so-called fixed functional appliances is the Herbst appliance, reintroduced by Pancherz (1979, 1981, 1985) after having originally been described by Herbst (1910). This type of pushing appliance is categorized as rigid because the Herbst bite-jumping mechanism is composed of two stainless steel plunger rod-and-tube assemblies that usually are attached at the upper first molar and lower first premolar regions. This type of rigid pushing appliance produces force vectors that are sagittal and also have been shown to be intrusive (McNamara et al, 1990; Pancherz, 1982, 1985) (Figure 17-3). In addition, the forces tend to produce transverse expansion and are more oriented along the down and forward direction of facial growth.

The treatment effects produced by the Herbst bite-jumping appliance (of banded, cast, or acrylic splint design) have

been well documented. The studies of Pancherz (1979, 1981, 1982, 1985), Wieslander (1984), and McNamara et al (1990) have shown that both skeletal and dentoalveolar effects are produced in patients with Class II malocclusions who have worn these appliances. In general the treatment effects produced are divided about equally between skeletal and dentoalveolar adaptations. The most common skeletal adaptation reported is an increase in mandibular length (approximately 2.0 mm) in comparison with untreated control subjects with Class II malocclusions (McNamara et al, 1990; Pancherz, 1985). Little maxillary skeletal change has been noted. The most pronounced dentoalveolar change has been a relative posterior movement of the upper buccal segment, with about 2.5 mm of distal maxillary first molar movement noted in comparison with untreated control subjects. Forward movement of the lower molars and proclination of the lower incisors also have been reported (McNamara et al, 1990; Pancherz, 1985).

One of the major advantages of the Herbst appliance and other fixed intermaxillary appliances is the relative speed with which treatment effects are achieved. Traditional approaches to treating patients with Class II malocclusions (e.g., extraoral traction, Class II elastics) often are hampered by problems with patient compliance. By anchoring the device intraorally, the clinician can substantially reduce the need for patient cooperation.

One of the disadvantages of the Herbst appliance is the rigidity of the Herbst bite-jumping mechanism. Although every attempt is made in construction to allow freedom of movement through enlargement of the attachment holes of the tube and plunger to the axles, the bite-jumping mechanism restricts lateral movements of the mandible.

In an attempt to overcome these problems, Jasper (1987)

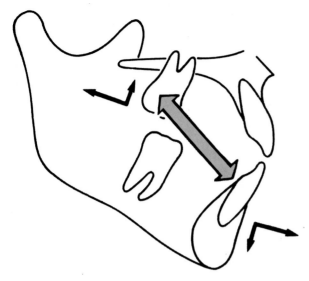

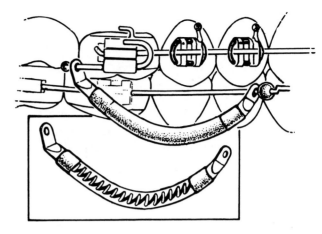

**Figure 17-4.** The attachment of the distal end of the force module to the maxillary dental arch through the use of a ball pin. The appliance can be activated by moving the ball pin anteriorly. The alignment of the spring within the jumper mechanism is shown in the inset.

**Figure 17-3.** Pushing vectors of force produced by the Herbst appliance and flexible force module. These bite-jumping mechanisms guide the mandible forward, producing protrusive and intrusive forces on the lower arch and retrusive and intrusive forces on the upper arch.

developed a new, flexible pushing device. This appliance produces both sagittal and intrusive forces (see Figure 17-3), as does the Herbst bite-jumping mechanism, and also affords the patient much more freedom of mandibular movement. These force modules also can be used in other applications and types of malocclusions, as discussed later in this chapter.

## Parts of the Appliance

This modular system, known as the *Jasper Jumper,* can be attached to most commonly used fixed appliances. The system is composed of two parts: the force module and the anchor units.

**Force module.** The force module, analogous to the tube and plunger of the Herbst bite-jumping mechanism, is flexible (Figure 17-4). The force module is constructed of a stainless steel coil or spring attached at both ends to stainless steel end caps in which holes have been drilled in the flanges to accommodate the anchoring unit. This module is surrounded by an opaque polyurethane covering for hygiene and comfort. The modules are available in seven lengths ranging from 26 to 38 mm in 2-mm increments. They are designed for use on either side of the dental arch.

When the force module is straight, it remains passive. As the teeth come into occlusion, the spring of the force module is curved axially as the muscles of mastication elevate the mandible, producing a range of forces from 1 to 16 ounces. This kinetic energy is then captured when the force module is curved, and the force is converted to potential energy to be used for a variety of clinical effects.

If properly installed to produce mandibular advancement, the spring mechanism is curved or activated 4 mm relative to

its resting length, thus storing about 8 ounces (250 g) of potential energy for force delivery. If less force is desired (e.g., force levels that produce tooth movement alone), the jumper is not activated fully. Increasing the activation beyond 4 mm does not yield more force from the module but only builds excessive internal stress in the module. The tendency to add more force for faster treatment results is to be avoided.

**Anchor units.** A number of methods are available to anchor the force modules to either the permanent or mixed dentitions. They are discussed in the following paragraphs.

*Attachment to the main arch wire.* The most common method of attachment of the force module to the dental arches in patients in the permanent dentition is through the use of previously placed fixed orthodontic appliances. When the jumper mechanism is used to correct a Class II malocclusion, the force module is attached posteriorly to the maxillary arch by a ball pin placed through the distal attachment of the force module; the module then extends anteriorly through the face-bow tube on the upper first molar band (Figure 17-5). The ball pin is anchored in position by having the clinician place a return bend in the ball pin at its mesial end.

The module is anchored anteriorly to the lower arch wire. Bayonet bends are placed distal to the mandibular canines, and small Lexan beads are slipped over the arch wire to provide an anterior stop. The mandibular arch wire is threaded through the hole in the anterior end cap and then ligated in place. The removal of the brackets on the lower second premolars in addition to the lower first premolars (as advocated originally) allows the patient greater freedom of movement.

*Attachment to auxiliary arch wires.* An alternative design incorporates the use of "outriggers" (Blackwood, 1991) (Figure 17-5). This .016 × .022 inch (.018-inch slot) or .018 × .025 inch (0.22-inch slot) auxiliary sectional wire al-

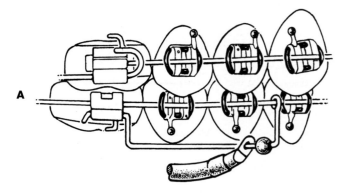

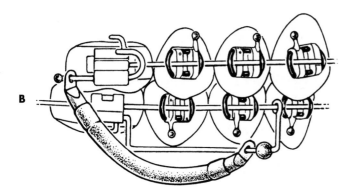

**Figure 17-5.** The use of outriggers for anchoring the force module. **A,** The rectangular auxiliary arch wire is looped over the main arch wire anteriorly and is cinched back through the auxiliary tube posteriorly. **B,** A ball pin is inserted through the distal hole in the jumper module, placed anteriorly through the facebow tube on the upper first molar band, and cinched forward to activate the module.

lows the clinician to leave the premolar bonds or bands in place by attaching the force module to a sectional wire anchored anteriorly to the main arch wire between the first premolar and canine (see Figure 17-5). Additionally, because freedom for the modules to slide is increased, a greater range of jaw movement is possible. Repairs and replacement of the jumper components are simplified with this outrigger modification.

The segmental arch wire is attached posteriorly through an auxiliary tube located on the lower first molar band (see Figure 17-5). The auxiliary wire can be bent so that the vestibular section is parallel to the occlusal plane (as shown in Figure 17-5), or a shorter vertical step can be placed posteriorly so that the inclination of the outrigger more closely approximates the down and forward growth direction of the patient's face. The posterior part of the jumper module is attached to the ball pin placed through the maxillary molar tube as described previously (see Figure 17-5).

If outriggers are used to anchor the module to the mandibular dentition, care must be taken to ensure that the sectional arch wire provides adequate space between the alveolus and gingiva to allow the module to slide without tissue impingement. Contouring the sectional arch wire and placing

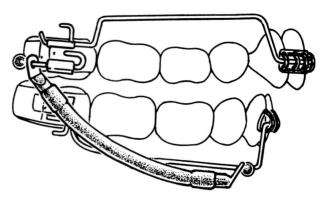

**Figure 17-6.** The use of the force module in a mixed dentition patient. In this instance a bayonet bend is placed distally to the canine, and a Lexan ball acts as a stop for the force module anteriorly. In this example, upper and lower rectangular utility arches connect the anterior and posterior teeth.

first order step-out bends in the arch wire may be helpful. After the module has been placed, it should slide smoothly along the sectional outrigger wire.

***Attachment in the mixed dentition.*** The force module also can be used in mixed dentition patients whose premolars have not yet erupted (Figure 17-6). The maxillary attachment is similar to that previously described in that the ball pin is used to attach the force module to the maxillary first molars. The mandibular attachment of the force module is through an arch wire that extends from the brackets on the lower incisors posteriorly to the first permanent molars, bypassing the region of the deciduous canines and molars (Figure 17-7). In a mixed dentition patient the use of a transpalatal arch and fixed lower lingual arch is mandatory to control potential unfavorable side effects produced by the appliance (e.g., molar and incisor tipping and flaring).

## Clinical Management

**Preparation of anchorage.** The most important aspect of the clinical management of this appliance system is the preparation of lower anchorage and the control of mandibular mesial tooth movement. As with the Herbst appliance, mesial movement of the lower incisors has been reported using this appliance system (Fraser, 1992; May et al, 1992). Unfavorable dentoalveolar adaptations can be minimized in the mandible through proper anchorage preparation.

Alignment of the upper and lower anterior teeth during the initial phases of orthodontic treatment must be completed. Full-sized (or nearly full-sized) arch wires should be inserted into the brackets in both arches before the placement of the force modules. The arch wires should be tied or cinched back posteriorly to increase anchorage (see Figure 17-7), including the second molars whenever possible. In addition, the clinician can place posterior tip-back bends in the mandibular arch wire to enhance anchorage.

If jumpers are anticipated in the treatment plan, anterior lingual crown torque can be placed in the arch wire. Alterna-

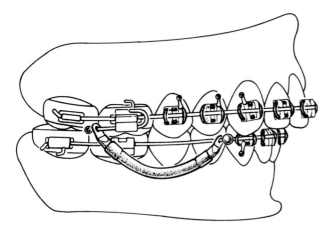

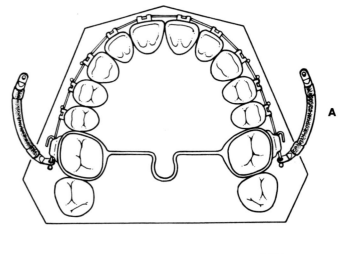

**Figure 17-7.** Maximal anchorage setup for the force module. The maxillary and mandibular arch wires extend to the second molars and are cinched back posteriorly. Tiebacks also can be used. The offset bend in the main arch wire (see Figure 17-8) is obscured by the Lexan ball.

tively, lower incisor brackets with 5 degrees of lingual crown torque incorporated into the slot also can be used to prepare anchorage. Lingually torqued lower incisor brackets are used in addition to, not as a substitute for, anchorage in the mandible.

**Use of stabilization wires.** Two types of auxiliary arch wires can be used to enhance anchorage: the transpalatal arch and the lower lingual arch. A transpalatal arch (Figure 17-8) can be used in instances in which distal maxillary molar movement is to be minimized and mandibular adaptations are to be maximized. A transpalatal arch is not incorporated into the appliance system if maxillary dentoalveolar movement is desired.

The use of a fixed lower lingual arch is strongly encouraged in most instances. This type of anchorage preparation is used routinely except when significant lower incisor proclination is desired as part of the overall treatment plan (e.g., in patients with mandibular dentoalveolar retrusion).

**Preparation of the arches.** As noted previously, the jumper mechanisms are not placed until the initial leveling and alignment of the dentition have been completed and full-sized or nearly full-sized arch wires have been placed in both arches. After the arch wires have become passive, the mandibular arch wire is disengaged and the brackets on the first and second premolars are removed bilaterally (see Figures 17-7 and 17-8). Unless outriggers are used, bayonet bends are placed in the arch wire distal to the lower canine bracket, and 3-mm Lexan beads are slipped over the ends of the arch wire and moved forward to rest against the bayonet bends bilaterally.

**Selection and installation of the modules.** To determine the proper length of the module, the clinician should measure from the mesial of the upper molar tube to the distal of the lower Lexan bead (Figure 17-9). Adding 12 mm to this measurement gives the appropriate length for the module. The

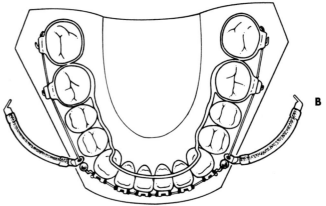

**Figure 17-8.** **A,** The use of the transpalatal arch combined with fixed appliances to enhance maxillary anchorage. **B,** The use of a lower lingual arch with fixed appliances to enhance mandibular anchorage.

arch wire then is threaded through the hole in the anterior end cap of the force modules. The mandibular arch wire is ligated in place, and the ends of the arch wire are cinched or tied back firmly to prevent proclination of the lower anterior teeth during treatment. Thus theoretically the force generated by the module is distributed throughout the mandibular dentition. The ball pin is then placed through the distal hole in the force module and inserted anteriorly into the face-bow tube on the maxillary first molar band and cinched forward as described previously (see Figure 17-4).

In high–mandibular plane angle patients the pin is cinched to achieve approximately 2 mm of module deflection (150 g per side). In normal or low–mandibular plane angle patients the ball pin is cinched forward to achieve 4 mm of module deflection (300 g of force per side). The patient should be coached to practice opening and closing movements slowly at first and told to avoid excessive wide opening during eating and yawning. The patient is cautioned to note any sticking of the module and is taught the way to move the module forward with the fingers to unlock them. The clinician must warn the patient against biting on the jumpers or "popping" them because these actions result in breakage.

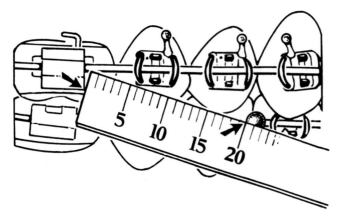

**Figure 17-9.** The determination of the proper length of the force module is performed by adding 12 mm to the measurement of the distance between the mesial aspect of the face-bow tube and the distal aspect of the Lexan ball. In this example the distance from the ball to the face-bow tube is 20 mm. Thus a 32-mm module should be selected.

**Activation of the module for orthodontic and orthopedic effect.** The protocol advocated here is based primarily on clinical experience. As described, the jumper modules initially are selected and placed so that the module assumes a mildly curved contour when the patient is holding the jaw in a comfortably retruded position. If molar distalization is desired (as can be accomplished in adult patients), a transpalatal arch is not placed and the maxillary arch wire is not tied or cinched back. In this case the jumper is placed so that only 2 to 4 ounces of force is produced by the module; a measuring gauge can be used to determine the precise amount of activation. In a growing individual in whom an orthopedic repositioning of the mandible is desired, higher force levels (6 to 8 ounces) are used continuously.

**Reactivation of the module.** If the Class II molar relationship is not corrected completely by the initial activation of the appliance, the modules should be reactivated 2 to 3 months after initial placement. The modular system is activated most easily by shortening the attachment to the maxillary first molar bands. The pin extending through the face-bow tube is pulled anteriorly 1 to 2 mm on each side to reactivate the module (higher–mandibular plane angle cases are activated 1 mm per side). The clinician should avoid shortening the ball pin excessively so that the jumper is not trapped against the distal aspect of the face-bow tube, thus preventing its rotation. A total of 2 to 4 mm of the pin should extend distally when the pin is activated maximally.

Activation of the force module also can be performed through adjustments in the lower arch. Crimpable stops of 1 or 2 mm placed mesially to the Lexan ball can produce a precise, controlled activation of the modules. Activation of the appliance in this manner is more accurate and easier to perform. It also prevents the possibility of damage to the ball pin–molar tube relationship and the necessity of replacing the module with a larger one.

At each appointment the clinician should check to be cer-

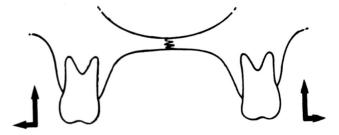

**Figure 17-10.** Expansive forces are positive side effects produced by the intrusive forces of the jumper mechanism.

tain that none of the anchoring bands or tiebacks have become loosened. Additionally the distal extensions of the ball pins often must be straightened so that they are parallel with the occlusal plane. If outriggers are used, the anterior portions must be adjusted so as not to contact the distal of the lower canine bracket. Increasing interdental spacing in the anterior segment indicates a breakdown of appliance integrity.

## Types of Forces Produced

Bilateral directions of force generated by the modules include sagittal, intrusive, and expansive forces. The sagittal forces distalize the posterior anchor unit (e.g., maxillary first molars, maxillary first and second molars) and apply anterior force to the mandible and mandibular dentition (see Figure 17-3). In addition, an intrusive force is produced in the maxillary posterior region and mandibular anterior region.

A buccal force also is produced by the module (Figure 17-10). An intrusive force applied along the buccal surface of a tooth produces maxillary arch expansion, a treatment response typically observed in using the jumper mechanism with fixed appliances. In addition, the modules curve toward the buccal, producing a modest vestibular shielding effect (Figure 17-11).

Expansive forces can be minimized or eliminated through the use of a transpalatal arch (see Figure 17-8) or a heavy arch wire that has been narrowed and to which buccal root torque has been applied. Indeed clinicians are encouraged to add buccal root torque if arch expansion and not molar tipping is desired. The expansive forces produced by the module can be contrasted to the lingual crown torque produced by extrusive pulling mechanics (e.g., Class II elastics).

## Treatment Effects

After the dental arches have been properly prepared, the modules can be used to produce numerous treatment effects.

### Maxillary adaptations

*Headgear effect.* One treatment effect produced most easily by force modules is distalization of the upper posterior segment, or the headgear effect. This type of movement is achieved by not cinching or tying back the maxillary arch wire and allowing the arch wire to remain straight and slightly extended past the buccal tubes. Light forces (2 to 4 ounces) can

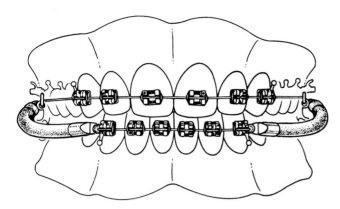

**Figure 17-11.** The force module curves to the buccal aspect, producing a shielding effect on the dentition. The offset bends in the main arch wire are not visible in this view.

then be expressed by the modules to distalize the upper molars. Because the forces are resisted by the entire lower dentition, minimal changes in mandibular dentition are noted. The headgear effect can be produced in not only actively growing patients but also some adult patients in whom maxillary molar distalization is desired (Cash, 1991). No evidence supports the hypothesis that this type of appliance can be used to promote mandibular growth in adult patients.

After the desired distal movement has been achieved, the module can be left in place to support the retraction of the premolars and canines. Segmental or continuous arch mechanics can be used to retract these teeth while maintaining molar anchorage. Alternatively the force module can be left in place to support the molars as the premolar and canine teeth spontaneously move posteriorly because of the pull of the gingival transseptal fibers between the teeth (the so-called "driftodontic" effect). A transpalatal arch or Nance holding arch also may be used to maintain the correction.

*Retraction of anterior teeth.* Canine teeth can be retracted in both extraction and nonextraction patients with the posterior maxillary dentition supported by the force module (Figure 17-12). In addition, a NiTi coil or an intramaxillary elastic attached to the pin through the face-bow tube can be used to retract the upper canines or six anterior teeth at once. The pull on the pin is resisted by the modules and mandibular dentition (Figure 17-13).

*Dental asymmetries.* The force module system also can be used in patients who have sagittal dental asymmetries. In a patient with a Class II subdivision type of malocclusion the maxillary arch wire can be tied back on the side of the existing Class I molar relationship. Asymmetric orthopedic effects also may be achieved.

**Mandibular adaptations.** As stated previously, the clinician should make every effort to incorporate maximal anchorage techniques when preparing the mandibular arch for this appliance system (see Figure 17-7). In growing individuals, changes in mandibular position (and presumably changes

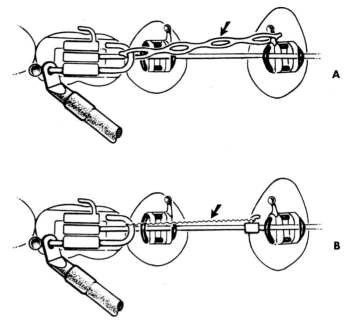

**Figure 17-12.** Retraction of the upper canine teeth using the ball pin and force module. A NiTi spring or an elastomeric chain can be attached from the ball pin anteriorly to either the canine bracket (**A**) or the maxillary arch wire (**B**). In this manner, anterior retraction is anchored posteriorly by forces generated against the mandibular dentition rather than against the maxillary dentition.

in mandibular length) are achieved after force module application. To date, no major prospective research has been conducted on this phenomenon. However, treatment effects produced by this flexible force module presumably are similar to those of the Herbst appliance because of the similarities in their mechanisms of action (see Figure 17-3).

In the attempt to produce mandibular advancement, the major variation in clinical management is the preparation of the maxillary anchor unit. The movement of the maxillary posterior dentition must be minimized to maximize mandibular change. The arch wire should be cinched or tied back as it is routinely in the mandibular dentition. In addition, a transpalatal arch (see Figure 17-8) should be used to obtain intraarch anchorage and minimize posterior tooth movement. A fixed lower lingual arch also is recommended.

As discussed, if mandibular advancement is desired, the level of force generated by the module is generally greater (6 to 8 ounces) than that generated if maxillary molar distalization is intended (2 to 4 ounces). By maximizing the force values produced by the module, patients tend to posture their jaws in a forward position. In contrast to the Herbst bite-jumping mechanism, however, the spring mechanism allows more freedom in both sagittal and lateral movements.

## Additional Applications

This chapter thus far has considered the use of the jumper mechanism primarily in the treatment of Class II malocclusion, the typical application of this type of appliance. This sys-

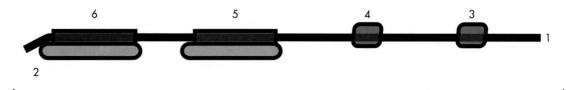

Extraction cases: .022-inch auxiliary lengthened

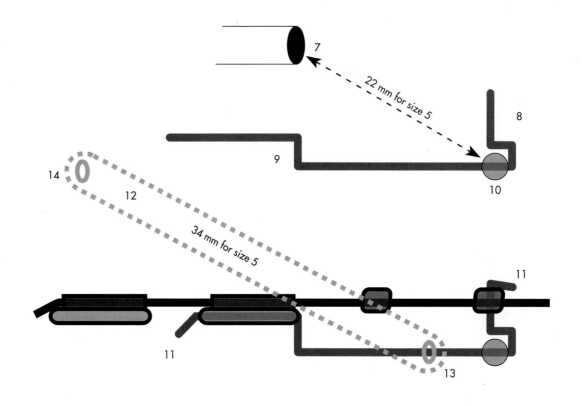

Nonextraction cases: .022-inch auxiliary shortened

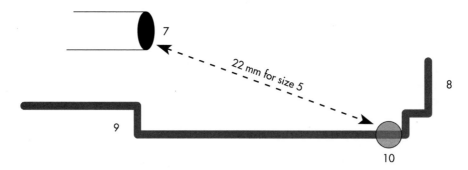

**Figure 17-13.** Arch wires. The thick horizontal line (*1*) represents the main lower arch wire. This wire must have appropriate labial root torque or a torquing auxiliary applied. The lower arch wire should be cinched at the distal of the lower second molar tubes (*2*). The canine bracket (*3*) must have a vertical slot large enough to hold the .022-inch auxiliary. Lower premolar brackets (*4*) should be left on for engagement of the lower arch wire. Lower first molar double tubes (*5*) are employed to hold the .022-inch auxiliary arch wire. Lower second molar double tubes (*6*) provide a more solid base to enhance arch-form stability, but they are optional. Upper headgear tubes (*7*) anchor the usual JJ ball-ended pins. The vertical part of the auxiliary (*8*) is placed in the vertical slot of the lower canine brackets. The molar part of the auxiliary (*9*) is pushed into the gingivally positioned accessory molar tube. The use of a plastic ball (*10*) is recommended. Cinching of the auxiliary ends (*11*) should be left until last. JJ (*12*). The JJ should be slipped onto the auxiliary (*13*) after trial placement and before final placement of the appliance in the mouth. The JJ is attached to the ball pin at the distal of the headgear tube.

tem of modules also has been used to support anchorage for the retraction of maxillary anterior teeth in patients with Class I occlusions.

Jumper modules also can be used in patients with Class III malocclusions. In contrast to the rigid bite-jumping mechanism of the Herbst appliance, the flexibility of the jumper mechanism allows its use in such individuals. This appliance should be used in patients whose malocclusions are characterized by maxillary skeletal retrusion rather than mandibular prognathism.

When using this system in patients with Class III malocclusions, the clinician should place the mandibular anchor points mesial to the permanent first molars. Bands that have auxiliary headgear tubes or lip bumper tubes are used to anchor the ball pin of the distal end cap of the force module. The Lexan ball is placed anteriorly distal to a bayonet bend just behind the bracket on the upper canine or on an appropriate place on the upper arch wire if the canines are not yet erupted. This appliance can be used with rapid maxillary expansion in patients with Class III malocclusions. Forces generated when the modules are used in this manner are usually light (2 to 4 g). This type of treatment should be discontinued immediately if any signs or symptoms of temporomandibular disorders develop. Other potential applications may include the correction of anterior crossbites in patients with functional (pseudo) Class III malocclusions, the postsurgical stabilization of Class II or III malocclusions, and presurgical muscle conditioning of patients with Class II malocclusions.

## Conclusions

The first part of this chapter has considered a flexible type of bite-jumping mechanism that pushes against the maxillary and mandibular dentitions. This module is a modification of the Herbst bite-jumping mechanism developed nearly 100 years ago (Herbst, 1910). The well-documented treatment effects of the Herbst bite-jumping mechanism appear similar to those produced by the force module described in this chapter. Both systems produce a relatively rapid correction of Class II malocclusion through the production of both sagittal and intrusive forces. Both skeletal and dentoalveolar adaptations have been observed with the jumper mechanism (Fraser, 1992; May et al, 1992).

This flexible force module system differs from the Herbst bite-jumping mechanism in a number of significant areas. First, the amount of force applied by the modules is more easily controlled by the clinician. The flexibility of the force module has been shown to increase patient comfort because greater lateral and sagittal movements are possible. In addition, the force module curves away from the dental arches in its activated position, making mastication and oral hygiene procedures easier to perform than they are with the Herbst appliance.

Another advantage of this auxiliary appliance system is that it can be added to existing appliances at virtually any point after arch preparation. The modules can be used as a primary method of treatment or added later after alternative treatments have proved unsuccessful (e.g., extraoral traction, functional jaw orthopedics). No need exists to remove the entire fixed appliance setup before the force modules are placed, nor is any additional laboratory cost required or time lost during treatment if the fabrication of lower lingual or transpalatal arches is not required.

As with any fixed force system, several disadvantages are associated with the use of these modules. The two most significant are breakage and unwanted tooth movement. The use of these modules on uncooperative patients increases the concern of breakage.

The appliance system has been improved over the past 10 years; the modules are now more resistant to fracture during wear. Patients should be instructed not to chew on the appliance or perform movements requiring wide opening of the mouth. Strict dietary controls are mandatory. The patient should be repeatedly cautioned not to "pop" the modules after yawning or excessive wide mouth opening.

As mentioned earlier, the clinician must prepare anchorage before the force module is placed against the lower arch. If the arch wire is full sized (or nearly so) and properly anchored posteriorly, forward movement of the lower dentition is minimized. The placement of lingual crown torque anteriorly and tip-back bends posteriorly further enhances anchorage. If the clinician is concerned about the mesial movement of the lower dentition, use of lighter forces is advocated.

As is usual with the incorporation of a new technique or appliance into an established regimen, clinical experience is necessary before the practitioner becomes comfortable with the manipulation and handling of the adjunct. Thus initial case selection is important for first-time users of the appliance. For example, a cooperative patient with mild Class II diagnostic features and minimal anchorage requirements is an ideal candidate. The treatment of uncooperative patients, "bail-out" patients, or patients who have severe skeletal Class II problems should be left to practitioners who have considerable experience in manipulation of the modules.

If employed appropriately, this appliance system provides the opportunity of minimizing the necessity of patient cooperation in the correction of sagittal discrepancies. If proper anchorage preparation is achieved and force values are kept within physiologic limits, successful treatment outcomes can be achieved.

# Assymetric Dentofacial Orthopedics with the Jasper Jumper

Barry Mollenhauer

## BASIC PRINCIPLES

Having an appliance available for use with noncompliant patients is most valuable because many studies in the health sciences have found less than 35% of the patient population to be compliant. Placing Jasper jumpers (JJs) not only overcomes noncompliance but also provides the best way to prove noncompliance to the parents during fixed appliance therapy. JJs have beneficial dentofacial orthopedic effects as well (Weiland, Bantleon, 1995).

Compared with most functional appliances, the JJs marry well with fixed appliances. Corrections of other malocclusions such as rotations, malalignment, and dysfunctional occlusion can be integrated with orthopedic therapy. In fact, reduction of occlusal dysfunction aids orthopedic effects. Thus all corrections may be accomplished in a one-phase management if the response is similar to the Fränkel function regulator (FR) II. McNamara et al (1985) found that mandibular response with the FR II appliance is better in patients older than 10 years and 6 months than it is in younger patients.

A subgroup of about one third of all cases requires unilateral use only of the appliance. This use may produce an asymmetric functional appliance effect, but this is unlikely because the majority of JJs are required for 4 to 6 weeks only, if installed according to the guidelines in this chapter. This period of JJ treatment is significantly shorter than the 6-month period suggested by Weiland and Bantleon (1995), whose team used two JJs for all cases but one. Such a regimen increases costs considerably and thus deters JJ use because many clinicians consider cost an important factor with this appliance. However, the JJ's cost is insignificant compared with the cost of prolonged treatment or overruns.

Little work has been done on asymmetric functional appliances. Nevertheless they are a necessary modality, even if only to correct the malocclused lower molars on the Class II side—the distinctive feature in Class II subdivision cases according to Rose et al (1994). The JJ is most suitable to correct asymmetries and improve facial appearance, both of which are in the domain of dentofacial orthopedics. The majority of patients requiring JJ therapy have a cant of the occlusal plane to the right side that can be viewed from the front. Because the majority of unilateral JJs are placed on the left side, this appliance aids in the correction of the cant of the occlusal plane in this majority by depressing the lower left canine segment.

Clinical observations in the use of this appliance highlight two insidious relationships of functional occlusion:

1. *Apparent noncompliance*—Much anecdotal evidence is available on the association of dysfunction with the rate of tooth movement. This association is particularly evident if simple round wires are used in molar tubes with tip-back bends for more than 6 months. All too often this method produces extrusion of the palatal cusps of the upper posterior teeth and may induce parafunction. A rarer but more severe reduction of tooth movement may result from working side interferences associated with excessive lingual tipping of lower molars caused by overly light lower arch wires. Many clinicians seem unaware of the association of tooth movement with parafunction and instead blame poor compliance for slow treatment progress.

2. *Unlocking of the occlusion*—Unlocking of the occlusion is evident in a different way to the clinician. This result may occur in cases in which JJs are required on one side only but in which orthodontic treatment started with the patient in a symmetric Class II relationship.

Alternately, the clinician may observe a change in Class II subdivision malocclusions. A bilateral buccal Class II malocclusion that was not present originally may occasionally develop a few months into treatment. This malocclusion may be confirmed by reviewing the patient's extraction or headgear requirements some months into treatment. Fixed appliances may unlock the occlusion in a manner similar to that produced by an occlusal splint or a bite plane; this result is presumably caused by induced interferences. Initially this malocclusion may be caused by bracket interferences, but later it may result from tooth movement. Thus all tubes and brackets required for JJs should be routinely incorporated in the fixed appliances setup because their need cannot always be predicted before treatment begins.

## Guidelines

The following guidelines can be used to overcome many of the inherent problems with JJs:

1. *Attachment with auxiliary arch wires has many benefits*—Apart from enabling compliance with many of the following guidelines, application of JJs by auxiliary arch wires allows quicker fitting and repair. Removal of the main arch wire or removal of brackets from the premolars is unnecessary. The use of an auxiliary arch wire requires lower accessory molar tubes, upper accessory tubes such as headgear tubes, and vertical slots in the lower canine brackets.

2. *The longest JJs provide the lightest forces*—Modern theory supports the assertion that very light forces produce orthopedic effects, whereas heavier forces produce dental effects. This assertion is contrary to former orthodontic theory, which was based on theories regarding the hyalinization of the periodontal membrane during intermittent headgear use. When JJs were first introduced commercially, most clinicians erroneously installed them in a manner similar to that used for the Herbst appliance. Faulty installation was associated with breakage and backward mandibular

rotation. Because the JJ is essentially a spring, longer variants provide lighter force. Longer JJs produce less lower incisor "dumping" (crowns tipped forward with the apices pivoted lingually) and backward mandibular rotation. The longest size previously available was 34 mm (size 5), with a headgear tube to plastic ball distance of 22 mm (Figure 7-13). Recently, however, JJs longer than 34 mm have become available; sufficient numbers of these have not yet been tried clinically to confirm their anticipated advantages. As for the use of a plastic ball, recent JJ practice indicates that it is not necessary with an auxiliary wire, but it may nevertheless be used for patient comfort. Its routine use seems to be a factor in reducing breakage.

3. *The correct balance of forces is essential for optimal effects*—The balance of forces between the forward thrust from the JJ and the labial root torque from the lower arch wire or torquing auxiliary is essential for ideal results. Unfortunately, predicting this balance before the fact is not possible. Too much labial root torque has the potential to produce gingival stripping, but insufficient torque allows dumping. The clinician should give great attention to achieving balance and continuously monitor patients to become comfortable with the optimal labial root torque for various clinical types.

4. *Use the longest JJ possible to prevent tensile breakage*—The most common cause of JJ breakage is over-opening of the mouth relative to the length of the JJ. Too-wide opening pulls the spring from its tube. Ideally the JJ should be long enough to prevent this, and the problem can be reduced somewhat by the use of a resilient auxiliary wire that can flex sideways and up as it is pulled from the molar tube. The length of the JJ should be checked carefully for each patient. Patients should be instructed to overcome this problem by opening the mouth slowly and gently after appliance installation.

5. *The auxiliary wire should be 0.022 inches*—Routinely using 0.022-inch high-tensile wire dramatically reduces breakage, except when the plastic ball is not used. Very high tensile wires are more useful as auxiliary wires. Soft wires deform and can cause irritation to the buccal mucosa. Previously 0.020-inch high-tensile wire was used for the auxiliary wire, but it broke occasionally. These modifications to the original design—especially to eliminate breakage—have many benefits. The dramatic decrease in breakage means that when the clinician who placed the JJ is unavailable, other clinicians who are not familiar with the appliances will not be called on to replace them. Because of increased wire strength, although patients are still instructed not to bite on the JJ tubes, this is no longer a significant a feature in breakage.

6. *The vertical slot should have sufficient patency.*—Some experimentation may be necessary to ensure that the patency of the vertical slot in the lower canine brackets is sufficient to allow placement of the 0.022-inch auxiliary wire. Edgewise brackets should have a vertical slot of sufficient aperture in the lower canine brackets to allow insertion of the auxiliary wire. Usually the slot is large enough, but it should be checked. The aperture in ribbon-arch brackets is not always sufficient with a ligature wire already included; in this case the ligature should be passed under (or lingual to) the arch wire and tied on the outside of the bracket. This maneuver leaves the vertical slot free for insertion of the auxiliary wire.

7. *Upper extractions shorten the JJ distance*—Upper extractions produce a short JJ distance, especially if the extraction spaces are closed or almost closed. A variation in size arises because JJs can be used in all stages of treatment. However, JJs should not be used if light aligning arch wires only are present. The management of JJ length is essential. The clinician should measure 22 mm from the front of the headgear tubes to several millimeters below the lower arch wire in the lower canine area. This position from the caliper should be noted; it is an essential step in the installation of the JJ because it indicates where the distal of the plastic ball is to be positioned. The clinician must decide whether the plastic ball is to be mesial or distal to the lower canine bracket. In cases requiring extraction it is often mesial to a vertical line down from the canine bracket. In nonextraction treatment of the upper arch in patients with large teeth, the 34-mm JJ may not be long enough to provide activation even when the jaws are closed unless the plastic ball is positioned quite distal to the canine bracket. Figure 17-13 shows this clearly. This measurement indicates the desired position to bend the auxiliary arch wire step-up to lengthen or shorten the forward run of the plastic ball. When extraction spaces have closed in the lower arch, a longer auxiliary wire produced by an extension mesial to the canine bracket provides flexibility to minimize breakage. However, the tensile strain on the JJ is the most common cause of its breakage.

8. *The appliance should be kept off the alveolar mucosa*—Obviously, the appliance should be kept clear of the buccal mucosa, but the correct amount of flare of the auxiliary as it comes out of the lower aspect of the canine bracket is even more important because the molar tube insertion cannot control this. A rectangular auxiliary in a rectangular tube can provide this control, but the device is more difficult to insert and remove. Trial placements may be necessary. Of course, "flaring out" also can be overdone, thus irritating the cheek rather than the alveolar mucosa.

9. *For extra stability, 2-ounce elastics can be worn over the JJs*—The application of 2-ounce elastics has been found to be a useful practice. It may be less threatening to the patient and produce fewer emotional reactions. The JJs do not appear as punishment but rather as supplements to the elastics. Class II elastics also keep the JJs in from the cheek. More important, they act only when the mouth is open because the JJs are

only effective near the rest or closed position of the mandible.

10. *The JJs should be applied before U7 tubes are attached*—The tubes on the upper second molars often get in the way, especially during removal of JJs.

11. *Class III traction has different requirements*—JJs applied for treatment of Class III malocclusions or anterior crossbite that is not resolved by the usual means can be just as effective as those applied in Class II malocclusions. However, the ball hook requires considerable room distal to the lower molar tube to prevent laceration of the soft tissues in this area.

12. *Partially preformed auxiliaries encourage use*—If appliances can be placed quickly, the decision to use them is usually not postponed. Normal principles of office procedures apply such as the availability of suitable bracket-table setups; quick placements also are enhanced if the auxiliaries are partly preformed. The posterior part of the auxiliary may be preformed and the plastic ball applied so that the measured step-up position may be marked and bent within seconds.

## Stock and Placement

These guidelines show that although most of the time the 34-mm JJ can be used, a full kit is desirable initially because the other paraphernalia must be available. The JJ kit is expensive but less expensive than the potential cost overruns of fixed appliance treatment.

A JJ can be placed in as little as 59 seconds. However, to ensure lighter forces, a slower pace may be necessary to place the JJs carefully with the lightest forces possible, while ensuring appropriate activation.

## Conclusions

The JJ appliance may prove an excellent instrument for dentofacial orthopedics because it can be applied and removed at any time the clinician desires. A national distributor of these appliances has stated that the appliance components are selling well, so a large database of cases must be available for study.

Large numbers of patients are necessary to overcome all the variables and complications involved in formally studying the capabilities of the JJ. For example, Rosenblum (1995) states that no "gold standard" exists for evaluating the anteroposterior positions of the maxilla and mandible. Bowden frequently shows lecture slides from his studies at the Melbourne Growth Unit that indicate the problems of quantifying functional appliance effects because of the large normal variation in the growth curves of untreated individuals.

Large numbers of patients and cases are most suitable for study by the newer complexity mathematics of chaos theory, neural networks (which highlight outliers or exceptions), and cognitive science. Stochastic resonance is particularly suitable for mathematically describing phenomena such as functional appliance treatment results because random noise (from influences such as seasonal and hormonal changes) can explain the varying responses of functional appliances (see Chapter 2).

Weiland and Bantleon (1995) found a 60:40 ratio of dental to orthopedic effects after 6 months' use of this appliance. No absolute answer is available yet concerning the duration a full-time appliance must be in place to have an orthopedic effect, but spectacular effects can be seen clinically after the JJs have been in place for 6 weeks.

In the recent literature, except for the accepted 10% of patients who need early treatment, a trend to one-phase treatment is being encouraged (Giannelly, 1995; Livieratos, Johnston, 1995). Thus if JJs overcome compliance problems—which they do most successfully—any favorable orthopedic effects are an added bonus.

O'Bryn et al's findings (1995) show that the position and dentoalveolar form of the mandible (rather than its size) are the significant long-term features in untreated patients with facial asymmetry. Wieslander (1994) also reports disappointing long-term findings, indicating that although the JJ has great potential, further research into its limitations is required.

# Chapter 18

# Combined Extraoral and Functional Appliances

T.M. Graber

## PHILOSOPHIC DICHOTOMIES

The great interest in removable appliances in the United States in the past 15 to 20 years has resulted in a melding of European and American methodologies. Traditionally, American orthodontists avoided the use of removable appliances, which are less exact in their accomplishments and offer less control of individual teeth. To many clinicians in the United States, removable appliances were synonymous with socialized dentistry and were derisively labeled "poor man's orthodontics." Many European orthodontists were not much more complimentary about the American systems with their complex wire configurations, heavy forces, high percentage of extractions, frequent root resorption and decalcification, and the orthodontists' lack of understanding about the potential of growth guidance and use of the neuromuscular components of the stomatognathic system in the establishment of normal occlusion.

The "either-or" and "all-or-none" approaches to mechanotherapy on both sides of the Atlantic failed to recognize that the essential facets of orthodontic care are case selection, diagnostic assessment, and treatment goals, regardless of the appliance used. The strong cultism and dogma that permeate the various systems and the cookbook approach to treatment reinforce antagonisms toward different modalities. Discretionary, cognitive, decision-making orthodontics based on the unique demands of each patient naturally suffers from this approach.

Despite the great interest in removable appliances in the United States in the recent past, enhanced by managed care and insurance inroads, an emotional, unreasoning rejection of certain biologically based and thoroughly researched technologies is still sometimes observed. This chapter describes the middle road between fixed and removable appliances. With proper diagnostic objectivity and discretion, the clinician can take advantage of the best parts of both appliance philosophies and reduce or eliminate many of their disadvantages. The combination or sequential use of removable and fixed appliances for certain malocclusion categories at specific times in the dental development can produce results superior to those achieved with either approach alone. Such an approach is based on the acronym KISS ("Keep it simple, sir!").

This approach has less iatrogenic potential and offers a superior and often less time-consuming methodology for correction of problems that should be approached in the mixed dentition period. Included among these problems are sagittal discrepancies and neuromuscularly induced types of malocclusions; the bulk of this chapter discusses the management of Class II problems. With the recent development of managed care, the use of the simplest and best approaches (i.e., KISS) is more important than ever.

### Need for Diphasic Therapy

A basic tenet of the combined fixed and removable appliance modality is the realization that two phases of therapy will likely be required, one during the mixed dentition phase of growth and one after the eruption of the premolars and canines. This is particularly true in patients with skeletal Class II and III malocclusions in which elimination of sagittal-basal malrelationships requires the harnessing of growth processes. Abundant source material already exists for a variety of appliances (e.g., Schwarz's *Lehrgang der Gesissregulung* [1961] offers many different designs for removable appliances that can be used alone or with fixed appliances. *Removable Orthodontic Appliances* by Graber and Neumann [1984] and the first edition of this book [1985] also discuss this combination).

**First phase therapy—functional appliances and extraoral force.** This chapter concentrates on the combination of functional orthopedic appliances and fixed appliances that use extraoral force to guide the anteroposterior and vertical growth of the maxilla and mandible to a more harmonious relationship and pleasing profile (Figure 18-1). Although Class I malocclusions are encountered most frequently in the general populace, a great number of patients have sagittal malrelationships, primarily in the Class II category. This is because both parents and patients are aware of the relative prominence of the maxillary incisors, the underdevelopment of the lower jaw, and the patient's inability to close the lips without strain because of abnormal perioral muscle function. The likelihood of enhancing the overjet by the deforming muscle activity (if the malocclusion is left unattended until the perma-

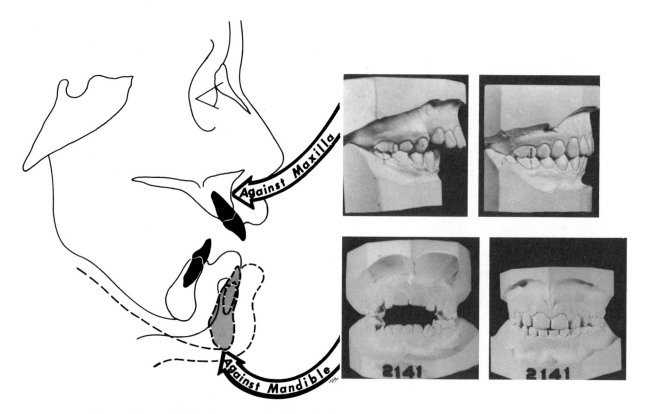

**Figure 18-1.** Traditionally, extraoral orthopedic force using fixed appliances has been directed against the maxilla and mandible in Class II and III and open-bite problems. Both retractive and protractive forces have been employed in the treatment of Class III malocclusions.

nent dentition stage) is sufficient reason to intercept the problem in the mixed dentition stage. However, added to this is the increased risk of damage to the protruding incisors if they are left unattended.

**Apical base dysplasia and neuromuscular involvement.** An essential requisite of treatment is the reduction of the apical base dysplasia. Paradoxically, many American orthodontists have been trained in the use of an appliance regimen based on placing full appliances on adult dentition. Only then can gnathologic precepts be implemented. The idea of instituting first-phase therapy too often runs counter to training and experience. Disregarding the obvious interplay between the three M's—muscles, malformation, and malocclusion—clinicians instruct parents to bring their children in when their permanent teeth erupt. Then with full multiattachment fixed appliances, intermaxillary elastics, headgear, and a greater likelihood of tooth sacrifice, the comprehensive treatment is carried to completion. No doubt exists that precise adjustments of arch wires and other features are capable of correcting individual tooth malpositions and producing the tooth-to-tooth relationships demanded by traditional gnathologists. Whether the result is completely stable, healthy, and noniatrogenic is sometimes another question. Detailing using fixed, multiattachment, light-wire mechanotherapy, with its obviously superior tooth position control is often needed in the second phase of therapy in the permanent dentition. This still

does not address the major concern—abnormality of the jaw relationship itself with adaptive, compensatory, deforming muscle activity, which worsens the problem. Too often the objective of the one-shot therapy approach has been to achieve a dental compromise for a skeletal and neuromuscular problem, ignoring the potential of growth guidance directed to the primary areas of concern.

Removable appliance adherents, particularly the many pediatric dentists who are usually the gatekeepers for orthodontic specialty referral, have been no less concerned about malocclusion characteristics. However, these clinicians have developed a greater awareness of neuromuscular involvement in malocclusion and a greater understanding of the way tooth relationships often reflect basal sagittal jaw malrelationships that are being enhanced by compensatory functional activity. They have begun to focus on the patient's physiologic processes and now attempt to harness the patient's growth and developmental processes instead of trying to make all the corrective maneuvers by shifting teeth into more "normal" relationships and then hoping the bone and muscle components will follow and adapt to the new occlusion.

**Functional appliance objectives.** Functional appliances (e.g., the Clark twin block activator, bionator appliance) attempt to correct sagittal abnormality by pushing the mandible forward with appliance guidance. The primary objective is to eliminate the deforming neuromuscular activity, which has a retrusive effect on the mandible and a tendency to increase the overjet by tipping the upper incisors further forward. The objectives of functional appliances also include an unloading of the condyle, with the research-supported expectation of enhanced condylar growth in a more favorable direction and some evidence of favorable adaptation of the articular fossa. The resultant reduction of the anteroposterior dysplasia, normalization of anterior face height, and favorable local changes in the dentition also have been documented.

**The treatment challenge.** In treatment decisions the importance of the clinician's diagnostic acumen comes to the fore. The orthodontic specialist is best qualified to make a diagnosis at earlier ages before the adult dentition erupts. If all Class II malocclusions were either maxillary protrusions or mandibular retrusions, the challenge would be clearer. However, many Class II malocclusions are combinations of both. The essential indicator of the sagittal discrepancy may well be the relative mandibular retrusion with localized maxillary dentoalveolar compensation (if the cephalometric research of McNamara [1989] is correct). Evidence suggests that abnormal muscle function in the classic Class II, division 1 malocclusion may extend to the suprahyoid and infrahyoid muscle groups and the posterior temporalis and deep masseter muscle fibers, all of which exert a restricting influence on the mandible through the muscle attachments. Permitting these aberrant functional forces to act on largely membranous bones, which are responsive to such forces, does not enhance normal growth and development or stimulate corrective compensatory tooth changes in the dental arches. Obviously the orthodontist should be the gatekeeper (decision maker) by virtue of superior training and experience.

The initial elimination of basal bone discrepancies and abnormal perioral muscle function before tooth straightening can significantly reduce the tooth-positioning challenge. A perceptive diagnostician first determines the area of greatest abnormality and then corrects the malocclusion, eliminating deforming neuromuscular factors that stand in the way of optimal development and stability in the process.

**Cephalometrics and growth guidance.** Cephalometrics has long permitted the clinician to determine the nature and degree of malrelationship and deficiency in the pretreatment analysis. Nevertheless, treatment objectives have reflected a fundamental compromise, an arbitrary clinical solution devoid of any suggestion of Popperian philosophy or cybernetic appreciation of the total problem, which is described in Chapter 2 by Petrovic. Despite evident mandibular underdevelopment, many of the multibanded, fixed-appliance treatment procedures are directed primarily at the maxilla instead of the major area of the abnormality. Distal driving of molars with extraoral force to permit retraction of maxillary incisors to a deficient mandible or extraction of premolars to make the same dental compromise is analogous to an orthopedic surgeon cutting off a good leg to make it shorter to match a clubfoot. If growth direction is unfavorable for sagittal correction, neither Class II elastics nor extraoral force application using a Kloehn cervical gear directed against the maxillary permanent

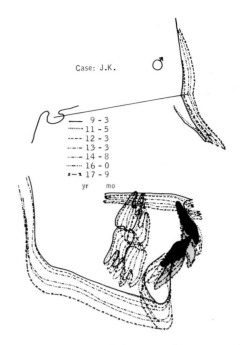

**Figure 18-2.** Vertical growth direction of a patient undergoing extraoral force orthopedics. Despite the withholding of forward maxillary growth, overjet remained excessive and mandibular retrusion dominated the profile.

first molars can cope with the problem (Figure 18-2). The major mandibular changes thus occur in the dentition with the lower incisors proclined, intentionally or unintentionally, to correct overjet and overbite. Apical base changes are evident in the anteroposterior position of point A in the maxilla, but point B in the mandible is actually rocked down and back by many techniques as the maxillary first molars are extruded by Kloehn headgear treatment.

## Role of Growth and Development

The principles of growth and development must be understood if the clinician is to adapt them to orthodontic treatment. Corrective procedures for Class II malocclusions must have as the objective all possible elimination of relative mandibular retrusion. Melvin Moss once commented, "Orthodontics is a 6 mm profession." He is correct in his analysis as far as sagittal discrepancy is concerned; such discrepancy is usually only a matter of 5 to 6 mm. Differential mandibular horizontal growth and elimination of functional retrusion are likely to make up only 2 to 3 mm of this increment. The balance comes from fossa change, vertical growth components, selective tooth movement, and alveolar bone compensation. Normally the mandible grows down the Y-axis or in a line from sella turcica to gnathion, as seen on a lateral cephalometric tracing. This is accomplished by combined horizontal and vertical growth. Maintaining equilibrium in a normal growing face requires adjustive and compensatory activities. Posteriorly the combined growth of the mandibular condyle and articular fossa balances the anterior components of maxillary sutural and septal growth and achieves tooth movement

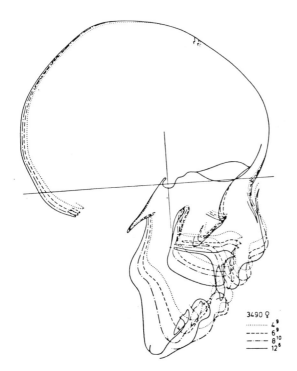

**Figure 18-3.** Tracings of lateral cephalograms showing the severe down and backward path of growth in a patient with muscular dystrophy. Both the maxilla and mandible are affected by this abnormal growth vector. A great increase in the mandibular plane inclination occurs under the influence of abnormal, selective, and deficient neuromuscular function.

(From Kreiborg S, Jensen BL, Møller E, Björk A: Craniofacial growth in a case of congenital muscular dystrophy: a roentgenographic and electromyographic investigation, *Am J Orthod* 74:207, 1978.)

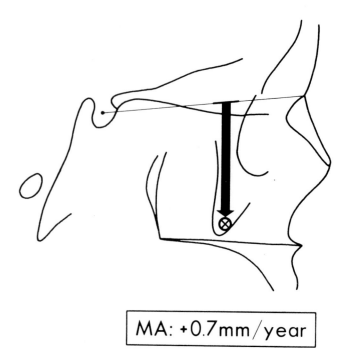

MA: +0.7mm/year

**Figure 18-4.** Approximate amount of basal maxillary vertical displacement per year (less than 1 mm) from the anterior cranial base to an implant in the zygomatic process, based on the work of Björk and Skieller. *MA,* Maxillary growth.

(Courtesy Paul Stöckli and Ullrich Teuscher, Zürich, Switzerland.)

and eruption and dentoalveolar compensation. Concentration of therapy on any one part of the dentofacial mosaic is seldom adequate to establish normal, stable, and balanced conditions and correct the problem.

In doctoral studies on congenital malformations, the author learned the truth of the maxim, "from the pathologic, we learn much about the normal" (1950). In Kreiborg's (1978) study of muscular dystrophy in which atrophy of temporalis and masseter muscles has occurred but continuing and adaptive function of suprahyoid and infrahyoid muscles is evident, the dramatic effect of this imbalance and the potential effect of function or malfunction on the mandible is clearly evident (Figure 18-3). The down and back growth pattern and opening of the Y-axis are in marked contrast to the normal down and forward vector seen with a relatively constant Y-axis. Compensatory maxillary and dentoalveolar growth struggle to maintain some semblance of an occlusal relationship, but the challenge is too great, and the tongue has become a detrimental factor, resulting in an anterior open bite. Maxillary orthopedics or dental compensations are obviously not going to solve the problem alone.

Nevertheless, maxillary growth is a consideration in the ultimate sagittal position of the chin point. If combined maxillary and alveolodental growth provides less vertical growth

than the contribution from the downward-moving glenoid fossa and mandibular condyle, the result is a more forwardly rotating mandible, a more horizontally placed chin point, and a closing of the Y-axis. This is the converse of the Kreiborg case described previously. Maxillary growth should be clinically manipulated to either open the Y-axis or close the Y-axis, thus influencing the horizontal position of point B on the mandible through mandibular autorotation.

## Incremental Expectations

In growth guidance the incremental change of the component parts is important. Björk (1955) has shown that the maxilla grows down from the cranial base at a rate of about 0.7 mm per year (Figure 18-4). Maxillary tooth eruption increases the dentoalveolar height about 0.9 mm per year (Figure 18-5). Mandibular eruption is about 0.75 mm annually (Figure 18-6). Therefore the nasomaxillary complex descends 1.5 to 2 mm per year. If eruption of the mandibular teeth is added to this figure, a total vertical development of between 2 and 3 mm occurs per year. According to Stöckli and Teuscher (1982), the counterpart development of the glenoid fossa and condyle must be considered. Because the fossa change is minimal (0.25 mm to 0.5 mm annually) (Figure 18-7), having followed the neural pattern of precipitate growth that is completed early, the condyle must provide the greatest increment of change, approximately 2.5 mm per year (Figure 18-8). The nasomaxillary complex growth, dentoalveolar growth, and fossa growth are

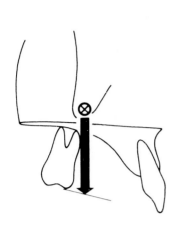

UA: +0.9mm/year

**Figure 18-5.** Average vertical dentoalveolar growth per year (slightly less than 1 mm) from an implant in the zygomatic process to the occlusal plane mesial to the first molars, according to Björk and Skieller. *UA,* Upper alveolar growth.
(Courtesy Paul Stöckli and Ullrich Teuscher, Zürich, Switzerland.)

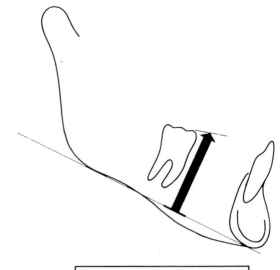

LA: +0.7mm/year

**Figure 18-6.** Average annual lower dentoalveolar vertical growth measured from the mandibular plane to the mesial cusp of the first permanent molar, according to Riolo et al and Teuscher. *LA,* Lower alveolar growth.
(Courtesy Paul Stöckli and Ullrich Teuscher, Zürich, Switzerland.)

largely membranous, as opposed to a secondary cartilage growth center in the condyle.

Current research indicates that the most susceptible areas of adjustment are the purely membranous structures (i.e., alveolodental compensation). However, condylar growth also is subject to environmental and appliance growth guidance influence, even though it is the dominant growth center of those units that comprises the maxillomandibular growth complex (see Chapter 2).

**Facial growth equilibrium—a fragile relationship.** The equilibrium established by the growing dentofacial parts is easily disturbed. This disturbance can be caused by the functional matrix—the normally functioning or abnormally deforming facial, masticatory, suprahyoid, and infrahyoid musculature as shown in the muscular dystrophy case of Kreiborg (1978). It also can be caused by orthopedic appliances such as a Milwaukee brace or by fixed or removable dentofacial orthopedics.

**Class II elastic traction and Kloehn headgear.** In an attempt to solve sagittal problems with Class II elastics, the orthodontist finds that vertical changes also are induced by the elevation of the lower molars with the net effect of rocking the mandible open. This maneuver moves point B into a more retruded position and often unfavorably influences anterior face height. The Y-axis angle opens (see Figure 18-2).

This undesirable response also can be produced by the indiscriminate use of the Kloehn cervical headgear. The maxillary first molars are driven distally into the "wedge" as the molars are *extruded* or *tipped down* and *back.* The mandible is ro-

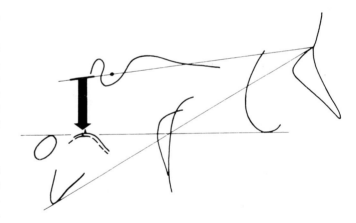

FO: +0.3mm/year

**Figure 18-7.** Vertical displacement of the articular fossa averages only 0.3 mm per year measured from the anterior cranial base line to the superior fossa surface, based on estimates by Björk et al. *FO,* Fossa growth.
(Courtesy Paul Stöckli and Ullrich Teuscher, Zürich, Switzerland.)

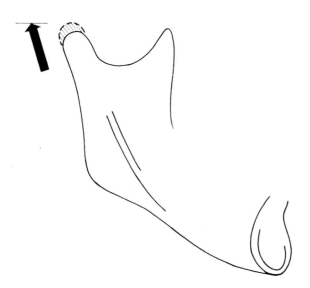

CO: +2.6mm/year

**Figure 18-8.** Average annual growth increments at the mandibular condyles, according to Ricketts, Luder, and Teuscher. This is normally about 2.6 mm per year, but the precise vector varies in direction. *CO,* Condylar growth.
(Courtesy Paul Stöckli and Ullrich Teuscher, Zürich, Switzerland.)

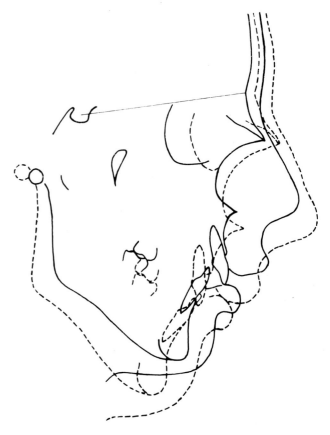

**Figure 18-9.** Clinical example of severe down and backward mandibular growth and rotation resulting from bimaxillary retropositioning and bodily movement of incisors aided by extraoral force. Note the increased angulation of the mandibular plane.
(Courtesy Paul Stöckli and Ullrich Teuscher, Zürich, Switzerland.)

tated down and back, increasing the apparent mandibular retrusion and allowing compensatory alveolodental growth to stabilize this undesirable sagittal change. The maxillary incisors are usually tipped down and back at the same time, restricting forward mandibular growth. This result has become so common that it is now known in orthodontic parlance as the *Kloehn effect.* Instead of horizontal withholding of the maxilla alone, a primary bite-opening tooth movement occurs that exacerbates instead of corrects the anteroposterior dysplasia. Even with good torque control and bodily lingual movement of upper incisors, molar extrusion can produce unfavorable sagittal consequences (Figure 18-9), lengthening the anterior facial height excessively and enhancing undesirable facial esthetics. Because normally only a 2.5 mm annual vertical height change occurs, not much extrusion of molar teeth needs to occur to create an unfavorable mandibular rotation with Class II elastic traction and conventional cervical extraoral force therapy directed against the maxillary first molars with a face-bow. Stöckli (1982) has demonstrated this change in Figure 18-10. The eruption of the upper and lower molars by 1 mm each results in an opening of the Y-axis by 2.5 degrees, a retrusion of the chin point, and a reduction of the sella-nasion-supramentale (S-N-B) angle by 2.5 degrees. As he observes, the claim of a poor growth pattern often is more likely because of an iatrogenic deflection of the natural growth path (Figure 18-11).

If this reasoning is correct, conventional multiattachment, fixed-appliance therapy using Class II elastics and Kloehn cer-

vical gear against the maxillary first molars and primarily attacking the maxilla in Class II malocclusions and ignoring basal mandibular retrusion is not likely to produce the best possible results (Figure 18-12). Nor does it provide optimal growth guidance, even though the mandible outgrows the maxilla by as much as 5 mm, as claimed by Lysle Johnston (1983). The way *mandibular* growth potential is controlled is the key to proper sagittal correction.

Can functional appliances alone provide the answer? Can they enhance the most favorable amount and direction of growth? These are primary objectives of functional jaw orthopedics. A common maneuver of all modifications of the Andresen activator, including the Fränkel, Clark, and Herbst appliances, is the forward posturing of the mandible by the appliance, moving the condyle forward in the glenoid fossa.

**Laboratory research versus clinical results.** The research of Breitner (1930) upholds the concept that condylar growth can be influenced with favorable fossa changes (as seen in primate studies) and sufficient basal maxillary, maxillary dentoalveolar, and mandibular dentoalveolar adjustments, all of which are needed to establish normal and stable occlusion.

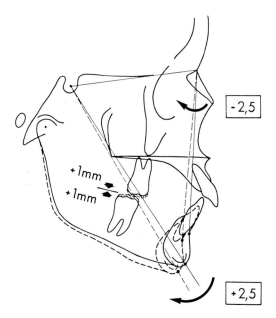

**Figure 18-10.** The effects of a 1-mm extrusion of the upper and lower molars during therapy are shown by a 2.5-degree decrease in the S-N-B angle and a 2.5-degree opening of the Y-axis angle. This can be interpreted as vertical growth, although in reality it is a bodily mandibular rotational translation.
(Courtesy Paul Stöckli and Ullrich Teuscher, Zürich, Switzerland.)

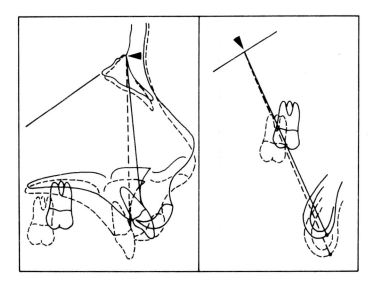

**Figure 18-11.** Rotational displacement of the maxilla with extraoral force also can elongate maxillary molars, and the net is downward and backward movement of the symphysis, increasing the Y-axis angle, as shown by Stöckli.
(From Ricketts RM et al: *Bioprogressive therapy,* Denver, 1979, Rocky Mountain Orthodontics.)

In spite of rather conclusive qualitative and quantitative laboratory evidence of enhanced prechondroblastic proliferation in the condyle, a changed angle of trabecular alignment (Stutzmann's angle) after mandibular advancement, increased mandibular length, and forward remodeling of the glenoid fossa from the laboratories of Petrovic (1981), Moyers (1977), McNamara (1975), Graber (1983), and others, controversy persists concerning the effects that take place in the human patient (see Chapter 2). Skeptics wonder whether results can be extrapolated from rat and monkey studies to human beings. Most of the skepticism, however, is based on two-dimensional, cephalometric measurements, which are suspect at the outset. Clinicians come in contact with an infinite variety of malocclusions. An astute observer learns to recognize the multifaceted nature of malocclusions grouped under a single heading such as Class II, division 1 (in which the primary qualifying factor is molar relationship). Treatment response is no less variable. Because the patient cannot be treated twice—once without condylar protraction and once with protraction—and the results compared, the clinician uses statistical means or norms and standards. Samples are small, and methods of posturing vary with different types of appliances and techniques, patient compliance, and different clinicians; some have larger horizontal increments in the construction bite, and some have larger vertical openings. Therefore no definitive answer is forthcoming. However, based on larger samples, researchers have observed greater condylar growth increments per year than the means given by the computerized data-processing companies; mandibular length also seems to be enhanced. Careful studies confirm the measurements and observations of Fränkel et al (1969).

## The Proper Case and the Proper Appliance at the Proper Time

Traditionalists from both the fixed-appliance multiattachment and the removable functional appliance schools point out that alveolodental compensations and maxillary reactions are largely responsible for skeletal and occlusal changes. Little doubt remains that this is partly true. However, case selection is essential for optimal success. The most dramatic changes occur in patients with forward rotating mandibular growth and deep-bite problems. Many of these cases present clear evidence of functional retrusion, mandibular overclosure, excessive posterior temporalis and deep masseter muscle activity, and tooth guidance. Posterior displacement can be as great as 2 mm in the average patient. An individual Class II, division 1 malocclusion may thus have a postural change, as do many Class II, division 2 cases.

In downward and backward rotating facial patterns, functional appliances are less likely to be successful. Untoward sequelae may occur such as proclination of the lower incisors, excessive anterior face height, poor facial esthetics, lack of lip seal, lack of stability, and dual bite (see Chapters 6 and 7). In these cases of unfavorable growth direction, the functional orthopedic concept alone is inadequate to correct the sagittal malrelationship, as are fixed appliances that direct their attentions primarily to distalizing the maxillary dentition. Optimal

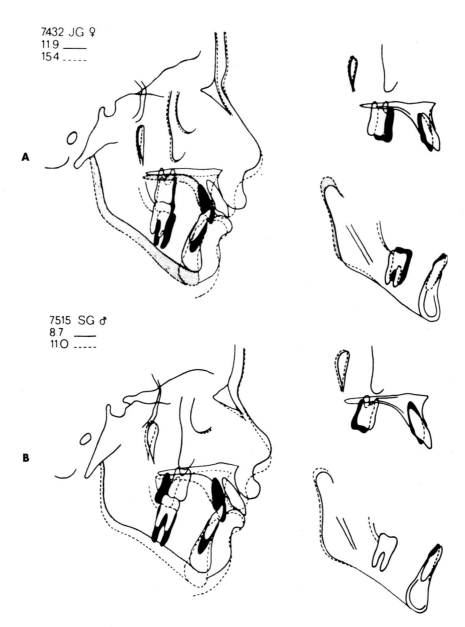

7432 JG ♀
119 ——
154 -----

7515 SG ♂
87 ——
110 -----

**Figure 18-12.**    Another clinical example of the effects of cervical extraoral force. **A,** Extraction case; **B,** nonextraction case. In both these patients the direction of change expressed at the symphysis is vertical as the mandibular plane is rocked open.

(From Meikle MC: Longitudinal changes during orthodontic treatment, *Am J Orthod* 77:184, 1980.)

response can be achieved only by combined orthopedic guidance of the maxilla and all possible forward positioning of the mandible. Orthognathic surgery may be the only solution. Orthodontic treatment must be directed toward relative depression of the maxillary alveolodental components in cases that start with excessive anterior face height and the greatest possible retardation of vertical basal maxillary growth. Success in these endeavors permits autorotation of the mandible, bringing the chin point upward and forward to improve the S-N-B relationship to sella-nasion-subspinale (S-N-A). High-pull extraoral force directed at the entire maxillary dentition is far more likely to accomplish these objectives than is any functional appliance alone.

**The potential of growth guidance.** Use of functional appliances does not routinely result in major changes in the nasomaxillary complex, as McNamara et al (1977) have shown. However, animal experiments by Droschl (1973), Graber (1983), Cederquist (1976), McNamara (1976), Moyers (1977), and others have shown significant retropositioning of the nasomaxillary complex. Both major sutural activity and dentoalveolar compensation are seen. Voluminous clinical material is available from the same sources. Delaire (1972) has shown dramatic success in forward protraction of the maxillary complex with fixed orthopedic appliances. Continuous heavy orthopedic force against the maxilla produces posterior rotation of the whole complex, as shown by Droschl (1973).

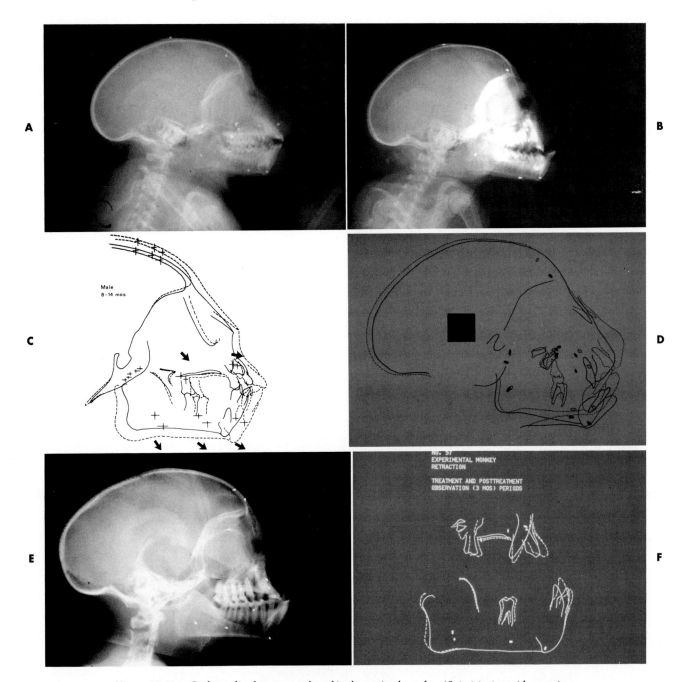

**Figure 18-13.** Orthopedic changes produced in the squirrel monkey (*Saimiri sciureus*) by continuous and intermittent forces in the Droschl (1973) and Cederquist (1976) studies. **A** and **B,** Severe maxillary retraction over a 3-month period with continuous orthopedic guidance. Superimposed implants contrast the normal pattern (**C**) with the tracings of the two top head films (**D**). Note the maxillary rotation around a point near the frontonasal suture with a rocking open of the mandible. Intermittent forces in the Cederquist study produced a marked maxillary retraction (**E** and **F**), but no maxillary rotation, with resultant minimal mandibular rotational compensation.

Delaire shows anterior maxillary rotation around the frontonasal suture with protraction. However, Cederquist (while at the University of Chicago [1976]) produced major orthopedic maxillary retraction in primates with no maxillary rotation by using heavy intermittent forces along the occlusal plane (Figure 18-13). Nevertheless, with conventional extraoral force, particularly from the cervical direction, downward rotation of the maxilla is a distinct likelihood, as shown by Wieslander (1974). Therefore the *direction* and the *method* of delivery of orthopedic force to the maxilla are important. Otherwise the increased anterior vertical dimension offsets the sagittal gain, rotating the mandible down and back, as discussed previously in this chapter. All efforts must be made to reduce both horizontal and vertical maxillary growth in these

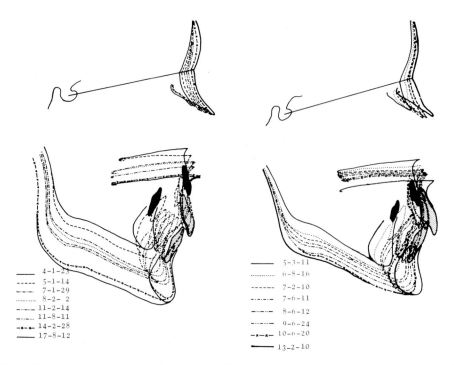

| | |
|---|---|
| —— 4-1-24 | —— 5-3-11 |
| ----- 5-1-14 | ........... 6-8-16 |
| —·—· 7-1-29 | ----- 7-2-10 |
| ........... 8-2- 2 | —·—· 7-6-11 |
| —··— 11-2-14 | —··— 8-6-12 |
| —···— 11-8-11 | —···— 9-6-24 |
| —x—x— 14-2-28 | —x—x— 10-6-20 |
| —— 17-8-12 | —— 13-2-10 |

**Figure 18-14.** Extraoral orthopedic growth guidance can be performed against the entire maxillary arch, not just the first molars, as is done with the Kloehn appliance. The maxilla has descended vertically, but the mandible has grown down and forward. These patients also wore maxillary biteplates that unlocked the occlusion and freed the mandible from any retrusive maxillary effects (see Figures 18-11 and 18-12). No maxillary first molar extrusion occurred (see Figure 18-10).

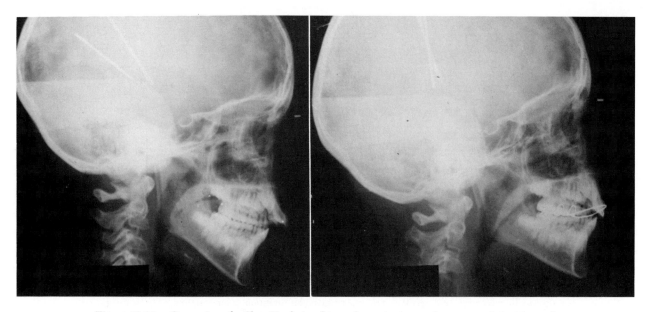

**Figure 18-15.** Correction of a Class II relationship and anterior space closure coupled with good mandibular growth over a 6-month period. Maxillary orthopedic treatment was directed against the entire dental arch. Because of the initial open bite tendency, no biteplate was needed.

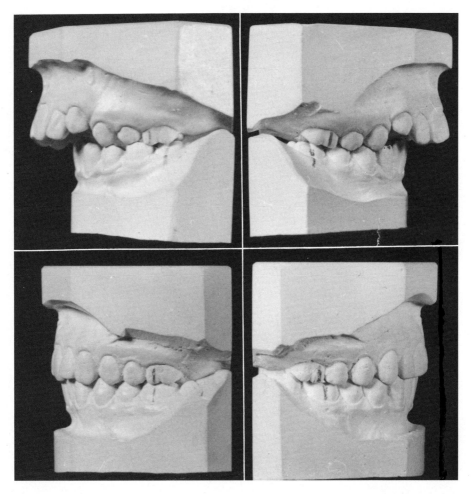

**Figure 18-16.** Dentoalveolar changes produced by maxillary extraoral orthopedics directed against the entire dentition, not just the permanent first molars. No appliances were worn on the lower arch.

unfavorable growth patterns. The combination of functional and dentofacial orthopedics provides the necessary force magnitude and vectors in such cases. Combination therapy may be used for all patients with Class II, division 1 or 2 malocclusions with significant benefit. Correction of the malocclusion by direct assault on the dysplastic relationships is the most desirable form of therapy.

Studies of the use of heavy intermittent force in primates and human beings in cases of cleft lip and palate show the viability of the technique for withholding both horizontal and vertical maxillary growth vectors. The appliance only needs to be worn 10 to 12 hours at night or at home (Figures 18-14 to 18-18). Maxillary rotation is almost nonexistent, as the Mills et al (1978) survey shows. Continuous heavy force produces maxillary rotation, as does the use of conventional Kloehn-type headgear against the maxillary molars (Wieslander, 1974), but if the force is directed against the entire dentition, as in the Cederquist (1976) and Mills et al (1978) studies, minimal extrusive tipping of the maxillary first molars occurs, even though the force is delivered from the cervical region. Research experience using a cast chromium-cobalt maxillary splint demonstrates that heavy, intermittent, orthopedic force

can be employed with removable appliances (Figure 18-19). However, acrylic functional appliances that posture the mandible forward at the same time can be used as "handles" on the maxilla and simultaneously remove any growth restrictions on the mandible (Figure 18-20). Even conventional retainers can be modified to accept high-pull orthopedic extraoral force (Figure 18-21).

**Functional appliances and extraoral force.** In patients with skeletal Class II, division 1 malocclusions with more vertical growth directions and excessive anterior face heights, the cast acrylic splint incorporates a mandibular acrylic component that postures the mandible forward, unloading the condyle. In addition, concomitant maxillary orthopedic force using high-pull headgear attached to the acrylic activator exerts a retarding force on horizontal and vertical maxillary growth vectors. This modified activator approach has been used successfully by a number of clinicians (Hasund [1969], Pfeiffer [1984], Grobety [1984], Stöckli [1982], Teuscher [1982], Hickham [1982], Stockfisch [1977], and others). The bulkiness of the original monobloc acrylic, or Andresen activator, can be reduced and still maintain the dual effectiveness

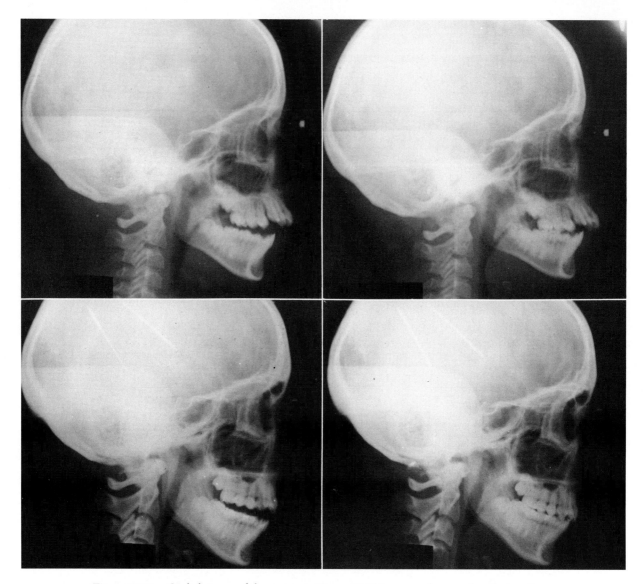

**Figure 18-17.** Cephalograms of the patient in Figure 18-16 in postural rest and occlusion. Some reduction of the excessive interocclusal clearance occurred, as well as sagittal correction. The change was effected by withholding horizontal maxillary growth, which encouraged unimpeded mandibular growth and favorable upward and forward mandibular dentitional eruption.

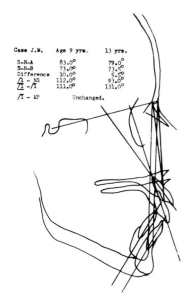

| Case J.M. | Age 9 yrs. | 13 yrs. |
|---|---|---|
| S–N–A | 83.0° | 79.0° |
| S–N–B | 73.0° | 73.5° |
| Difference | 10.0° | 5.5° |
| $\underline{1}$ – NS | 112.0° | 93.0° |
| $\underline{1}$ –/$\overline{1}$ | 111.0° | 131.0° |
| /$\overline{1}$ – MP | Unchanged. | |

**Figure 18-18.** Tracings of before and after lateral cephalograms in occlusion for the patient in Figures 18-16 and 18-17. The maxillary plane was not tipped down anteriorly as is often the case with Class II elastic traction and the use of Kloehn headgear. This result was confirmed by the Mills, Holman, and Graber (1978) longitudinal study of 120 treated patients.

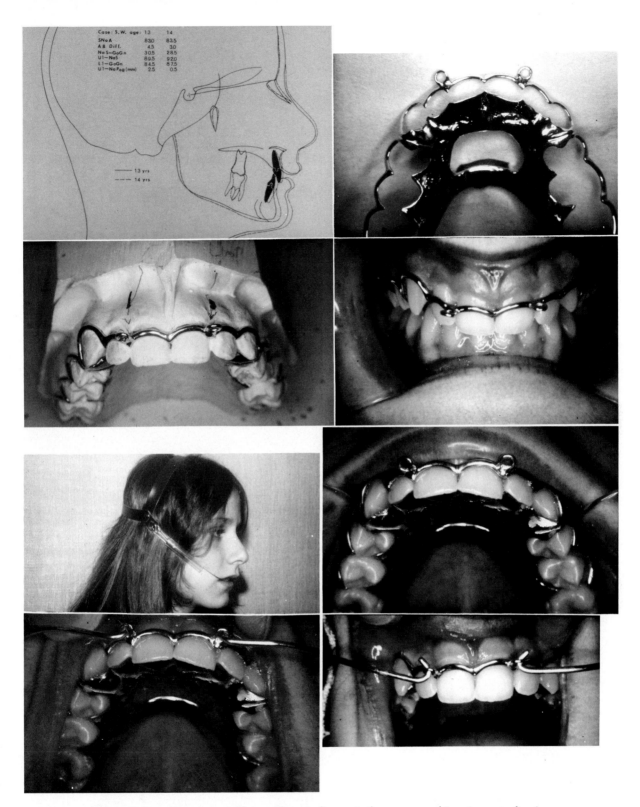

**Figure 18-19.** A cast removable maxillary appliance similar to one used in primate studies (see Figure 18-13) provides good anchorage on the maxilla and attachment for extraoral orthopedic force directed along the Y-axis. No palatal plane or mandibular plane rotation occurs. The primary effect is to withhold horizontal and vertical maxillary downward translation and eruption of the maxillary teeth. This effect permits some favorable autorotation of the mandible, which is desirable in vertically growing faces. Acrylic may be added behind the maxillary incisors as a biteplate or slightly inclined plane to unlock the occlusion and prevent inhibition of mandibular growth and positioning by maxillary retraction. This is recommended in patients with deep bite problems.

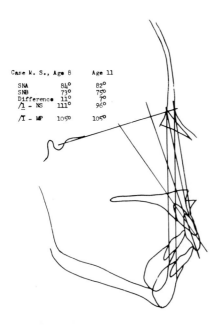

Case M. S., Age 8     Age 11

| | Age 8 | Age 11 |
|---|---|---|
| SNA | 84° | 82° |
| SNB | 73° | 75° |
| Difference | 11° | 7° |
| /1 – NS | 111° | 96° |
| /1 – MP | 105° | 105° |

**Figure 18-20.** Class II, division 1 malocclusion treated with an activator. Slight maxillary horizontal withholding is combined with optimal mandibular growth increments and is unrestricted by maxillary retractive and incisal forces.

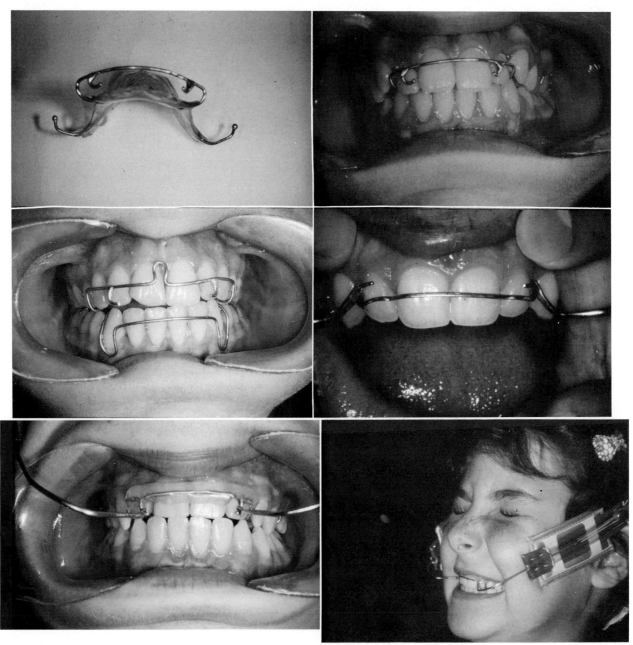

of the appliance. A transpalatal coffin spring–shaped wire can be used, as can the bionator or Fränkel appliance. If indicated, even buccal shielding wires and lip pads can be incorporated to break up abnormal perioral muscle function and the well-known lower lip trap (see Figure 18-36). The orthodontic problems at the source of the abnormality can then be attacked. Trying to solve all problems with fixed appliances and putting the teeth in proper occlusion at the expense of a correct tooth–to–basal bone relationship, which often results in uncorrected basal jaw dysplasias and neuromuscular problems, is more mechanical than biologic, no matter the effectiveness of the appliances. With root resorption, sheared alveolar crestal bone, occasional periodontal problems, and possible decalcification among the hazards of treatment, some observers have asked whether the punishment fits the crime.

## COMBINATION THERAPY

### Maxillary Retraction Splints and Extraoral Force Combinations

**Margolis acrylic cervicooccipital anchorage (ACCO).** Fixed appliances have no monopoly on the use of extraoral force. Clinicians such as Margolis (1976) and Spengeman (1967) incorporated extraoral force with removable appliances a long time ago for patients with Class II malocclusions, using them both in active and retention phases of treatment. Spengeman devised several varieties of removable appliances to hold back relapsing maxillary arches (Figure 18-21). The Margolis appliance is called an *ACCO*. Hundreds of orthodontists in the United States have used this appliance in one form or another, particularly as a means of active retention (Figure 18-22). The addition of acrylic over the labial wire of the Hawley-type retainer lends added stability and better retention (Figure 18-23). Elimination of mild incisor irregularity is possible with these appliances. The teeth are cut off the working model and rearranged in wax before the labial wire is formed and the acrylic is added. The Harry Barrer spring retainer does the same thing. Interproximal stripping is used during appliance wear to improve the alignment. Margolis (1967) used the ACCO to hold the torque correction already achieved by fixed appliances; the broad labial acrylic surface holds the incisor inclination better than does the conventional round labial wire of the Hawley retainer. The regular removable upper retainer also is not capable of maintaining the sagittal correction achieved. The slight closing of the vertical loops of the labial wire to close incisor spaces left from active treatment can actually offset the torque adjustment already achieved. However, this tendency is reduced with the labial acrylic construction of the ACCO, which exerts a greater bodily force on the incisors.

Margolis (1967) also modified the appliance further by adding 1-mm buccal tubes to the labial wire and soldering them vertically at the canine–lateral incisor embrasure to receive the J-hook extraoral force arms. An inclined plane may be incorporated to eliminate functional retrusion and free the mandible for all possible forward growth.

An unwanted retrusive force on the lower jaw is sometimes created by tipping the maxillary incisors lingually with a conventional Hawley-type upper retainer; an acrylic table behind the maxillary incisors provides a bite opening that prevents this undesirable consequence. Acrylic can be carried over the occlusal surfaces of the posterior teeth to give added support for reception of extraoral force arms if no tooth movement is desired in this area. Occlusal cover also may be needed to prevent overeruption of the posterior teeth and the creation of an open bite. Such a splint is sometimes used in temporomandibular joint (TMJ) therapy.

The use of a bite plane alone, engaging only the lower incisors with no posterior occlusal cover, keeps the upper and lower posterior teeth apart, stimulating eruption of the molar teeth. The appliance can be modified to produce differential eruption, as recommended by Harvold and Woodside (1974), by freeing the lower posterior teeth but covering maxillary posterior teeth with a thin acrylic layer in addition to the anterior biteplate. This method or the use of metal spurs that act as occlusal rests reduces the curve of Spee while allowing vertical and horizontal movement of the lower buccal segment teeth. If indicated, acrylic is cut away from the lingual side of the maxillary posterior teeth to permit finger-springs to distalize molar and premolar teeth (Figure 18-22). One side is distalized at a time with the Margolis ACCO. Ball clasps or passive finger-springs on the other side enhance retention of the appliance. A new ACCO is made after extraoral force and finger-spring adjustments have created a Class I relationship on one side. The new acrylic configuration and clasps on the completed side provide anchorage to correct residual Class II tendencies for the other side of the arch, a maneuver that is completed with combined extraoral force and distalizing finger-springs.

The ACCO should be worn both day and night with a minimum of 12 hours of nocturnal extraoral force. Fixed appliances are often used before using the ACCO to correct individual tooth malpositions, which is similar to the methodology in other functional appliance procedures. A short period of fixed-appliance mechanotherapy using direct-bonded attachments and flexible arches for incisor rotation and depression also may be needed. Auxiliaries may provide a very limited degree of axial inclination control or torque. The ACCO can continue to be used as a retainer after the treatment objectives have been achieved. Extraoral force can again be applied to the ACCO, as indicated, to treat any residual sagittal abnormality or tendency to return to the original Class II relationship.

**Figure 18-21.** Modified maxillary removable Hawley-type appliances that permit the use of extraoral force against the maxillary dentition. Multiple ball clasps or occlusal cover can increase the resistance to dislodgment by extraoral traction.

(From Graber TM, Neumann B: *Removable orthodontic appliances,* ed 2, Philadelphia, 1984, WB Saunders.)

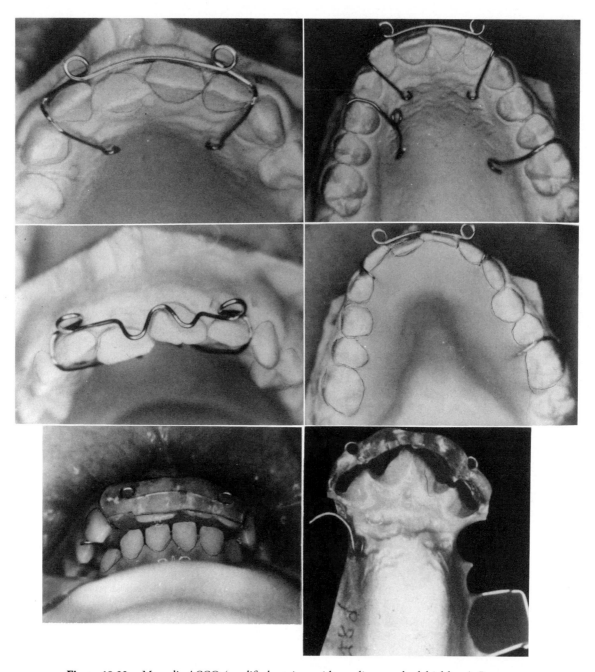

**Figure 18-22.** Margolis ACCO (modified retainer with acrylic over the labial bow). Loops are bent in the labial bow to receive J hooks from the extraoral appliance. The labial bow can be notched or undulated for better retention of the adapted acrylic. The teeth can be moved distally to a mild degree by cutting away contiguous palatal acrylic and using finger springs. This is usually done on one side at a time.

(From Graber TM, Neumann B: *Removable orthodontic appliances,* ed 2, Philadelphia, 1984, WB Saunders.)

**ACCO modifications.** Another modification of the ACCO is its use as an active retainer in patients with Class II, division 1 malocclusions in which a tendency exists for relapse of the overjet because of the original maxillary protraction. The initial therapy is accomplished with multi-attachment fixed appliances and any necessary auxiliary appliances in addition to extraoral force. The ACCO is then placed with or without a jackscrew for transverse control, depending on the need for expansion (Figure 18-23). The occlusal surfaces of the maxillary posterior teeth are covered for retention and the added stability needed when extraoral force arms are attached to the labial wire and acrylic assemblage. The acrylic cover for the posterior teeth frees the intercuspal interdigitation in Class II cases and eliminates any retrusive action of anterior or

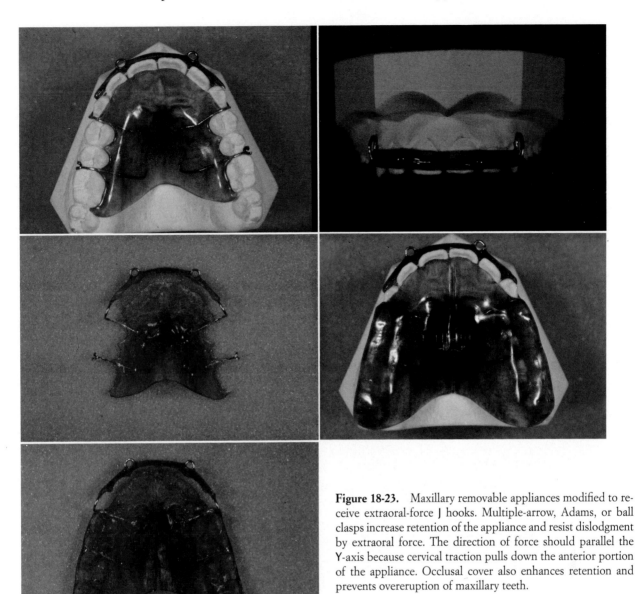

**Figure 18-23.** Maxillary removable appliances modified to receive extraoral-force J hooks. Multiple-arrow, Adams, or ball clasps increase retention of the appliance and resist dislodgment by extraoral force. The direction of force should parallel the Y-axis because cervical traction pulls down the anterior portion of the appliance. Occlusal cover also enhances retention and prevents overeruption of maxillary teeth.

posterior tooth guidance. The appliance also may continue to be used as a biteplate to reduce any excessive overbite by allowing only the lower incisors to contact the bite plane on the anterior aspect of the palatal acrylic. The lower buccal segments are free to erupt, whereas the upper posterior teeth are prevented from doing so by the acrylic cover. This allows differential eruption, and the sagittal relationship also is improved. If eruption of both upper and lower posterior segments is desired, the acrylic is cut away from the upper posterior teeth as well.

**Jacobson splint.** Jacobson (1967) has used a splint similar to the ACCO with some success for correction of mild Class II problems or for first-phase therapy or pre–fixed-appliance

guidance. The reduction of overjet and the sagittal discrepancy reduce the deforming action of abnormal perioral muscle function. The splint eliminates sagittal overjet problems that enhance abnormal perioral muscle function (Figures 18-24 and 18-25).

The force magnitude of this type of removable maxillary appliance must not be too great or the appliance will be dislodged. Figure 18-25 shows that the direction of pull should coincide roughly with that of the Y-axis or a line extending from the symphysis to a point 1.5 cm in front of the external auditory meatus. This reduces the potential for unfavorable basal maxillary tipping and extrusion of teeth, as noted earlier; the orthopedic potential is thus limited. Figure 18-26 depicts a soft acrylic version of the Jacobson splint.

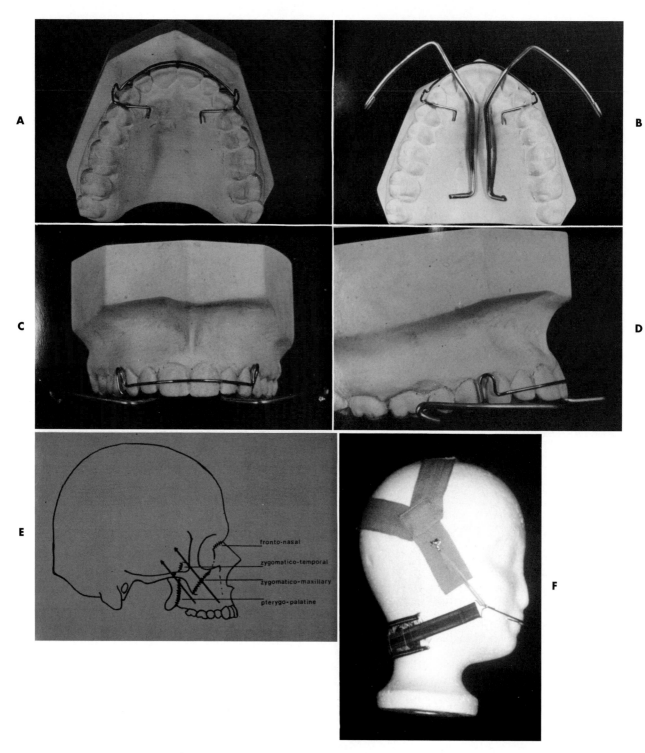

**Figure 18-24.** The Jacobson craniomaxillary appliance. **A** through **D,** Extraoral force arms are incorporated directly in the palatal acrylic. A conventional labial bow is used. Retention of the appliance can be increased with arrow, ball, or Adams clasps. The direction of extraoral force is shown in **E** and **F.** According to Sicher (1954), this should have a direct effect on the maxillary sutures. (Courtesy Alexander Jacobson, Birmingham, Alabama.)

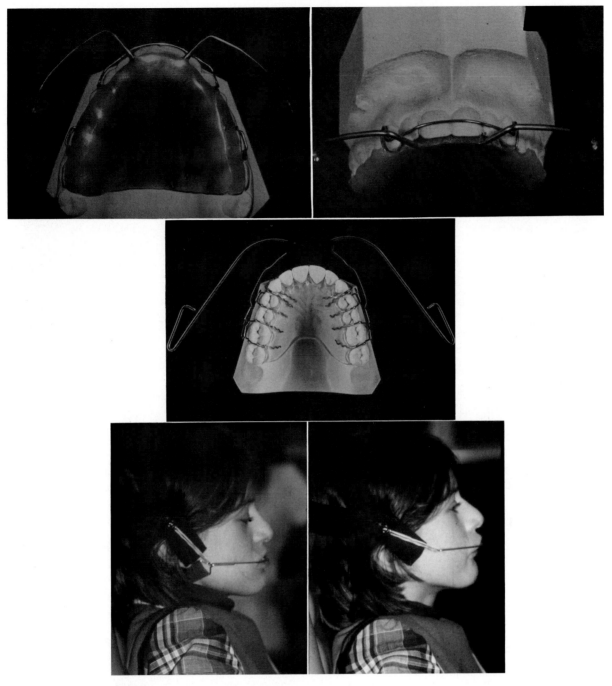

**Figure 18-25.** The Jacobson craniomaxillary splint with occlusal cover to enhance retention and prevent maxillary eruption while allowing unimpeded upward and forward eruption of the mandibular buccal segment teeth to assist in sagittal correction. The extraoral force arms also can be soldered to molar clasps. A combination of cervical and occipital force or occipital traction only can be used.

(Courtesy Alexander Jacobson, Birmingham, Alabama.)

**Verdon combination appliance.** Verdon has had demonstrable success with a similar appliance design (Figures 18-27 and 18-28). The basic appliance of choice is usually a modified active plate, but it can just as easily be a modified activator if mandibular protraction is desired as subsequent illustrations demonstrate. As with other purely maxillary splints, the major objective of the Jacobson and Verdon splints is to effect a change through a distalizing influence on the maxillary arch, leaving the mandibular arch alone. The magnitude of force is moderate at best because of the risk of dislodging the appliance, despite the excellent retention provided by the Adams clasps. Nevertheless, a surprising amount of force can

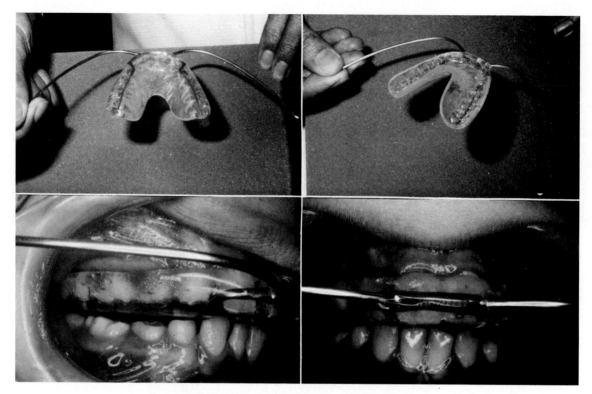

**Figure 18-26.** Another version of the Jacobson splint. This splint is made of soft positioner-type plastic with the labial bow anchored differently in plastic.
(Courtesy Alexander Jacobson, Birmingham, Alabama.)

be used toward an occipital headcap if the direction of the force is sufficiently high. As Stöckli and Jacobson point out, this is the best direction, roughly paralleling the Y-axis, to prevent tipping down the anterior end of the palatal plane. A cervical strap can be used, but the force amounts are significantly smaller, producing more dentoalveolar and less basal effects.

### Bimaxillary combination appliances

*With and without fixed appliances.* The first part of this chapter discussed maxillary splints and their combined use with extraoral force. Some mandibular guidance is possible through the use of biteplates for selective eruption of mandibular posterior teeth, inclined planes to posture the mandible forward slightly as the lower incisors glide up and forward in an attempt to reach full posterior occlusal contact, and guiding loops built into the palate to engage the lingual mucosal tissue beneath the lower incisors as a proprioceptive trigger, eliciting 1 to 2 mm of forward posturing to avoid the contact. The major emphasis in the past, however, has been on the use of the maxillary splint as a "handle" on the maxilla which receives extraoral force to restrict horizontal and vertical dentomaxillary development.

Maxillary splint–extraoral force combinations are indicated primarily for maxillary protraction malocclusions, although withholding horizontal maxillary growth allows the mandible to catch up and reduce the sagittal discrepancy. However, the potential for incremental change is limited to

2 to 3 mm unless a functional mandibular retrusion is to be eliminated. In this case, 1 to 1.5 mm of additional sagittal correction is possible. To achieve total sagittal correction of a full Class II, division 1 malocclusion, the clinician should enlist all possible force contributions from the area in which the greatest deficiency lies—the mandible. The condyle experiences 2.5 mm of growth per year. By eliminating any restriction of this growth from neuromuscular environmental assaults; optimizing the direction of condylar, mandibular, and fossa growth; and enlisting differential upward and forward mandibular dentitional eruption of the lower buccal segments, sagittal correction can be increased to 6 mm in the average case. Forward posturing of the mandible can not only accomplish these treatment objectives but also can eliminate functional retrusion and overclosure problems and attendant TMJ sequelae.

*Posturing the mandible forward.* In many cases, postural hyperpropulsion alone may be sufficient to achieve sagittal and vertical correction. The posturing appliance may be modified to make the necessary transverse correction.

A generation of European orthodontists thought this treatment was sufficient at a time in which functional orthopedics dominated therapeutics, but orthodontic research and experience have shown that all Class II, division 1 malocclusions are not the same, do not grow in the same amounts or direction, and do not have the same expectations of treatment success. No single arbitrary appliance exists into which all malocclu-

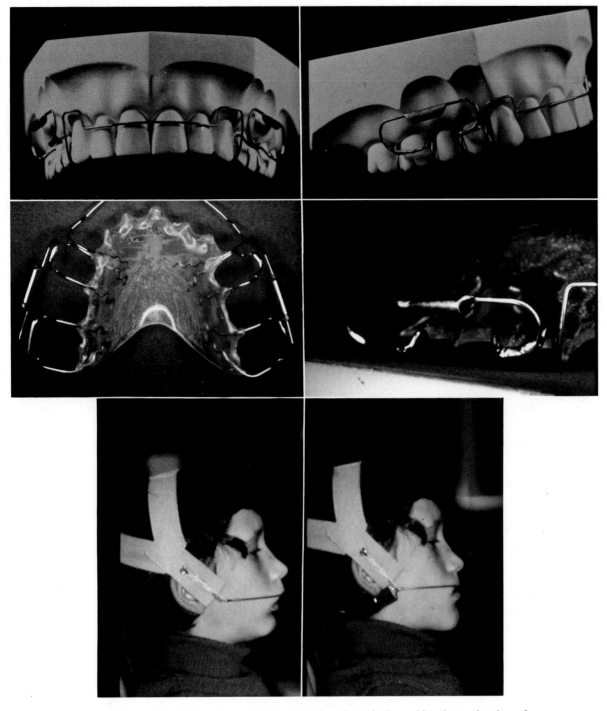

**Figure 18-27.** Maxillary appliance with extraoral force buccal tubes soldered to molar clasps for the face-bow. Either occipital or combined occipital-cervical extraoral anchorage can be used. (Courtesy Pierre Verdon, Tours, France.)

sions can be forced. Morphogenetic and functional factors, growth potential and direction, tooth size and shape, anterior and posterior face height proportions, and patient compliance are just some of the characteristics that must be considered in decisions regarding the treatment of malocclusions. Orthodontists must have an armamentarium at their command that permits them to modify their therapeutic efforts to take into account this multiplicity of factors before and during the treatment regimen. Although treatment of the maxilla using maxillary splints or extraoral force alone may prove inadequate in attaining full correction, so may the use of functional appliances. The logical treatment response is a bimaxillary as-

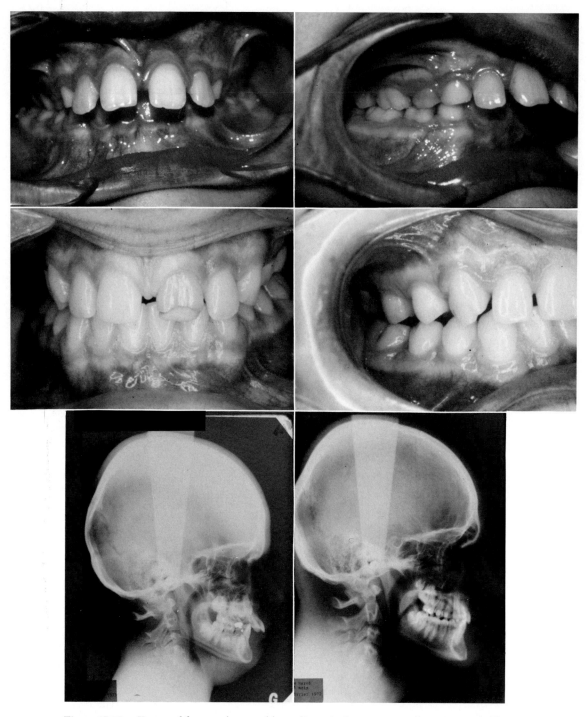

**Figure 18-28.**    Extraoral force and removable appliance in the treatment of a patient with Class II maxillary protraction. The final appliance incorporates an anterior bite plane to allow eruption of the mandibular posterior teeth.

(Courtesy Pierre Verdon, Tours, France.)

sault on the three-dimensional problem with intraoral appliances alone or with extraoral combinations.

**Tränkmann approach.** Depending on the morphogenetic pattern and severity of the initial malocclusion and the role of environmental compensations, different appliances may be se-

lected. For less severe problems, conventional removable appliances that have been modified to achieve the treatment objectives may be adequate. Orthodontic overkill with multiple attachments, loops, and elastics and extraoral force is not always necessary or indicated. This is particularly true when the iatrogenic potential is considered.

A                                                    B

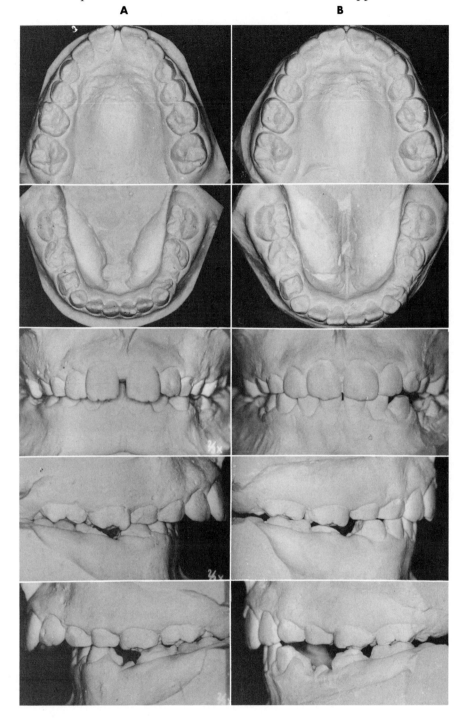

**Figure 18-29.** Class II, division 1 malocclusion treated with removable appliances. **A,** Before therapy; **B,** after therapy.

(Courtesy Joachim Tränkmann, Dresden, Germany.)

Figure 18-29 shows a patient with a mixed dentition, Class II, division 1 malocclusion treated with simple removable appliances (Figure 18-30). The use of forward posturing loops on the maxillary appliance, which engage the lingual acrylic surface of a lower removable appliance, eliminated functional retrusion and provided an initial activator effect as the maxillary and mandibular arches were slightly expanded by jackscrews to correct the minor space deficiency.

A functional appliance was then placed to complete sagittal and vertical correction with the aid of local finger-springs. If this procedure had not been sufficient to provide the anteroposterior and vertical correction needed, an extraoral appliance could have been attached to the functional appliance for added maxillary withholding or retraction. Figures 18-31 and 18-32 show the results achieved without the need for a total assault on the problem. The axial inclination of the lower in-

A

B

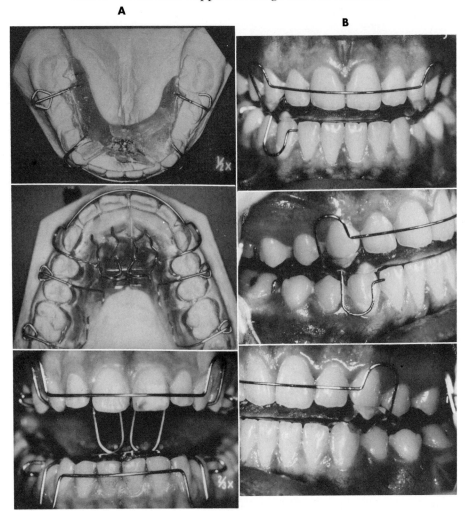

**Figure 18-30.** Appliances used in correction of the case in Figure 18-29. Maxillary and mandibular active plates have expansion screws and efficient arrow clasps for retention. The maxillary appliance has two sagittal guiding loops that engage the lingual mandibular acrylic on closing, protracting the mandible (**A**). Minor arch length problems are corrected by judicious use of expansion screws. A functional appliance is then placed to correct the residual sagittal problems. If maxillary protraction is evident, horizontal buccal tubes can be added to the molar clasps or incorporated directly into the interocclusal acrylic to permit use of extraoral force (**B**).

(Courtesy Joachim Tränkmann, Dresden, Germany.)

cisors remains at 90 degrees, and the potential proclination of these teeth has not materialized. The spontaneous regression of epipharyngeal lymphoid tissue is a clear sign of the restoration of normal nasal breathing and an expected developmental process.

## Pfeiffer, Grobety, Stöckli-Teuscher, Stockfisch, Hanson, and Hickham Techniques

Dentofacial orthopedic procedures performed on the maxilla are indicated most often in maxillary protrusion problems. Sagittal correction is possible, but any treatment effect on the mandible is indirect unless a biteplate or Class II elastics are used. However, most Class II, division 1 malocclusions are primarily mandibular underdevelopment problems with lo-

calized premaxillary protrusion. Therapy requires an attack on the mandibular retrusion. A deficiency appliance is needed; holding back horizontal growth of the maxilla is not enough. Indeed, as Mills, Holman, and Graber (1978) show, maxillary withholding can transmit force to the mandible and actually prevent full mandibular growth, and the mandible may achieve a correct position and size even after treatment.

Significant growth may occur in the mandibular dentoalveolar areas, mandibular condyle, and temporal fossa region. A frequent postural functional retrusion may occur, particularly in patients with Class II malocclusions with deep bites and premature incisal guidance, which can restrict full mandibular growth pattern accomplishment. Significant factors here are the abnormal retrusive forces of the posterior temporalis, deep masseter, and suprahyoid and infrahyoid musculature.

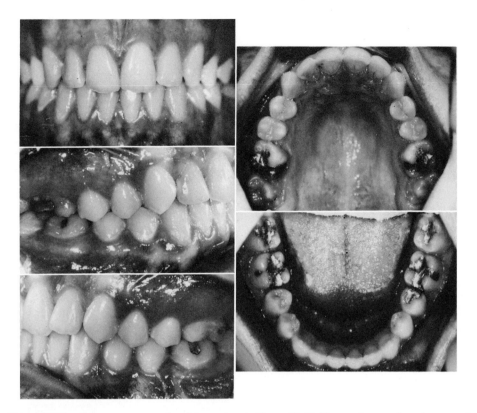

**Figure 18-31.** Posttreatment results of the patient in Figure 18-29. No attachments have been used to correct individual tooth malpositions.

(Courtesy Joachim Tränkmann, Dresden, Germany.)

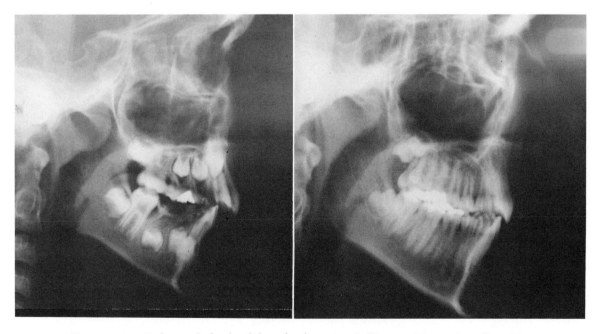

**Figure 18-32.** Before and after headplates for the patient in Figures 18-29 to 18-31. Proper incisor inclination has been retained. If sufficient mandibular growth had not resulted, even with the unlocking of the occlusion and positional retraction achieved in the construction bite, extraoral force could have been used to withhold horizontal maxillary growth.

(Courtesy Joachim Tränkmann, Dresden, Germany.)

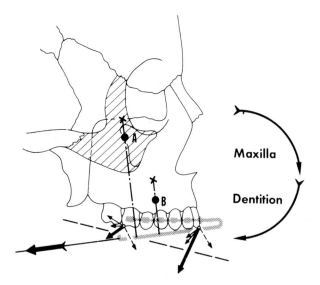

**Figure 18-33.** If the teeth are banded and stabilized with an arch wire in the maxillary arch, a cervical pull appliance (e.g., Kloehn-type) produces a force direction below both the center of resistance of the maxilla *(A)* and the center of resistance of the dentition *(B)*. The distances of the force vector to *A* and *B* determine the corresponding centers of rotation *(x)*. Thin arrows indicate the reactive movement vectors of the dentition and maxilla at particular points. A posterior rotation of the maxilla and dentition must be expected from the analysis. As the thicker arrows show, the incisors move down and back more than the molars. This tips the occlusal plane down, as the interrupted line shows, blocking open the mandible and moving the symphysis down and back.

(Courtesy Paul Stöckli and Ullrich Teuscher, Zürich, Switzerland.)

The early elimination of restrictive muscle forces if at all possible is biologically and therapeutically sound. This requires a mixed-dentition, first-phase assault on the problem or even earlier treatment in the deciduous dentition in carefully selected cases. As Stöckli and Teuscher write (1994):

> The prime target of the treatment concept employing the activator-headgear combination is to restrict developmental contributions that tend toward a skeletal Class II and to enhance developmental contributions that tend to harmonize the anteroposterior relationship of maxillomandibular structures. It is of paramount concern that no untoward deflections of growth displacement vectors be introduced when a treatment device is used to interfere with facial growth.

**Deflections of growth—favorable and unfavorable.** *Untoward deflections of growth* refers to not only the possible restrictive effect of maxillary orthopedics if the occlusion is not unlocked but also the direction of orthopedic force.

As Wieslander, Merrifield, Cross, and many clinicians have observed, the direction of extraoral force affects the maxillary and palatal planes. In many cases, tipping the anterior end of the palatal plane down is counterproductive. Nevertheless, conventional Kloehn headgear procedures are likely to do this in any protracted therapy, as Stöckli (1985) shows (Figure 18-33). With the face-bow directed against the maxillary molars, the combined tipping of the anterior end of the maxillary arch and the posterior tipping and extrusion of the molars

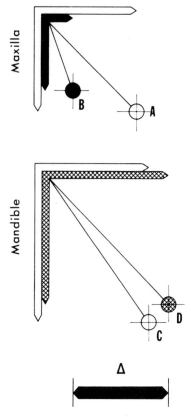

**Figure 18-34.** Restriction of both horizontal and vertical growth increments can be a desirable orthopedic effect on the maxilla, as recommended by Harvold. If successful, the maxillary position can effectively move from *A* to *B* in the facial profile. With a normal mandibular growth amount and direction *(C)*, reduced maxillary growth allows favorable autorotation of the mandible to *D*, further reducing the sagittal malrelationship in Class II malocclusions. This effect has been shown by Graber et al (Droschl, Cederquist, Mills, and Holman).

(From Stöckli PW, Teuscher UM: Combined activator-headgear orthopedics. In Graber TM, Vanarsdall RL, editors: *Orthodontics: current principles and techniques,* ed 2, St Louis, 1994, Mosby.)

produce a rocking open of the mandible that moves the chin down and back. These results may be quite acceptable in deepbite, forward-rotating growth patterns but are contraindicated in vertical or down and backward growing faces because they increase the sagittal discrepancy and mandibular retrusion.

Therefore an analysis of the initial pattern and probable growth direction is imperative before the clinician arbitrarily places a cervical extraoral device, with or without the activator combination, in patients with unfavorable growth patterns. Excessive anterior face height indicates the need for depression of posterior teeth and the use of all possible efforts to stimulate upward and forward mandibular rotation. The direction of force should essentially be along the Y-axis or above or through the center of resistance of the maxilla. The desirable orthopedic effect on the maxilla is the restriction of horizontal and vertical growth increments. As Stöckli and Teuscher (1985) show in Figure 18-34, effective restraint of maxillary growth and translation permits favorable autorotation of the mandible up and forward even if no effort is made to interfere

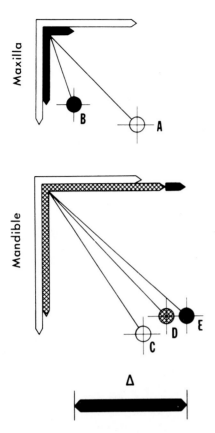

**Figure 18-35.** If the improved sagittal relationship provided by proper horizontal and vertical extraoral orthopedic control (with favorable mandibular autorotation) is further enhanced by a forward-posturing mandibular appliance, condylar growth is optimized, and the normal growth vector and amount as exemplified by *C* are changed to a more forward direction and amount by autorotation *(D)*. Stimulation of condylar growth also occurs *(E)*. Such a reaction is particularly desirable in patients with excessive anterior face height and unfavorable anterior to posterior height ratios.

(From Stöckli PW, Teuscher UM. Combined activator-headgear orthopedics. In Graber TM, Vanarsdall RL, editors: *Orthodontics: current principles and techniques*, ed 2, St Louis, 1994, Mosby.)

with the normal mandibular growth pattern. This finding is the opposite of the Kloehn effect illustrated in Figure 18-33. Furthermore, if the favorable autorotation of the mandible is enhanced by forward posturing of the mandible and optimizing of condylar growth increments and direction, the profile improvement potential is even more favorable (Figure 18-35).

**Pfeiffer and Grobety combination therapy.** Pfeiffer and Grobety also have great experience in combination therapy (Graber, Neumann, 1984):

Since 1967, we have combined the action of these two appliances (Activator and headgear), thinking that one would not be detrimental to the other. To our great surprise, we discovered that not only were their actions complementary but also their respective effects increased until they represented a highly efficient combination of therapies.

**Treatment goals.** The treatment goals of Pfeiffer and Grobety mirror their expectations for the mixed dentition

combination approach in Class II, division 1 malocclusions. The activator (1) prevents, intercepts, and if necessary, corrects pernicious habits (thumb sucking, lip sucking, abnormal swallowing, mouth breathing); (2) acts as a space maintainer; (3) expands if necessary; (4) starts to correct individual positions of teeth; (5) starts to correct deep bites (within freeway space limits); and (6) helps correct the Class II relationship in three different ways. It prevents vicious habits and reorients physiologic forces thus allowing for the normal growth of the mandible; under the influence of the muscles of mandibular retraction, promotes mesial movement of the lower teeth and distal movement of the upper teeth; and possibly inhibits growth of the maxilla by means of the same muscles as they try to return to rest position. The activator does not significantly incite activation of mandibular growth; however, this is a genetically defined potential that cannot be quantitatively altered.

**Recent clinical research findings.** Clinical opinion may have been altered slightly since this last article appeared in 1983 because of the overwhelming evidence from the Petrovic laboratory concerning histologic validation of condylar growth enhancement by the activator. Additional research by Elgoyhen, McNamara, Droschl, Cederquist, Graber, and others on nonhuman primates and human beings shows the potential of growth direction alteration and growth increment change. This important (and still controversial, if the work of Gianelly et al is correct) work is covered extensively in Chapter 2 of this book by Petrovic and in the Rakosi chapters.

These time-honored concepts regarding mesial movement of the mandibular teeth and distal movement of the maxillary teeth call attention to another controversial aspect of activator effects. One of the strongest criticisms of these appliances is that they tend to slide the mandibular teeth forward on the basal bone and procline the mandibular incisors, as Björk noted in 1952. This occurs in spite of various appliance modifications. Case selection is again a critical factor. Starting treatment on a patient with procumbent lower incisors is different from starting it on a patient with retroclined lower incisors. A discretionary decision is needed to determine whether a functional appliance should be used and the steps that should be taken to prevent further proclination. At best, the hope is that forward movement of the mandibular teeth is minimal in most cases and that the various construction bites in Class II malocclusions stimulate all possible forward mandibular growth and result in changes in morphology to help establish a normal sagittal maxillomandibular basal relationship. The restrictive effects of mandibular overclosure, functional retrusion, and excessive activity of the retractor muscles of the mandible are now considered significant factors in preventing the attainment of optimal lower jaw growth. The appliance intercepts the effects on the growth pattern, permitting a free expression of the morphogenetic blueprint.

**Cervical extraoral effects occurring with activator use.** Pfeiffer and Grobety listed the following probable effects of cervical appliance use combined with an activator: (1) slowed or interrupted maxilla growth; (2) initiation of distal movement of the anchor molars and to some extent the adjacent teeth; (3) tipping of the anchor teeth either way, if desired;

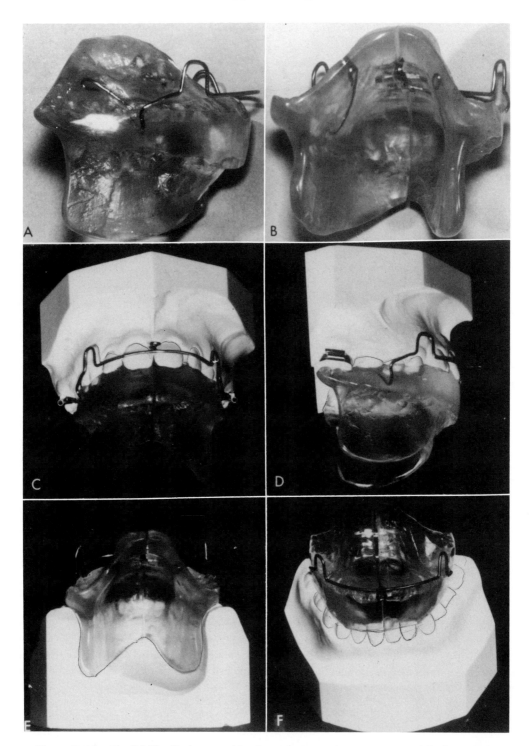

**Figure 18-36.** The Pfeiffer-Grobety combination technique using a conventional Andresen-type activator (**A** and **B**) with cemented molar bands and buccal tubes for the extraoral face-bow (**C** and **D**) and producing an orthopedic effect on the maxilla. The lingual flanges are extended as far into the floor of the mouth as possible to give maximal anchorage and a basal bone-guiding effect on the mandible (**E**). Lower incisors are usually capped with acrylic, as are the posterior teeth, to enhance appliance stability and maintenance of the protracted mandibular construction bite (**F**). A jackscrew is incorporated for any needed expansion. The spur on the labial bow controls the extraoral face-bow position. The occlusal acrylic can be cut to allow differential eruption as indicated. No clasps are used; the appliance is loose and free floating with this method, unlike in the Stöckli-Teuscher approach.

(From Pfeiffer JP, Grobety D: Simultaneous use of cervical appliance and activator; an orthodontic approach to fixed appliance therapy, *Am J Orthod* 61:353, 1972.)

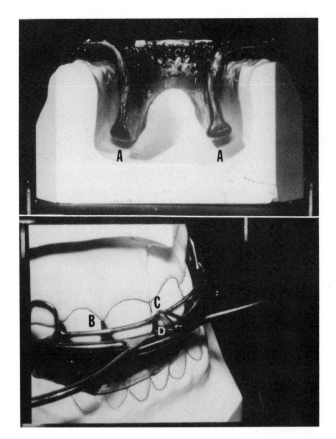

**Figure 18-37.** The Pfeiffer-Grobety activator has an unusually long and rolled lower lingual periphery *(A)* to enhance the basal bone effect on the mandible. The labial bow *(B)* has a spur *(C)* to hold the face-bow *(D)* and prevent it from moving and dislodging the activator.

(From Pfeiffer JP, Grobety D: Simultaneous use of cervical appliance and activator; an orthodontic approach to fixed appliance therapy, *Am J Orthod* 61:353, 1972.)

(4) extrusion of the molars, thereby opening the bite and rotating the mandible down and back; and (5) tipping down of the anterior part of the palate.

As mentioned previously, whether all these effects are desirable is debatable. Case selection and growth direction are important factors. Distalizing maxillary molars may have an impact on second and third molars later, as is the case with Kloehn-type therapy in which an increase in maxillary second molar crossbite occurs. Cephalometric studies indicate that the upper first molar position is essentially the same for Class I, II, and III malocclusions, meaning that the sagittal problem is not in the forward positioning of the molars in most instances. The posttreatment stability and permanence of the results have been questioned in cases in which molars are driven distally by extraoral forces primarily directed against them. Serial cephalometric studies demonstrate that this is largely a tipping and extrusive reaction, and the net result is a partial relapse when appliances are removed; the molars return to an upright position later by relapsing forward.

Many deep-bite problems need molar eruption to reduce the vertical deficiency, but buccal segment eruption is better served by withholding maxillary eruption and stimulating all possible mandibular buccal segment eruption. Harvold and Woodside have noted repeatedly that this differential eruption also has a favorable mesializing component that reduces the sagittal discrepancy. Extruding maxillary molars tip the mandible down and back, increasing anterior face height, facial convexity, and apical base difference. Stöckli and Teuscher (1985) note that as little as 1 mm of extrusion of upper and lower molars can reduce the subspinale-nasion-supramentale (A-N-B) angle 2.5 degrees and open the Y-axis by a similar amount. The more the mandible is tipped down, the more procumbent the lower incisors are to the facial plane. This procumbency makes these teeth more susceptible to proclination by the activator (see Figure 18-10).

Despite these limitations, the evidence is clear that significant improvement can be achieved in properly chosen cases (Figures 18-38 through 18-40). Figure 18-36 shows six different aspects of the Pfeiffer-Grobety activator. The method of ensuring maximal retention and basal bone effects with long and rounded lingual flanges is shown in Figure 18-37. By distributing the force over a larger basal bone area, the undesirable tooth-tipping effects are reduced. Because of the wedging effect on the basal bone supporting the V-shaped buccal segment morphology, this area absorbs the pressure from the forward posturing. The proprioceptive feedback from the mucosal tissue indicates that the mandible should be kept forward and any unpleasant sensory responses should be reduced. The means used for insertion and control of the extraoral face-bow with a spur on the labial bow of the activator should be noted. No clasps are used in the free-floating Pfeiffer-Grobety activator to retain the appliance on the maxilla, but the maxillary occlusal surfaces are covered with acrylic to prevent eruption.

The before and after models of a patient with a treated, severe, Class II, division 1 malocclusion are shown in Figure 18-38; the molar bands are in place and the activator is inserted between the models to show the amount of vertical opening. This is similar in concept to the use of the Herren and Harvold-Woodside activators. With a relatively large sagittal discrepancy, some clinicians prefer a smaller vertical opening for comfort and ease of patient acceptance, or the advancement can be done as Fränkel recomends, in two stages (see Chapter 10). The dramatic dental and facial changes indicate successful treatment (Figures 18-38 and 18-39). Figure 18-40 shows before and after cephalometric tracings with a significant reduction of the apical base dysplasia and excessive overbite and overjet and restoration of normal profile contours.

**Stöckli and Teuscher combination therapy.** Stöckli and Teuscher recognize the problems of the long-misused Kloehn cervical traction and the fact that different types of extraoral force can be used to depress maxillary molars, thus preventing undesirable tipping while exerting a restrictive influence on the horizontal growth component of the maxilla. Both vertical and horizontal withholding are valid treatment objectives because the Stöckli-Teuscher activator-headgear combination achieves the desired changes in three planes of space without

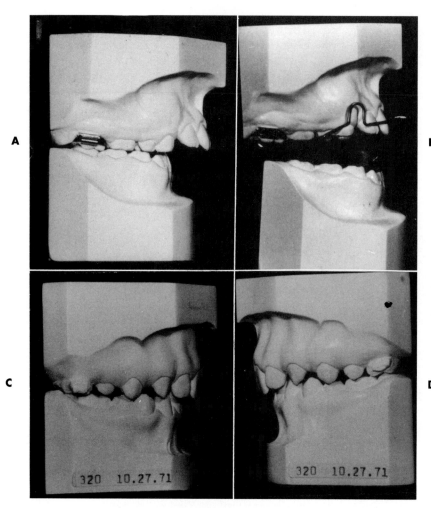

**Figure 18-38.** Beginning models (**A** and **B**) of a patient with a Class II, division 1 malocclusion with molar tubes in place and an activator inserted between the upper and lower models. **C** and **D,** Results after 30 months of treatment. Some detailing remains (i.e., space control, axial inclination of the upper incisors).

(From Pfeiffer JP, Grobety D: Simultaneous use of cervical appliance and activator; an orthodontic approach to fixed appliance therapy, *Am J Orthod* 61:353, 1972.)

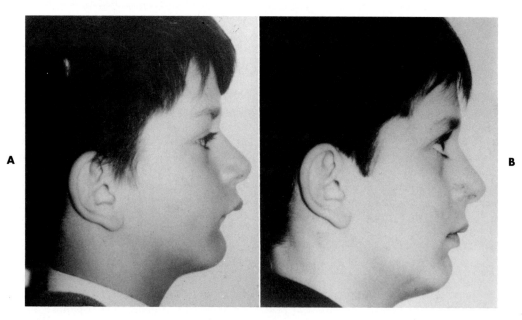

**Figure 18-39.** **A,** Before treatment; **B,** after treatment. Note the dramatic facial change that results from combined therapy. In this case, cervical therapy was beneficial because it elongated the maxillary molars and tipped the palatal plane down and back, opening the bite in a vertically deficient malocclusion.

(From Pfeiffer JP, Grobety D: Simultaneous use of cervical appliance and activator; an orthodontic approach to fixed appliance therapy, *Am J Orthod* 61:353, 1972.)

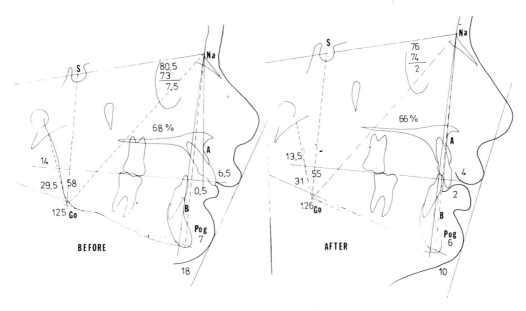

**Figure 18-40.** Before and 30 months after removal of combination activator–extraoral force appliances for the patient in Figures 18-38 and 18-39. A 5-degree decrease in the apical base difference and an improvement in the anterior facial height and the relationship of the incisors to the facial plane are evident. The 1.5-degree increase in the mandibular plane inclination resulted from cervical traction, which elongates the first molars as it tips them distally. The whole maxilla usually rotates down and back with such a force vector. That the molars were moved distally is evident from the residual spacing in the finished models in Figure 18-38.

(From Pfeiffer JP, Grobety D: Simultaneous use of cervical appliance and activator; an orthodontic approach to fixed appliance therapy, *Am J Orthod* 61:353, 1972.)

some of the disadvantages previously listed. A high-pull headgear can be used for depression and for cases in which the extraoral force is directed through the potential center of rotation of the maxilla—the maxilla maintains its position without tipping the palatal plane down and increasing the anterior face height, as the cervical extraoral appliance is more likely to do. A high-pull headgear also does not tip up the anterior end of the palatal plane, which tends to enhance maxillary incisor protrusion and upper lip prominence (Graber, Vanarsdall, 1994) (Figures 18-41 to 18-43).

**Stockfisch, Janson, and Hickham approaches.** Stockfisch has similarly combined his kinetor functional appliance with extraoral force, banding the maxillary first molars with 1.2-mm buccal tubes to receive the extraoral force face-bow. The kinetor is a skeletonized elastic activator that is easier for the patient to wear during daytime, which is desirable. Stockfisch has incorporated an interocclusal elastic tube arrangement that stimulates functional activity in the construction bite position. He writes, "In about 60% to 70% of all anomalies, full multi-banded therapy can be avoided by combination therapy—headgear and Kinetor" (Graber, Neumann, 1984). Although further fixed attachment guidance is necessary, the first period of combination therapy during the mixed-dentition stage usually reduces fixed appliance treatment time as much as 50%. Stockfisch used cemented first molar bands with double tubes for reception of extraoral force face-bows and any future fixed attachment treatment needed for individual tooth malposition correction. The clasp

of the kinetor snaps above the buccal tube assemblage, locking the functional appliance on the maxilla. This modality is entirely in agreement with the philosophy of Fränkel, who has stressed so often with his function regulator the essential importance of anchoring the functional appliance on the maxilla to prevent free float and its deleterious effects (see Chapter 10). The cemented molar bands with their buccal horizontal tubes do this very well in combination.

Janson encourages a combined approach using functional appliances and extraoral force, following the further development of the bionator by Ascher. She too resolves basal dysplasias and abnormal perioral muscle problems with therapy in the mixed-dentition stage and then turns to comprehensive fixed-attachment edgewise therapy for finishing therapy in the permanent dentition (Figures 18-44 and 18-45).

A similar combined activator–extraoral force approach to the correction of sagittal problems in patients with mixed dentition Class II, division 1 malocclusions has been used by Hickham (1980) with consistent success. He also "indexes" or caps the lower incisors, making sure that the labial capping of these teeth is extended gingivally enough to discourage all possible labial tipping by the forward posturing of the mandible. Instead of applying extraoral force to cemented molar bands, he solders hooks to the labial wire of the activator to receive the extraoral force of the J-hook arms. The same up and backward occipital direction recommended by Stöckli and Teuscher is used to control downward maxillary rotation, while still permitting a restrictive effect on horizontal and vertical maxillary basal and dentoalveolar components. Selective

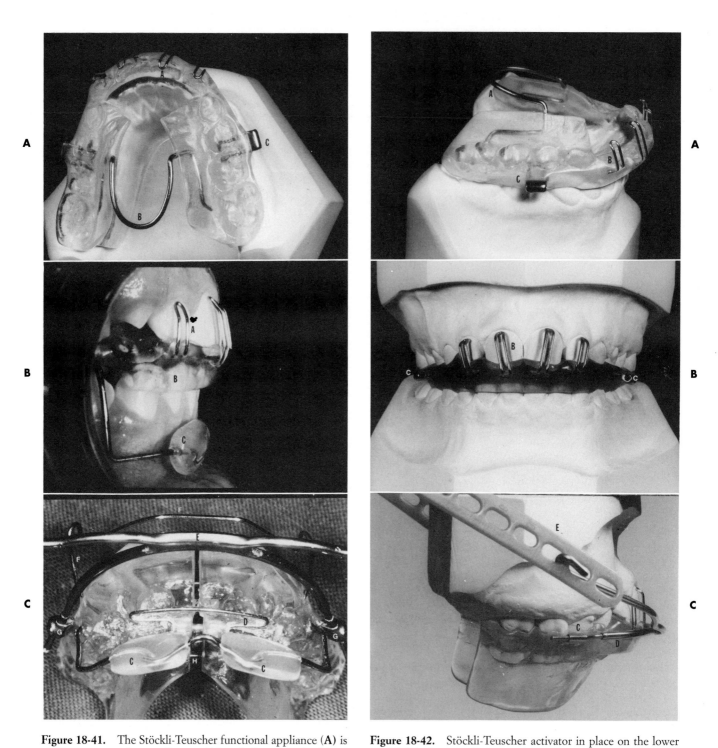

**Figure 18-41.** The Stöckli-Teuscher functional appliance (**A**) is similar to open-palate appliances. Although the transpalatal loop (*B*) is often considered a tongue-control mechanism, it also may be used for expansion by splitting the appliance in the midline between the incisors. Incisor guiding or torquing loops (*A*) can be activated or deactivated, and buccal tubes (*C*) may be incorporated in the interocclusal acrylic. **B,** The acrylic capping (*B*) may be cut away to allow upper or lower incisors to be proclined or retroclined. Fränkel lip pads (*C*) can be added to enhance establishment of normal perioral muscle function. **C,** A protrusion bow (*D*) may be added to assist in labial tipping of both upper and lower incisors. The face-bow (*E*) is already in place in the buccal tubes (*G*). Instead of labial guiding wires, a conventional labial bow (*F*) can be used, if desired. A jackscrew (*H*) is occasionally added for controlled expansion.

(Courtesy Paul Stöckli and Ullrich Teuscher, Zürich, Switzerland.)

**Figure 18-42.** Stöckli-Teuscher activator in place on the lower model (**A**), showing the transpalatal coffin-type spring (*A*), anterior incisal guidance loops (*B*) instead of a conventional labial bow, and horizontal molar tubes (*C*) to receive the extraoral force face-bow arms. **B,** Functional appliance in place between the maxillary and mandibular working models, with both maxillary and mandibular incisors capped in acrylic. The vertical opening is smaller than those in the Woodside, Herren, Hamilton, or Shaye activators. **C,** Insertion of the face-bow (*D*) into the molar tube (*C*). The headgear (*E*) is hooked to the directionally adjusted outer bow (*E*). Note the long lingual flanges in the lower portion to enhance the basal guiding effect on the mandible.

(Courtesy Paul Stöckli and Ullrich Teuscher.)

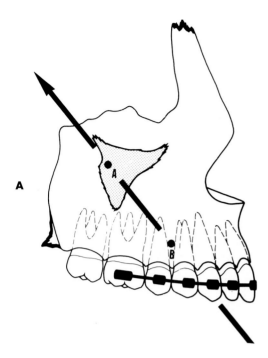
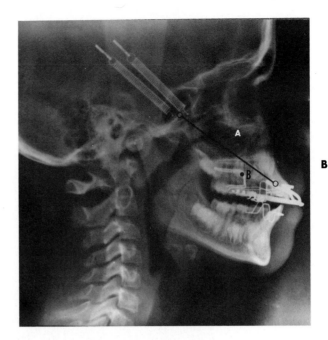

**Figure 18-43.** **A,** Theoretically, to achieve maximal retractive and intrusive mechanics with extraoral force and prevent the Kloehn effect of molar eruption and downward pull on the anterior end of the palatal plane, extraoral force should be directed as close as clinically feasible through both the center of rotation of the maxilla *(A)* and the center of rotation of the dentition *(B)*. **B,** Activator-headgear combination in place. The direction of the occipital pull headgear is between both centers of rotation *(A and B)*. This produces a small amount of maxillary posterior rotation and somewhat more anterior offsetting dentitional rotation. From a practical point of view, however, these forces may offset each other.

(Courtesy Paul Stöckli and Ullrich Teuscher.)

grinding of the activator results in a biteplate effect that frees the mandibular buccal segments for upward and forward corrective eruption while withholding the maxillary basal and dentoalveolar complexes; it can also exert a slight distal force on the mandibular buccal segments by virtue of the interproximal projections that engage the mesiobuccal aspects of the maxillary buccal segment teeth.

## Miscellaneous Combination Appliances

A constant problem with any removable appliance is lack of patient compliance; if other components such as extraoral force arms and a headcap are added to a bulky acrylic activator, patient cooperation is even more of a concern. For this reason, skeletonized activators are preferred by many clinicians. The bionator is a favorite appliance because it does not have palatal acrylic coverage and can be worn during the day. Care must be exercised in the use of extraoral force so the appliance will not become dislodged. Fixed molar bands are more stable, but direction of force then becomes a factor, as Stöckli has stressed. Undesirable molar tipping and extrusion, unwanted tipping of the anterior end of the palatal plane, down and back rotation of the mandible to increase a vertical growth direction vector, and equally undesirable labial tipping of lower incisors and lingual tipping of upper incisors should be considered in any design modification. Many variations are possible such as

not using acrylic caps for the lower incisors if they are lingually inclined, labial capping if resistance to forward incisor tipping is desired, or using a lower labial bow instead of items such as acrylic caps or maxillary acrylic occlusal covers or spurs and rests. Different horizontal and vertical construction bite registrations can be used, depending on the original malocclusion, the preferences of the operator performing the procedure, and the tolerance of the patient; nothing in orthodontics better illustrates the descretionary nature of mechanical therapy than do these myriad factors. Research by Petrovic et al (1981), reported in Chapter 2 of this book, shows that some activators are more effective when worn full time, and others can be worn for shorter periods for optimal tissue response. This chapter should be read carefully by the clinician who wishes to introduce a series of modifications.

## CONCLUSIONS

In keeping with the KISS principle, a number of appliances and modifications have been presented in this chapter to correct sagittal, vertical, and transverse malocclusion problems. Their use is based on current research in the biomechanic field and depends heavily on careful qualitative and quantitative histochemical studies by Reitan (1984), Rygh (1977), Petrovic and Stutzmann (1972), Petrovic et al (1982), McNamara

*Continued on p. 416*

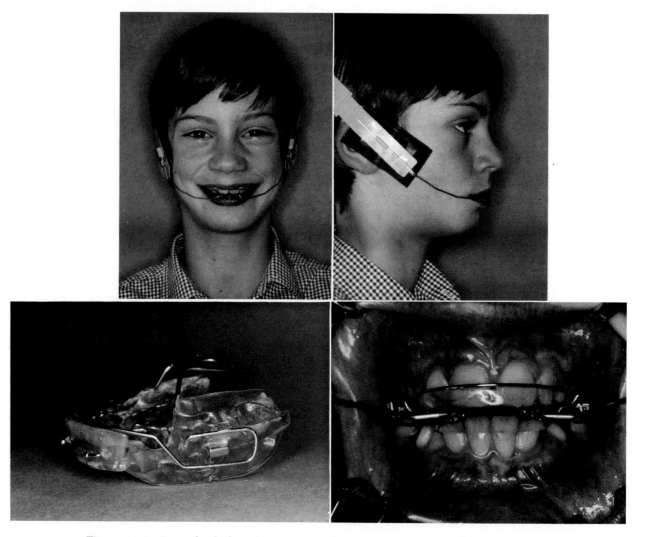

**Figure 18-44.** Janson has had much experience with the bionator, as used by Ascher. In a retrospective study of the bionator, she concluded that most of the sagittal change is a result of dentoalveolar compensation. However, after the incorporation of circular loops anteriorly in the capping acrylic, J hooks may be attached to a headcap to augment maxillary retraction as the mandible is postured forward and the vertical dimension is opened by the bionator.

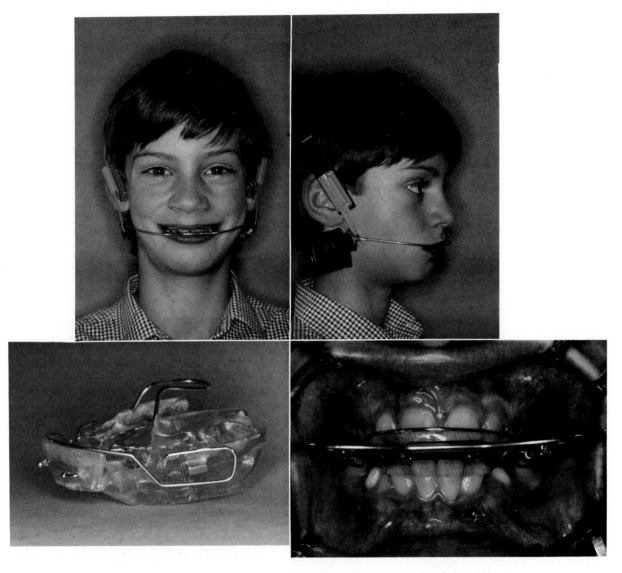

**Figure 18-44, cont'd.**   Horizontal molar tubes also may be embedded in the posterior interocclusal acrylic to receive the face-bow ends, and either a regular oblique-pull headgear or a combination high-pull low-pull type can be used to augment the restrictive effect on the maxillary complex. The operator may alternate anterior or posterior extraoral force attachment as desired, if both anterior loops and posterior molar tubes are incorporated.

(Courtesy Ingrid Janson, Munich, Germany.)

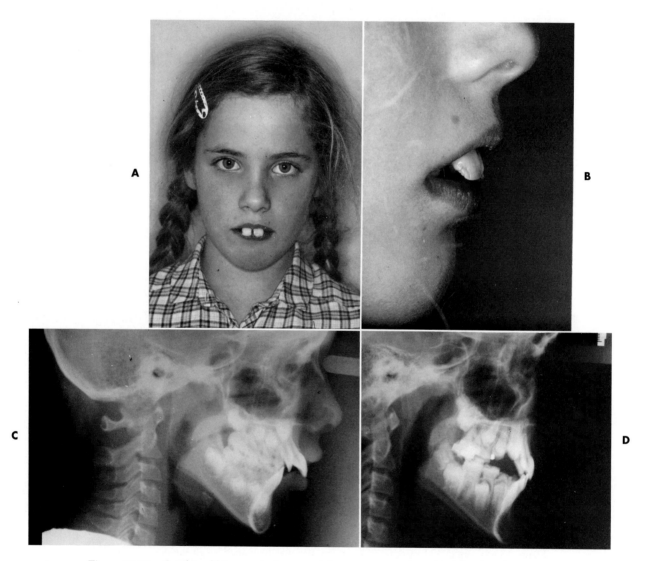

**Figure 18-45.**   Combined bionator and extraoral force treatment. **A** to **C,** Malocclusion. **D,** Appearance 14 months later after combined headgear is applied to the banded maxillary first molars and a bionator is used as modified by Ascher.

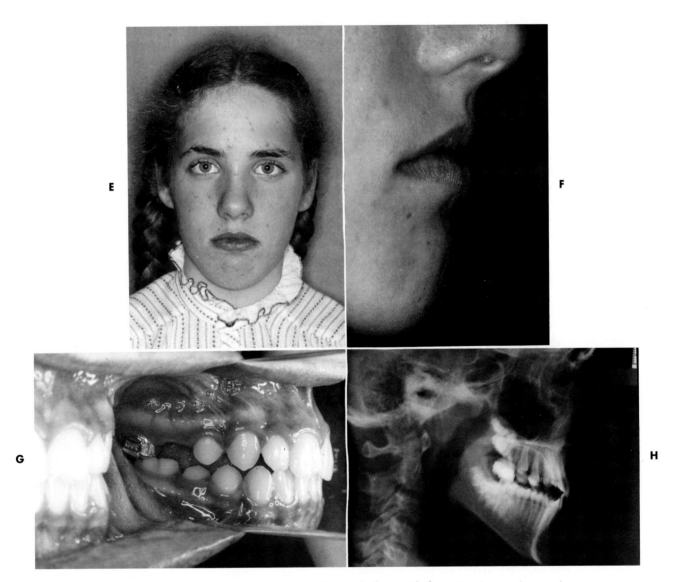

**Figure 18-45, cont'd.** **E** to **G,** Appearance 22 months later, with the patient in retention, awaiting eruption of the maxillary second premolars. **H,** Result achieved. Note the banded first molars, which help hold the bionator in as a retainer and which formerly received the extraoral face-bow.
(Courtesy Ingrid Janson, Munich, Germany.)

(1981), Moyers (1981), Graber (1983b), and others on both experimental animals and human beings and on clinical research by Ahlgren (1979), Bimler (1965), Fränkel, Schmuth (1983), Rakosi (1982), Sander (1983), Stöckli, Teuscher (1982), McNamara (1981), Moss (1981), Shaye (1983), Hamilton (1983), Graber (1984), Björk (1983), Woodside (1983), and others. The therapy described here is not the only approach to achieving treatment objectives. It may be simpler, but it most certainly does not require less diagnostic study and acumen. Proper case selection is imperative for success with this mechanotherapy or any other therapy. No treatment results are automatic, and no perfect appliance has yet been developed.

Criteria for case selection are covered in other sections of this book, particularly in Chapters 6 and 7 and 19 through 22. As discussed in these chapters, diagnosing patients is a continuing process that begins with the patient coming in for routine adjustment and treatment assessment. An emphasis on growth and development sounds appealing, but simply talking about these developmental phenomena is not enough. The clinician must have a thorough knowledge of the principles of growth and development before instituting therapy. A proper means of assessing the growth process during treatment also is essential. Although untrained neophytes may wish to use functional orthopedic therapeutics because appliance fabrication and treatment mechanics seem simpler, the best qualified operators to employ removable appliances are orthodontic specialists who have sufficient training, experience, and background to know the cases to select, the way to assess treatment results, and the proper time to *change* direction or appliances.

## No Uniform Blueprint for Treatment

Years of teaching have made the author aware of the keen desire of clinicians for a step-by-step set of instructions for therapy. With 8 to 64 types of Class II malocclusions and multiple factors contributing to dentofacial morphology at any time, any attempt to create a generalized, generic treatment plan for all patients does a disservice to the profession. This constant desire to fit all patients into one treatment mode has led to the cultism and dogma that have permeated orthodontics for the past 50 years. Johnston exuded supreme confidence as he said of twin-wire therapy, "Don't worry, it is automatic. Put it on and the wires do the rest" (1957). The clinician who follows the philosophy of Begg fits all patients into the same mechanical straitjacket, and the Bull technique uses a different but equally regimented bear trap. All three systems have been tossed into the historical wastebasket by straight-wire disciples, who hold all removable appliances in disdain because of lack of torque, tip, or in-and-out adjustment potential. Surely the proponents of removable appliances are advanced enough to recognize that optimal therapy for tooth alignment, jaw relationship, neuromuscular balance, tissue tolerance, patient compliance, treatment time, and ease of manipulation is not possible with one set of brackets and arch wires, no matter the level of their engineering or the capabilities of their wire memory. Different approaches and appliances are needed for different types of malocclusions, and clinicians should now understand (especially in treating pa-

tients with skeletal problems) that using several appliances for the same patient during different dental developmental stages may be the best treatment. Furthermore, even the best clinician may have to change appliances in the middle of treatment because one appliance approach has worked or not worked. Results cannot always be predicted. Continually diagnosing patients at each visit is the key to success. Orthodontists should always have alternative treatments from which they can choose. Combination activator-headgear therapy may seem deceptively simple to neophytes or nonspecialists; they may be lulled into a sense of false security by traveling salesmen, orthodontic supply representatives, and clinicians who earn royalties on prodontals. (Even Edward H. Angle was paid $90,000 by SS White for the ribbon arch patent and $145,000 for the edgewise bracket, according to Sam Lewis.) Appliances are simple, but their misuse is easy without a proper diagnostic assessment at each visit. Treatment planning is not likely to be so simple. In light of the current emphasis on health maintenance organizations (HMOs), preferred provider organizations (PPOs), and independent practice associations (IPAs) and managed care pressures, a paragraph that addresses the issue of appliance use and misuse may be pertinent (Graber, Neumann, 1984):

It is hoped that those who embark on the use of these fixed-removable combinations will have the ethical, moral and professional concerns so that the patient is always served best. Providing less than optimal orthodontic guidance for a child simply because the dentist does not have the skill and training for the job violates the oath of Hippocrates. In addition, weasel-wording and rationalizing about lesser fees and the supposed inability of orthodontic specialists to take care of all the patients will not make the situation any better. The proliferation of orthodontics of all types being done by ill-trained pedodontists and general practitioners whose level of "business" has dropped in other areas is no coincidence. Peer review in this area of dental practice is practically non-existent. Orthodontic consultation from specialists is always available in most cities, but few dentists emulate their medical confreres and seek it out. Only in those instances in which orthodontic specialty guidance or consultation is unavailable, as in many small towns or rural areas, might the dentist feel justified to take on this kind of treatment, even though it is likely to be of a lesser caliber than could be provided by a trained orthodontic specialist. For here, the alternative for the patient is nothing at all. Such a responsibility should not be taken lightly because of the iatrogenic potential of some orthodontic therapy. And we need not wait for the pressures applied by consumer advocacy and a litigious society to do some self-policing. The dentist should educate himself as completely as possible in the fields of craniofacial growth and development and in all aspects of diagnosis, if he plans to embark on orthodontic guidance. Continuing education courses are a must. As a Director of one of the more successful programs of this type in the United States, I am proud to see the number of dentists availing themselves of this type of indoctrination, following the G.V. Black maxim, "The professional man cannot be other than a continuous student."

Continuing dental education courses are no substitute for a bona fide, 3-year, full-time graduate degree. The clinician's ultimate responsibility is to the patient. The clinician's moral duty is to provide the best possible orthodontic care. If the clinician cannot render the highest level of service, he or she should make sure that the patient sees a practitioner who can. This is why medical and dental specialties exist.

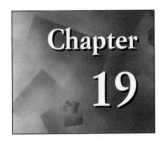

# Chapter 19

# Treatment of Class II Malocclusions

Thomas Rakosi

## DEVELOPING TREATMENT CONCEPTS

Any description of Class II malocclusions is difficult at best because this arbitrary categorization includes various types of malocclusions. In the original and strictest interpretation the designation of Class II essentially defines the sagittal relationship between the upper and lower first permanent molars as propounded by Edward H. Angle. Subsequent clinical experience and the development of more sophisticated diagnostic assessments such as gnathostatics by Simon and cephalometrics by Broadbent and a host of workers in the field delineated the broad range of types of Class II malocclusion. Particularly important was the recognition of the dysplastic skeletal sagittal relationship of the maxilla and mandible to each other and the cranial base. Equally important has been the assessment of vertical components and their roles in the horizontal malrelationships forming further subclasses of Class II malocclusion. Finally, an essential facet of differential diagnosis in these cases has been the functional adaptation to horizontal and vertical dysplasia, which results in posterior (and occasionally anterior) condylar displacement or rocking open of the mandible in an autorotational maneuver because of excessive anterior or deficient posterior facial height.

As a result of these findings, Class II malocclusions are usually diagnosed on the basis of the habitual occlusion and first molar relationship. The malocclusion may result from a spatial, sagittal abnormality of the maxilla or mandible or a combination of both and may be influenced by a vertical dysplasia of the maxilla, mandible, or both. The condylar position in the fossa in habitual occlusion may be normal, posterior, or anterior, depending on occlusal guiding forces and neuromuscular adaptation. Transverse discrepancies abound.

These potentially variable malocclusion characteristics and means of recognizing and treating them are discussed more fully in Chapter 6. This chapter describes the means used in coping with the different characteristics. The many past attempts to find a universal appliance to treat all Class II malocclusions have not succeeded. Some proposed biomechanic treatment procedures were aimed at the mixed dentition, and others were aimed at the permanent dentition. These treatment procedures can be divided into three broad groups based on the philosophy or working hypothesis espoused:

1. The concepts that bone morphology is presumably inherited and functional environment adapts to this form are fundamental to one group of orthodontic therapies. According to this philosophy, growth and development are independent processes that cannot be influenced. Corrective procedures may be implemented after the eruption of the permanent teeth to move them to achieve dentoalveolar correction, but the hereditarily linked skeletal pattern cannot be influenced. Thus the only therapeutic possibility is a dentoalveolar compensation of the Class II skeletal relationship (Figure 19-1). This philosophy as exemplified by the Begg technique and some forms of the current straight-wire philosophy asserts that a causal approach to treatment is possible only in dentoalveolar malocclusions, and correction can be achieved only within the framework of the original malocclusion. The mode of therapy is instituted in the adult dentition. The skeletal discrepancy can be compensated for with the aid of extraction or altered by orthognathic surgery.

2. According to the second philosophy every patient has the potential to achieve perfect occlusion. Any deviation from ideal occlusion is attributed to the environment. The first supporter of this hypothesis was Angle. However, the classic edgewise approach as espoused by Brodie (1940) and his students was a combination of hereditary determinism and ideal occlusion philosophies. According to this philosophy, establishing the full dentition in an ideal intercuspal relationship leads to normal function and maintenance of the treated result. A modification of this empiric approach was fostered by Andresen and his followers. They assert that form adapts to function, and the influence of the muscles is the primary etiologic basis and environmental factor in the development of malocclusion. By altering environmental factors, the clinician thus can stimulate mandibular growth, inhibit maxillary growth, and alter growth direction.

Many proponents of a so-called universal appliance are convinced that using the activator or some other device can stimulate growth of the mandible and position it anteriorly in all Class II malocclusions.

417

3. The third and most recent orthopedic and orthodontic philosophy is based on a large amount of primate research and clinical experience. It seeks a middle ground in the form versus function and heredity versus environment struggle. Function is not identical with environmental influences. Certain aspects of function also can be inherited, especially the posture and morphology of the muscles and soft tissues. The functional influences conditioned by heredity have been designated as *epigenetic factors* by van Limborgh (1968). Hereditary influence does not arise from the cells but is guided indirectly by function. According to this hypothesis, a range of normal accomplishment is possible. Under the best possible circumstances, the achievement of an optimal growth potential within the scope or range of the individual genetic pattern is possible. This is the basic principle of modern functional orthopedic therapy for Class II malocclusions during the growth period. An essential task of differential diagnosis is to assess the scope of the genetic pattern in each case.

## THERAPEUTIC CONSIDERATIONS

The location of the skeletal dysplasia is decisive in determining therapy. Not only is the differential diagnosis between skeletal and dentoalveolar malocclusion characteristics important, but also an exact determination of the specifics of the skeletal abnormality is essential. The Class II skeletal relationship, for example, can be caused by a posteriorly positioned mandible or an anteriorly positioned maxilla (Figure 19-2).

Growth promotion in the temporomandibular joint (TMJ) area is indicated in mandibular retrusion, whereas growth inhibition is required for maxillary protrusion. If possible, growth inhibition should be directed at the sutural hafting zone of the craniofacial complex. These two objectives require different biomechanic treatment procedures. Even the limitations imposed by the differential growth accomplishment of the maxilla and mandible require discretionary therapeutic decisions.

Growth stimulation of the secondary cartilaginous condylar growth center is more difficult than it is for purely membranous bone because the structures are made to resist com-

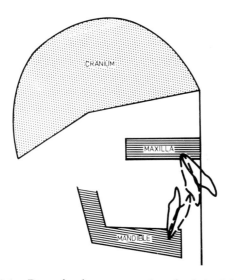

**Figure 19-1.** Dentoalveolar compensation of a skeletal Class II relationship. The lower incisors are tipped labially, and the upper incisors are tipped lingually.

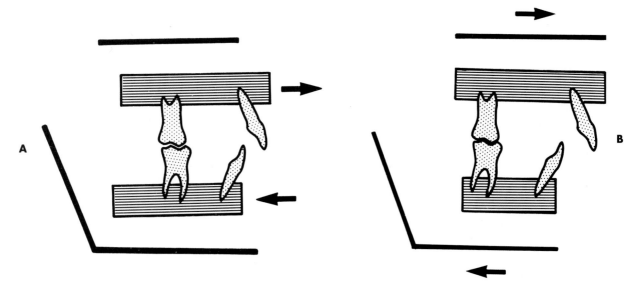

**Figure 19-2.   A,** Dentoalveolar Class II relationship. The upper dental arch and alveolar process are positioned anteriorly, and the lower dental arch and alveolar process are positioned posteriorly. **B,** Skeletal Class II relationship. The upper jaw bases are positioned anteriorly, and the lower jaw bases are positioned posteriorly.

pression and other functional stresses. Although it is not as resistant as primary cartilaginous centers such as the epiphysis and diaphysis of long bones, the unique prechondroblast-chondroblast cycle of this growth center is timed in its development so that only certain cells are responsive to external stimuli at precise stages in their maturation. Vascularization also is less efficient than it is with membranous bone, although recent research by Biggerstaff shows an extensive subcondylar plexus. Therapeutic growth guidance can be performed only during the active growth period (Figure 19-3).

The membranous bone sutures of the maxilla respond well to external stimuli, with many undifferentiated cells and a high fibroblast turnover in the sutures. Vascularization is good; it expedites the local response. Inhibitory action on membranous bone sutures is particularly effective because fibroblasts hyalinize and die within 4 hours after the application of orthopedic pressures, whereas a chondroblast may take as long as 160 hours to succumb to even greater pressures. Clearly, different treatment responses occur in the maxilla and mandible. Therapeutic inhibition of maxillary growth is not limited to active growth spurts, although it is more effective at this time. Some treatment response is possible at a later period when condylar response is minimal or nonexistent.

Mandibular growth alone does not correct all Class II problems. A case in point is a 9-year-old patient with Class II malocclusion associated with abnormal tongue function. Cephalometric analysis showed no basal skeletal discrepancy and indicated a probable horizontal growth pattern (Figure 19-4). The maxillary and mandibular bases were short, and the ascending ramus was long. Both upper and lower incisors were procumbent. No orthodontic therapy was performed, and the tongue dysfunction persisted. After 3 years the patient had a definite sagittal discrepancy with a reduced sella-nasion-supramentale (S-N-B) angle despite a high growth increment of the mandibular base. The lingual tipping of the lower incisors may be attributed to a change in the perioral functional pattern. A confirmed lip trap with hyperactive mentalis muscle function arose during this 3-year period. If therapy had been instituted during the high growth period, the result might have been good and stable. Lack of treatment enhanced the skeletal discrepancy and intensified the adaptive and deforming neuromuscular activity.

## TREATMENT PLANNING

Before starting to treat a patient with a Class II malocclusion, the clinician must ascertain a number of important facts:

1. The clinician must assess whether the malocclusion is of

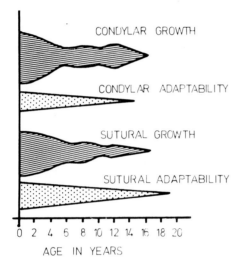

**Figure 19-3.** Respective adaptability of condylar and sutural growth, depending on the age of the patient.

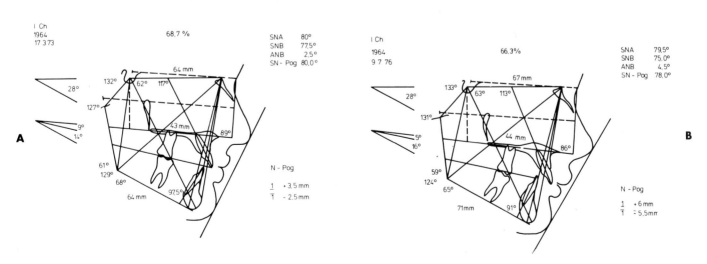

**Figure 19-4.** Patient with a Class II malocclusion at, **A,** 9 and, **B,** 11 years. Despite an increased mandibular growth rate, the skeletal relationship became worse.

skeletal or dentoalveolar origin. Causal treatment can be successful only during the growth period.

2. The clinician also must distinguish whether the malocclusion is a functionally true one, with a normal path of closure from postural rest to habitual occlusion, or a functional retrusion, with the condyle moving up and back from postural rest to habitual occlusion. Normally, condylar action in the lower joint cavity is primarily rotary from rest to occlusion. Translatory condylar movement not only jeopardizes the normal condyle-disk-eminence relationship but also produces a retruded spatial mandibular malposition on full occlusion. A primary treatment objective must be to eliminate the retruded condylar position, harmonizing it with the more anterior postural rest position. This can be done quite successfully using functional orthopedic procedures. If the path of closure is normal, with only rotary condylar function from postural rest to occlusion, and the malocclusion is a true sagittal skeletal discrepancy, the treatment challenge is different. Not only the occlusal position must be changed, but also a neuromuscular adaptation to the new postural position of the mandible must occur, as the condyle grows up and backward to its correct relationship with the fossa structures. Achieving a permanent neuromuscular adaptation to the appliance-oriented mandibular postural position can be difficult. If the original postural resting position persists, a functional disturbance, "Sunday bite," or dual bite is the consequence.

3. Accurate forecasting of the probable growth direction is important in the assessment of therapeutic possibilities. With a horizontal growth pattern, therapeutic control of the vertical dimension is difficult, just as control of the horizontal dimension is problematic with a vertical growth vector.

4. Growth increments over time are crucial considerations. Questions of the size of the growth potential and when it can be expected are important in the clinician's choice of a therapeutic method. Treatment timing is crucial. The forecast may indicate major growth increments in the future, but if appliances are worn during a quiescent growth period, failure to accomplish treatment objectives is likely even though significant growth increments may occur after treatment.

5. Etiologic considerations in differentiating hereditary malocclusions and the consequences of neuromuscular dysfunctions are important in assessing the scope of functional appliances and their efficacy in therapy.

To obtain more detailed and needed information, the clinician should obtain both functional and cephalometric examinations before starting treatment.

## Functional Criteria

The most important functional criteria for treatment planning for Class II malocclusions are as follows:

1. The assessment of the relationship between rest posi-

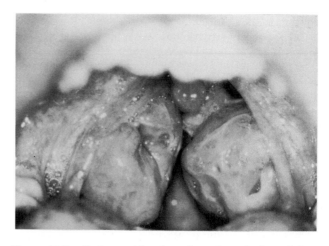

**Figure 19-5.** Patients with enlarged tonsils and adenoids have difficulty wearing activators. Growth direction is more vertical.

tion and occlusion to differentiate a functionally true and a forced-bite malocclusion is crucial.

2. The examination of the relationships between overjet and function of the lips is another important procedure. If the lower lip postures and functions in the incisal gap created by the excessive overjet and if hyperactive, adaptive, and exacerbative mentalis muscle function is present, these deforming activities should be eliminated during the day if the functional appliance of choice is worn only at night.

3. The posture and function of the tongue should be assessed. In some malocclusions, abnormal tongue function needs to be controlled with accessory elements or appliances.

4. The mode of breathing is important because patients with disturbed nasal respiration or enlarged tonsils and adenoids are not able to retain functional appliances in the mouth as prescribed (Figure 19-5).

## Cephalometric Criteria

A complete analysis is necessary before orthodontic therapy begins. This analysis is no less important for removable appliances than it is for fixed appliances. The following considerations are of particular interest to the clinician planning treatment:

1. The relationship of the maxilla to the cranial base must be considered. In patients with prognathic maxillas, a maxillary withholding or a distal driving of the 6-year molars is usually indicated. Functional appliances are not very effective in such cases.

2. The position and size of the mandible are important factors. In patients with retrognathic mandibles, the therapeutic requirements are different, depending on the size of the mandible.

3. The clinician should note the axial inclination and position of the incisors before deciding on the mode and amount of movement of these teeth.

4. The growth pattern is important in decisions on the design and construction of the appliance.

Cephalometric analysis requires a value judgment as to whether in a specific Class II malocclusion the maxilla is prognathic and large or the mandible is retrognathic and small. (See Chapter 6.)

## CLASSIFICATION OF CLASS II MALOCCLUSIONS

### Morphologic Classification

A number of classifications of Class II malocclusions can be made. One of the simplest divides the malocclusion into the following four groups:

1. The first group is Class II dental malocclusions caused only by tooth migration (i.e., dentoalveolar malocclusions).
2. The second group consists of Class II malocclusions with the fault in the mandible; the mandible is retrognathic, and the maxilla is orthognathic. This category comprises most of the Class II malocclusions encountered in orthodontic practice.
3. The third group is Class II malocclusions with the fault in the maxilla; the maxilla is prognathic, and the mandible is orthognathic. As McNamara's study (1981) has shown, the malocclusions form a relatively small percentage of cases treated (see Chapter 17).
4. The fourth group consists of combinations of groups 2 and 3. Both groups are likely to have local tooth malpositions in addition to the basal malrelationship as the incisors adapt sagittally to the perverted perioral musculature. Maxillary arch width also is subservient to neuromuscular compensations. Whether the maxilla is prognathic or orthognathic and whether the mandible is orthognathic or retrognathic are important considerations as long as a sufficient basal malrelationship exists to elicit abnormal buccinator mechanism activity.

### Cephalometric Classification

A more sophisticated categorization is possible with the help of increasingly detailed cephalometric criteria. If these criteria are used, five basic groups of Class II malocclusions can be recognized.

1. Some Class II malocclusions are based on Class II sagittal relationships without skeletal components. The subspinale-nasion-supramentale (A-N-B) angle can be normal. Usually the upper and lower jaw bases are both retrognathic and the sella-nasion-subspinale (S-N-A) and S-N-B angles are reduced. A labial tipping of the upper incisors is likely; the lower incisors can be tipped either labially or lingually, depending on local neuromuscular compensation for the excessive overjet. Labial tipping of the lower incisors reduces the overjet but

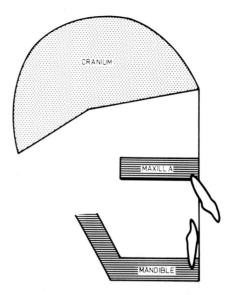

**Figure 19-6.** Dentoalveolar Class II relationship with labial tipping of the upper incisors and lingual tipping of the lower incisors.

makes orthodontic correction more difficult because uprighting of the lower incisors also is a necessary treatment objective. This uprighting is often quite difficult if no spaces are present (Figure 19-6).

2. Functionally created Class II malocclusions, with forced mandibular retrusion in habitual occlusion but with normal postural rest relationships, are another important category. The path of closure may be abnormal or forced because of an excessive overbite and infraocclusion of the buccal segment teeth. The S-N-B angle is smaller in habitual occlusion but improved in the postural resting position. Usually the mandibular base is of normal size, and no growth deficiency is present. In such cases, early interceptive functional therapy is the method of choice (Figure 19-7).
3. Class II malocclusions with the fault in the maxilla also are common. The profile convexity of the upper jaw can be basal (with a larger S-N-A angle), dentoalveolar (with an increased sella-nasion-prosthion [S-N-Pr] angle), or dental (with an increased upper incisor to S-N plane angle signifying labial incisal tipping) (Figure 19-8).

Therapeutic mechanisms and possibilities depend on the axial inclination of the incisors and the type of maxillary prognathism. Simple tipping of the incisors can be corrected with removable appliances, but torque and bodily movement should be done with fixed appliances. Maxillary basal prognathism requires heavy orthopedic force.

The maxillary base can be normal in size and positioned anteriorly, or it can be too long. When evaluating the maxillary base, the clinician also should consider its inclination. An upward and forward inclination aggravates the maxillary protrusion (Schwarz [1958] calls this a *pseudoprotrusion*). A retroinclination (palatal plane tipped down anteriorly) can actually compensate for maxillary prognathism. The control of the vertical

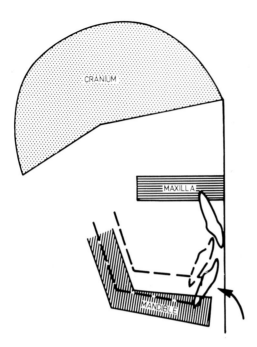

**Figure 19-7.** Functional Class II relationship with a distally forced bite. From an anterior rest position the mandible glides into a posterior habitual occlusion, usually under the influence of tooth guidance.

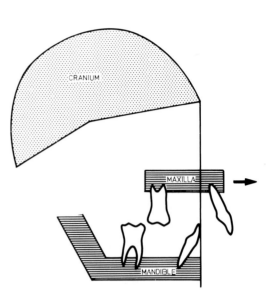

**Figure 19-8.** Skeletal Class II relationship with fault in the maxilla. The upper jaw base is prognathic, and the lower jaw base is orthognathic.

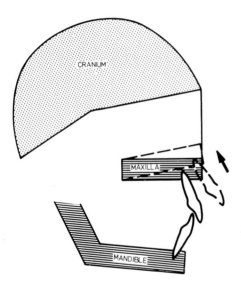

**Figure 19-9.** Class II relationship with prognathism and anteinclination of the maxilla (anterior end tipped up).

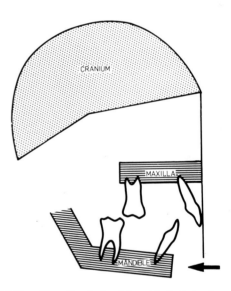

**Figure 19-10.** Class II relationship with fault in the mandible. The maxilla is orthognathic, and the mandible is retrognathic.

dimension in this type of malocclusion often depends on the inclination of the maxillary base, especially if it is combined with either a deep overbite or an open bite. Combined therapy (headgear and activator) is required to influence the maxillary prognathism (Figure 19-9).

4. Class II malocclusions with faults in the mandible dominate. In these cases a smaller S-N-B angle is present, as is mandibular retrognathism. The retrognathic mandible can be small or normal and is posteriorly positioned in the facial skeleton. If the size is normal, the saddle angle is larger and flatter, with the condylar fossa in a relatively posterior position (Figure 19-10).

Treatment possibilities depend on growth increments and growth direction. In cases exhibiting horizontal or neutral growth vectors, conventional activator therapy is likely to be successful. In patients with vertical growth vectors, anterior positioning of the mandible is not likely to take place permanently, although in certain cases the so-called vertical activator can be used. Amounts of growth during appliance wear are a consideration, as indicated above.

5. A combination of the four previously designated patterns is possible, particularly a combination of 3 and 4. Class II malocclusion with retrognathic upper and lower jaws also is possible. In such cases, treatment follows a combined functional and fixed appliance approach, and success depends on the growth pattern, direction, and increments during appliance wear.

## GROWTH POTENTIAL

As already indicated, growth direction is quite important, but the amount of growth (or growth potential) is equally important. The size of the jaw bases can be assessed in correlation with the nasion–sella midpoint (N-Se) length, as recommended by Schwarz (1958). The growth rates for the different growth patterns can be evaluated with the help of previously derived tables. (See Chapter 6.) If a particular dimension is too short with respect to the other measurements, increased growth rates can usually be anticipated in the area of apparent deficiency. An exception is the short mandibular ramus observed in a vertically growing face.

## THERAPEUTIC METHODS

The objectives of mixed dentition treatment for Class II malocclusions vary, depending on the type of malocclusion, as outlined previously. The following therapeutic methods have been found useful:

1. The elimination of abnormal perioral muscle function is feasible using inhibitory therapy. Neuromuscular dysfunctions should be corrected in the first phase of treatment. Most often a lower lip screen can be used in combination with other methods.

2. Anterior positioning of the mandible by elimination of functionally induced retrusions and concomitant growth stimulation is a valid objective, with the activator serving as a primary corrective device.

3. Growth inhibition of the maxilla for prognathic maxillary problems, with distalization of upper buccal segment teeth using extraoral force, is a useful therapeutic method. Active plates can sometimes be used for minor problems in this category.

Experience has shown that a combination of therapeutic tools is necessary to produce the optimal result.

## APPLIANCES USED IN THE TREATMENT OF CLASS II MALOCCLUSIONS

Different treatment objectives demand different appliances. Appliances used for anterior positioning of the mandible include the vestibular screen for functional retrusion and lip-trap problems; activators and occasionally bite planes or guide planes also can be used. The activator and its various modifications are clearly the appliances of choice in most instances.

The bite plane has not been described in this book because it is not a typical functional appliance. However, as Hotz (1961) has shown with his *Vorbissplatte,* the bite plane can be used in specific cases in which difficulties are likely to arise with the use of the conventional activator (e.g., in the presence of occluded nasal passages, allergic manifestations, mouth breathing) (Figure 19-11). The appliance is similar in appearance to a modified Hawley retainer; it provides acrylic palatal coverage to which an anterior inclined plane has been added to engage the lower incisors and cause the mandible to slide anteriorly. Anchorage is obtained with Adams or arrowhead clasps and labial bows. The prognosis is more favorable with the so-called *Deckbiss* (deep bite), forced-bite type of problem. The postural change potential is adequate, but its growth-stimulating potential as far as condylar growth is concerned is clearly less than that of the activator. The *Vorbissplatte* can be used under the following conditions:

1. The first premolars (at least) must have erupted to provide good anchorage for the appliance. The use of Adams clasps on the first premolars and first molars is usually recommended. Arrowhead clasps are often used after the second premolars have erupted.

2. The upper and lower dental arches should be reasonably well aligned. Because anchorage is a critical matter, additional tooth movement tasks are not feasible; they reduce appliance efficiency.

3. The maxillary incisors should not be tipped much to the labial. Appreciable uprighting of these teeth with an intramaxillary appliance such as the biteplate has had only limited success.

4. The lower incisors should be upright or lingually inclined. Appliances tend to tip these teeth labially, which can be beneficial in some instances. However, if these

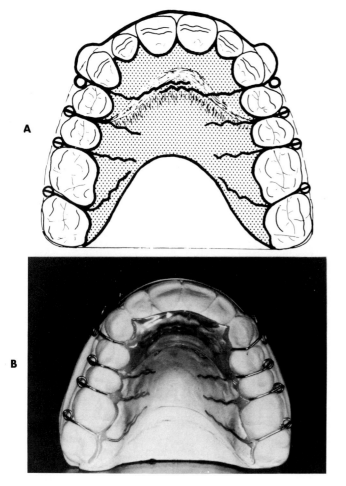

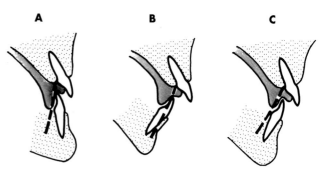

**Figure 19-12.** **A,** Construction of the inclined bite plane is difficult with lingual tipping of the lower incisors. **B,** The plane tips the lower incisors labially. **C,** It also guides the mandible anteriorly.

**Figure 19-11.** Anterior bite plane. **A,** Schematic. **B,** On the cast.

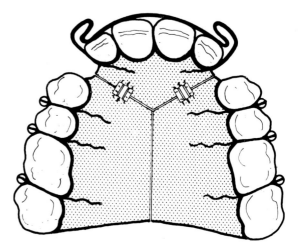

**Figure 19-13.** The Y plate with double jackscrews and arrowhead clasps for retention.

teeth are already labially inclined and are further tipped labially, full correction is not possible because of incisor interference, and the patient will have increased difficulty wearing the appliance (Figure 19-12).

Normally the guide plane has an angulation of approximately 45 degrees, with a seating groove for the lower incisors to reduce the labial tipping tendency that occurs with the anterior mandibular posturing.

Appliances for relative distalization or withholding of maxillary buccal segment teeth may be used in certain cases. Extraoral force delivered by properly designed headgears can produce both skeletal and dentoalveolar responses. After the permanent dentition has erupted, fixed multiattachment appliances can be used with both headgear and elastic traction. Removable Y plates with jackscrews incorporated for distal movement of the maxillary molars may be used in the mixed dentition after eruption of the first premolars.

The Y plate (Figure 19-13) is an active, removable-plate type of appliance that moves teeth under certain conditions.

Its appearance is similar to that of the biteplate, and it is anchored on the maxillary arch with Adams or arrowhead clasps. The labial bow inserts into the acrylic in the lateral incisor–canine embrasure. The plate has two jackscrews placed in oblique position at the canine areas. The opening of the jackscrews exerts a distalizing component on the buccal segment teeth, and a reciprocal force is delivered to the anterior palatal contour and maxillary incisors. To reduce the mesial force component, which tends both to tip the incisors labially and dislodge the appliance, the screws are activated alternately and unilaterally. Under the following conditions, the plate can be used to distalize buccal segment teeth:

1. The first premolars have already erupted, giving increased anchorage.
2. The upper incisors are fairly upright, and a slight labial tipping of these teeth is beneficial or at least not undesirable.
3. No extensive bodily movements are required.
4. The second permanent molars have not yet erupted.

## Indications for the Various Treatment Methods

No one method can be used to treat all Class II problems. Various methods and appliances are required, depending on the specifics of the malocclusion. Using only functional appliances for all Class II malocclusions would help only those cases with forced-bite functional retrusion or retrognathic mandibles and would do little for problems caused by prognathic maxillas. Therefore fixed appliances and extraoral force are clearly indicated in cases demanding repositioning of the maxillary base and dentition, but such appliances have limited influences on the position of the mandible and the elimination of neuromuscular abnormalities.

**Dentoalveolar therapeutic measures.** The primary objective of functional appliances is the forward positioning of the mandible. However, these appliances also can be used for functional retrusion in cases in which a forced distal bite is evident and for some dentoalveolar malocclusions resulting from abnormal perioral muscle function. Not only can the eruption of teeth be controlled (e.g., in deep-bite cases) but also various tooth movements can be performed. The following types of tooth movement can be attained with the activator:

1. Buccal tipping during transverse expansion adjustments
2. Labial and lingual tipping
3. Extrusion
4. Aligning of abnormally tipped teeth
5. Correction of eccentric rotations

Other types of movement can be performed with more limited success. These include intrusion and mesial or distal movement. Some kinds of movement cannot be performed with an activator; these include bodily movement, centric rotations, and torque. Fixed appliances must be used for these objectives. A distalization of the maxillary teeth and an orthopedic effect on the maxilla are possible with extraoral force. The withholding of downward and forward growth is a valid and achievable objective in cases of maxillary prognathism. In vertical growth patterns, inhibition of maxillary growth also is a viable treatment goal.

The movement of teeth with an activator depends on the stage of eruption and the nature of the tooth movement required. The intraoral eruption process can be divided into two phases or steps (Figure 19-14).

1. The first stage is a stage of drift that occurs while the tooth is erupting into the oral cavity; the movement of the teeth is under the influence of contiguous muscle forces. This eruption can be guided using the acrylic planes of the activator itself.
2. The second stage is a stage of interarch influence as the teeth contact their antagonists; equilibrium is established by the occlusal force during this stage. Acrylic guide plane control by the activator is limited in this stage.

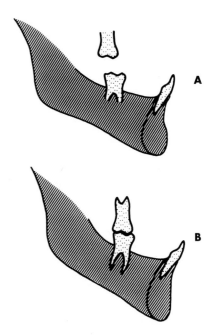

**Figure 19-14.** Two stages of the intraoral phase of tooth eruption. **A,** No tooth contact. **B,** Occlusal phase (contact with the antagonists).

The dentoalveolar type of Class II malocclusion also can be created using screening appliances and activators that have been trimmed to provide the acrylic guiding planes. These therapies are in addition to the traditional use of headgear force applied to the permanent first molars. Purely active nonfunctional removable appliances, as designed by Schwarz, Korkhaus, and others, can be used in the treatment of simple problems, but skeletal effects from these appliances are minimal. Nevertheless, they may provide all the therapeutic force needed in dentoalveolar problems.

**Skeletal therapeutic measures.** Growth direction is decisive in determining the mode of treatment for skeletal malocclusions. In the treatment of a Class II relationship with a horizontal growth pattern during the mixed dentition and a retrognathic mandible, a conventional activator (H activator) is recommended. If a prognathic maxilla is the cause of the Class II relationship, as is frequently the case for African-American patients, positioning of the mandible anteriorly for a causal correction of the anomaly is not possible. Instead, growth inhibition is indicated in the midface region. Extraoral force attached to fixed appliances is usually the most likely mechanism for treatment, although removable-fixed combinations can be used in properly chosen cases (i.e., in combined basal sagittal dysplasias with prognathic maxillas and retrognathic mandibles). If abnormal perioral neuromuscular activity also occurs in these combined cases, a lower lip screen may be used simultaneously. In extraction cases the maxillary second molars are often used in this type of treatment, allowing a dental compensation by moving the maxillary buccal segments distally. Only with this method can a deep overbite be opened; the buccal segment teeth are moved distally into the V, autorotating the mandible down and back. Because of the tendency for the chin point to move into a more retrusive position, the clinician must exercise care in such cases and choose only the most favorable mandibular growth direction cases. Maxillary second molar extraction should be considered only if the developing third molars are normal in size and position. After premolars have been extracted, the posterior segments move mesially to some degree regardless of appliance efforts to prevent it. This movement closes the bite more, making the correction of a deep bite case difficult with such an approach; the relapse tendency is significant. In the most severe problems, some compromise of the result and orthognatic surgery are the only avenues of therapy.

In the treatment of vertical growth patterns with retrognathic mandibles, a specially designed activator (the V activator) should be constructed. The prognathic maxilla is corrected by high-pull extraoral force or compromised by first premolar extraction. Sometimes both measures are required.

The extraction of only the two maxillary first premolars may be required in Class II malocclusions with vertical growth patterns and prognathic maxillas. The control of the deep overbite in such cases is not difficult because of the vertical growth pattern. A lower lip screen also may be incorporated to eliminate perioral muscle dysfunction. If the maxillary first premolars have been removed, however, multiattachment fixed appliances are usually required.

**Functional criteria for determination of mode of therapy.** Functional analysis is imperative before the clinician chooses a specific type of mechanotherapy.

In functional retrusion cases in which the mandible moves up and back from rest into a forced retrusive habitual occlusion, the clinician does not need to attempt to alter the postural rest position of the mandible. In such cases the Class II relationship is largely of a dental nature and caused by improper intercuspation. Screening types of appliances or activators can be used with occlusal equilibration in the later stages of therapy.

In true Class II malocclusions with normal up and forward paths of closure from postural rest to occlusion, not only the occlusal position but also the postural rest position should be altered by anterior positioning, which is accomplished by proper bite construction. Such neuromuscular adaptation is more difficult and not always successful. In any event, such treatment must be done by the practitioner during the growth period.

Occasionally the postural rest position is actually more retruded than is the occlusal position in a Class II malocclusion. Tooth guidance slides the mandible forward into what appears to be a less severe skeletal malrelationship than actually exists. Treating the sagittal malrelationship by anterior positioning of the mandible is difficult in such cases. Dual-bite conditions may persist even after treatment, however, with possible TMJ problems during or after active treatment. In such cases a distal vector of force must be exerted on the maxilla and maxillary teeth, usually with more effective extraoral force methods either separately or with functional appliance therapy.

## Treatment of Various Types of Class II Malocclusions

The systematic, definitive methods of treatment previously described are possible only in typical cases having the cephalometric and functional criteria elucidated. Many borderline cases require a discretionary combination of the various methods. Such modifications of classic functional appliance therapy are often called *midstream correction,* or therapeutic diagnosis. In other words the response of the patient to a predetermined treatment plan is a major consideration in achieving the ultimate correction. Similar malocclusions often respond differently, and such responses should be continually observed by the clinician in making the necessary therapeutic alterations. Clinicians treat individuals, not malocclusion categories, and exact cookbook procedures do not work for all patients. The perceptive clinician resorts to therapeutic diagnosis and therapeutic modifiability as treatment progresses and is always alert to the need to change treatment plans as treatment response or lack of response dictates.

**Treatment with the conventional activator.** An 8½-year-old girl with a Class II, division 1 malocclusion and a maternal hereditary pattern is shown in Figure 19-15. The patient still has a thumb-sucking habit and the retained infantile deglutitional pattern that is so often associated with prolonged finger sucking.

The growth pattern is average, and the facial type is retrognathic. The Class II relationship is apparently caused by a small mandible ( −3.5 mm), short ascending ramus ( −3 mm), and larger cranial base angle ( +7 degrees), which results in a more posterior position of the temporomandibular fossa. The maxillary base is of average length with a slight upward inclination. The A-N-B difference is 5 degrees. The initial pattern shows the lower incisors tipped somewhat labially, diminishing the overjet. This is often the case in retained infantile deglutitional patterns because of forward tongue posture and function. The path of closure is normal, with a rotary action of the condyle from postural rest to habitual occlusion.

Because the mother's own severe Class II malocclusion provided strong motivational assistance, the clinician decided to begin treatment as soon as the incisors erupted. The clinician felt that the hereditary pattern and deforming perioral neuromuscular activity would enhance the dysplasia if left alone for a long time. The treatment objectives of elimination of the dysfunction and stimulation of all possible favorable condylar growth stimulation at this early age had a more favorable prognosis because of the small, retrognathic mandible.

A larger growth spurt can usually be expected; after elimination of restrictive and deforming perioral malfunction, good sagittally directed mandibular growth is likely. This is because of the favorable morphology of the mandible. With such early and simple treatment guidance, the individual optimal outcome is achieved.

All skeletal relationships in this case were favorable for conventional activator treatment, but the labial inclination of the lower incisors should have been considered when the cli-

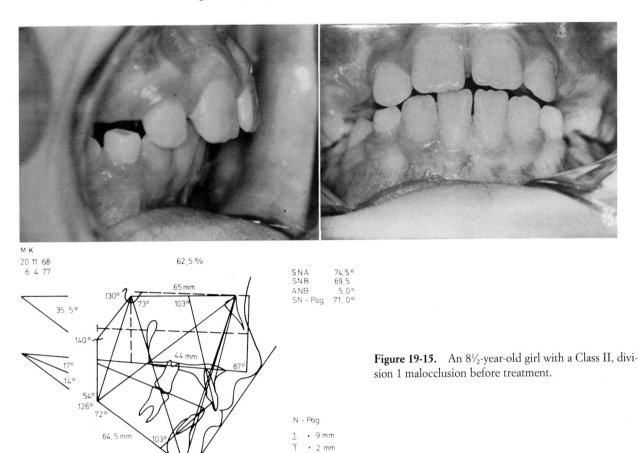

M K
20 11 68
6 4 77

62,5 %

130°  73°  103°
65 mm

35,5°

140°

17°
14°

44 mm

87°

54°
126°
72°

64,5 mm  103°

SNA    74,5°
SNB    69,5
ANB     5,0°
SN - Pog  71,0°

N - Pog

$\underline{1}$  ↗ 9 mm

$\overline{1}$  ↗ 2 mm

**Figure 19-15.** An 8½-year-old girl with a Class II, division 1 malocclusion before treatment.

nician postured the mandible anteriorly. Therapy began with a vestibular screen to eliminate the lip trap and hyperactive mentalis function. The activator was constructed 4 months later with a 7-mm mandibular advancement to an end-to-end incisal relationship. The vertical dimension was opened 3 mm.

Both upper and lower labial bows were active, contacting the teeth at the incisal thirds of the labial surfaces. The incisal edges were supported with acrylic. The acrylic was trimmed away from the lingual aspect of the lower incisors to help tip the teeth lingually. The acrylic was trimmed away from the lingual side of the upper incisors in the coronal region only, because the clinician desired to tip these teeth only slightly lingually to partially compensate for the uprighting of the lower incisors. The appliance was trimmed in the buccal segments to effect distal movement of the upper molars. Stabilizing wires were incorporated mesially to the permanent first molars. In the lower buccal segments, trimming was performed to stimulate slight extrusion of the lower molars and assist in achieving a Class II relationship. The upper molars had a distalizing force against them but were prevented from extrusion.

After 4 years of treatment and retention (also using the activator) the Class II relationship was improved by anterior positioning and growth of the mandible. The retrognathic profile persisted despite a reduction of the A-N-B difference to 2.5 degrees. The growth increment of the mandibular base was 7.5 mm, or 3.5 mm more than the average values. Maxillary and ramal growth increments were average. The basal difference articulare-pogonion (Ar-Pog) to articulare-subspinale (Ar-A) point improved from 11 to 18 mm. The growth direction became more horizontal. The lower incisor inclination improved with anterior positioning of the mandible and pressure from the labial bow (Figure 19-16). As the illustrations show, early treatment for this patient resulted in elimination of abnormal environmental influences, normalization of function, and an undisturbed growth process. The growth increments of the mandible were quite high. Guessing the amount of growth without therapy is a conjectural exercise, but the elimination of disturbing and restrictive factors and synchronization of growth processes did lead to a harmonious occlusion with no skeletal discrepancy. The skeletal discrepancy probably would have increased without treatment, with continuous restrictive suprahyoid and infrahyoid activity combined with excessive posterior temporalis and deep masseter function preventing the full accomplishment of an optimal pattern. This result could have occurred despite growth and would have enhanced the difficulty of causal therapy at a later date.

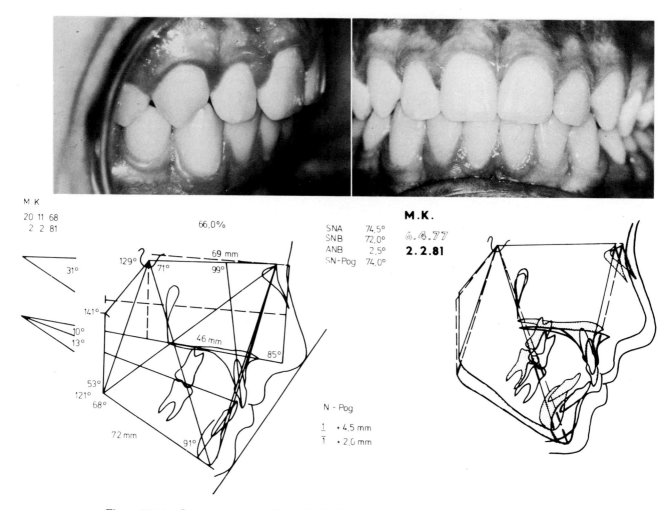

**Figure 19-16.** Same patient as in Figure 19-15 after treatment. *Bottom right,* Superimposition of before and after tracings.

**Compensation of the Class II excessive overjet by labial tipping of the lower incisors.** The 9½-year-old patient illustrated in Figure 19-17 has a Class II skeletal relationship with a retrognathic mandible. The maxillary and mandibular bases are of average length, but the ramus is short (−7 mm). The growth forecast is neutral. The axial inclination of the upper incisors is good, but they are 9 mm in front of the nasion-pogonion (N-Pog) line. The lower incisors are tipped labially, decreasing the apparent overjet. The Class II sagittal relationship is more severe in the rest position, and the mandible slides anteriorly into habitual occlusion during the path of closure. This convenience deflection and labial tipping of the lower incisors mask the true severity of the malocclusion. The patient has abnormal perioral muscle function with a lower lip trap and hyperactive mentalis function.

The objectives of therapy here are to eliminate the lip dysfunction and position the mandible anteriorly to stimulate all possible favorable mandibular growth. Treatment was started with a lower lip screen during the day and an activator at night. The construction bite was taken with the mandible positioned anteriorly 6 mm and the bite opened 5 mm. The upper incisors were held with the labial bow and complete acrylic contact on the lingual and incisal surfaces. The lower labial bow was active, with acrylic in contact on the incisal edges but cut away from the lingual surfaces of the incisors. The acrylic was trimmed in the buccal segments to distalize the maxillary teeth, holding the permanent first molars with stabilizing wires at the mesial embrasure. Because the holding of the forward position of the mandible is difficult in this mesial, occlusal-guidance type of Class II malocclusion, the acrylic was trimmed in the lower posterior teeth to encourage their mesial movement.

After 3 years, no forward positioning of the mandible could be observed, despite a good growth increment of the mandibular base. Only slight ramus growth occurred, and the neutral growth pattern persisted. The malocclusion was compensated for by the extreme labial tipping of the lower incisors. A primary reason for this tipping was the grinding of the activator acrylic to encourage mesial movement of the lower posterior teeth and the fact that these teeth were already labially tipped at the beginning of treatment. The lower lip screen, which removed the hyperactive mentalis muscle's retrusive effect on the incisors and eliminated the lip trap, also enhanced the labial tipping. Clinical experience shows that

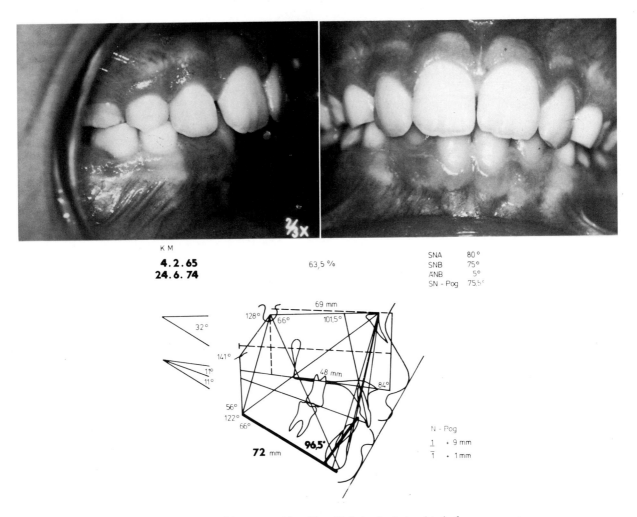

**Figure 19-17.** A 9½-year-old patient with a Class II skeletal relationship before treatment.

protracting and maintaining a retrognathic mandible of average base length to nasion to the midpoint of the sella (N-Se) in a normal path of closure problem is very difficult, even when the mandible slides anteriorly into habitual occlusion. The dental compensation of a Class II problem with labial tipping of the lower incisors is a poor result in the mixed dentition period, except in cases with vertical growth patterns (Figure 19-18). In this case, the S-N-B angle remained at 75 degrees, and the S-N-A angle remained at 79 degrees, with an apical base difference of 4 degrees. Because the treatment result was considered unstable, a new activator was made for the retention period. The construction bite was advanced only 2 mm and opened 3 mm. Both upper and lower labial bows were activated. The acrylic was trimmed contiguously to the upper posterior teeth to encourage distalization, whereas the upper incisors were held with acrylic contact. The lower posterior teeth were held and loaded occlusally, whereas the lower incisors were relieved of acrylic in the lingual and incisal areas. The appliance was worn another 18 months. Reexamination 2 years out of retention showed only slight improvement of the mandibular retrusion in spite of the increased growth rate of the mandibular base and a swing toward a more horizontal growth direction. The axial inclination of the lower incisors improved and ended at the same value as at the beginning of treatment.

In this mixed dentition case the unfavorable functional relationship in the original malocclusion (the anterior guidance into occlusion) made positioning the mandible anteriorly difficult, particularly because the retrognathic mandible was already of average basal length or longer in relation to the N-Se length. The only exception is in functional retrusion cases with abnormal paths of closure from postural rest position up and back into a forced habitual occlusion. In cases with long mandibular bases, treatment by attempts to stimulate growth is difficult because of the usual low growth potential and the fact that the mandible has already achieved its age-dependent individual optimal size. The basic tenet of this working hypothesis is that differential diagnosis using a multifaceted set of diagnostic criteria that only the orthodontist, with years of intensive specialty training, can provide is essential; growth stimulation is possible only in cases of growth restriction or deficiency (Figure 19-19).

This patient had a large incremental growth change in the second period of treatment, with a more favorable growth di-

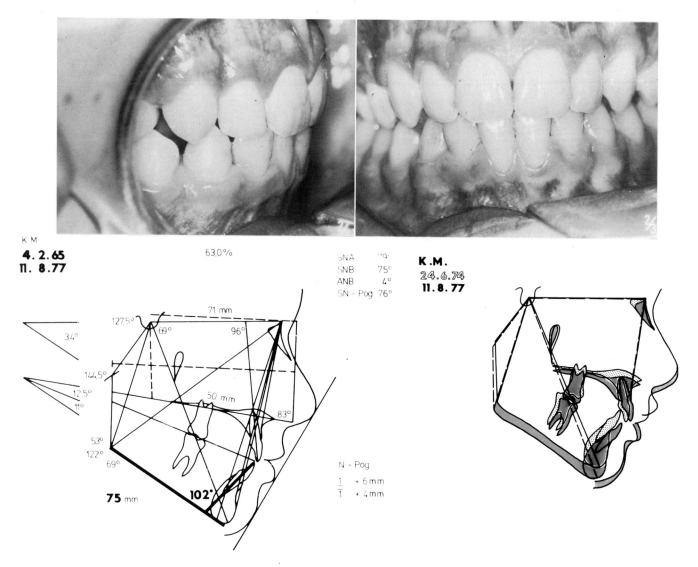

**Figure 19-18.** Same patient as in Figure 19-17 after the first phase of treatment. *Bottom right,* Superimposition of before and after tracings.

rection. The growth increment of the mandibular base, however, was not affected by treatment because the appliance did not activate the muscles and soft tissues because of the slight forward positioning of the mandible and a low construction bite. The endogenous growth pattern and change in growth direction to a more horizontal vector were supported by the appliance as it prevented the lower molars from erupting and relieved the lower incisors on the lingual side. Any differentiation of the natural growth processes and those stimulated by treatment is hard to ascertain. Mandibular growth can be stimulated under certain conditions, but not every Class II malocclusion can be treated by growth stimulation of the mandible using an activator. Even in the more difficult cases, however, the abnormal environmental influences can be eliminated, and more harmonious occlusal relationships can be achieved, providing more favorable conditions for optimal and synchronous development of the stomatognathic system.

**Treatment of the side effects of extraoral force therapy.** Unfavorable or partial response is always possible with any form of orthodontic guidance. The case illustrated in Figure 19-20 illustrates this point. The patient, a 9-year-old girl, had a Class II malocclusion with a slight maxillary prognathism and mandibular retrognathism. The maxillary base and ramal height measurements were larger than average, whereas the mandibular basal length was 2 mm less than were the average values. In such cases an increased growth rate of the mandible can usually be expected, resulting in a more favorable horizontal growth direction to help correct the Class II relationship. On the other hand, control of the vertical dimension to correct a deep overbite can be difficult.

The upper incisors were labially inclined 9 mm in front of the N-Pog line, whereas the lower incisors were well positioned and only 1.5 mm ahead of the N-Pog plane. The patient had a lip dysfunction because of the excessive overjet.

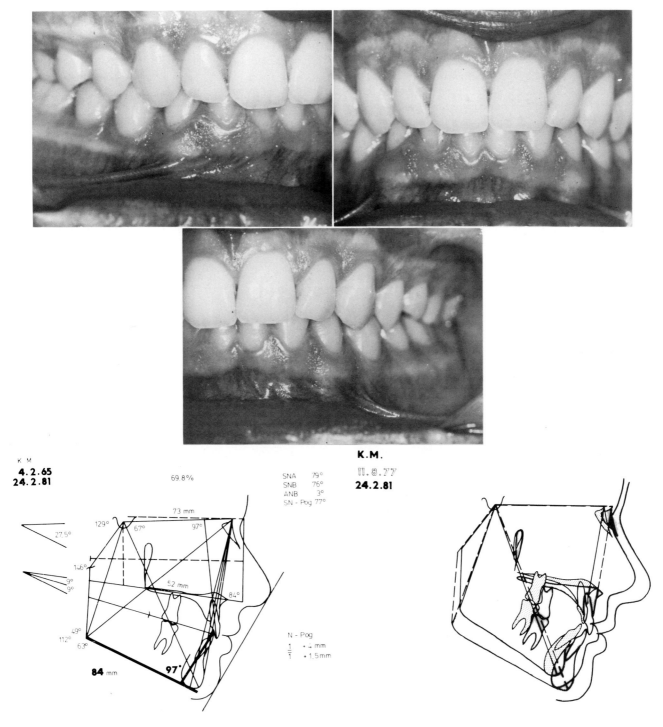

**Figure 19-19.** Same patient as in Figure 19-17 2 years out of retention. *Bottom right,* Superimposition of tracings after the first treatment phase and after retention.

Treatment was started with cervical headgear because the maxillary base was slightly protruded, and the clinician felt that distalization and the extrusive effects of extraoral force could favorably influence the deeper than normal overbite. Also, if the first permanent molars receive headgear therapy before activator treatment, the mesial embrasure is opened and the stabilizing wires readily move into open contact and

continue the favorable eruption guidance of these teeth. A lower lip screen also was used in the initial stages of treatment to eliminate the untoward effects of the lower lip trap.

After 1 year of treatment the skeletal relationship had improved. A growth increment of 3 mm occurred in the mandibular base, but no measurable change was observed in the maxillary or ramal area. The S-N-A angle decreased, and the S-N-B angle increased, with a resultant A-B difference of 2.5 degrees. An unexpected finding was the labial tipping of the incisors, particularly the uppers. The original axial inclination of 110 degrees increased inexplicably to 121 degrees. The most probable explanation is that both the inner labial bow of the headgear and the lower lip screen resisted the restraining effect of the labial musculature, whereas the tongue continued to posture and function in a forward position, exerting a labial vector of force. The clinician should check tongue function ahead of time for this possible iatrogenic effect, but compensatory tongue malfunction also can occur during treatment; continual vigilance is essential. In this case, both the headgear and vestibular screen were discontinued, and an activator was made with an anterior positioning of 2 mm and an opening of 3 mm in the construction bite to permit the uprighting of the incisors. The objective at this time

was to upright the incisors, guide eruption of posterior teeth, and eliminate the deleterious effects of tongue pressure (Figure 19-21). Both upper and lower labial bows were activated. The appliance design permitted a lingual sliding of the upper incisors along an acrylic inclined plane that contacted the incisor labial surface but had the acrylic cut away in the dental and palatal areas. The lower incisors were held on the incisal surface but were allowed to move lingually because the acrylic had been ground away from the lingual tooth surfaces.

A good axial inclination of the incisors had been achieved 2½ years later. Mandibular growth continued, improving the anterior positioning of the mandible and increasing the S-N-B angle. The articular angle was reduced (Figure 19-22).

This case is particularly interesting because of the untoward and unexpected side effects of the headgear treatment. Despite favorable initial conditions and projections that the

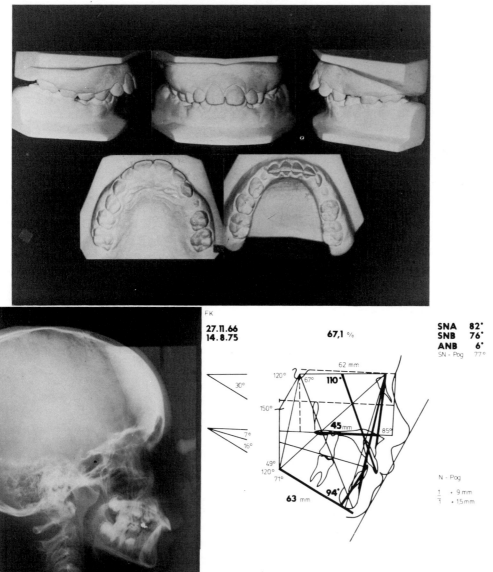

**Figure 19-20.**   A 9-year-old girl with a Class II malocclusion before treatment.

skeletal discrepancy would be solved within 1 year, the change in muscle balance induced unfavorable axial inclination changes in both upper and lower incisor segments. A good lesson can be learned here concerning the need for continuing therapeutic diagnosis.

**Combined treatment of an incisal biprotrusion.** Figure 19-23 shows a 6-year-old boy with a Class II skeletal pattern with a prognathic maxilla and retrognathic mandible. The maxillary base was average in length but positioned anteriorly. The distance from sella to pterygopalatine fossa was 18 mm larger than average. The mandibular base was short (−4 mm), and the ramus was long (+2 mm). The growth pattern was projected as horizontal, with a slight open bite caused by an upward tipping of the anterior terminus of the palatal plane. Both upper and lower incisors were tipped labially, and a def-

inite tongue and lip habit could be seen. Despite the evidence of complete diagnostic records, treatment was not started immediately. The patient returned 15 months later, and new records were taken. No change had occurred in the skeletal discrepancy. Growth increments were slight in both maxillary and mandibular bases. Ramal growth had been significant, however, and the growth direction had become more horizontal. The abnormal perioral muscle function was still present, and the incisors were more labially tipped. Potential lip incompetency was likely (Figure 19-24).

Despite the likely need for later extraction of the four first premolars and full multiattachment fixed appliance control if no treatment was instituted until the full permanent dentition, therapy was begun with removable appliances and without extraction because of the persistence of the abnormal deforming muscle forces on both the labial and lingual aspects,

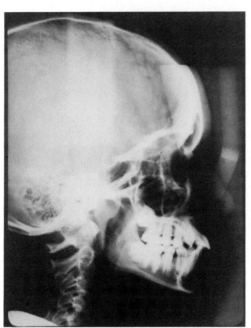

**Figure 19-21.** Same patient as in Figure 19-20 after the first phase of treatment. *Bottom right,* Superimposition of before and after tracings.

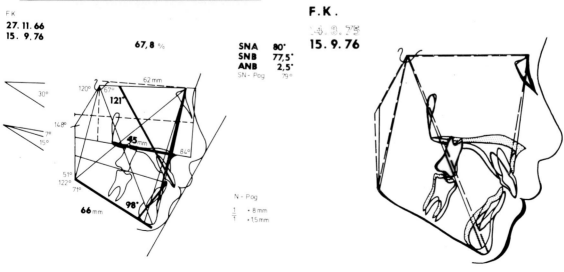

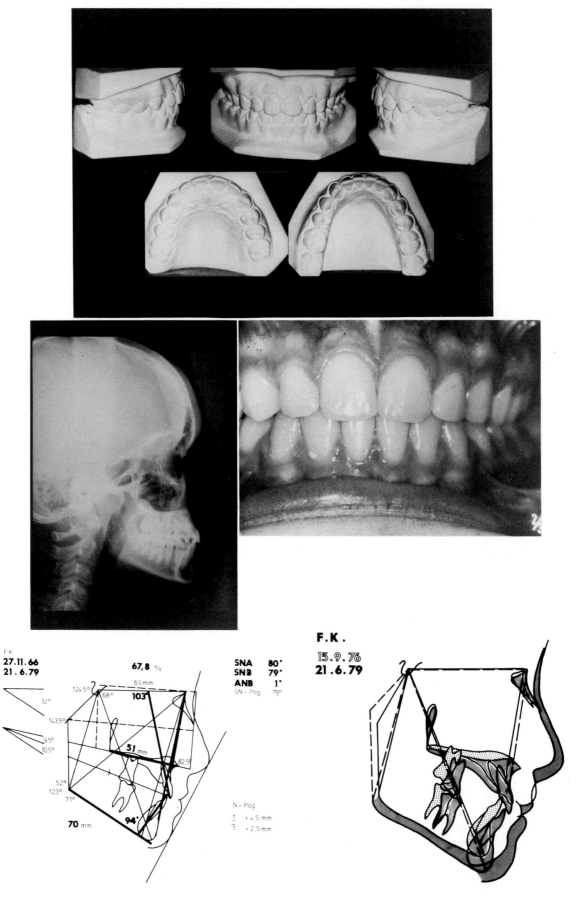

**Figure 19-22.** Same patient as in Figure 19-20 after treatment. *Bottom right,* Superimposition of tracings after the first phase and after completion of treatment.

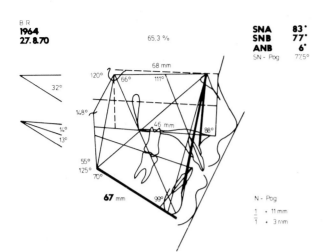

B R
1964
27.8.70

65.3 %

SNA 83°
SNB 77°
ANB 6°
SN - Pog 77.5°

68 mm
120°
32°
66°
111°
148°
14°
13°
46 mm
88°
55°
125°
70°
67 mm
99°
N - Pog
1/1 · 11 mm
1/1 · 3 mm

**Figure 19-23.** A 6-year-old boy with a Class II skeletal pattern 1½ years before treatment.

which were exacerbating the malocclusion. Also, an assessment of the profile showed a relatively normal configuration. Extraction of the four first premolars might have produced a dished-in face. Only a slight dental discrepancy existed, with spaces present between the upper incisors, and a good relation existed between the lower incisors and the N-Pog line.

The treatment objectives were to eliminate the dysfunction, distalize the upper posterior teeth and upright the upper incisors, and achieve a slight anterior positioning of the mandible. This treatment approach sought to harmonize the intermaxillary relationship even if the incisor protrusion could not be eliminated completely.

Therapy was initiated with a vestibular screen to eliminate or at least inhibit the dysfunction. Because of the tongue thrust and incisor protrusion, the screen was constructed with a tongue crib. After reduction of the potential lip incompetence, a distalizing force was applied to the upper molars with extraoral force. The occlusion was then stabilized and retained with an activator. The construction bite moved the mandible anteriorly some 5 mm and opened the bite 3 mm. The upper incisors were tipped lingually, whereas the lower incisors were held in place. Incisal edges were supported by acrylic contact; both labial bows were activated.

After 4 years of treatment and retention, the A-N-B angle of 3 degrees showed an improved skeletal sagittal relationship, but the upper and lower jaws both had become prognathic. The jaw bases were of average length, but the ramus length had increased (+7 mm). The incisal protrusion persisted, but the profile was improved (Figure 19-25).

Although the patient could have been treated with first premolar extraction later and fixed multiattachment appliances, a reasonably good result was achieved by early interception and guidance and no extraction, using relatively simple appliances.

**Treatment with a vertical activator.** A case report of a 9-year-old boy illustrates the use of the vertical activator (Figure 19-26). The patient showed a strong vertical growth pattern and a large lower gonial angle measurement on the lateral cephalogram. Both upper and lower jaw bases were retro-

gnathic, with an A-N-B angle of 6 degrees. The mandibular retrognathism was accentuated by the large articular angle. Maxillary and mandibular bases were of average size, but the ramus was quite short (−11 mm). The palatal plane inclination was average, inclined neither up nor down. The axial inclination of the incisors was within normal limits, but they were positioned ahead of the N-Pog line. The maxillary incisors were rotated and crowded.

The unfavorable growth direction is a contraindication for conventional activator therapy. Anterior positioning of the mandible is not possible because of the vertical growth vector. Distalization of the upper molars would rock the mandible down and back, increasing the retrognathism. The following therapeutic alternatives can be considered:

1. Extraction of the upper first premolars and retrusion of the anterior teeth may be necessary. However, this therapeutic approach is likely to overincrease the retrognathism and elongate the incisors significantly, producing a gummy smile.
2. Attempting a slight anterior positioning of the mandible, with a retroinclination (tipping down) of the maxillary base to compensate for the excessive overjet, is another treatment possibility. Some dental compensation by tipping the upper incisors lingually and the lower incisors labially might be necessary.

The second method of treatment was chosen. The crowding of the upper incisors was first corrected with an anterior expansion plate (Figure 19-27). A vertical activator was then fabricated with a construction bite that positioned the mandible only 2 mm anteriorly but opened the bite 8 mm. The acrylic was extended labially on the upper incisors to the area of greatest convexity, whereas an inclined plane was made incisally. The acrylic was ground away on the lingual side. The cervically positioned labial bow was activated. The lower incisors were held in their present position with no trimming of the acrylic, although the labial bow was activated. The acrylic was trimmed in the upper posterior regions to distalize the posterior teeth, and stabilizing wires were placed mesial to the upper first molars.

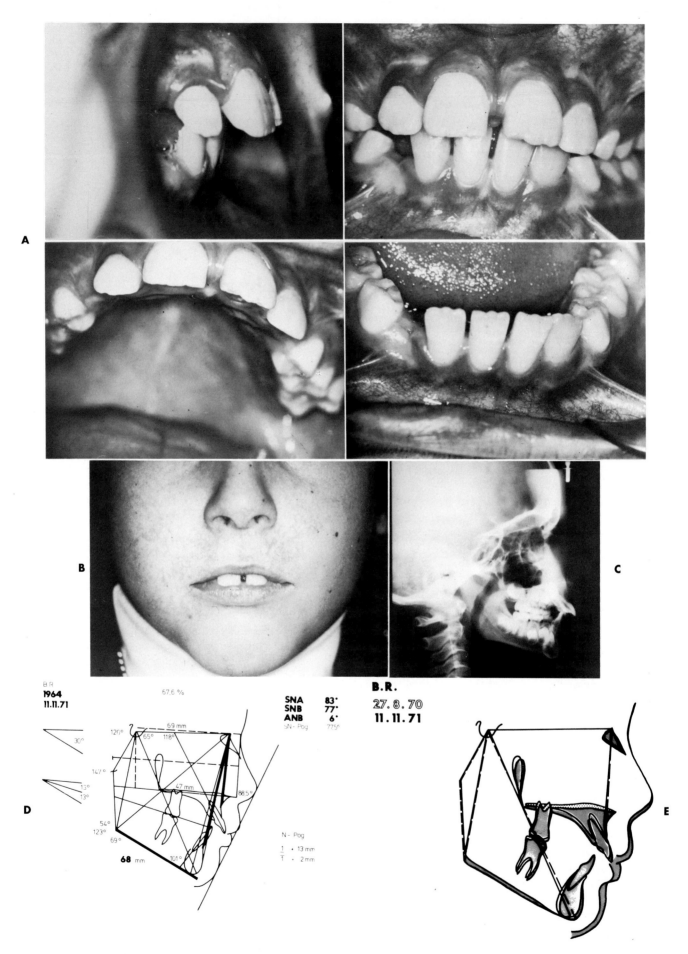

**Figure 19-24.** Same patient as in Figure 19-23 immediately before treatment. Note the incompetent lip seal, **B,** and the superimposition of tracings from 1½ years before and at the start of

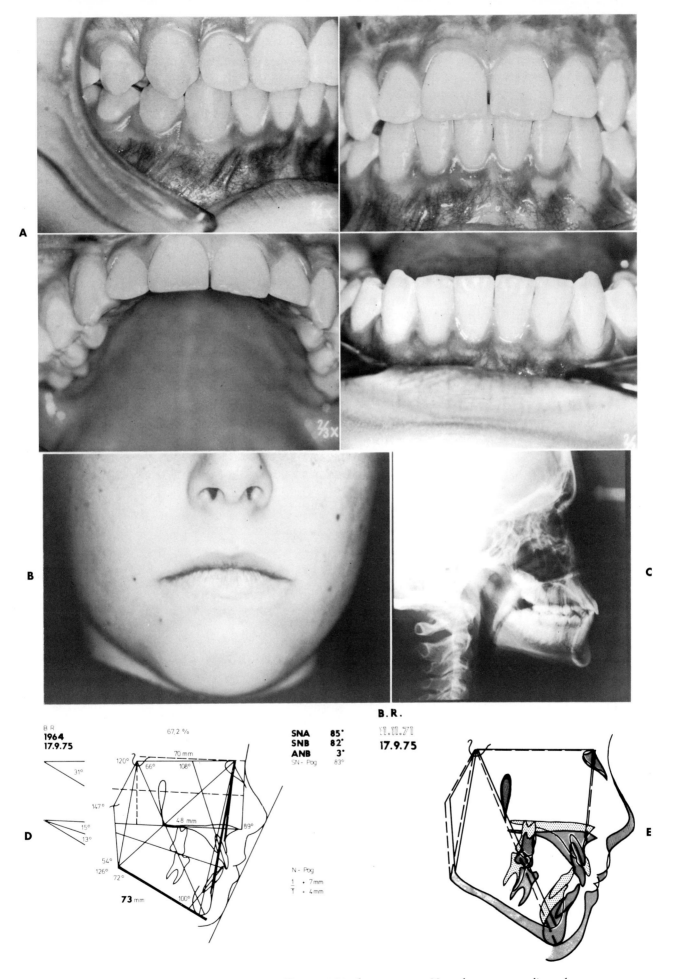

**Figure 19-25.** Same patient as in Figure 19-23 after treatment. Note the competent lip seal, **B**, and the superimposition of before and after tracings, **E**.

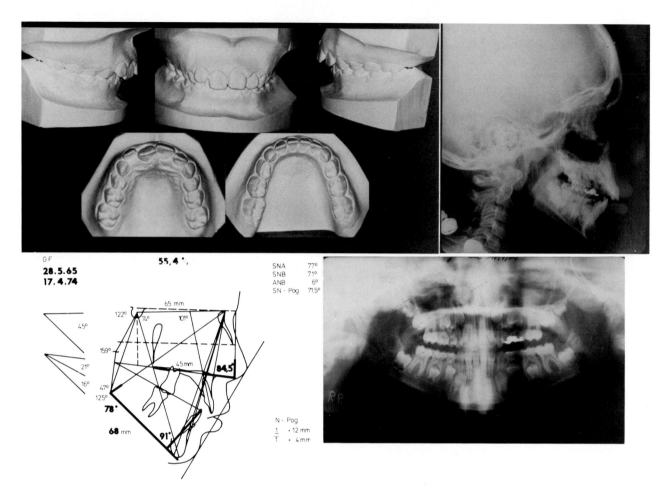

**Figure 19-26.** A 9-year-old boy before treatment.

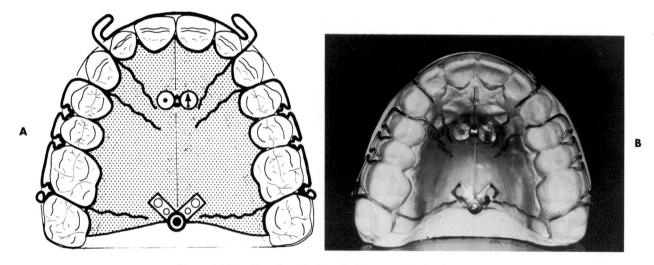

**Figure 19-27.** Fan-shaped plate. **A,** Schematic. **B,** On the cast.

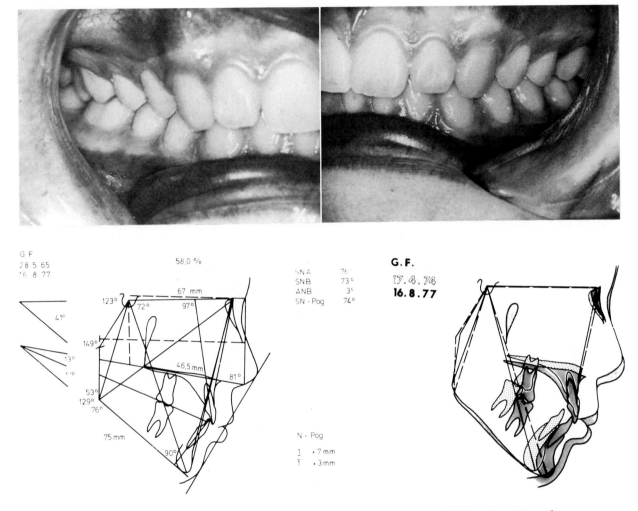

**Figure 19-28.** Same patient as in Figure 19-26 after treatment. *Bottom right,* Superimposition of before and after tracings.

After 3 years of treatment, the Class II relationship had improved. The mandible had been positioned somewhat anteriorly, and a high growth increment (+7 mm) with a reduction of the articular angle was evident. However, the S-N-B angle increased to only 73 degrees, leaving the A-N-B angle at 3 degrees. A retroinclination of the maxillary base was achieved (3.5 degrees), indicating an adaptation of the maxillary base to the vertically growing mandible. The upper incisors had been tipped lingually as planned to reduce the overjet (Figure 19-28).

In this case, successful treatment of the Class II vertical growth pattern with an activator was possible because the inclination of the maxillary base was favorable (the anterior portion was not tipped up) and a high growth increment of the mandibular base was evident during treatment. The patient was reexamined out of retention 3 years later. Some growth in the maxillary and mandibular bases could be observed in this postretention phase. The mandibular base was of average length, the maxillary base was slightly longer (+3 mm), and the ramus was still short (−6.5 mm). Both jaw bases were retrognathic. The S-N-A and S-N-B angles were increased, at

least partly because of maxillary base growth. The compensation of the overjet resulted from the labial tipping of the lower incisors. The vertical growth pattern persisted (Figure 19-29).

**Therapy to effect changes in the inclination of the maxillary base.** Unfortunately, too many orthodontists do not realize that the tipping of the anterior end of the maxillary base has a significant effect on the ultimate treatment result. The following case of a girl 8 years and 4 months old with a Class II malocclusion caused by a large maxillary prognathism illustrates this problem (Figure 19-30).

The initial examination revealed a large S-N-A angle and an average S-N-B angle, with an A-N-B angle of 6 degrees. The growth projection was average, both saddle and gonial angles were small, and the articular angle was large. Both jaw bases were long, but the ramus was short (−5 mm). The maxillary base was tipped up anteriorly 6 degrees, and the upper incisors were procumbent. An open bite was present as a result of the tipped palatal plane. A prolonged finger-sucking habit was present until the patient reached 6 years of age, and a compensatory tongue malfunction persisted.

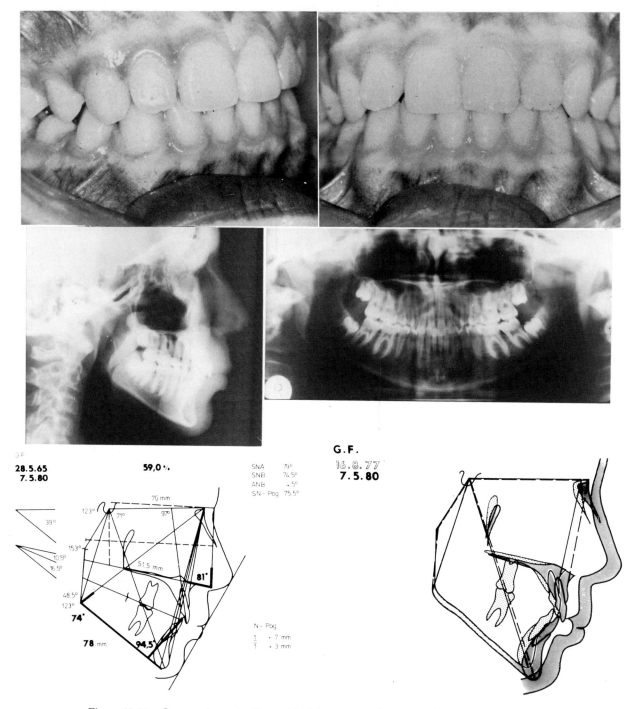

**Figure 19-29.** Same patient as in Figure 19-26 3 years out of retention. Note the intercuspation on both right and left sides (*top*) and the superimposition of tracings after treatment completion and after retention (*bottom right*).

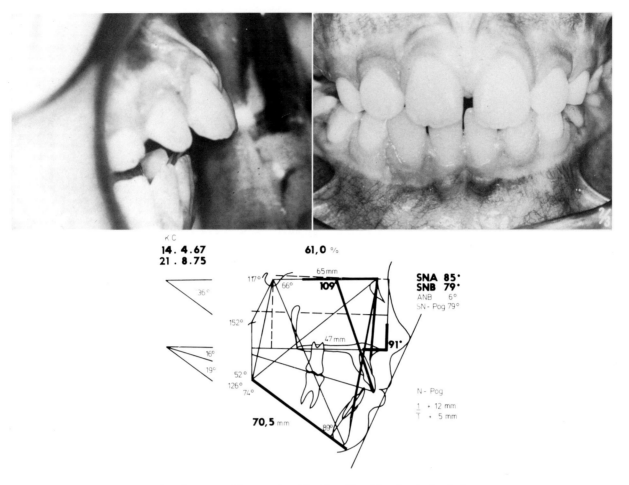

**Figure 19-30.** A girl 8 years and 4 months old with a Class II malocclusion before treatment.

The following treatment plans were considered:

1. Because the Class II relationship was caused largely by the anterior position of the maxilla, with an orthognatic mandible, conventional activator treatment was contraindicated. Distalization of the upper first molars could be attained with extraoral force, but this would tip the mandible down and back, unfavorably influencing the vertical dimension in an original open-bite case. To treat the malocclusion, the four first premolars could have been removed and full multiattachment fixed mechanotherapy could have been instituted, maintaining maximal anchorage in the maxilla and reciprocal anchorage in the mandible as spaces were closed. However, the patient was too young for this approach, and further enhancement of the malocclusion by abnormal perioral muscle function was likely if treatment was postponed for the eruption of the permanent dentition.

2. Because of the worsening malocclusion, a functional approach could be used immediately; this approach would at least eliminate the deforming effects of the lip and tongue dysfunctions. The upward tipping of the palatal plane and labial inclination of the upper incisors were thought to be caused by the abnormal perioral muscle function initiated by the longtime finger-sucking habit that had depressed the maxillary anterior segment and allowed overeruption of the posterior teeth.

The treatment objectives were as follows:

1. The prognathic maxilla should be adapted to the orthognathic mandible by tipping down of the palatal plane and retropositioning of the maxilla.
2. A compensation could be achieved in the dentoalveolar region by lingual tipping of the maxillary incisors.

A vertical activator was constructed, opening the bite 8 mm with no mandibular advancement. The mandibular acrylic portion of the appliance was not trimmed. The lower teeth were held, and the acrylic plate was extended with flanges in the molar region. The acrylic also was extended as high as possible in the labial area of the upper incisors but trimmed away incisally and lingually to permit these teeth to be extruded and move lingually under the influence of an active labial bow. To eliminate the abnormal tongue function, an active plate with a tongue crib was worn during the day during the first months of treatment.

After 4 years of therapy, both sagittal and vertical relationships had been improved, although the maxillary prognathism

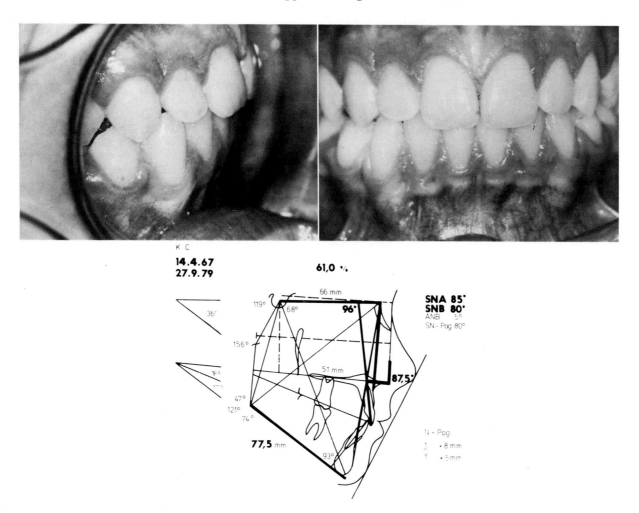

**Figure 19-31.** Same patient as in Figure 19-30 after treatment.

was still present. The maxillary base had rotated inferiorly in the anterior region some 3 degrees without posterior relocation. The upper incisors had tipped lingually 13 degrees, and partial skeletal and dentoalveolar compensation existed. Both maxillary and mandibular basal growth increments were high. The ramus remained short, and the projected average growth direction persisted. As indicated previously, the maxillary prognathism was not affected (Figure 19-31). If headgear therapy had been used, the S-N-A angle could have been decreased, but an unfavorable bite opening with an accentuation of the open bite and mandibular retrognathism also could have occurred. The vertical dimension was improved by the therapy of choice, although it was not completely corrected.

A compensation of the malocclusion enables vertical activator treatment to influence the inclination of the maxillary base. This is especially important in thumb-sucking problems that create deficient midface vertical dimensions. Prognosis for successful therapy is good in these cases if the habit is caught early enough. Patients with average growth patterns and tipping up of the maxillary bases are treated similarly to patients with vertical growth patterns because of the greater

need to stress correction of the vertical components of the malocclusion.

**Treatment of Class II malocclusions with divergent growth rotation of the jaw bases.** Class II malocclusions with divergent growth rotation of the jaw bases, first described by Björk (1969) and later elaborated by Lavergne and Gasson, should be recognized early. Nevertheless, the 9-year-old patient illustrated in Figure 19-32 provides an example of a classic contraindication for activator therapy. The girl still sucked her finger when seen and had an anterior open bite. The malocclusion also was caused by a skeletal discrepancy (i.e., divergent rotation of the jaws during growth). This type of open bite cannot successfully be treated with screening therapy because of this unfavorable growth process. In addition to the open bite, a maxillary prognathism was present, with an S-N-A angle of 86 degrees. The total discrepancy in the upper arch was 11 mm, divided as follows:

1. A sagittal discrepancy of 8 mm was evident. The upper incisors were 12 mm ahead of the N-Pog line and

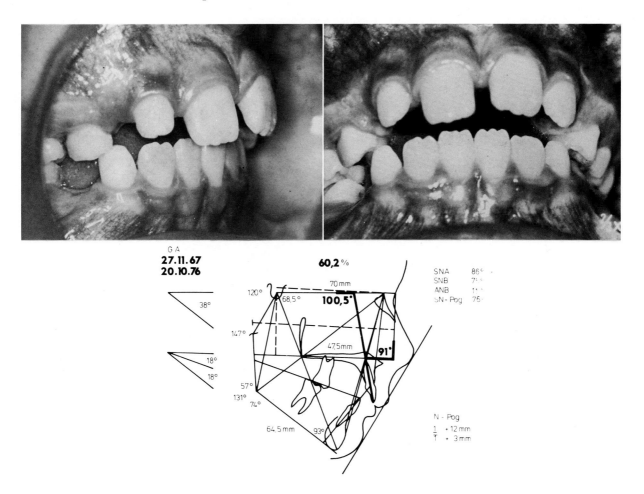

**Figure 19-32.** A 9-year-old girl with a Class II malocclusion before treatment.

needed to be moved to about 4 mm ahead of this line. Any anterior positioning of pogonion by future growth increments and proper direction, improving the sagittal relationship and the N-Pog line, was not likely in this case because of the down and back mandibular growth.

2. The dental discrepancy was 3 mm per quadrant. Spaces existed between the incisors but were inadequate in the canine region. The gaining of space by distalization of the posterior segments would not be possible because of the divergent jaw bases and the wedging open of the bite. Adaptation of the mandible to the prognathic maxilla also was not possible. The mandible was only slightly retrognathic, with no dental discrepancy and a good relationship of the lower incisors. The maxillary base was relatively long compared with the short mandibular base and ramus length.

The treatment decisions were as follows:

1. The correction of the malocclusion was postponed because retrusion of the upper incisors and canines was required. The only treatment available was extraction of two upper first premolars followed by fixed multiattachment control.

2. Because of the finger sucking and perioral neuromuscular compensation and exacerbation, a pretreatment phase of guidance with a vestibular screen was recommended to prevent further deformation and eliminate the deleterious environmental influences.

3. The upper first premolars were to be removed at the beginning of the second, or active, treatment phase, with fixed appliances applying maximal anchorage to the maxillary posterior teeth and retracting and extruding the anterior segment to correct the open bite and excessive overjet.

These approaches were implemented. No lower appliances were used. By 3½ years later the overjet was reduced, but the Class II skeletal and buccal segment relationship remained. The maxillary base and ramus were of average length, and the mandibular base was small and retrognathic. The maxillary prognathism had decreased, but the upward tipping of the

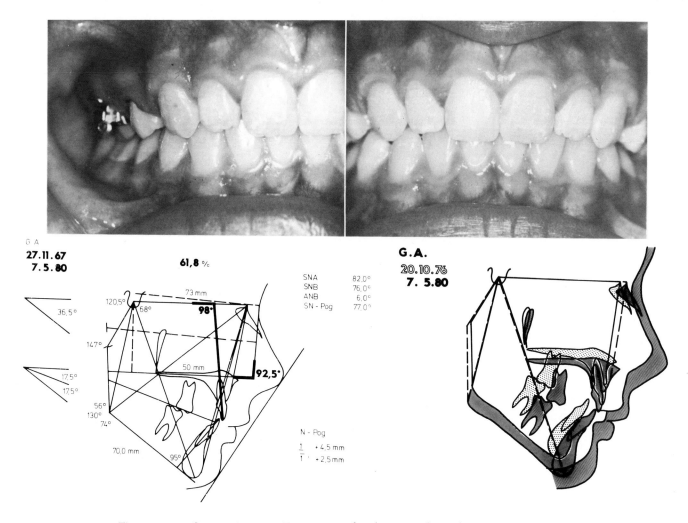

**Figure 19-33.**    Same patient as in Figure 19-32 after the active phase of treatment. *Bottom right,* Superimposition of before and after tracings.

maxillary base was even more pronounced. The upper incisors had been moved lingually and torqued; the lower incisors had tipped slightly labially. The divergent growth pattern and maxillary prognathism were compensated by the dentoalveolar adjustment (Figure 19-33).

This type of Class II malocclusion, with a maxillary prognathism, divergent or at least vertical growth patterns, and a well-aligned lower arch, is probably the only indication for extraction of the two upper first premolars. Functional methods cannot be expected to influence such a skeletal dysplasia much, even though Fränkel has described *selected* cases that seem to indicate a change in growth direction under rigorous function regulator (FR) wear and a stringent exercise discipline. The use of the interceptive vestibular screen in the first phase of treatment reduces the local neuromuscular deformational potential only until full mechanotherapy can be instituted (see Chapter 12).

**Multiattachment treatment after failure of activator therapy.** The following case illustrates the fixed appliance alternatives after unsuccessful early functional appliance attempts.

The patient was an 11-year-old boy with a Class II sagittal relationship, horizontal growth pattern, and deep overbite. The boy's developmental age was 12 years, although the permanent second molars had not yet erupted (Figure 19-34). The patient had a lower lip-sucking habit and a marked mentolabial sulcus. The postural rest position was posterior as the mandible slid anteriorly into habitual occlusion. Despite the deep bite the interocclusal clearance was small.

Cephalometric evaluation indicated that the Class II relationship was probably caused by maxillary prognathism, because only slight mandibular retrognathism was present. The growth direction was markedly horizontal for this age group. The jaw bases and ramus were of average length. The upper incisors were tipped slightly labially and 12 mm ahead of the N-Pog line; the lower incisors were in good position. The slight labial tipping of the lower incisors, despite the confirmed lower lip habit and no evidence of tongue thrust, could be explained by the case history. The patient had been treated with an activator. Unfortunately, no original records were available to assess the original malocclusion. The motivation of the patient seemed to be good, but he was disappointed with the failure of activator therapy and wondered why the

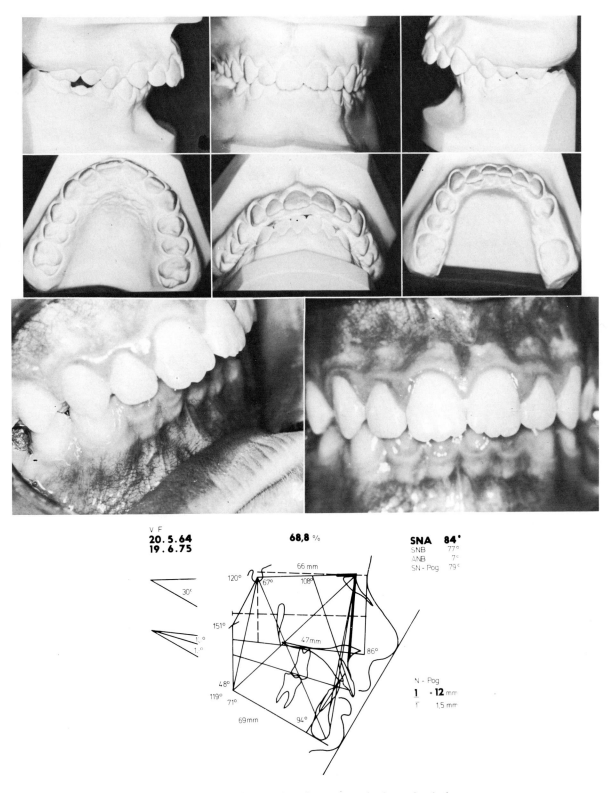

**Figure 19-34.** An 11-year-old boy with a Class II sagittal relationship before treatment.

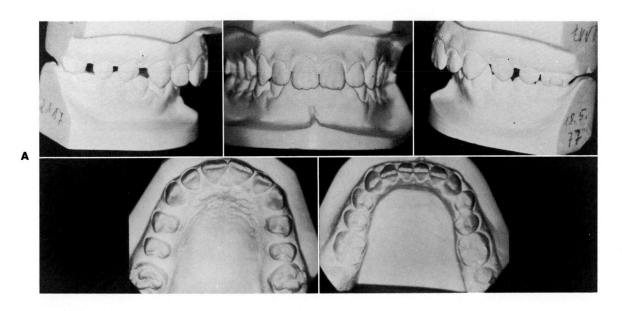

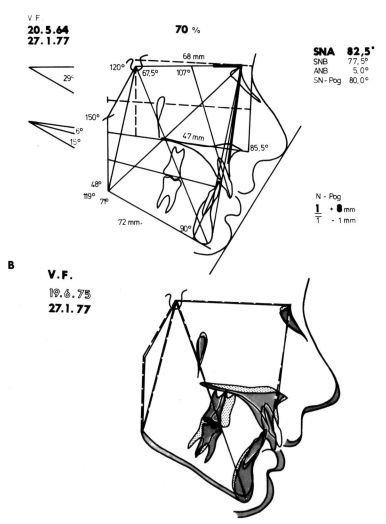

**Figure 19-35.**   **A,** Same patient as in Figure 19-34. **B,** Appearance after the first phase of treatment (*top*) and superimposition of before and after tracings (*bottom*).

activator not been successful despite the horizontal growth direction. The answer seems to be that the morphologic and functional relationships were unfavorable for activator treatment.

In treating cases of maxillary prognathism, the clinician should institute therapy with extraoral force. Even in cases with horizontal growth patterns, adaptation of the mandible to a prognathic maxilla is not possible. Reexamination of activator therapy cases that have not been successfully treated reveals that many of them show a larger than normal S-N-A angle. In such cases, particularly with full Class II relationships, the clinician should start treatment with a headgear for maxillary orthopedic retraction (see Chapter 18).

The functional pattern in this case was not favorable for activator treatment. The posterior rest position was masked by the anterior habitual occlusion, which resulted from cuspal guidance. The small interocclusal clearance also was a contraindication. The lower lip habit increased the excessive overjet.

Treatment was begun with maxillary extraoral force and a lower removable appliance with lip pads to intercept the lip habit. The labial bow of the lower appliance stabilized the lower incisors, whereas the pads eliminated the perverted function and established a normal lip seal. The acrylic lingual to the lower incisors was trimmed away.

After 1½ years of this second phase of treatment the upper molars had moved distally and were extruded some, opening the bite slightly. The lower incisors had uprighted. The S-N-A angle and overjet were reduced (Figure 19-35). An activator might have been used in the second phase, but the deep bite and functional pattern would have hindered its success. Without leveling of the excessive curve of Spee the deep overbite could not be completely controlled. After the eruption of the premolars this type of leveling is not possible with functional methods. Significant extrusion of the lower posterior teeth and the use of intrusive forces on the lower anterior teeth is required for the best possible correction.

After distalization of the upper first molars, spaces were present in the upper buccal segments. Only careful control of fixed appliances allows the proper closure of these spaces by distalization of the remaining buccal segment teeth with torque and intrusion of the incisors. In this case the upper arch was aligned and spaces were closed with elastic traction and extraoral force.

After 1½ years of second-phase active treatment the Class II relationship had been corrected and the overbite and overjet reduced. Continued mandibular growth and a more anterior position were evident. The S-N-A angle was reduced to 81 degrees. The incisor relationship was partially compensated by a light labial tipping of the lower incisors (Figure 19-36). Leveling of the curve of Spee (compensating curve) was accomplished as planned. Over the course of treatment the growth increments of the mandibular base and ramus were average, although the ramus was overly long from the beginning of therapy. Maxillary basal growth was minimal—1 mm.

This case might have been treated more successfully in the mixed dentition if therapy had been initiated with extraoral force to reduce the maxillary prognathism. With early correction of the Class II molar relationship, the maxillary buccal segment teeth migrate distally in their eruption. This movement can be well guided with an activator. The mistake may have been beginning treatment with an activator instead of a headgear.

**Multiattachment fixed mechanotherapy with maxillary second molar extraction after unsuccessful early activator treatment.** One more method is available to achieve partial activator correction of Class II malocclusions. This method is illustrated in a 15-year-old girl with a mature, 17-year-old developmental age and a horizontal growth pattern (Figure 19-37).

Diagnostic records taken at 15 years showed long and prognathic jaw bases in relation to the cranial base. The A-N-B difference was 4 degrees. The incisors were tipped labially. The lower incisors were excellent relative to the N-Pog line, but the upper incisors were still 9 mm ahead of this plane. The teeth were well aligned in the lower arch, but slight crowding existed in the upper arch. The path of closure from postural rest to occlusion was up and forward, with a normal hinge or rotary condylar movement. The interocclusal space was 3 mm. The patient had been treated between 9 and 12 years with an activator. The likely reason for failure was the initial and continuing maxillary prognathism. In retrospect, maxillary withholding and distalization with extraoral force would have adapted the protrusive maxilla to the mandible.

Because the developmental age of 17 years allowed only dental compensation for skeletal malrelationships, and because extensive distalization of maxillary posterior teeth (about 6 mm) was still required, tooth sacrifice offered the only possibility for lasting correction. Premolar extraction was contraindicated because of the horizontal growth pattern and the possibility of residual spacing distal to the canines. Also, no appreciable help in control of the overbite was available with such an approach. Only by distalization of all the maxillary buccal segments could the bite be opened and corrected sagittally at the same time. Maxillary incisor intrusion alone would be limited at this stage and would not provide enough correction of the incisor overbite. The only approach left, with third molars present and in good position in the tuberosity area, was to remove the maxillary second molars after assurance of good patient compliance (see Chapter 18).

In such cases, first distalizing the maxillary first molars with extraoral force and then placing the remaining multiattachment appliance to complete the correction is a quite effective treatment approach. This two-phase approach shortens the treatment time. With continued use of stabilizing headgear to hold the molars in the Class I relationship, distalization of the remaining teeth can be accomplished by intramaxillary elastics and power chains. Retrusive, intrusive, and torque adjustments are necessary to gain the best possible incisor relationship. Class II elastics also are necessary on a part-time basis to assist in this maneuver and slightly elevate the lower molars for overbite control. The clinician must take care not to flare the lower incisors labially. A lower headgear can be used to bolster lower anchorage, if desired.

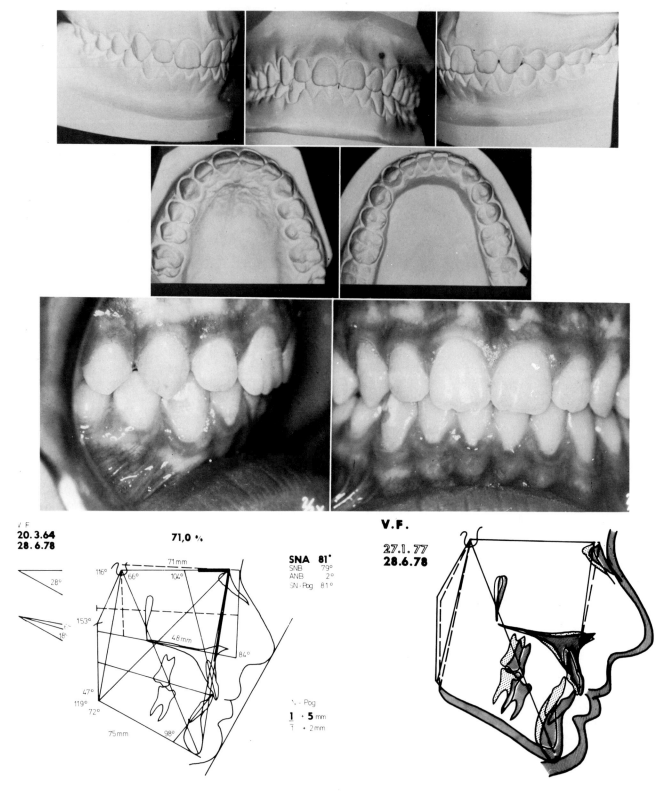

**Figure 19-36.** Same patient as in Figure 19-34 after treatment. *Bottom right,* Superimposition of tracings after the first phase and after the completion of therapy.

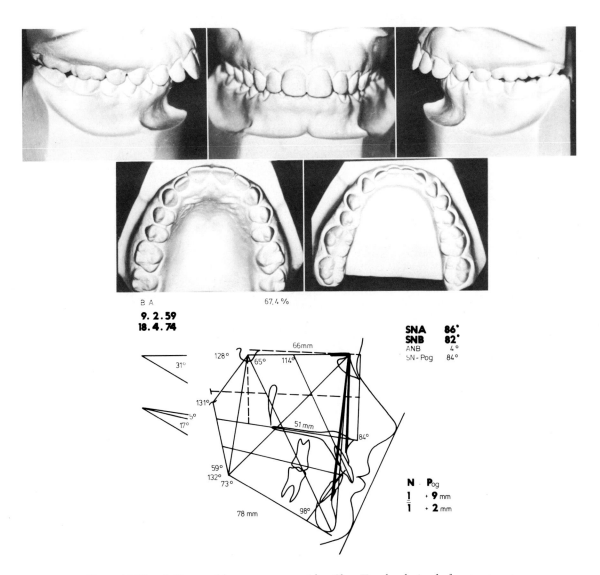

**Figure 19-37.** A 15-year-old young woman with a Class II malocclusion before treatment.

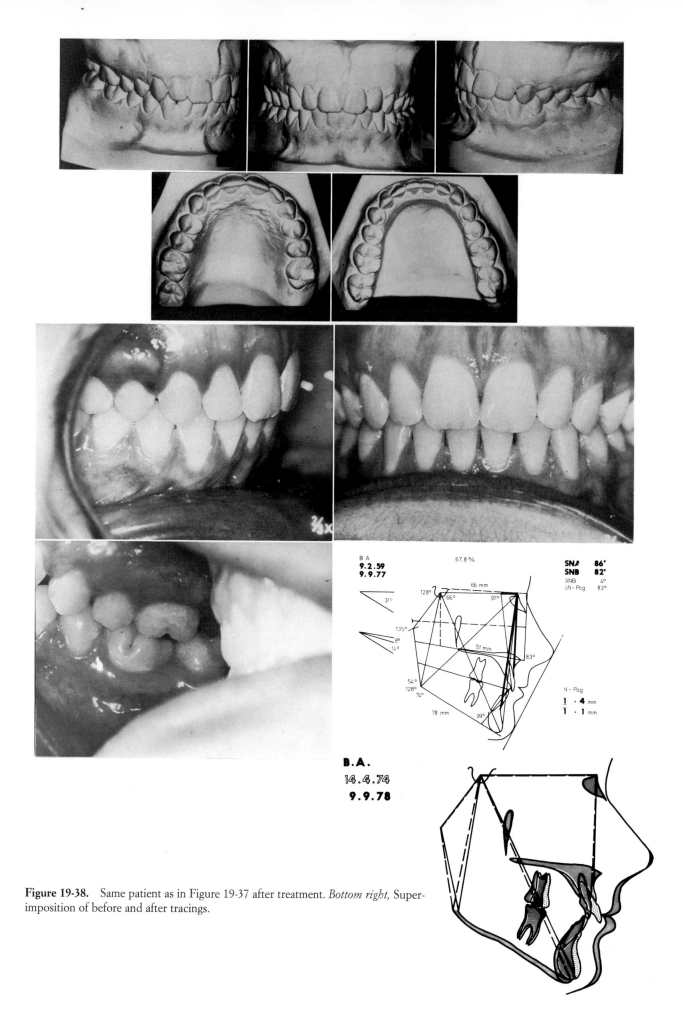

**Figure 19-38.** Same patient as in Figure 19-37 after treatment. *Bottom right,* Superimposition of before and after tracings.

After 2 years of active treatment, no skeletal change was noted, but the dentoalveolar relationships were improved and the deep overbite was corrected (Figure 19-38). Profile improvement also was accomplished with an improved lip line. No success had been achieved with early, first-phase activator treatment, although early treatment could have prevented the increasing severity of the malocclusion. If extraoral force had been used, the orthopedic changes would have been greater in the area in which they were needed most—in retracting the prognathic maxilla. After growth is complete, only dental compensation is possible, as this case illustrates.

## SUMMARY

A number of methods are available to attempt the correction of Class II malocclusions. The method chosen depends on a series of factors that must be carefully evaluated before therapy is instituted:

1. The developmental age of the patient
2. The location and etiology of the malocclusion
3. The functional relationship
4. The specific morphologic characteristics in both the skeletal and dental areas
5. The motivation and likely continuing cooperation of both the patient and the patient's parents

No universal appliance or cookbook formula is available for Class II therapy. All patients cannot be fitted into the same appliance, any more than the mythical Procrustes could fit all his guests into the same bed. Only a careful and complete diagnosis, a continued diagnostic monitoring during treatment, a careful step-by-step accomplishment of the treatment objectives, a number of appliances in the armamentarium, and a willingness to change appliances as changing situations dictate will ensure the best possible treatment.

# Chapter 20

# The Deep Overbite

Thomas Rakosi

In treating a deep overbite, the clinician should be concerned with more than the vertical dimension. The clinician must consider the sagittal relationship and the direction and amount of growth to be expected for the patient.

Most of the problems concerning treatment objectives have already been discussed in Chapter 19. However, some types of Class II malocclusions have horizontal growth patterns in which the correction of deep overbite problems is more difficult than is the correction of the sagittal Class II relationship. In many adults, orthognathic surgery is the only method for complete correction, not so much because of the sagittal malrelationship as because of the vertical dimension deficiency, a deficiency dependent on growth guidance, which is not possible in the adult patient. Excessive overjet can be corrected by the removal of two upper premolars and the therapeutic retrusion of the incisors. In most adults this means an actual deepening of the bite as the incisors are uprighted during space closure.

The overbite problem and the entire vertical dimension should be considered in the treatment of every malocclusion. The vertical dimension is unique in that the growth rate is highest and lasts the longest in this vector. Because growth tends to increase the vertical distance between the jaw bases, performing treatment during this period is most advantageous. Nevertheless, the vertical dimension is not stable. Even in adults who have never had any orthodontic treatment, significant changes can occur. Abrasion or loss of teeth can close down the vertical dimension. Tooth elongation or overeruption also can occur, increasing the vertical dimension. The stability of tooth position depends on the eruption or elongation tendency of the teeth and on the opposing forces. If the occlusal forces are altered, the equilibrium is disturbed and the teeth migrate in the direction of the occlusal plane.

## ETIOLOGIC CONSIDERATIONS

From an etiologic standpoint, overbite can be differentiated into the developmental deep bite and the acquired deep bite. Two types of developmental or genetically determined deep overbites have been described:

1. The skeletal deep overbite with a horizontal growth pattern is a common malocclusion.
2. The dentoalveolar deep bite caused by supraocclusion of the incisors also is common. In these cases the interoc-

clusal clearance is usually small, meaning the overbite is functionally a pseudo–deep overbite.

Therapeutic correction of a developmental deep overbite is very difficult and is usually successful only with active mechanical methods.

An acquired deep overbite may be caused by the following factors:

1. A lateral tongue thrust or postural position frequently can produce an acquired deep overbite. This type of dysfunction produces an infraocclusion of the posterior teeth, which in turn leads to a deep overbite. A classic Class II, division 2 malocclusion is a good example of this type of case. The freeway space is usually large, which is favorable for dentofacial orthopedic functional appliance treatment.
2. Premature loss of deciduous molars or early loss of permanent posterior teeth can cause an acquired secondary deep overbite, particularly if the contiguous teeth are tipped into the extraction sites.
3. The wearing away of the occlusal surface or tooth abrasion can produce an acquired, secondary deep overbite in some patients.

## THE MORPHOLOGIC CHARACTERISTICS OF THE DEEP OVERBITE

The deep overbite can be localized in either the dentoalveolar or skeletal areas. The area affected determines the type of treatment.

### Dentoalveolar Deep Overbite

The dentoalveolar deep overbite is characterized by infraocclusion of the molars and supraocclusion of the incisors (Figure 20-1). The growth pattern usually is average or tends toward the vertical.

The deep overbite caused by the infraocclusion of molars has the following symptoms:

1. The molars are partially erupted.
2. The interocclusal space is large.
3. A lateral tongue posture and thrust are present.
4. The distances between the maxillary and mandibular basal planes and occlusal plane are short.

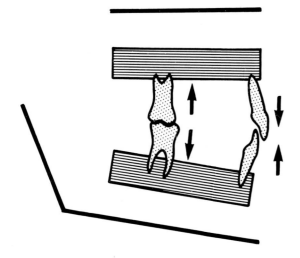

**Figure 20-1.** Dentoalveolar deep overbite caused by infraocclusion of the molars and supraocclusion of the incisors.

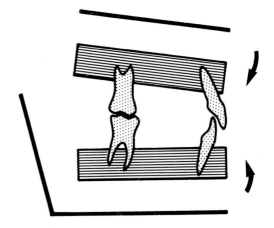

**Figure 20-3.** Skeletal deep overbite caused by convergent rotation of the jaw bases.

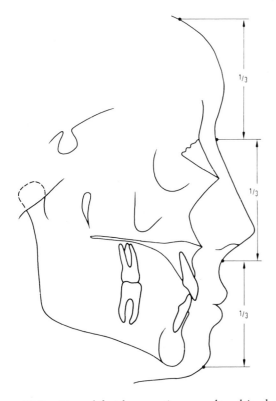

**Figure 20-2.** Normal facial proportions are altered in skeletal deep overbite malocclusions. The anterior lower face height is shorter.

The deep overbite caused by overeruption of the incisors has the following characteristics:

1. The incisal margins of the incisors extend beyond the functional occlusal plane.
2. The molars are fully erupted.
3. The curve of Spee (compensating curve) is excessive.
4. The interocclusal space is small.

## Skeletal Deep Overbite

The skeletal deep overbite is characterized by a horizontal type of growth pattern. The anterior facial height is short, particularly the lower facial third, whereas the posterior facial height is long. Although the normal ratio of upper to lower anterior facial height is 2:3, it is reduced in the skeletal deep overbite to a ratio of 2:2.5 or 2:2.8. The horizontal cephalometric planes (sella-nasion, palatal, occlusal, and mandibular) are approximately parallel to each other. The interocclusal clearance is usually small (Figure 20-2).

The inclination of the maxillary base is significant in the evaluation of the treatment plan for this type of problem. An extreme horizontal growth pattern can be at least partially compensated by an up and forward inclination of the maxillary base (anteinclination). On the other hand, the combination of a horizontal growth pattern with a down and forward inclination (retroclination) of the maxillary base results in a more severe skeletal deep overbite (Figure 20-3).

## TREATMENT PLANNING

Problem-specific therapeutic measures can be taken, depending on the skeletal or dentoalveolar nature of the deep overbite. In skeletal problems, therapy should be directed toward enhancement of the divergent rotation of the jaw bases, using whatever appliances (fixed or removable) are available. In dentoalveolar problems, intrusion and labial inclination of the incisors are desirable, as are extrusion of the posterior segment teeth and leveling of the occlusal plane to reduce the curve of Spee (Figure 20-4).

An important consideration is whether therapy is performed during or after the growth period. During the growth period, tooth eruption can be stimulated in the posterior segments and inhibited in the anterior segments. The vertical growth component in the condylar and sutural areas also is amenable to favorable therapeutic influence. Extrusion of the

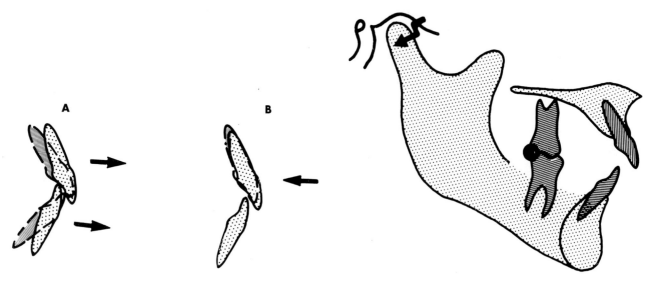

**Figure 20-4.** A deep overbite in the incisal region can be treated by labial tipping of the upper and lower incisors, **A,** or distal driving and intrusion of the upper incisors only, **B.**

**Figure 20-5.** Distal driving of the upper molars can result in a molar fulcrum and premature contact, with levering of the condyles.

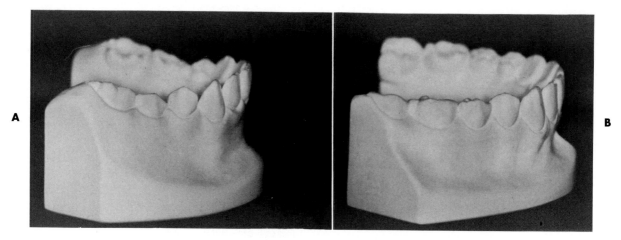

**Figure 20-6.** Leveling of the compensating curve is the precondition for correction of a deep overbite. Compensating curve before, **A,** and after, **B,** treatment.

molars and premolars also implies a skeletal growth stimulus with vertical rotation of the mandible, rocking the mandible down and back. Such a maneuver, of course, can accentuate the sagittal discrepancy in a Class II malocclusion, increasing the angle of facial convexity.

If treatment is performed in the adult dentition after all growth has ceased, the extruded molars can create a molar fulcrum without additional growth or developmental adaptation. The molars thus act as premature occlusal contacts for mandibular rotation (Figure 20-5). This rotation can occur in either an anterior or a posterior direction and has potent temporomandibular joint (TMJ) implications.

During anterior rotation the condylar and TMJ structures can be damaged by subluxation or distraction of the associated ligaments, retrodiscal pad, or capsule. Subluxation may be needed for acute TMJ dysfunction syndromes, but this should be handled carefully, particularly in light of nocturnal parafunctional activity. TMJ problems can be created by such

maneuvers in patients in whom they did not exist before, inciting nocturnal bruxism and clenching.

During a posterior rotation the bite opens, creating occlusal interferences and disturbances. Although bite opening may be desirable as a therapeutic objective, the clinician must keep in mind that occlusal equilibration may likely be needed because growth compensation is minimal or nonexistent. Without constant attention to the establishment of proper exteroceptive and proprioceptive occlusal contact, TMJ dysfunction, bruxism, and clenching can occur.

A variety of therapeutic measures are available to the clinician, depending on the age and developmental status of the patient and the etiologic basis and location of the malocclusion. In the growing individual, growth stimulation is a valid treatment objective with functional appliances. In the true deep bite problem, with a large interocclusal clearance, lateral tongue posture and function, and infraocclusion of posterior teeth, functional appliances are valid tools.

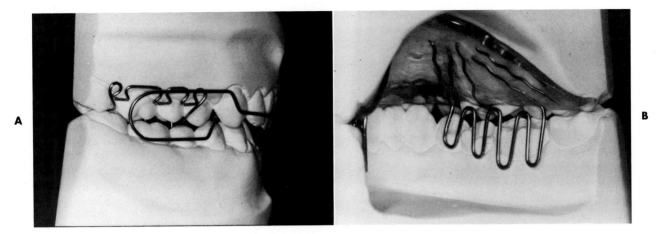

**Figure 20-7.** Palatal plate construction for screening of lateral tongue thrust and cheek sucking. **A,** Labial bow with buccinator loops. **B,** The lateral tongue crib permits extrusion of the molars.

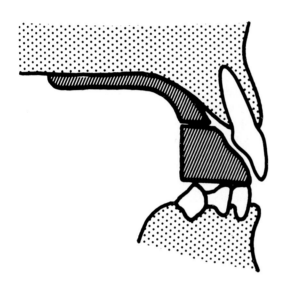

**Figure 20-8.** Bite plane for intrusion of the lower incisors and simultaneous extrusion of the molars.

In all other types of deep overbite, after the possibility of growth stimulation is gone, fixed or removable mechanical appliances are needed to achieve the optimal treatment response. Causal treatment is possible in the dentoalveolar type of problem through intrusion of the incisors and leveling of the curve of Spee (Figure 20-6). However, the skeletal discrepancy can be compensated for only by dentoalveolar orthodontic or orthognathic surgical methods.

## Treatment of the Dentoalveolar Deep Overbite

Treatment mechanics depend on the specific malocclusion characteristics. In cases of true deep overbite the goal of treatment is extrusion of the molars and premolars. During eruption of the posterior teeth the therapy can be performed with an activator to guide the eruption. In cases of extreme lateral tongue thrust a palatal plate with a lateral tongue crib can be

used to discourage the habit. If an additional cheek-sucking habit is evident, it can be eliminated with a modified labial bow (Figure 20-7). The bow, which is similar in construction to the bionator, has buccinator loops. Use of this type of plate may be alternated with an activator, the plate being worn during the day and the activator worn at night.

Elongation or further eruption of the posterior teeth also can be achieved with biteplates. This type of plate loads the incisors for intrusive effect but leaves the posterior segments free to erupt, leveling the curve of Spee. Actual intrusion is minimal, but a relative intrusion occurs with the extrusion of the posterior teeth.

The use of the biteplate has not yet been described because it is not a true functional appliance (Figure 20-8). However, it can be used in deep-bite cases in late mixed, transitional, or early permanent dentitions. The method of anchoring or clasping—arrowhead, Adams, or crib clasps—depends on the stage of dentitional development. Arrowhead clasps have the advantage of contacting the teeth at the gingival third of the embrasure, with a wedging effect that stimulates eruption. The labial bow helps stabilize the biteplate and contacts the teeth at the incisal third. The most important part is the acrylic bite plane or block immediately behind the maxillary incisors. By acting as a premature incisal stop, usually within the confines of the interocclusal clearance, the block frees the posterior teeth from occlusal contact and allows them to erupt. To stabilize the position of the mandible if no change is desired, the clinician should cut a seating groove for the lower incisors in the acrylic plane. Because the plate is not trying to position the mandible anteriorly, the angle of the plane is 90 degrees to the long axis of the lower incisors. After full eruption of the permanent teeth, treatment usually requires completion with fixed appliances, except the original problem was solely one of dysfunction.

The treatment of pseudo–deep overbite is more difficult. The primary objective here is the intrusion of the incisor teeth, which can be achieved with only limited success by an activator or biteplates. However, a slight intrusion in the mixed dentition and some labial tipping of the incisors may be achieved, which has the effect of reducing the overbite. Multibanded control is still necessary in the more severe cases.

The treatment of the acquired deep overbite usually requires multiattachment fixed appliances for optimal correction, although treatment also can be improved with plates and pull-springs. The uprighting of tipped molars has a significant effect on the reduction of the overbite. Fixed appliances do this best.

The steep curve of Spee must be leveled for maximal correction of the deep overbite. This leveling can be performed during the eruption of the posterior teeth by eruption guidance with an activator that has been properly ground in the interocclusal area. Again, leveling in the permanent dentition requires fixed appliances with individual tooth control and intermaxillary elastic traction or vertical elastic stimulus of eruption.

## Treatment of Skeletal Deep Overbite

As pointed out initially in this chapter, the treatment of a skeletal deep overbite requires consideration of the sagittal dimension. Most skeletal deep overbites are combined with Class II sagittal intercuspation.

The treatment of a deep overbite combined with a Class II sagittal malrelationship can be handled with several therapeutic approaches. Growth inhibition of the upper jaw and growth promotion in the lower jaw combined with dentoalveolar changes should result in the improvement of a deep overbite. Treatment can be performed using a headgear in combination with an activator. Treatment may proceed as follows:

1. Distalization and elongation of the upper first permanent molars is the first step. The eruption of the teeth in the posterior segments can then be guided by a properly trimmed activator.
2. The unfavorable inclination of the jaw bases should be opened if at all possible in convergent growth rotation patterns. This can be achieved at least partly with an activator of special design or by the use of extraoral force.
3. Dentoalveolar compensation for a deep bite is needed, especially in skeletal deep overbite treated after the growth period is completed. This compensation can be achieved by extrusion and distalization of the maxillary molars, sometimes aided by second molar extraction. Intrusion and labial tipping of the lower incisors with leveling of the curve of Spee further benefit the dentoalveolar compensation.

## Early Treatment of Deep Overbite

Treatment started in the early mixed dentition has the possibility of influencing the skeletal characteristics of the deep overbite malocclusion. A case in point illustrates the potential.

A patient 6 years and 3 months old had a severe overbite with demonstrable gingival impingement (Figure 20-9). Evidence of constant traumatic irritation of the impinged gingival margin because of the deep bite was clear. The objective of early treatment was to relieve the gingival impingement and

support the overbite dentally. Treatment of this tissue-impingement type of deep bite is indicated later; however, without growth, orthognathic surgery may be the only mode of correction to prevent early loss of incisor teeth.

The growth direction in this patient was horizontal despite a short and retrognathic mandibular base. This retrognathism was accentuated by the posterior position of the temporal fossa (a large cranial base angle). The ramus was long, however, as was the maxillary base. Functional analysis indicated a large interocclusal clearance and lateral tongue thrust and posture symptoms. This malocclusion configuration is usually amenable to correction by functional appliances.

The objectives of treatment were as follows:

1. Distalization of the upper molars to reduce both the sagittal and vertical dysplasia, opening the bite as the teeth were moved posteriorly and extruded into the wedge was a primary goal. This task was to be performed with extraoral force.
2. Extrusion of the partially erupted buccal segment teeth as the second phase of orthodontic guidance was another important objective. An activator was fabricated and trimmed to stimulate extrusion of the posterior segments and exert an intrusive force on the anterior teeth to level the curve of Spee.
3. Elimination of the lateral tongue posture and thrust that created much of the problem by preventing full eruption of the posterior teeth also was a priority. This maneuver was controlled by a removable plate–type appliance incorporating lateral tongue cribs; the appliance was worn during the day. The labial bow of the plate incorporated buccal loop extensions similar to those used in the bionator to prevent the cheeks from interposing between the occlusal surfaces.

The period of treatment, including retention, continued beyond the eruption of the first premolars and lasted $4\frac{1}{2}$ years. An examination 2 years after retention showed an improvement of both the mandibular retrognathism and deep overbite. The molars had been extruded, whereas the incisors were intruded (Figure 20-10). The relationship between the eruption height of the incisors was thus altered favorably. According to Schwarz, the relationship in a normal case should be a ratio of 5:4 for the incisor to molar height (Figure 20-11). In this case, before treatment the molar infraocclusion resulted in a ratio of 5:3.7 in the upper dental arch and 5:3.8 in the lower dental arch. Therapeutic correction changed this ratio to 5:4.4 in the upper jaw and 5:4.1 in the lower jaw.

## Early Treatment of Class II, Division 2 Malocclusion

A Class II, division 2 problem in an 8-year-old boy is used to illustrate the possibilities for early treatment. The initial habitual occlusion relationship involved a deep, gingivally impinging overbite (Figure 20-12). Despite this deep bite the interocclusal clearance was not overly large, and a normal path of closure from rest to occlusion was evident. The growth projection was markedly horizontal, but the mandibular base was

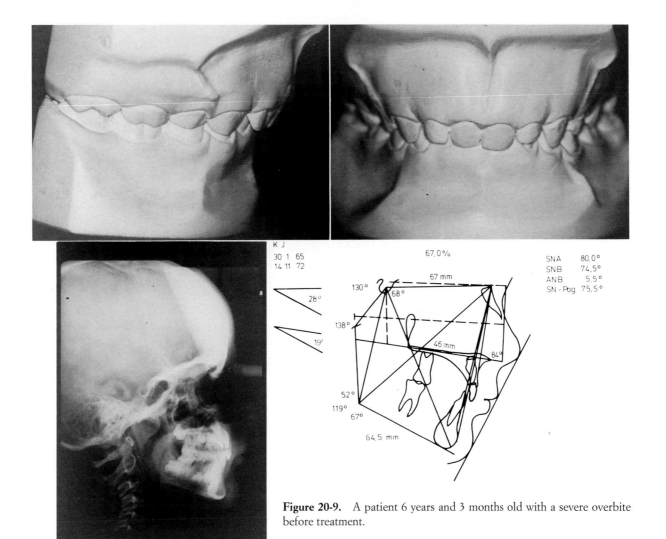

**Figure 20-9.** A patient 6 years and 3 months old with a severe overbite before treatment.

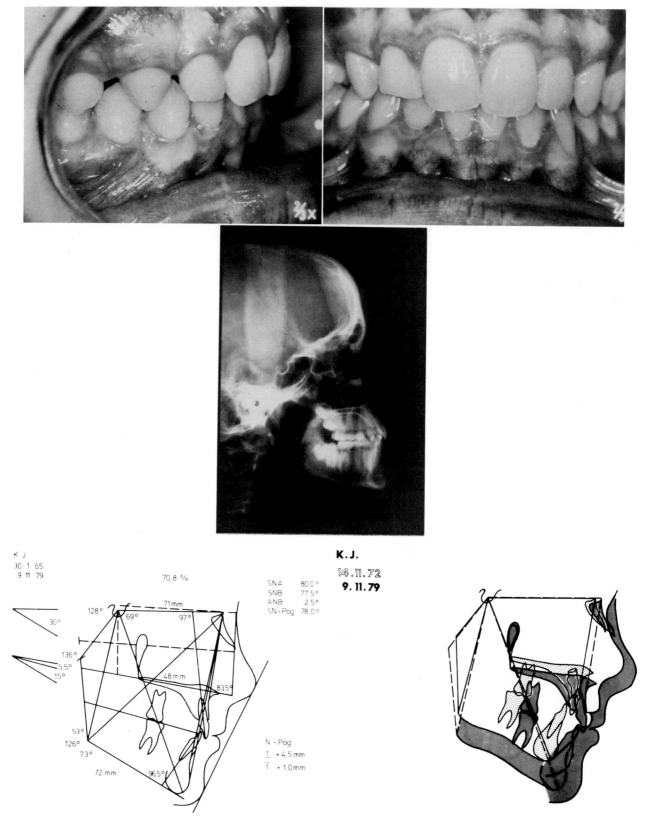

**Figure 20-10.**   The same patient as in Figure 20-9 after treatment. *Bottom right,* Superimposition of before and after tracings.

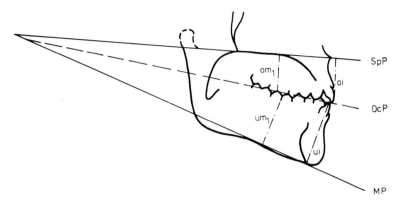

**Figure 20-11.** Measurement of anterior and posterior alveolar heights. *oi,* Upper incisor; *om,* upper molar; *ui,* lower incisor; *um,* lower molar. *SpP,* palatal plane; *OcP,* occlusal plane; *MP,* mandibular plane.

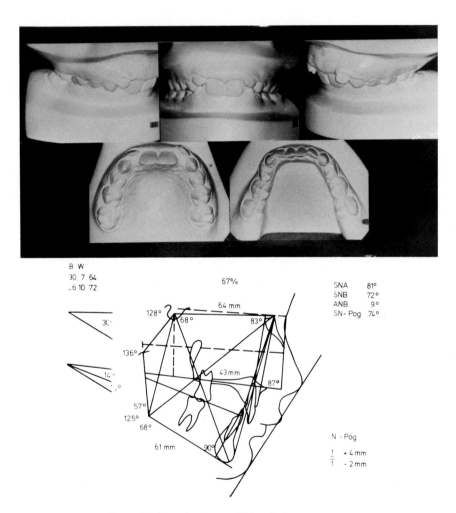

**Figure 20-12.** An 8-year-old boy before treatment.

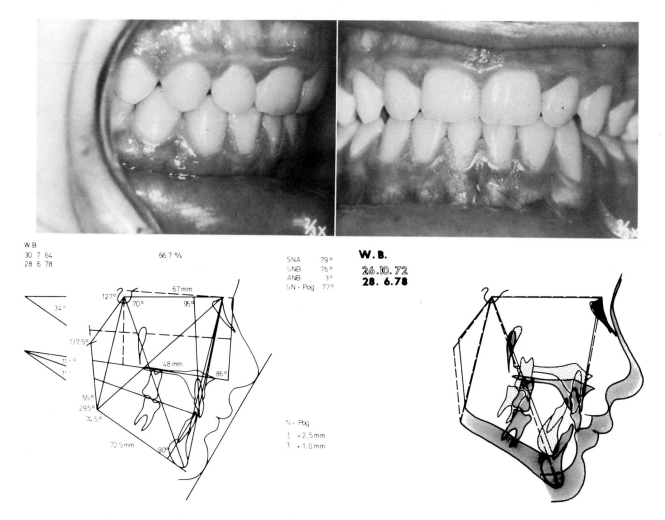

**Figure 20-13.**   The same patient as in Figure 20-12 after treatment. *Bottom right,* Superimposition of before and after tracings.

short and retrognathic, whereas the ramus height and maxillary base were both of average size. The maxillary central incisors were lingually tipped, and the lateral incisors were labially tipped. The upper molars had migrated mesially. The first priority in treatment was to distalize the upper molars using extraoral force. In the second phase of treatment, an activator was placed to fulfill the following treatment objectives:

1. Anterior posturing of the mandible
2. Intrusion of the incisors and extrusion of the buccal segments
3. Protrusion of the upper central incisors

The reciprocal force from the last adjustment was transmitted through acrylic stabilizing projections at the mesial embrasure of the upper first molars, enhancing the distalization of these teeth. The alignment of the maxillary incisors in these cases is often achieved in the initial stage through the use of extraoral force, particularly if a functional retrusion is present. Alignment requires only a short period of direct-bonded attachments on these teeth. Double buccal tubes on the upper first molars permit the use of light wires for tooth alignment and

the reception of the inner bow of the headgear face-bow at the same time.

By 5 years later, when the patient was out of retention, the deep overbite and Class II relationship had been improved. A change in the inclination of the maxillary base, tipping the anterior end up or withholding it as the posterior end continued to descend and opening the Y axis, all were important maneuvers to increase the chances of stability. The change in the dentoalveolar region was not as extensive as it was in the previous case (Figure 20-13). The incisor to molar height ratio was improved in the upper arch from 5:3 to 5:3.6 and in the lower arch from 5:3.8 to 5:3.9. The relatively normal overbite at the end of treatment was caused by skeletal alteration during the growth period.

Most deep overbite malocclusions are combined with Class II relationships and horizontal growth patterns. The treatment of these malocclusions has already been described in Chapter 19. In adults, combined therapy is usually needed, with strong reliance on extraoral traction and possible removal of maxillary second molars. The treatment challenge is beyond the capabilities of functional appliances alone.

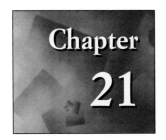

# Chapter 21

# Treatment of Class III Malocclusions

Thomas Rakosi

The factors creating and influencing true Class III malocclusions are quite different from those seen in Class II relationships. Although both types of malocclusions may be morphogenetically determined, most Class III problems have strong hereditary components. This fact implies that the endogenous developmental pattern is dysplastic and becomes increasingly so from infancy to maturity. Functional influences play only secondary or adaptive roles in the etiology of Class III malocclusion.

The differentiation of the various types of Class III malocclusion is important; some types can be successfully treated in the early stages with functional appliances, whereas other Class III skeletal relationships can be corrected only by orthognathic surgical procedures. The limitation of activator therapy is reached much sooner in Class III cases than it is in mandibular retrognathism patients.

## ETIOLOGIC CONSIDERATIONS

As indicated previously, environmental factors are less important in the genesis of the Class III malocclusion. Regardless of functional activity, the progressive severity of the maxillomandibular malrelationships can usually be observed. This dysplasia is thus linked to age. In a study by Rakosi (1966a) (Figure 21-1), mandibular length was correlated with the nasion-sella distance on lateral cephalograms in patients between the ages of 6 and 19 years. In patients younger than 7½ years, the mandibular base length was relatively short. Many practitioners have noted that after this age the base length became progressively longer in relation to the average values. This curve expresses the genetically linked development of the Class III relationship.

Functional factors and soft tissue also can influence these inexorable malocclusion patterns. A flat, anteriorly positioned tongue that lies low in the mouth is considered by van Limbourg and others to be a local epigenetic factor in Class III malocclusion. This factor should be eliminated during therapy, if possible. Whether tongue posture is a compensatory, adaptive phenomenon or a primary etiologic factor, inherited in a similar mode as are bone size and shape, is controversial. Some patients have compulsive habits of pro-

truding the mandible, which seems to support the development of mandibular prognathism. This phenomenon has been observed with some types of mental disease. As has been pointed out by Moyers and others, enlarged tonsils and nasorespiratory difficulties also may result in anterior tongue posturing, with the tongue dropping down and flattening as this strong reflex action maintains a patent airway. Linder-Aronson has alluded to the compensatory tongue position change with excessive epipharyngeal lymphoid tissue and autonomous improvement observed over a 5-year period after the removal of the occluding mass. Other researchers have made similar findings.

Occlusal forces created by abnormal eruption also may produce unfavorable incisal guidance and promote Class III relationships. The anterior displacement of the mandible by incisal guidance produces what is called a functional or pseudo–Class III malocclusion. If this result is left unattended, in many cases it can become a functionally and skeletally true Class III malocclusion in the later dentofacial developmental stages (Figure 21-2). Premature loss of deciduous molars also may cause mandibular displacements with occlusal guidance from maloccluded teeth or lingualized maxillary incisor teeth. If the mandible loses its posterior proprioceptive and functional support in habitual occlusion, it may be extended anteriorly in an attempt to establish full occlusal contact during chewing. Such neuromuscular compensation can result in a permanent prognathic mandibular position and subsequent eruption of teeth into positions that support this malrelationship (i.e., labially tipped lower incisors, lingually tipped maxillary incisors, interference with the full eruption of the maxillary teeth). Indeed, lack of eruption of maxillary buccal segments, a phenomenon sometimes caused by tongue thrusting or postural activity, permits the mandible to close through an excessive interocclusal space, autorotating into a Class III malocclusion because of abnormal vertical development. In open-bite problems this autorotational maneuver is sometimes created to close the bite by removing teeth, letting the mandible close further and reducing a Class II tendency. Overclosure can thus accentuate a Class III malocclusion even as it can enhance a Class II problem under tooth guidance. Maxillary vertical height is usually deficient in Class III cases.

461

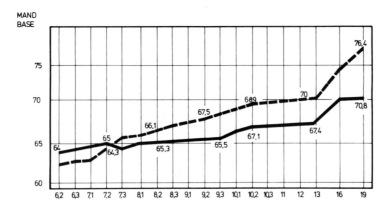

**Figure 21-1.** Increments of mandibular base length between 6 and 19 years in patients with Class III malocclusions. Broken line denotes average length.

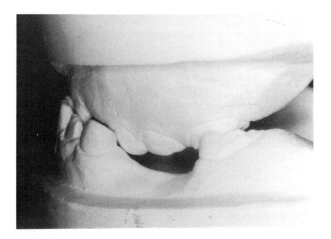

**Figure 21-2.** Anterior crossbite that arose after loss of deciduous teeth.

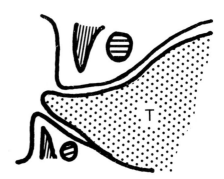

**Figure 21-3.** Persistence of embryonic prognathism in the neonatal period, associated with the suckle-swallow function. *T,* Tongue.

## FREQUENCY OF CLASS III MALOCCLUSIONS

The frequency of Class III malocclusions is only 1% to 3%, a figure quite low compared with that of Class II problems. This figure depends on ethnic and geographic factors and age. The midface deficiency so often seen in Asian societies results in a high percentage of Class III malocclusion problems. Scandinavian percentages for Class III problems are higher than those of the Italian populace. A lesser incidence of Class III malocclusion (and more bimaxillary protrusion) is seen among African-Americans. Occasionally in isolated geographic areas in which inbreeding exists, the frequency can rise significantly. One age-dependent Class III relationship, for example, is neonatal mandibular protrusion. This embryonic condition occurs during the second month and usually disappears after the fifth month. In isolated cases, however, especially in premature infants, it can persist (Figure 21-3).

An age-conditioned growth characteristic is the great mandibular growth spurt between 2 and 6 years, when the mandible literally emerges from its seemingly retruded position at birth. Some observers attribute this early growth spurt to the suckling or nursing posture in which the mandible is thrust forward constantly to grasp the nipple. This infantile suckle-swallow pattern usually disappears by 2 years.

Most Class III malocclusions become apparent during or after the eruption of the deciduous teeth. Before 6 years an increase in the frequency of the Class III malocclusion may be seen, especially in dentitions abraded by nocturnal bruxing associated with anterior positioning of the mandible. Because the malocclusion is progressive, it should be treated early. One study of 2000 preschool children done in Germany (Rakosi, 1970b) reports that the Class III malocclusion accounts for 18% of all malocclusions seen before the exfoliation of the deciduous teeth. This number decreases to 3% during the first phase of the mixed dentition period. Of these cases, one third result in the development of severe dysplasia and are treated in conjunction with surgery (orthognathic procedures) or by surgery alone.

## MORPHOLOGIC AND FUNCTIONAL CONSEQUENCES

The sequelae associated with this malrelationship are varied:

1. Incorrect loading of the teeth
2. Disturbances in the functional equilibrium
3. Impairment of chewing and speech functions
4. Difficulty of prosthetic restoration
5. Cosmetic and occasional psychologic considerations

These manifestations may occur singly but are usually associated with varying degrees of severity, depending on dentofacial and behavioral compensation.

### Initial Symptoms of Class III Malocclusion

Early signs of true, progressive mandibular prognathism occasionally can occur in infancy. A protruded mandible with an anteriorly positioned tongue can be seen only in cases of very severe dysplasia before the eruption of the incisors. In the first months of life a sequential development of the Class III condition may be observed. This step-by-step progression is described as follows (Figure 21-4):

1. Eruption of the maxillary central incisors in a lingual relationship and the mandibular incisors in a forward position with no overjet
2. Development of an incisal crossbite during the eruption of the lateral incisors into a normal relationship
3. Full incisor crossbite some weeks later
4. Flattening of the tongue as it drops away from palatal contact and postures forward, pressing against the lower incisors
5. Habitual protraction of the mandible by the child into the protruded functional and morphologic relationship

About 10% of all Class III cases originate during infancy. This mode of development is of interest for several reasons. The etiology of the malocclusion determines or should assist in outlining the corrective treatment procedures. The skeletal growth pattern and growth centers of the maxilla and mandible are not the only factors in treatment decisions. The functional environment also is quite important. As indicated previously, most Class III malocclusions become apparent during or after eruption of the deciduous teeth or during eruption of the permanent incisors.

In evaluating the Class III relationship during the deciduous dentition period, the clinician must consider whether the problem will progress or correct itself. The possibility of therapy at this time must be weighed carefully for certain cases. To make a proper determination, the clinician must undertake a careful analysis of all possible signs for future development. In the deciduous dentition these include such symptoms as a scissors bite with facets of wear on specific teeth, spaces between the teeth, tooth buds in the mandible, and underdevelopment of the maxilla. In the mixed dentition, other possible signs may be evident (e.g., crossbite of individual teeth, minimal overjet, lower incisors lingually inclined to reach back to

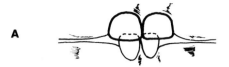

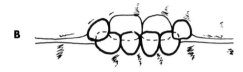

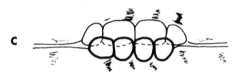

**Figure 21-4.** Development of a Class III relationship during eruption of the deciduous incisors. **A,** Eruption of the centrals. **B,** Incisal crossbite of the centrals. **C,** Crossbite of all incisors.

achieve a normal overjet, selected skeletal symptoms apparent from cephalometric examination; see Chapter 6).

## DIAGNOSTIC CONSIDERATIONS

As with any type of dentofacial abnormality, the diagnostic assessment of a Class III malocclusion should be thorough and complete. Diagnostic procedure comprises clinical examination, functional analysis, radiographic examination, cephalometric analysis, study model analysis, and soft tissue examination. Because these procedures are discussed in detail in other chapters, only the most salient factors for treatment planning for Class III malocclusions are discussed here.

### Clinical Examination

The clinical examination comprises the usual general medical and dental background details, anamnestic information that might demonstrate a predisposition to malocclusion, and specific dentofacial details associated with particular problems. Blood dyscrasias jeopardize future surgery and should be noted. Juvenile diabetes and other diseases increase surgical preparation time and also the general risk if surgery is indicated.

**The general examination.** The general examination comprises the following procedures:

1. An assessment of general physical attributes
2. Height and weight comparisons with normal standards
3. Visual and digital examination of the morphology of the face and head
4. Evaluation of the biologic age of the patient
5. Projection of the growth potential

As noted previously, the shape of the face and skull can be of value in predicting future dysplastic relationships (Figure 21-5). The skull can be dolichocephalic, brachycephalic, or mesocephalic. The face can be leptoprosopic,

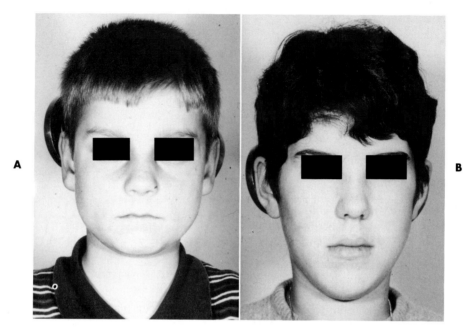

**Figure 21-5.** The shape of the face should be considered before the introduction of expansion treatment. **A,** Mesoprosopic face. **B,** Leptoprosopic face.

### TABLE 21-1. • ASSESSMENT OF THE DENTAL AGE

| Erupting Tooth | Dental Age* | | | | | | | |
|---|---|---|---|---|---|---|---|---|
| Canine | | | | | | | | |
| Boys | 10:08 | 11:06 | 12:02 | 12:06 | 10:00 | 10:07 | 11:02 | 11:10 |
| Girls | 9:10 | 10:02 | 11:03 | 11:08 | 9:02 | 9:10 | 10:05 | 11:02 |
| Central incisor | | | | | | | | |
| Boys | 6:08 | 6:10 | 7:00 | 7:11 | † | † | 6:08 | 7:04 |
| Girls | 6:06 | 6:10 | 7:04 | 7:08 | † | † | † | 7:01 |
| Lateral incisor | | | | | | | | |
| Boys | 7:04 | 8:04 | 8:10 | 9:00 | 6:11 | 7:03 | 7:11 | 8:06 |
| Girls | 7:05 | 7:08 | 8:06 | 8:07 | 6:07 | 7:00 | 7:05 | 8:00 |
| First molar | | | | | | | | |
| Boys | 6:00 | 6:04 | 6:08 | 6:10 | † | † | † | † |
| Girls | 6:03 | 6:03 | 6:08 | 6:10 | † | † | † | † |
| Second molar | | | | | | | | |
| Boys | 12:09 | 12:10 | 13:06 | 14:00 | 10:09 | 11:02 | 11:09 | 12:05 |
| Girls | 11:11 | 11:11 | 12:10 | 13:05 | 10:05 | 10:10 | 11:04 | 12:00 |
| First premolar | | | | | | | | |
| Boys | 10:05 | 10:08 | 11:10 | 12:00 | 9:01 | 9:08 | 10:04 | 11:01 |
| Girls | 9:02 | 10:02 | 10:05 | 11:03 | 8:11 | 9:04 | 9:11 | 10:05 |
| Second premolar | | | | | | | | |
| Boys | 10:10 | 11:11 | 12:05 | 13:00 | 10:01 | 10:07 | 11:02 | 11:10 |
| Girls | 10:05 | 11:01 | 11:05 | 12:02 | 9:10 | 10:02 | 10:09 | 11:03 |

*Age is provided in years:months.

†Eruption took place earlier than could be determined clinically.

euryprosopic, or mesoprosopic. The dolichocephalic and leptoprosopic configurations are accompanied by long face syndromes and have dominant vertical growth patterns. Tooth extraction is likely to be more frequently indicated in these cases, and rapid palatal expansion is more likely to be feasible. In the brachycephalic and euryprosopic combination, a short face with a more horizontal vector of growth is evident. Expansion treatment is possible, but extractions are seldom indicated.

To evaluate the age and growth potential, the clinician must consider not only chronologic but also biologic age, which depends on skeletal maturation, morphologic evaluation, and an estimate of the likely onset of puberty. The prepubertal and pubertal growth peaks must be considered. The adolescent growth potential often causes difficulties for reten-

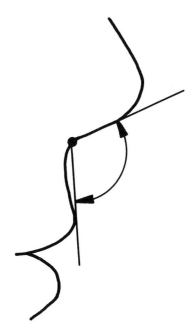

**Figure 21-6.** The nasolabial angle.

tion procedures in corrected Class III malocclusions. Assessment of biologic age helps determine whether the major increments of growth have been accomplished or still lie ahead. If the developmental age of the patient is younger than the chronologic age, higher growth rates lie ahead and surgery should be postponed. Retention is easier in a developmentally mature patient after treatment; surgery, if necessary, can be performed earlier. Hand and wrist x-ray films may provide information on relative maturity and whether growth has ceased or will continue in significant amounts.

The dental age of the patient should be determined. The growth rate varies depending on the number of erupted teeth. If the teeth are still erupting, a greater growth rate can be expected, and greater potential treatment changes are possible than if the developmental age is precocious with regard to chronologic age (Table 21-1). Cephalometric examination also can help in forecasting the growth potential. Thus the clinical growth projection is based on the relation between chronologic, developmental, and dental ages and on the parental and sibling history. If growth acceleration or retardation is evident in the genetic pattern, the likelihood of it being repeated in the patient is considerable.

**The clinical examination.** The clinical examination is the same as it is for other malocclusions, with assessment of the craniofacial and oral soft tissues and dentition being performed.

The configuration and form of the forehead and nose in relation to the lower face are significant for esthetic evaluation and prognosis. A well-formed nasolabial angle is important for esthetic improvement. If the angle is acute, the premaxillary segment can be retracted; if the angle is obtuse, the segment must be protracted to improve facial esthetics (Figure 21-6). The soft tissue of the chin can compensate for or accentuate a skeletal Class III relationship, depending on its thickness. Gingival retraction or dehiscence can often be seen in an early Class III malocclusion. This damage is irreversible and is an indication for early treatment (Figure 21-7).

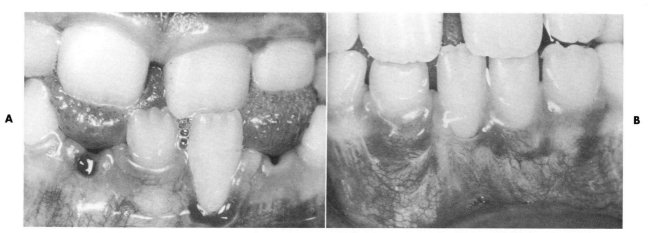

**Figure 21-7.** **A,** Gingival damage after eruption of the central incisors in a crossbite relationship. **B,** Even after the relationship is corrected, the gingival retraction remains irreversible, requiring a surgical flap.

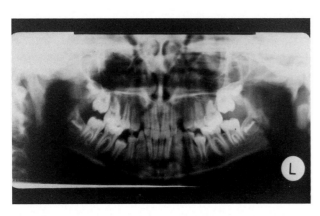

**Figure 21-8.** Anodontia of the upper canines makes the treatment of a Class III relationship more difficult.

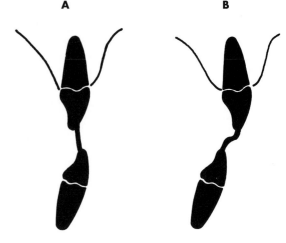

**Figure 21-10.** Functional relationships in Class III malocclusion. **A,** True malocclusion. **B,** Forced bite.

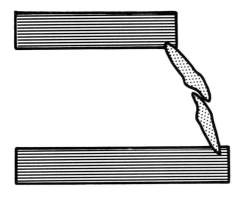

**Figure 21-9.** Labial tipping of the upper incisors and lingual tipping of the lower incisors indicate dental compensation in a Class III skeletal relationship. Orthodontic treatment of this condition is difficult because the condition cannot be corrected with removable appliances.

The next step is examination of the dentition, including the morphology and number of teeth. Congenital absence in the maxilla (e.g., missing canine or first premolar teeth) makes treatment more difficult (Figure 21-8). When evaluating the axial inclination of the teeth, the clinician should note certain disadvantageous irregularities such as labial tipping of the upper incisors and lingual tipping of the lower incisors still in anterior crossbite. A concavity of the lingual alveolar structure in the mandible also is a clue to future difficulties in the correction of Class III malocclusion (Figure 21-9). Crowding of maxillary teeth also enhances treatment problems; treatment may require extraction of the counterpart teeth in the lower arch, leading to great difficulty in closing spaces and maintaining proper incisor axial inclination. To make treatment easier if extractions are required, the clinician should perform extractions in the mandible before proceeding to those in the maxilla. Depending on the state of development, enucleation or germectomy may be feasible for the lower first premolars. The molar occlusal relationship is usually Class III, but the plane of occlusion also should be evaluated because its correction may be necessary before surgery.

## Functional Analysis

Functional analysis is obviously an important part of the assessment. The path of closure from the postural rest position to occlusion must be carefully studied. The mandible may slide anteriorly into a forced protrusion because of premature contact and tooth guidance when the jaw closes into full occlusion. Such anterior displacements have more favorable prognoses. In contrast, patients with problems caused by an anterior rest position with respect to habitual occlusion are difficult to treat and usually require orthognathic surgical teamwork for correction (Figure 21-10).

In addition to true Class III poor prognosis cases and functional Class III good prognosis cases, a pseudo–forced bite category also exists. This is a skeletal Class III malocclusion with a dental compensation arising from labial tipping of the upper incisors on a deficient maxillary base and lingual tipping of the lower incisors on an excessively long mandible. Orthodontic presurgical treatment must decompensate these malpositions before surgical procedures can be performed. Preorthodontic and postorthodontic treatment assistance is almost always necessary. Attainment of the achievable optimal result often requires surgical adjustment of the apical bases.

**Temporomandibular joint assessment.** Examination of the temporomandibular joint (TMJ) also is important. Some Class III characteristics predispose patients to future TMJ problems (e.g., premature contacts, traumatic occlusion, mandibular functional displacement [particularly asymmetric opening], tongue malfunctions). If the condyle occupies the most posterior position in the temporal fossa, the likelihood of its riding over the posterior periphery of the articular disk is increased, with concomitant clicking and later crepitus. Impingement on the retrodiscal pad may produce undesirable objective symptoms. However, predicting future TMJ problems in asymptomatic Class III patients is difficult because of the variable circumstances. Their age distributions may be the same as are those for other TMJ patients, but Class III patients have usually undergone years of orthodontic-orthopedic treatment, and the surgical treatment does not always produce correct bilateral condylar function. These are predisposing causes, but patients with TMJ problems often seem better able psychologically to adjust to their chewing problems because of their long history of functional difficulties.

Abnormal tongue function, size, shape, and posture must be considered at all ages. Whether an abnormality is a primary etiologic factor or a compensatory secondary characteristic is controversial and often hard to ascertain. It may be a combination of both. The tongue may be postured low in the mouth and be flat and elongated, especially in cases of mouth breathing. In cases of macroglossia the tongue is not contained within the dentition, and the scalloping effect of tooth contact may be visible on the periphery.

**Radiographic assessment.** In addition to the clinical examination of tongue size, a cephalometric evaluation is important. The tongue position can be examined palatographically both before and after treatment to determine the effectiveness of therapeutic measures. The differentiation of tongue position problems is extremely important. These problems often involve tongue shape. If the tongue is too big, it can influence the dental arch, resulting in both tooth impressions on the tongue and spacing in the dental arches. Active tongue thrusting may be noted during swallowing and should be checked. Such activity may be associated with the so-called infantile or visceral swallow. This type of swallow is frequently a retained infantile pattern that has not matured, but it also can be a compensatory activity.

**Lip function and morphology assessment.** Finally, lip size, posture, and function should be assessed. A short, hypotonic upper lip is often seen in combination with a heavy, redundant, everted lower lip. Correction of the skeletal and dental aspects of the malocclusion is not guaranteed to correct soft tissue abnormality.

## Cephalometric Examination

The goal of the cephalometric examination is the same as is that for any skeletal malocclusion: to evaluate the facial type, relationship of the jaw bases, growth pattern, dentoalveolar relationship, localization of the malocclusion, soft tissues and their relationships to etiologic and prognostic considerations, functional relationships, and scope of therapeutic possibilities.

The facial type is completely different in the patient with a Class III malocclusion compared with that seen in a patient with a Class I or II problem. In a study by Rakosi (1982b), Class II and III malocclusions were compared (Figure 21-11). In Class III cases the prognathic pattern began in the cranial base area. Localization of the Class III malocclusion in one craniofacial area was not possible. The sella angle and articular angle were smaller in Class III problems, moving the

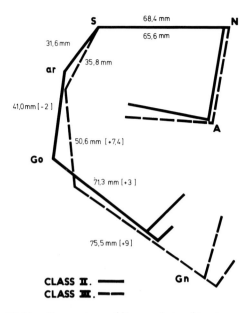

**Figure 21-11.**  Comparison of linear relationships in a group of 50 patients with Class II and III malocclusions.

mandible anteriorly in relation to the cranial base. The gonial angle was not large in all Class III malocclusions. The study also showed that the mandibular bases in both classes of malocclusion were larger than normal—3 mm in the Class II group and 9 mm in the Class III sample. Coupled with the anterior positioning of the mandible, this extra length created the sagittal discrepancy. Soft tissue changes also differed. These changes were amenable to significant change after orthognathic surgical intervention, both clinically and cephalometrically. A small alteration in soft tissue proportions is able to change the whole facial image impression of observers. In patients in whom orthognathic surgery has been performed on the ascending ramus to correct prognathism, the face appears larger. Measurements, however, show that the face is not larger after Class III surgery; only the facial length is shortened. This shortening averages only 2% and occurs mostly in the lower third of the face. If the osteotomy is performed in the mental region, the distance between subnasion and the oral commissure appears larger. This may be because of the lengthening of the lip after the upward rotation of the mandible. If the orthognathic surgery involves setting the maxilla forward, the visual impression is again different, depending on any procedure performed on the mandible. The clinician should study carefully these potential changes in profile before choosing a particular surgical technique.

## Cephalometric Classification of the Class III Malocclusion

The scope and possibilities of treatment depend on the localization of the malocclusion and characteristics in the skeletal and dentoalveolar areas. The following distinctions can be used in categorizing the Class III sagittal relationship:

1. Class III malocclusion caused by a dentoalveolar malrelationship

2. Class III malocclusion with a long mandibular base
3. Class III malocclusion with an underdeveloped maxilla
4. Class III skeletal malocclusion with a combination of an underdeveloped maxilla and a prominent mandible; horizontal or vertical growth pattern
5. Class III skeletal malocclusion with tooth guidance, or pseudo–forced bite

**Class III malocclusion caused by a dentoalveolar malrelationship.** In the dentoalveolar Class III malocclusion (Figure 21-12), no basal sagittal discrepancy is apparent. The subspinale-nasion-supramentale (A-N-B) angle is within normal limits. The problem is primarily concentrated in the incisal relationship, with the maxillary incisors tipped lingually and the mandibular incisors tipped labially.

All that is usually needed to treat these patients is correction of the incisal malrelationship. This is a simple procedure that may be performed at any age. Most Class III malocclusions are in this category in their initial stages. However, during the eruption of the permanent teeth, the problem can become more severe. Some observers feel that prolongation of this malrelationship can exacerbate the sagittal discrepancy with an activator-like functional effect that enhances the mandibular prognathism and may retard the maxillary horizontal development. This result would be more likely in the anterior crossbite or forced bite categories, however. Hence treatment should be instituted early, establishing a normal functional engram and stimulus in the developing face.

If a dentoalveolar Class III malocclusion is encountered in the adult, it can still be successfully corrected with orthodontic procedures alone if the symptoms are purely local. Prediction at an early age of which cases will maintain the primarily dentoalveolar discrepancy and which will become more progressive, involving the basal structures is not easy. Hereditary pattern is a strong clue, however. Early detection is sometimes possible by looking at the lateral cephalogram. In some cases a long mandibular base with spaces between the developing unerupted teeth can be a clue to future prognathism. The

maxilla is a crucial area in these cases. If it adapts to the strong mandibular growth, the relationship can remain harmonious; if not, the facial skeleton shows an apparent mandibular overgrowth. Not all Class III malocclusions are the fault of the mandible. Particularly in some Asian patients, manifest midface underdevelopment is a major factor.

**Class III malocclusion with a long mandibular base.** As Figure 21-13 shows, both the mandibular base and ascending ramus are large. The sella-nasion-subspinale (S-N-A) angle is normal, but the sella-nasion-supramentale (S-N-B) angle is larger than normal, creating a negative A-N-B difference. The gonial angle is usually large, and the articular angle is usually small, but this is not always so. The mandible is not only longer but also usually anteriorly positioned. The tongue's morphology is flattened, whereas the tongue is postured forward and lies lower in the mouth. Often a cupping out of the lingual alveolar bony support below the lower premolars is seen in association with this postural adaptation.

The axial inclination of this type of Class III malocclusion is the opposite of that seen in the dentoalveolar Class III problem. The upper incisors are tipped labially, and the lower incisors are inclined lingually. This kind of relationship is an indication of a partial dentoalveolar compensation and limits the therapeutic possibilities. In these cases a lateral crossbite often is evident, and the maxillary arch appears to be narrowed. Actually, part of the problem is that a wider part of the mandibular dental arch is moved anteriorly to relate with a narrower maxillary width dimension. Many malocclusions in this group can be treated only in the early mixed dentition period. Orthognathic surgery combination treatment is the best answer for severe dysplasias or for treating older patients. This type of malocclusion can be designated as one caused by fault within in the mandible.

**Class III malocclusion with an underdeveloped maxilla.** In some Class III malocclusions the maxillary base is small and retrognathic (Figure 21-14). A smaller than normal S-N-A angle is combined with a normal S-N-B angle. Patients with

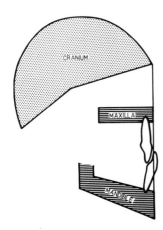

**Figure 21-12.** Class III dentoalveolar malocclusion. The bases are normally related.

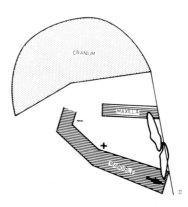

**Figure 21-13.** Class III skeletal relationship with a large mandibular base.

cleft palates are good examples of this category, as are certain Asian groups with midface deficiencies. Early treatment can be successfully performed by growth guidance during the eruption of the maxillary incisors in cases with favorable initial lingual inclination of the upper incisors, which permits their labial tipping. Actual growth stimulation or a change in maxillary growth direction in the middle face can be accomplished by extraoral orthopedic protraction procedures using appliances such as the Delaire mask (Figure 21-15).

**Class III malocclusion with a combined underdeveloped maxilla and a prominent mandible.** In the retrognathic maxilla–prognathic mandible combination, the S-N-A angle is small and the maxillary base is short (Figure 21-16). The

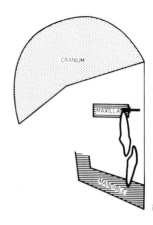

**Figure 21-14.** Class III skeletal relationship with an underdeveloped maxilla.

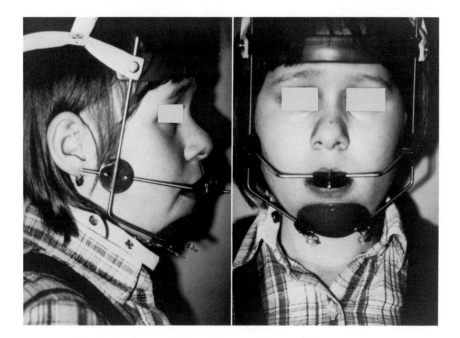

**Figure 21-15.** Modified Delaire mask for maxillary protraction.

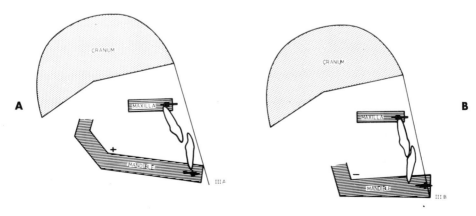

**Figure 21-16.** Class III skeletal relationship with an underdeveloped maxilla and a prominent mandible. **A,** Vertical growth pattern. **B,** Horizontal growth pattern.

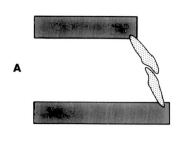

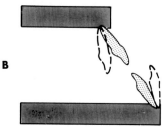

**Figure 21-17.** Class III skeletal relationship with a pseudo–forced bite. **A,** Compensation of a Class III relationship. **B,** Uprighting of the incisors.

S-N-B angle is large, and the mandibular base is long. The ramus can be short or long. Depending on the ramal length, the two variations in this category may be differentiated.

In a patient with a short ramus, the growth pattern is vertical and the gonial angle is large. A Class III sagittal relationship often is combined with an open bite. Sometimes crowding also occurs in the upper arch that may require extraction during correction. Treatment is possible in the more moderate cases, usually only with four first premolar extractions and fixed multiattachment appliances. If the problem is severe, orthognathic surgery is the only answer.

In a patient with a long ramus, the growth pattern is horizontal, the gonial angle is small, and a reversed overbite is apparent. In early treatment, correction of the overbite and control of mandibular development is possible in many cases by the use of occlusal force. However, the maxilla also may become prognathic if treatment is performed during the eruption of the incisors. In other cases the overbite may remain stable, but the mandible becomes more prognathic. Prediction is more difficult in these problems.

**Class III skeletal malocclusion with a pseudo–forced bite or anterior displacement.** Pseudo–forced bite or anterior malocclusions (Figure 21-17) have already been discussed in Chapter 7. The condition known as Class III skeletal dysplasia is partially compensated by the labial tipping of the upper incisors and lingual inclination of the lower incisors. This tooth malposition results in additional anterior guidance of the mandible on the path from postural rest to habitual occlusion as the lingual aspect of the lower incisors rides on the maxillary incisor margins after initial contact. Although the full occlusal relationship gives the appearance that the mandible is even further forward than it is, this type of case is very difficult to treat orthodontically because of the unfavorable axial inclination of both upper and lower incisors and the

true sagittal basal malrelationship. In these cases, therapy consists mostly of uprighting the incisors and then instituting an orthognathic surgical regimen to correct the anteroposterior basal jaw relationship.

## TREATMENT PLANNING FOR CLASS III MALOCCLUSIONS

The therapeutic possibilities depend on the developmental age of the patient and the nature of the malocclusion. For example, dentoalveolar Class III malocclusions and forced bite, anterior displacement cases without skeletal involvement may be treated at any time. The treatment objectives include uprighting labially tipped lower incisors and lingually inclined upper incisors. Expansion also is sometimes necessary in the upper arch. This kind of treatment can be performed easily with active plates (with jackscrews and fingersprings), inclined planes, and activators, without multiattachment fixed appliances in the mixed or permanent dentition. For example, Figure 21-18 shows a 31-year-old patient who had an incisor crossbite corrected with an inclined plane before prosthetic rehabilitation. The malocclusion was dentoalveolar.

Skeletal Class III malocclusions may be divided into three groups with regard to therapy:

1. The malocclusion fault is in the mandible, and the mandible is prominent, with a long body. Treatment is concentrated primarily on the mandibular base. A posterior repositioning of the mandible is possible during the growth period with functional or extraoral orthopedic procedures. However, growth can only be effectively inhibited or redirected in cases treated during the deciduous dentition or early mixed dentition.
2. The malocclusion fault is in the maxilla, and the maxillary base is retrognathic and short. Stimulation of maxillary development is possible. Treatment is more effective, particularly during the eruption of the upper incisors. As with the mandible, maxillary growth can be redirected only during the growth period.
3. The malocclusion fault is in both the maxilla and mandible; this type of dysplasia requires a combined approach, often leading to ultimate orthognathic surgical correction.

Investigations show that the actual difference in jaw base length in maxillary retrusion and mandibular retraction is not as significant in the permanent dentition as it is in the deciduous or mixed dentition. If the mandible is at fault, a maxilla of normal size can be retarded in its further development, whereas in a malocclusion in which the fault lies in the maxilla, an average size mandible can become large with increasing age (Table 21-2).

The length of the maxillary base can be increased with treatment; the younger the patient, the more significant is the potential for correction. Clinical research demonstrates that the length of the upper jaw base can be influenced with treatment until 10 years. In older age groups the maxillary base no longer shows any change during treatment (Figure 21-19).

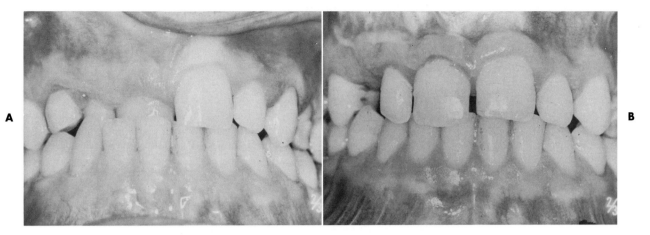

**Figure 21-18.** A 31-year-old patient with forced bite of the incisors. **A,** Before treatment. **B,** After treatment.

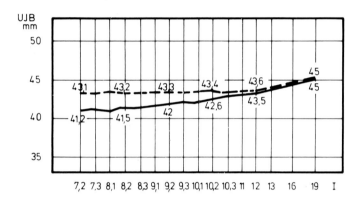

— UJB - LENGTH BEFORE TREATMENT
-- UJB - LENGTH AFTER TREATMENT

**Figure 21-19.** Increments of maxillary base length between 6 and 19 years in patients with Class III malocclusions. Broken line denotes average length.

**TABLE 21-2. • EXTENT OF THE MANDIBULAR BASE, MAXILLARY BASE, AND ASCENDING RAMUS IN CASES OF MANDIBULAR PROGNATHISM**

| Dentition | Mean Duration of Treatment in Months | Extent of Mandible in mm | | | Ascending Ramus in mm | | Extent of Maxilla in mm | |
| --- | --- | --- | --- | --- | --- | --- | --- | --- |
| | | Ideal | Found Before Treatment* | Found After Treatment† | Found Before Treatment* | Found After Treatment† | Found Before Treatment* | Found After Treatment† |
| Primary dentition | | | | | | | | |
|   Fault in mandible | 7.0 | 61.6±1.1 | +2.0±1.0 | +0.9±1.8 | 0 ±2.3 | +2.6 | +0.2±1.0 | +0.5 |
|   Fault in maxilla | 18.0 | 65.7±1.9 | −4.2±2.4 | +1.5±1.2 | −2.7±1.3 | +2.0 | −5.0±1.0 | +4.21±1.2 |
| TOTAL | 13.0 | 64.0±1.7 | −1.4±2.1 | −0.9±2.0 | −1.5±1.8 | +2.2 | −2.8±1.2 | +2.8±1.4 |
| Mixed dentition | | | | | | | | |
|   Fault in mandible | 6.2 | 64.0±2.2 | +4.9±2.3 | +0.6±1.0 | −0.4±1.5 | +1.4 | −0.3±1.4 | +0.7 |
|   Fault in maxiilla | 10.0 | 67.6±2.6 | −2.1±2.2 | +1.0±1.0 | 0.0±1.6 | +0.7 | −3.0±2.4 | +0.7 |
| TOTAL | 9.0 | 65.7±2.1 | +1.4±2.4 | +0.6±1.0 | −0.4±1.5 | +1.4 | −1.4±2.0 | +0.7±2.3 |
| Permanent dentition | | | | | | | | |
|   Fault in mandible | 15.0 | 66.2±1.2 | +6.4±3.4 | ∅ | +6.5±3.2 | +0.6 | 0.0±1.0 | ∅ |
|   Fault in maxilla | 8.0 | 70.5±3.1 | +0.5±3.0 | ∅ | +4.6±3.6 | ∅ | −2.0±2.2 | ∅ |
| TOTAL | 14.0 | 68.5±3.5 | +0.5±3.0 | ∅ | +6.0±2.5 | ∅ | −1.5±1.5 | ∅ |

*Relative to ideal values.

†Relative to found values before treatment.

**Scope and limitation of treatment in the various dentitional periods.** As the age of the patient increases, the amount of growth to be expected decreases and the skeletal Class III relationship becomes more permanent. As has been pointed out before, influencing the growth process and tooth eruption as early as clinically feasible in the initial stages of the dysplastic relationship is advantageous. Treatment is possible in the different stages of dentitional development, but early treatment is more likely to be successful.

*Treatment in the deciduous dentition.* Early malocclusion symptoms are usually apparent in the deciduous dentition. The patient often postures the mandible habitually in an anterior relationship, with the tongue also posturing low and forward as the dorsum flattens out. If these symptoms are observed, orthopedic control using a chincap may be the method of choice to hold the mandible in a posterior position. Treatment can be started as early as 1 year and can be continued until the age of 4 or so as the only growth guidance procedure. Combination treatment with an intraoral appliance is usually necessary later. Only treatment done on the deciduous dentition has the potential of being completely successful in most cases with any significant degree of potential mandibular prognathism. Treatment begun later is more likely to leave residual signs of mandibular prognathism or maxillary retrusion, even though the dental result can be quite successful. Obviously the magnitude of the original insult and the dominance of the morphogenetic pattern are qualifying factors. After eruption of all the deciduous teeth, three types of Class III relationship can be differentiated.

FUNCTIONAL CLASS III RELATIONSHIP. In this category, no skeletal Class III signs are present. The mandible slides anteriorly into an edge-to-edge or crossbite relationship. Usually the tooth guidance is in the canine region. Often careful equilibration of these teeth is all that is needed to correct the problem. In other cases, decreased intercanine distance, which might be caused by chronic nasorespiratory problems, and low tongue posture may be dominant factors in the creation of the morphology that results in tooth guidance. In such cases, expansion of the maxillary arch without canine equilibration is indicated. Canines that have been needlessly ground down do not retain well in these cases. However, a functional Class III relationship may be a beginning sign of a true Class III malocclusion. Patients with such malocclusions need to be followed continuously, and orthopedic guidance may be needed at any time.

CLASS III RELATIONSHIP WITH THE FAULT IN THE MANDIBLE. A fault in the mandible can become manifest in the deciduous dentition despite the fact that the mandible appears retrognathic in the early years for most children. In these cases the mandibular basal measurement and the S-N-B angle can be large. However, the mandibular base can be of average length or even short in the deciduous dentition, and the mandible can be prominent or anteriorly positioned. The maxilla is usually normally developed in these cases. Growth inhibition or redirection and posterior positioning of the mandible is a valid treatment objective here. A chincap or a reverse (Class III) activator can be used to exert a retrusive force on the mandible in patients who fall in this group.

CLASS III RELATIONSHIP WITH THE FAULT IN THE MAXILLA. Patients with the fault in the maxilla show a retrognathic maxilla or midface even though the mandible is orthognathic or essentially normal. The tooth buds of the upper incisors are often rotated and crowded. Treatment can usually be accomplished with an activator or Fränkel appliance in mild cases, although extraoral orthopedic protractive force using a Delaire-type face mask is required in severe problems. Treatment of this type of problem during the eruption of the incisors before the maxillary incisors become locked behind the mandibular counterparts is advantageous. Loading the palatal area behind the upper incisors while relieving the labial muscle forces with lip pads, as recommended by Kraus (1956), Fränkel (1967), and others, is often effective.

A combination of these two types of Class III malocclusions (retrusive maxilla and protrusive mandible) of course is possible and logically requires therapeutic control of both areas via maxillary protraction and mandibular retractive growth guidance. To illustrate treatment in a case that employs these principles, Figure 21-20 shows a 6-year-old boy with a developmental age of 5 years. His mother had a severe Class III malocclusion. She had come for a prognostic evaluation of the problem in the boy's deciduous dentition because of her concern. Clinically the patient already exhibited an edge-to-edge incisal relationship and a prominent symphysis. Cephalometric examination showed prognathic tendencies in both jaws, more in the upper than in the lower jaw. The growth pattern was projected as horizontal, but the up and forward tipping of the maxillary base (anteinclination) was opening the bite anteriorly. The maxillary base was 1.5 mm longer than average, the ramus 3 mm shorter, and the mandibular body 4 mm larger than average, which is extremely large for this age and a good sign of genetically determined mandibular prognathism. Assessment of the axial inclination of the incisors is not of much value at this time because these teeth are naturally quite upright in the deciduous dentition.

Treatment was postponed for $1\frac{1}{2}$ years until the eruption of the incisors. In the meantime the prognathism increased, especially in the mandible. The A-N-B angle was now −3 degrees. Both the mandibular base and the ramus height were large, whereas the maxillary base was of average length. The horizontal growth pattern and the anteinclination of the maxillary base persisted. Comparison of the serial cephalograms showed increasingly severe malocclusion. The functional analysis showed a normal path of closure with no tooth guidance, making this a true Class III problem.

Treatment was started with a Class III activator. The construction bite was opened 4 mm to achieve an edge-to-edge relationship after all possible retrusion of the mandible was achieved. A tongue crib was used in the lower anterior region instead of the usual acrylic material. The lower incisors were guided lingually with a labial bow. Lip pads were incorporated in the appliance in the upper anterior segment to hold off any pressure from the contiguous musculature, and the upper incisors were guided labially by adding successive thin layers of self-curing soft acrylic. Therapy was continued in this manner until all incisors had erupted.

After $1\frac{1}{2}$ years of mechanotherapy a good overbite had

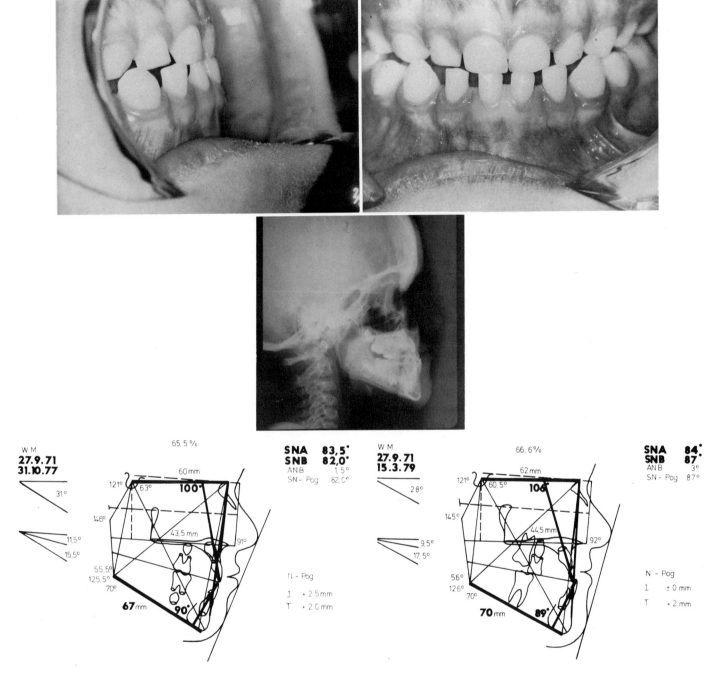

**Figure 21-20.** A 6-year-old boy with a Class III malocclusion before treatment. Tracing on bottom right was taken 1½ years after the tracing on bottom left.

been achieved (Figure 21-21). The prognathism of the maxillary base had increased, whereas the mandibular prognathism was decreased, resulting in a posterior positioning of the mandible despite an increased growth rate of the maxillary base. The skeletal discrepancy was partially compensated for by the labial tipping of the upper incisors and the lingual tipping of the lower incisors. During the course of further development the intermaxillary relationship remained stable because of the adaptation of the maxillary complex to the prognathic mandible.

*Treatment in the mixed dentition.* Even in the mixed dentition a posterior position of the mandible can still be achieved. The goal of early treatment is to gain proper incisal guidance as soon as possible, which may lead to harmonious growth of the jaw bases if the dysplasia is not severe. Obviously, treatment undertaken at the earliest possible time when only minor Class III symptoms are present is likely to be the most successful and stable.

In patients in whom the problem is primarily dentoalveolar, the upper incisors are tipped lingually initially, and the

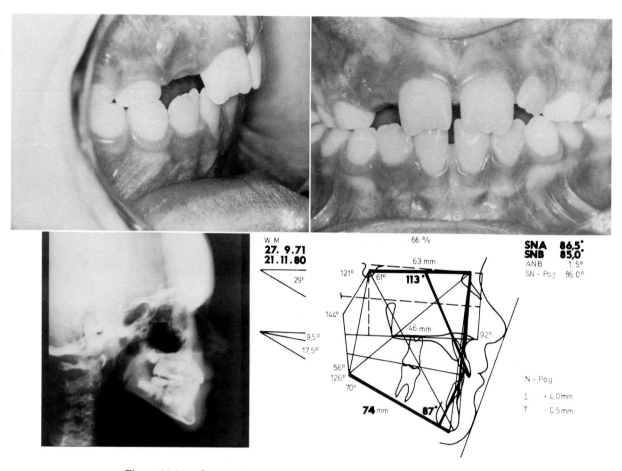

**Figure 21-21.**    Same patient as in Figure 21-20 after eruption of the incisors.

lower incisors are tipped labially. The first objective of treatment is to correct the incisor crossbite and upright these teeth. As previously noted, treatment can be performed with variations of the active plate, inclined planes, or activators. During treatment, some skeletal symptoms of the Class III malocclusion often arise (i.e., a long mandibular base or a forward positioned mandible). Continued observation of the developing dentition is necessary in these cases; the clinician should pursue long-term follow-up and have a readiness to intercede with the proper orthopedic or fixed attachment guidance as indicated. Often an activator can be used as a retainer, or a chincap may be necessary to control the mandibular prognathism tendency. Treatment (or at least supervision) is essential in mixed dentition cases until the full eruption of the permanent teeth.

In Class III malocclusions with the fault in the mandible in mixed dentition cases, the same treatment objectives of growth inhibition and posterior mandibular positioning are indicated. An activator can be used to alter the incisal guidance and attempt to position the mandible posteriorly. Sometimes in the early mixed dentition, extraction of the lower deciduous canines and deciduous first molars can be performed to facilitate the correction of the incisal guidance. In some carefully selected cases, enucleation of the lower first premolars is possible, decreasing lower arch length and providing dental compensation for the skeletal problem as the six lower

anterior teeth are retracted into the extraction sites. Germectomy also limits alveolar growth.

Treatment of a Class III malocclusion with a vertical growth pattern is more difficult than is treatment with a horizontal pattern. Achieving a good overbite is difficult with a vertical growth vector. Excessive anterior face height is evident; it compensates for the growth but usually is not enough. In these cases a chincap or a low- or high-pull headgear may be helpful to control posterior eruption, depending on the growth direction.

In Class III malocclusions in the mixed dentition with the fault in the maxilla, all efforts should be made to promote growth and protract the maxillary complex. Both horizontal and vertical growth should be encouraged because maxillary vertical deficiency enhances the apparent mandibular protrusion with its autorotation into an overclosed habitual occlusion. Many of these cases have excessive interocclusal clearance, and stimulation of maxillary vertical growth also enhances eruption of the posterior teeth, rotating the mandible down and back into a more normal sagittal relationship. An improvement in the midface concavity can be seen if treatment is performed during the eruption of the maxillary incisors. The eruption can be channelled as desired by the guiding planes of the activator, with simultaneous relief of labial muscle force provided by the lip pads at the depth of the vestibule. Simultaneously the mandible can be put under a

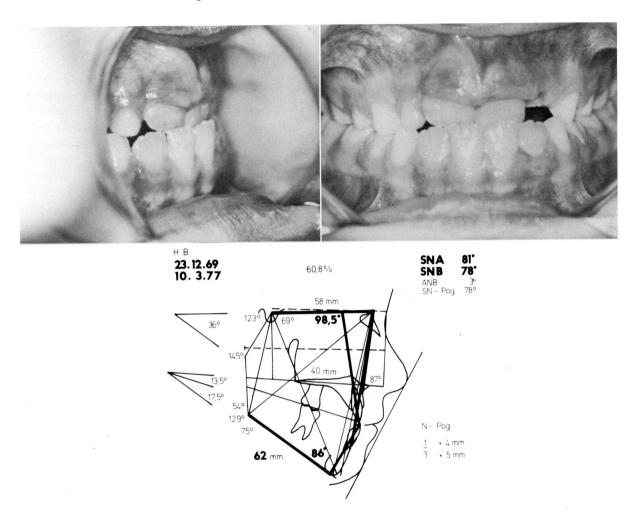

**Figure 21-22.**    An 8½-year-old girl with an incisor crossbite before treatment.

retrusive chincap force to reduce the sagittal discrepancy. An alternate approach is to align the maxillary arch with a short period of direct-bonded attachments or active plates; the midface can be favorably influenced by the orthopedic protraction of a Delaire mask. If the crowding of the maxillary arch is too severe, extraction may be required in the maxillary arch. In such a case the lower first premolars also must be removed to allow proper dentitional adjustment. Clearly, fixed multiattachment therapy and possible orthognathic surgery may be the therapies of choice, depending on the severity of the problem and the age-linked expressivity.

To illustrate management of a mixed dentition problem, Figure 21-22 shows an 8½-year-old girl with an incisor crossbite. The growth pattern projected was average; the jaw bases were of average length for her age; the basal relationship was normal, despite a short ramus; and the A-N-B angle was 3 degrees. The upper dental arch was crowded, but the lower arch was well aligned and wide.

Treatment was started with a Class III activator to guide the upper incisors labially and move the lower incisors lingually. The lower deciduous canines were extracted to assist in this correction. After full eruption of the incisors and all four first premolars, the upper arch was expanded with an active plate. Subsequently the lower arch also was expanded to align and position upright the teeth. A good overbite was achieved after 15 months of activator treatment, although the lower incisors were tipped lingually (Figure 21-23). The basal relationship as evidenced by the A-N-B angle remained stable, despite a large growth increment of 3.5 mm in the mandibular base. The maxillary base and ramus height were both short. The growth rate of the mandibular base was characteristic of a morphogenetically dominant Class III pattern. Because of early incisal control and development of a normal engram of proper incisor proprioception during the transitional dentition period, the mandible did not slide into a prognathic relationship. The effects produced on the temporomandibular fossa as a result of retrusive stimulus on the mandible are matters for speculation. However, because this area is membranous bone, it is susceptible to potential morphologic change and adaptation, as primate studies have shown. Therefore the possibility exists that part of the correction seen in some of these Class III cases under orthopedic influence is caused by a distalizing of the fossae and by some minimal mandibular change.

In another example, Figure 21-24 shows a 7½-year-old girl with an anterior crossbite and maxillary arch crowding.

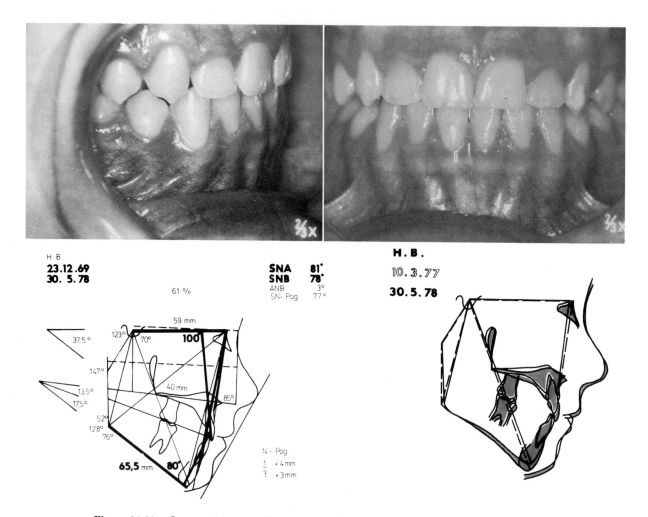

**Figure 21-23.**   Same patient as in Figure 21-22 after activator and fixed appliance treatment. *Bottom right,* Superimposition of before and after tracings.

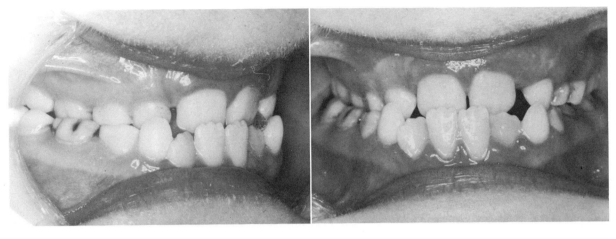

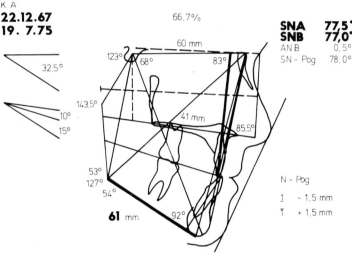

**Figure 21-24.** A 7½-year-old girl with an anterior crossbite and maxillary arch crowding before treatment.

The arch length deficiency was large above with no room for the lateral incisors. Both upper and lower jaw bases were retrognathic in position. The A-N-B angle was almost a straight line at 0.5 degree. The length of the jaw bases was average.

The correction of the incisor crossbite was not considered a problem because of the lingual inclination of the maxillary centrals, which could be tipped labially. The crowding was so severe, however, that extraction of the first premolars would be necessary later. Because treatment began in the early mixed dentition period, a program of serial extraction and simultaneous correction of the anterior crossbite were possible.

Treatment was carried out with two activators. The upper incisors were tipped labially and the mandible was held in a retruded position with the first activator. The clinician attained these results by adding layers of self-curing soft acrylic on the lingual surfaces of these teeth and the contiguous alveolar process; the lower incisors had an active labial bow retrusive effect. Serial extraction procedures were carried out, with removal of the lower first premolars occurring first followed by removal of the upper first premolars as these teeth erupted. The removal of the lower premolars before the upper teeth is almost always advantageous in Class III maloc-

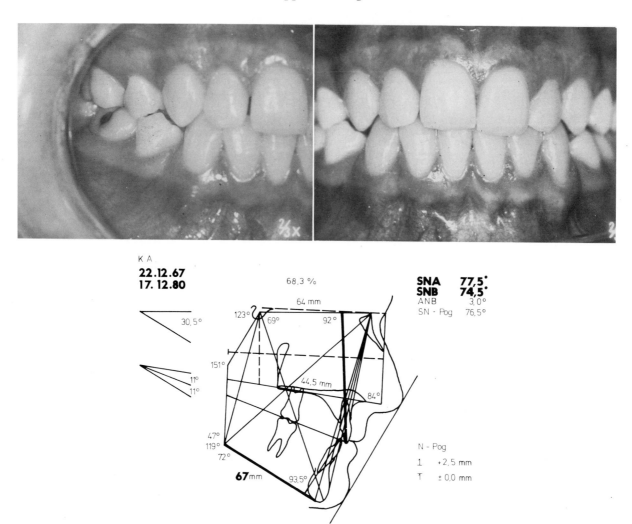

K A
**22.12.67**
**17.12.80**

68,3 %

64 mm

30,5°

123°    69°    92°

151°

44,5 mm    84°

47°
119°
72°

**67** mm    93,5°

11°
11°

**SNA    77,5°**
**SNB    74,5°**
ANB    3,0°
SN - Pog    76,5°

N - Pog

1    + 2,5 mm

T    ± 0,0 mm

**Figure 21-25.**    Same patient as in Figure 21-24 after treatment.

clusions. The second activator was used for retention and to seat the occlusion.

After 4½ years of treatment and retention a good incisal and skeletal relationship had been achieved with a normal 3-degree A-N-B angle (Figure 21-25). The growth increments were average. The early initiation of therapy allowed the use of functional appliances. Later appliance introduction meets with more severe tooth malalignment, and fixed appliances become the mechanisms of choice. They may be necessary anyway as a final phase of treatment to align malposed teeth after establishment of a proper skeletal sagittal relationship.

In another case report, a 9-year-old girl had a Class III malocclusion with the maxilla at fault and an A-N-B angle of −2 degrees (Figure 21-26). The growth pattern was projected as vertical. The maxillary base was small and retrognathic. The upper arch had crowding and rotations present.

Treatment was provided with multiattachment fixed appliances and extraction of four first premolars. The Class III relationship was compensated for by dentoalveolar adjustment (Figure 21-27).

*Treatment in the permanent dentition.* By the time the permanent teeth have erupted, treatment for a Class III malocclusion can be successful only if the problem is primarily dentoalveolar and not a true skeletal malrelationship. The skeletal type of Class III malocclusion can be compensated for by tooth removal and surgery. The method of choice depends on the severity of the problem and a projection of residual sagittal growth changes still possible in the terminal developmental period. A thorough diagnosis and a projection based on a likely growth pattern are most important. If the problem is too severe for orthodontic correction alone (with or without extraction), the proper preparations should be made for surgery. Clinical histories show many examples of patients wearing orthodontic appliances for 4 to 6 years before the clinician decides to resort to orthognathic surgery. In many of these cases a proper diagnosis at the beginning would have provided the necessary information indicating the likelihood of a need for orthognathic procedures.

Sometimes presurgical therapy means decompensating for natural adjustments that have been made. This requires posi-

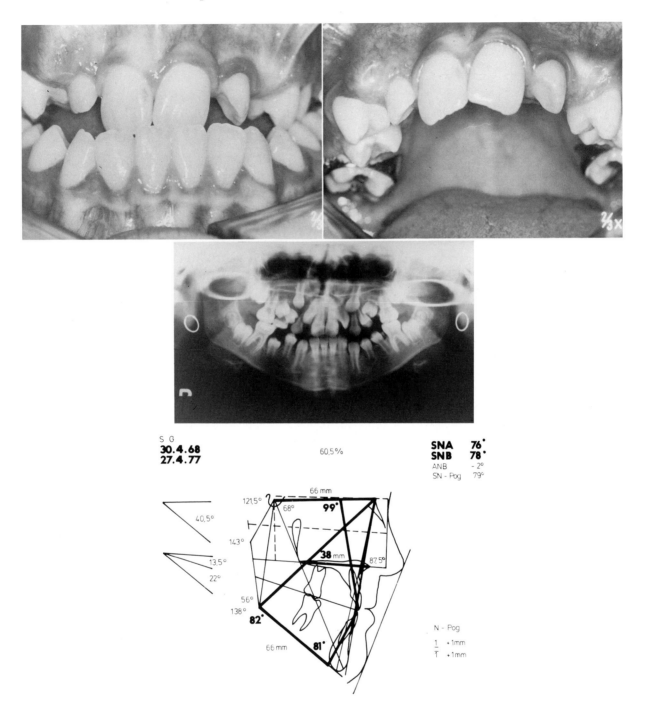

**Figure 21-26.** A 9-year-old girl with a Class III malocclusion before treatment.

tioning lingually inclined mandibular incisors and labially inclined maxillary incisors upright to reduce excessive eruption of incisors and level the curve of Spee. The patient is treated to regain an anterior crossbite because the skeletal change affected by surgery reestablishes a normal overbite and overjet. All these treatment procedures require fixed multiattachment therapy and are beyond the scope of functional appliances (Figures 21-28 and 21-29).

The activator can be used for retention after orthognathic surgical correction. The amount of disturbance, mode of nat-

ural adaptation to changed muscle pull after surgery, and functional adaptation are often unknown quantities. The changing of the origins or insertions of muscles during the course of orthognathic surgery requires adaptation in both these muscles and the bony tissues in which they insert. Retention is strongly indicated to help guide posttreatment adaptation in the most favorable direction. An activator is ideal for this muscle training. The appliance is fabricated with the mandible in the most retruded position and a slight opening of the vertical dimension. The lower incisors are held with

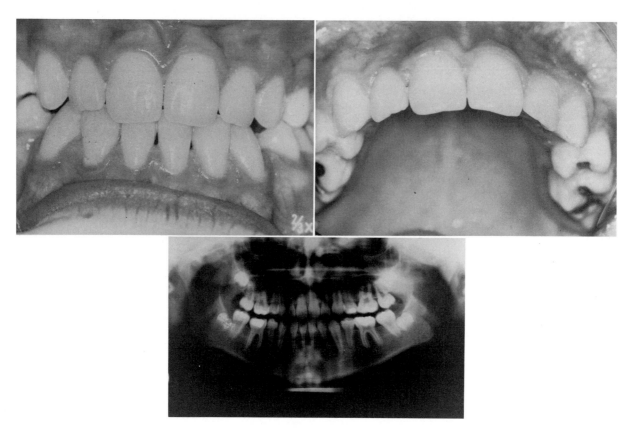

**Figure 21-27.** Same patient as in Figure 21-26 after treatment.

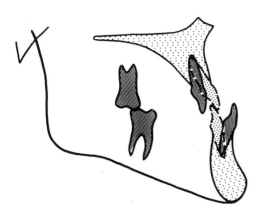

**Figure 21-28.** Dental compensation of a Class III skeletal relationship by labial tipping of the upper incisors and lingual tipping of the lower incisors.

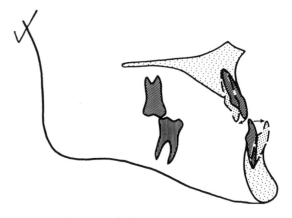

**Figure 21-29.** Presurgical decompensation of a Class III relationship by upright positioning of the tipped incisors.

acrylic capping or indexing. The acrylic is not trimmed away in the molar area because it is supposed to hold the teeth in position.

Removable functional appliances can be used successfully in the treatment of Class III malocclusions if they are introduced early, even in the deciduous dentition of selected cases. Use in mixed dentition when the incisors are erupting and the skeletal characteristics are not yet blatantly manifest is highly desirable, and the results attained are more likely to be stable. In all other cases the range of use of functional appliances in the treatment of Class III malocclusions is limited, and these appliances can be used effectively only with other fixed appliance methods and orthognathic surgery. Use of a functional appliance as a retainer is recommended in many instances because muscle adaptation is slower and the activator serves as a training appliance.

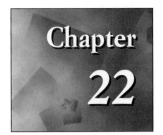

# Chapter 22

# The Open-Bite Malocclusion

Thomas Rakosi

The treatment of an open-bite malocclusion is partially described in Chapter 5. This section discusses the general concepts of open-bite therapy.

## ETIOLOGIC CONSIDERATIONS

Epigenetic and environmental factors are both of concern in the etiology of open bite. Epigenetic factors include posture; morphology and size of the tongue; skeletal growth pattern of the maxilla and mandible, particularly the lower jaw; and vertical relationship of the jaw bases. These characteristics are genetically determined. A vertical deficiency generally occurs in the amount of basal and alveolar bone growth in a specific area.

Of the environmental factors, abnormal function and improper respiration are the most significant. Most children (91% in Rakosi's study [1966c]) have some sort of abnormal functional pattern or potentially deforming habit. The significance of tongue dysfunctions in the etiology of open bite has already been discussed in Chapter 7. Disturbed or occluded nasal respiration can cause a change in the posture or function of both the tongue and mandible, which can lead to an open-bite malocclusion (see Chapter 1).

## ESTHETIC CONSIDERATIONS

The dentoalveolar open-bite malocclusion is esthetically unattractive, particularly during speech when the tongue is pressed between the teeth and lips. In evaluating the esthetics, the following relationships are of special interest:

1. Balance between the nose, lips, and chin profile is essential for optimal esthetics.
2. The nasolabial angle also is important. If this angle is small or acute, a retraction of the upper incisors is likely to improve esthetics after a premolar extraction. If the nasolabial angle is obtuse or large, proclination of the upper incisors may enhance facial appearance. However, the change is not caused by changes in the nasal contour but rather by changes in the draping of the lip.
3. The configuration of the lips—the space between the lips at rest and the relation of the lip line to the underlying teeth and gingival tissue—plays an important role in esthetics. A short upper lip that reveals excessive amounts of maxillary gingival tissue is not esthetically appealing.
4. The length of the lower third of the face (Figure 22-1) and the relative prominence or retrusion of the chin affect appearance. Of particular concern is the distance between stomion and subnasale, which is often short with respect to the total maxillomandibular profile height.

## FUNCTIONAL CONSIDERATIONS

Tongue posture and function should be primary considerations in open-bite problems. Differentiation between primary causal and secondary adaptive or compensatory tongue

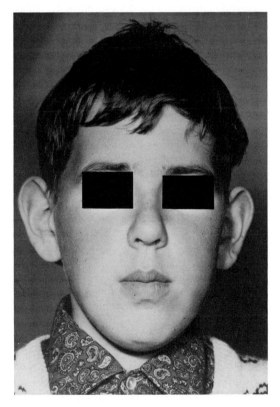

**Figure 22-1.** The lower facial third is elongated in patients with skeletal open bites.

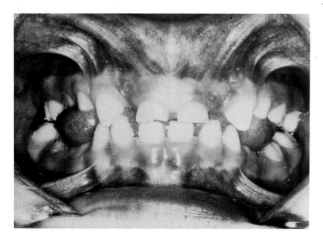

**Figure 22-2.** Bilateral open bite in which the tongue was a factor in the deciduous dentition.

dysfunction is essential. Functional analysis also must assess the magnitude of force (i.e., simple pressing versus strong protractive action). Cephalometric analysis can localize the nature of the open bite and determine whether it is skeletal or dentoalveolar. Hence correlation of the functional and cephalometric analyses is necessary when the clinician determines the role and effect of tongue activity.

According to Bahr and Holt, four varieties of tongue-thrust activity may be differentiated:

1. Tongue thrust without deformation is a common phenomenon. Despite the abnormal function, no deformation ensues.
2. Tongue thrust causing anterior deformation (i.e., anterior open bite, sometimes coupled with bilateral narrowing of the arch and a posterior crossbite) also may occur. Moyers (1964) terms this a *simple open bite.*
3. Tongue thrust causing buccal segment deformation with a posterior open bite is often seen clinically. Lateral tongue thrust activity also can be responsible for a functional deep bite, a variation of the posterior open bite (Figure 22-2). Some Class II, division 2 malocclusions fit this category. Invagination of the cheek into the interocclusal space also may be a factor in this dysfunction.
4. Combined tongue thrust, causing both an anterior and a posterior open bite, is another common dysfunction. This is called a *complex open bite* by Moyers and is more difficult to treat.

Tongue posture is as important as tongue function. The retained infantile deglutitional pattern usually produces a forward posturing of the tongue as a vestige of the nursing posture. Finger-sucking habits often prolong this infantile protractive tongue posture, with the tip of the tongue between the anterior teeth. In the normal maturational cycle, the tip of the tongue drops back as the incisors erupt. After the anterior space is created by interference with normal incisor eruption, compensatory function is evident during deglutition as the individual tries to effect a seal during the swallowing cycle.

## CLINICAL CONSIDERATIONS

Various forms of anterior open bite may be observed, depending on the severity of the malocclusion:

1. Cases with an overjet combined with an open bite of less than 1 mm can be designated as pseudo–open bite problems.
2. A simple open bite exists in cases in which more than 1 mm of space may be observed between the incisors, but the posterior teeth are in occlusion.
3. A complex open bite designates those cases in which the open bite extends from the premolars or deciduous molars on one side to the corresponding teeth on the other side.
4. The compound or infantile open bite is completely open, including the molars.
5. The iatrogenic open bite is the consequence of orthodontic therapy, which produces atypical configurations because of appliance manipulation or adaptive neuromuscular response.

In the mixed dentition period, various therapeutic measures may cause an open bite:

1. An open activator with a high construction bite can cause a tongue thrust habit and resultant anterior open bite. During intrusion of the posterior teeth a posterior open bite also may be created, especially in the deciduous molar area.
2. In expansion treatment the buccal segments can be tipped excessively buccally, with elongation of the lingual cusps. This creates prematurity and effectively opens the bite.
3. In distalization of maxillary first molars with extraoral force the molars are often tipped down and back, elongating the mesial cusps. This creates a molar fulcrum that can open the bite and is of particular concern in downward and backward growing faces that already have excessive anterior face heights.

## CEPHALOMETRIC CRITERIA

A proper cephalometric analysis enables a classification of open-bite malocclusions.

The extent of the dentoalveolar open bite depends on the extent of the eruption of the teeth. Supraocclusion of the molars and infraocclusion of the incisors can be primary etiologic factors. In vertical growth patterns the dentoalveolar symptoms include a protrusion in the upper anterior teeth with lingual inclination of the lower incisors. In horizontal growth patterns, tongue posture and thrust may cause proclination of both upper and lower incisors.

A lateral open bite may be considered dentoalveolar in combination with infraclusion of molar teeth. Contributing causal factors include cheek sucking, lateral tongue thrust, or lateral postural tongue spread in the postural resting position. Interruption of the abnormal function with appliances

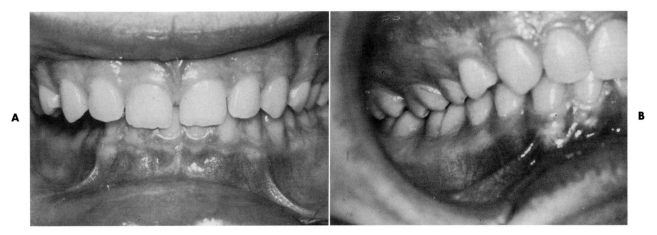

**Figure 22-3.** Lateral open bite in a 14-year-old boy with nonocclusion of the right premolars. **A,** Before and, **B,** after screening of the dysfunction.

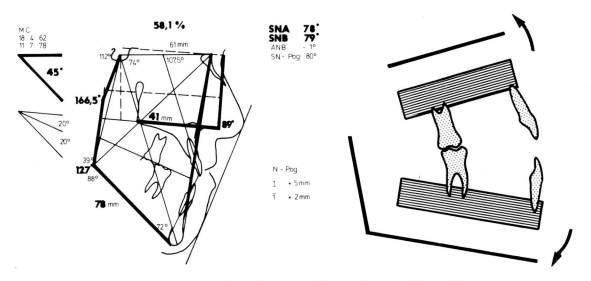

**Figure 22-4.** Vertical growth pattern with anteinclination of the maxilla.

(screening therapy) can bring about improvement.

An example is shown in Figure 22-3. A 14-year-old boy had a severe cheek-tongue dysfunction that was eliminated with therapy; the posterior open bite also was eliminated.

In skeletal open bite the anterior face height is excessive, particularly the lower third, whereas posterior face height (ramus height) is short. The mandibular base is usually narrow, and antegonial notching is often present. The symphysis is narrow and long, and the ramus is short. The gonial angle, particularly the lower section, is large, and the growth pattern is vertical. Depending on the inclination of the maxillary base, or palatal plane, the following variations may be observed:

1. A vertical growth pattern with upward tipping of the

forward end of the maxillary base is a common phenomenon. This can provide a condition in certain patients in which unfavorable sequelae complement each other to cause severe skeletal open bite (Figure 22-4).

2. A vertical growth pattern with downward tipping of the anterior end of the maxillary base also may be seen. This can combine with an offsetting relationship to compensate the open bite (Figure 22-5).

3. A horizontal growth direction with an open bite caused by upward and forward tipping of the maxillary base is another variation (Figure 22-6). This type of problem is designated a decompensated deep overbite by orthodontic practitioners.

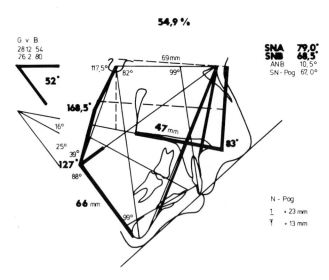

**Figure 22-5.** Vertical growth pattern partially compensated by a slight retroinclination of the maxilla.

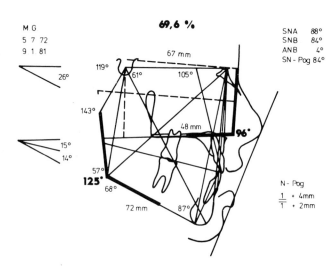

**Figure 22-6.** Horizontal growth pattern with anteinclination of the maxilla. This is the dominant cause of the open bite.

## THERAPEUTIC CONSIDERATIONS

Therapy depends on the localization and etiology of the malocclusion. Habit control and the elimination of abnormal perioral muscle function are causal therapeutic approaches in the treatment of the dentoalveolar open-bite problem. In skeletal open-bite problems a redirection of growth is possible during the active growth period. Later, only compensatory therapy with extraction and tooth movement or orthognathic surgery is possible.

In addition to the dentoalveolar and skeletal open-bite categories, a combined skeletodental type exists that requires a combined therapeutic approach. Even in a dentoalveolar treatment approach the growth pattern should be considered because of the different reactions of individual growth pat-

terns to various neuromuscular abnormalities, and vice versa. In the latter case a bimaxillary protrusion can occur in a horizontal growth pattern, whereas lingual tipping may result in a vertical growth pattern.

The proper time to institute treatment depends on the etiology of the malocclusion. If the causal factor can be eliminated, early interceptive therapy is indicated; dysfunctions should be eliminated as quickly as feasible. On the other hand, skeletal problems can be solved or at least compensated for at a later age.

Various treatment regimens are possible during the various developmental periods of the dentition. Many of these problems are discussed in Chapter 5. Only a summary of the different treatment approaches is given here.

## Open-Bite Treatment in the Deciduous Dentition

Control of abnormal habits and elimination of dysfunction should be given top priority in the deciduous dentition. In many instances the open bite improves as soon as the habit is stopped. Autonomous improvement can be expected only if the deforming muscle activity is terminated and the open bite is not complicated by crowding of the upper arch or crossbite. Treatment with screening appliances or activators is indicated in such open-bite cases.

A skeletal open bite is seldom observed in the deciduous dentition. Habit control is of only secondary consideration in these cases, retarding the increasing severity of the dysplasia. Extraoral orthopedic appliances such as chincaps can be used effectively to redirect growth.

## Treatment of Open Bite in the Mixed Dentition

Three types of open-bite malocclusion may be differentiated in the mixed dentition period:

1. Dentoalveolar open-bite malocclusion may occur as a consequence of various dysfunctions. In the early mixed dentition period, screening therapy (as described in Chapter 5) is indicated. In the late mixed dentition, however, with a severe tongue thrust or posture problem, screening therapy may be unsuccessful. In such cases the open bite may respond favorably to multiattachment fixed appliances, but a long posttreatment retention phase is necessary until abnormal perioral muscle function can be reduced. Swallowing exercises (i.e., swallowing without thrusting, putting the tip of the tongue behind the upper or lower incisors) may reinforce the establishment of a mature deglutitional and functional pattern for the tongue during both treatment and retention.

    The example shown in Figure 22-7 is an 8-year-old girl with a developmental age of 9½ years. An open bite with a tongue posture–dysfunction problem was evident. The maxillary and mandibular bases were prognathic, the maxillary base was of average length, and

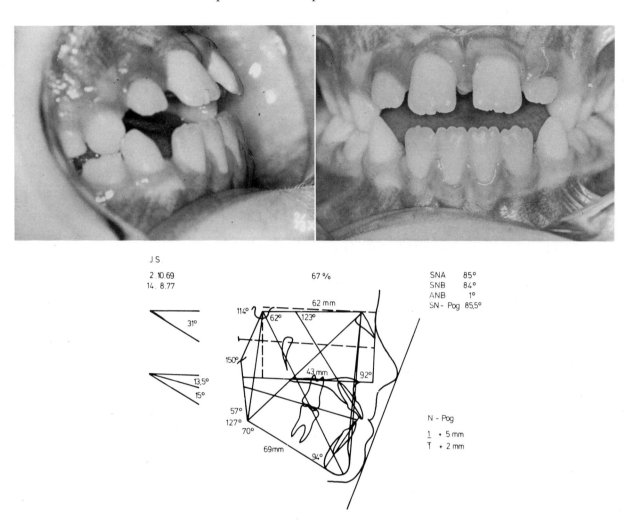

**Figure 22-7.** A 8-year-old girl with an open bite before treatment.

the mandibular base and ramus were long. Interocclusal space was minimal or nonexistent. The growth pattern was extremely horizontal, as might be expected from the skeletal configuration. The tongue thrust had apparently caused a double protrusion. Because of the abnormal function and the small size of the incisors, generalized spacing existed between the teeth. The open bite was complicated by the upward and forward inclination of the maxillary base. Inhibitory treatment was initiated using a double screen but was unsuccessful. The severe tongue pressures prevented upright positioning of the incisors and closing of the spaces. The open bite was corrected with fixed appliances, intermaxillary elastics, and other methods after eruption of the canines and premolars. Even with the closure of the open bite, a slight protrusion of the upper incisors persisted (Figure 22-8). This protrusion also was a compensation for the Class III basal relationship tendency, as shown by the subspinale-nasion-supramentale (A-N-B) angle of zero degrees. Growth increments were predictably high in the mandibular base as opposed to average increments in the maxilla.

Inhibitory treatment failed in this case because correction of a double protrusion is difficult using screening appliances alone; the tongue problem cannot be completely eliminated. Complementary active force was required to position the incisors upright, although the growth vector was horizontal. The bite was open because of the strong anteinclination (upward and forward tipping) of the maxillary base. Lack of a normal freeway space probably indicates overeruption of the posterior teeth.

2. Skeletal open-bite malocclusion also may occur. Treatment of skeletal open bite depends on at least two factors—the severity of the malocclusion and the possibility of dental alveolar compensation.

The growth pattern in this type of problem is almost always vertical. Not only the extent of this vertical growth pattern but also the inclination of the maxillary base is decisive in treatment planning. If the rotation of the jaw bases is divergent, the prognosis is poor. If the maxillary base is tipped down and forward (retroclined), functional therapy may sometimes be successful.

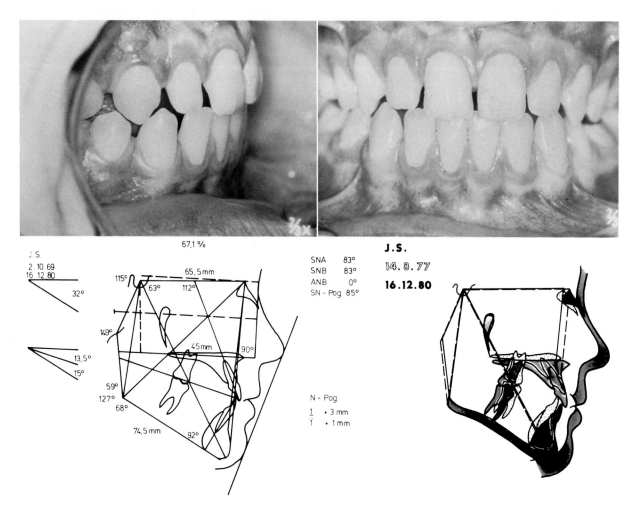

**Figure 22-8.** Same patient as in Figure 22-7 after treatment. *Bottom right,* Superimposition of before and after tracings.

In addition to intrusion of buccal segments and extrusion of the incisors, mesial movement of the posterior teeth also is a beneficial dentoalveolar measure to help close the bite. Moving teeth forward in the **V** by the removal of the four first premolars often makes closure of the bite possible despite the skeletal nature of the problem. Treatment can be undertaken with activators combined with extraction and extraoral force application. In extreme cases, with divergent rotation of the jaw bases, removal of four premolars and fixed appliance therapy constitute the best approach to treatment. Severe cases require orthognathic surgery, with impaction of buccal segments and even sagittal split osteotomy in some cases to close the bite and provide stable correction.

Figure 22-9 shows an 8-year-old girl with a long face syndrome, extremely vertical growth pattern, and slight anterior open bite. Her jaw bases were retrognathic and short, with an A-N-B difference of 4 degrees and reduced ramus length (−13.5 mm). The posterior to anterior height ratio was 49%, which is quite low. The lower gonial angle was large at 93 degrees. Crowding was present in the upper arch. The slight open bite was considered secondary. The maxillary base was retroclined at an angle of 83 degrees, which was considered favorable for therapy. Treatment began with the removal of four premolars, and fixed appliance therapy was planned for later in hopes of preventing the need for surgical correction. Because habit control was not deemed necessary, therapy was postponed to 11½ years. In the interim the upper incisors had uprighted somewhat, possibly because of acquired abnormal lip function. The growth pattern persisted in a vertical direction, with the ramus remaining short (−10 mm).

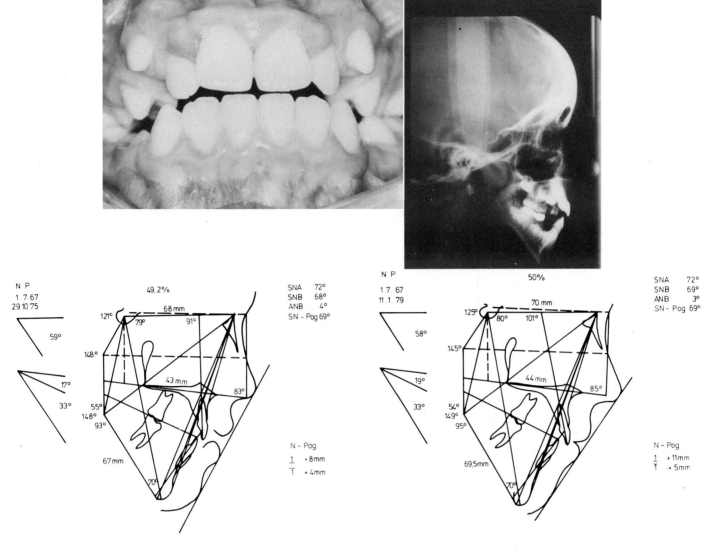

**Figure 22-9.** An 8-year-old girl with a long face syndrome and an open bite before treatment.

After 2½ years of multiattachment mechanotherapy, the dental arches were aligned and the open bite was closed, but no improvement of the skeletal relationship was observed (Figure 22-10). A study of three siblings showed the hereditary nature of the long face syndrome that dominated the family facial pattern. Because the malocclusion was not caused by a functional aberration, functional appliance therapy was not justified.

In some cases of extreme vertical growth patterns, lip-sealing ability is significantly disturbed. To achieve a better neuromuscular environment, a surgical resection of the mentalis muscle can be performed to reduce the "golfball chin" effect (Figure 22-11). This operation is indicated in the mixed dentition period after eruption of the lower canine teeth, according to Schilli. After the growth period, cosmetic plastic surgery of the chin area may be necessary (Figure 22-12). This type of transpo-

sition of the mentalis muscle attachment permits greater extension of the lower lip to effect a lip seal and can enhance the stability of the treatment result and bite closure.

3. Combined open bite is a third possibility. Most skeletal open-bite cases are probably at least partially attributable to abnormal perioral muscle function. The work of Rolf and Christine Fränkel (1983) supports this observation. Because of the dual nature of the etiology, a combined treatment approach is recommended. Treatment follows two possible combinations—elimination of abnormal perioral muscle function and improvement of skeletal relationships.

The abnormal perioral muscle function is eliminated or at least intercepted in the early mixed dentition period, and the required serial extraction procedures, if indicated, are performed. Tooth eruption can be guided

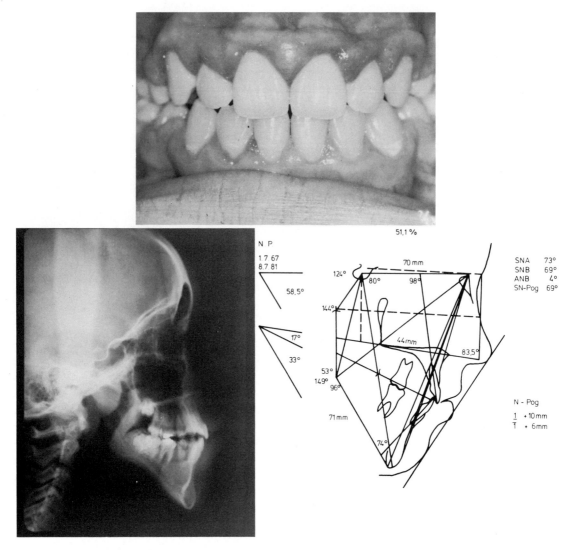

**Figure 22-10.** Same patient as in Figure 22-9 after fixed appliance treatment. *Bottom right,* Tracing 3½ years after removal of the first molars.

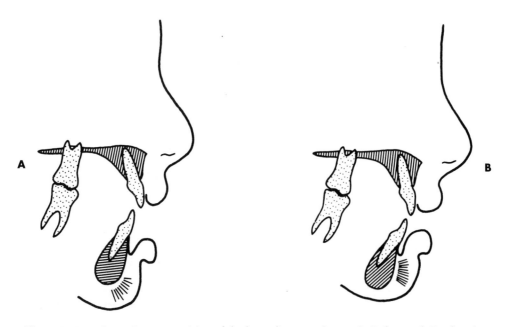

**Figure 22-11.** Operative transposition of the lower lip musculature. **A,** Before and, **B,** after the mentalis resection.

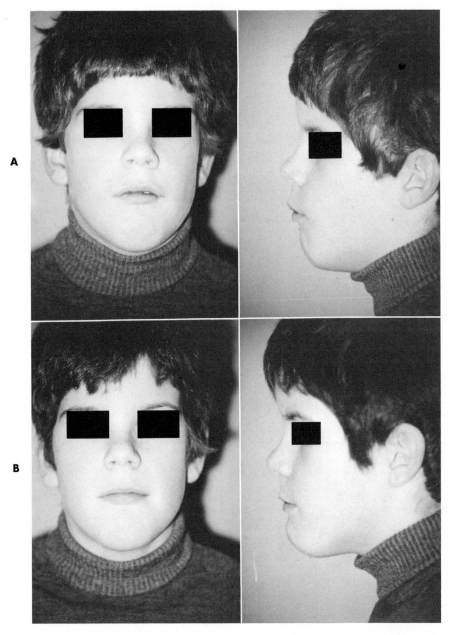

**Figure 22-12.** A patient at 10 years. **A,** Before mentalis resection. **B,** After the transposition of muscle attachments.

and the habit pattern can be controlled fairly well with an activator. After the eruption of the permanent teeth the remaining malocclusion can be reduced by compensatory tooth movement, usually performed with fixed appliances.

CASE STUDY

An example of this combined treatment is shown in Figure 22-13. The patient, a 7½-year-old girl, had an open bite and a severe vertical growth pattern. The mother and one sibling had the same morphogenetic pattern. Both jaw bases were retrognathic, and the maxillary base and ramus particularly were short (−15 mm). The vertical growth pattern was par-

tially compensated by a down and forward inclination of the maxillary base. The axial inclination of the incisors was average. Crowding was apparent in the upper and lower dental arches. A tongue problem had persisted with a finger-sucking habit until 6 years.

Serial extraction procedures (including first premolar sacrifice) were instituted with concomitant placement of an activator. The construction bite was established at 5 mm vertically, but the mandible was positioned only slightly anteriorly (2 mm). The treatment objective was to control the neuromuscular malfunction while loading the posterior teeth that had overerupted, freeing the incisors for further eruption un-

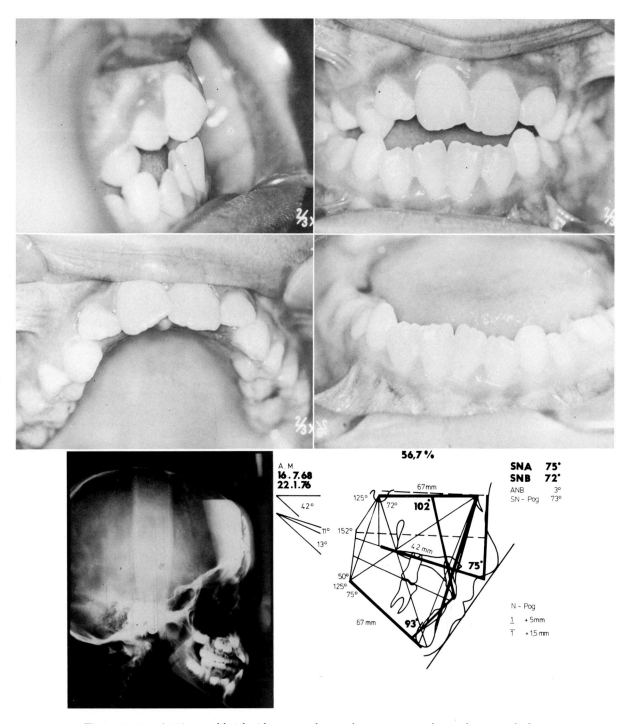

**Figure 22-13.** A 7½-year-old girl with an open bite and a severe vertical growth pattern before treatment. Down and forward tipping of the palatal plane has partially compensated the open bite.

der the guidance of the labial wire of the activator. After the eruption of the canines and premolars, the remaining spaces were closed with fixed multiattachment therapy and intermaxillary traction for the open bite.

At the end of active treatment 3½ years later, despite the dentoalveolar improvement, only a slightly better skeletal relationship had developed. The growth rate of the mandibular base was high, but the ramus remained short (−13.5 mm). The maxillary growth increments were aver-

age. The retroclination of the maxillary base persisted and aided the alveolodental compensation for the original malocclusion (Figure 22-14).

The achievable optimal result of therapy was possible in this case only because of the favorable inclination of the maxillary base and the compromise decision of tooth removal that allowed dentoalveolar compensation. Early interceptive habit control at least prevented exacerbation of the malocclusion by the potentially deforming abnormal function.

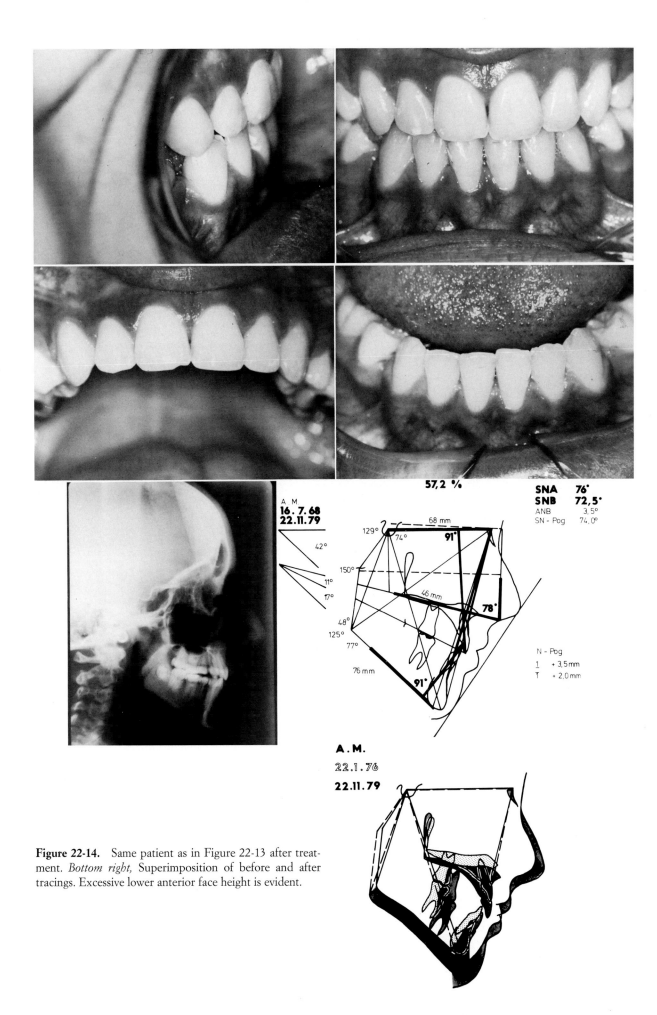

**Figure 22-14.** Same patient as in Figure 22-13 after treatment. *Bottom right,* Superimposition of before and after tracings. Excessive lower anterior face height is evident.

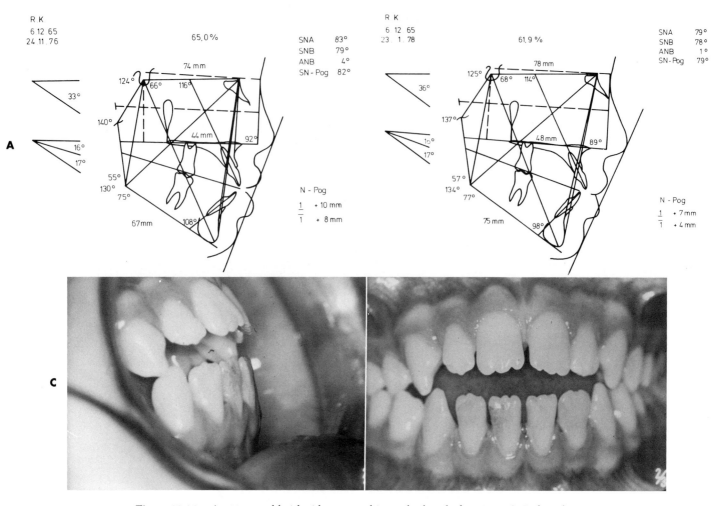

**Figure 22-15.** An 11-year-old girl with an open bite and other dysfunctions. **A,** Before therapy. **B,** After treatment with functional appliances. **C,** Before fixed appliance therapy.

Another example of combined treatment is the attempt to achieve some skeletal improvement and correct dental malrelationships in the second phase of treatment. To illustrate this approach, an 11-year-old girl with an open-bite malocclusion, severe tongue dysfunction problems, and a double protrusion of the incisors is shown in Figure 22-15. The maxilla was prognathic, but the mandible was orthognathic. Although the growth pattern was horizontal, the up and forward inclination of the maxillary base contributed to the open-bite relationship. Treatment was started with an activator, with the following objectives:

1. To intercept and control the abnormal neuromuscular influences
2. To influence the unfavorable upward tipping of the maxillary base and reduce its relative prognathism

The treatment of the double protrusion and the final correction of the open bite were planned for a later treatment phase. A vertical activator was constructed that extended the acrylic over the labial surfaces of the upper and lower incisors

(indexing) and was trimmed away from the acrylic linguoincisally. The posterior teeth were loaded and an occlusal acrylic cover interposed for a depressing action; this procedure was performed because the interocclusal clearance was minimal and the viscoelastic properties of the muscles and the stretch reflex action could be enlisted. After 14 months of activator treatment the protrusion and inclination of the maxillary base were reduced. Labial tipping, of the lower incisors in particular, also was reduced. Posterior segment eruption was thereby withheld.

A second phase of this combination approach required fixed appliances to achieve the final adjustments. This second phase of correction took less than 7 months (Figure 22-16).

## Treatment of Open Bite in the Permanent Dentition

The use of functional methods is limited in the permanent dentition. Usually, multiattachment fixed mechanotherapy is the method of choice, with guided extraction procedures to

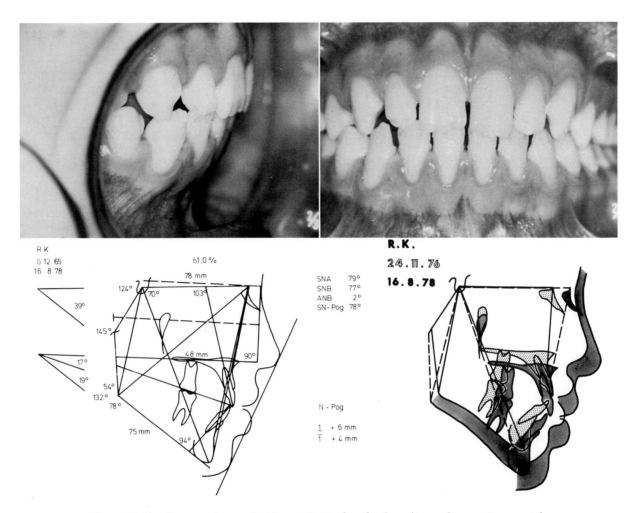

**Figure 22-16.** Same patient as in Figure 22-15 after fixed appliance therapy. *Bottom right,* Superimposition of tracings taken before activator therapy and after fixed appliance therapy.

correct dentoalveolar problems and compensate for any skeletal problems that exist. If the dysfunction persists, functional therapy can play only a subordinate role.

Some minor improvement in the dentoalveolar region can be achieved; for example, a posterior open bite can be closed by screening the tongue from interposing between the occlusal surfaces. A slight anterior open bite also may be reduced, if no crowding is present. A combination of screening and active extrusive force on the incisors (e.g., by using a tongue crib on a palatal plate with an active labial bow) reduces the open bite. Intrusion of posterior teeth is very difficult, however, although initial success with repelling magnetic force appliances appears promising (see Chapter 14).

Functional appliances are helpful in the retention phase of therapy. Interocclusal cover of the posterior teeth prevents relapsing overeruption of the buccal segments, whereas aber-

rant neuromuscular activity is effectively screened from deforming the dentoalveolar region.

Diagnosis is still the primary challenge in these open-bite problems. Indications for any mode of therapy should be determined during the diagnostic period. Both functional and cephalometric analytic assessments are needed before treatment planning is completed. Therapy for some open-bite malocclusions is very simple, and self-improvement may be evident after the elimination of abnormal perioral muscle function. The diagnostic assessment determines whether the case satisfies the criteria for screening therapy. Cases with unfavorable morphogenetic patterns, growth vectors, or patient ages do not respond adequately to functional appliance treatment. Indeed, they are likely to become progressively worse despite appliance wear. However, the fault does not lie with the appliance but with improper diagnosis.

# References and Selected Readings

Adams CP: *The design and construction of removable appliances,* ed 5, Bristol, England, 1984, John Wright & Sons, Ltd.

Adams CP: An investigation into indications for and the effects of the functioning regulator, *Eur Orthod Soc Rep Cong* 45:293, 1969.

Adams CP: Kieferorthopädie mit Herausnehmbaren Geräten, *Berlin Quintessenz Verlag* 1988.

Adams CP: The modified arrowhead clasp, *Trans Br Soc Stud Orthod,* pp. 50-52, 1949.

Adran B, Kemp F: A radiographic study of the movement of the tongue in swallowing, *Dent Prac* 5:252, 1955.

Ahlgren J: Early and late electromyographic response to treatment with the activator, *Am J Orthod* 74:88-92, 1978.

Ahlgren J: An electromyographic analysis of the response to activator (Andresen-Haupl) therapy, *Odontol Rev* 11:125, 1960.

Ahlgren J: A longitudinal clinical and cephalometric study of 50 mal-occlusion cases treated with activator appliances, *Eur Orthod Soc Rep Cong* 48:285, 1972.

Ahlgren J: The neurophysiologic principles of the Andresen method of functional jaw orthopedics. A critical analysis and new hypothesis, *Svensk Tandlak Tidskr* 63:1, 1970.

Ahlgren J: Tongue function during activator treatment. A cephalometric and dynamometric study, *Eur J Orthod* 55:1251, 1979.

Ahlgren J, Posselt U: Need of functional analysis and selective grinding in orthodontics, *Acta Odontol Scand* 21:187, 1963.

Altuna G, Woodside DG: Die Auswirkung von Ausbissblocken in Oberkiefer bei Macaca Rhesus (Vor Laufige Ergebnisse), *Fortschr Kieferorthopädie* 38:391-402, 1977.

Altuna G, Woodside DG: Response of the midface to treatment with increased vertical occlusal forces—treatment and posttreatment effects in monkeys, *Angle Orthod* 55(3):252-263, 1985.

Amoric M: Thermoformed Herbst appliance, *J Clin Orthod* 29:173, 1995.

Andresen V: *Funktions-Kieferorthopädie,* ed 2, Lepzig, 1939, Hermann Meusser.

Andresen V: The Norwegian system of functional gnatho-orthopedics, *Acta Gnathol* 1:5, 1936.

Andresen V: The Norwegian system of gnathological functional orthopedics, *Acta Gnathol* 4:1, 1939.

Andresen V: Über das sogenannte Norwegische System der Funktionskieferorthopadie, *Dtsch Zahnärtzl Wschr,* 1936.

Andresen V, Häupl K: *Funktions-Keiferorthopädie,* Leipzig, 1936, Hermann Neusser.

Andresen V, Häupl K: *Funktionskieferorthopädie. Die Grundlagen des norwegischen Systems,* ed 4, Leipzig, 1945, Johann Ambrosium Barth.

Andresen V, Häupl K, Petrik L: *Funktionskieferorthopädie, VI. Umgearbeitete and erweiterte Auflage von K. Häupl und L. Petrik,* Munich, 1957, Johann Ambrosium Barth.

Andrew RJ: Evolution of facial expression, *Science* 142:1034, 1963.

Andrews LF: The six keys to normal occlusion, *Am J Orthod* 62:296, 1972.

Angelopoulos G: Long-term stability of temporomandibular joint remodeling following continuous mandibular advancement in the juvenile Macaca fascicularis: a histomorphometric, cephalometric and electromyographic investigation, master's thesis, Toronto, 1991, University of Toronto.

Angle EH: Orthodontia, *Dent Cosmos* 11, 1920.

Armstrong MM: Personal communication, 1993.

Ascher F: *Praktische Kieferorthopädie,* Vienna, 1968, Urban & Schwarzenberg.

Auf der Maur HJ: Elektromyographische Befunde am musculus pterygoideus externus während der Distalbisstherapie mit dem Activator, *Schweiz Monatsschr Zahnheilkd* 88:1085, 1978.

Bachraty A, Bachraty L: Klinische Studie zur wirkung des starren offenen Aktivators, *Fortschr Kieferorthop* 55:228, 1994.

Baker J: The tongue and the dental function, *Am J Orthod* 40:927, 1954.

Bakke M, Paulsen HU: Herbst treatment in late adolescence: a clinical, electromyographic, kinesiographic, and radiographic analysis of one case, *Eur J Orthod* 11:397-407, 1989.

Ballard CF: A consideration of the physiological background of mandibular posture and movement, *Dent Pract* 6:80, 1955.

Ballard CF: Some observations on variations of tongue posture as seen in lateral skull radiographs and their significance, *Eur Orthod Soc Trans* 35:69, 1959.

Ballard CF: The significance of soft tissue morphology in diagnosis, prognosis and treatment planning, *Trans Eur Orthod Soc* 29:143-175, 1953.

Ballard CF: Variations of posture and behaviour of the lips and tongue which determine the position of the labial segments: the implications in orthodontics, prosthetics and speech, *Eur Orthod Soc Rep Cong,* p. 67, 1965.

Balters W: *Eine Einführung in die Bionatorheilmethode: ausgewählte Schriften und Vortrage,* Heidelberg, Germany, 1973, H. Herrmann Verlag.

Balters W: Ergebnis der gesteuerten Selbstheilung von kiefer-orthopädischen Anomalien, *Dtsch Zahnaerztl* 15:241, 1960.

Balters W: In Ascher F, editor: *Praktische Kieferorthopädie,* Munich, 1968, Urban & Schwarzenberg.

Balters W: Die Technik und Ubung der allgemeinen und und speziellen Bionator-therapis, *Quintessence* 1:77, 1964.

Baron R: Remaniements de l'os alvéolaire et des fibres desmodontales au cours de la migration physiologique, *J Biol Buccale* 1:151, 1973.

Baume LJ, The post-natal growth activity of the nasal cartilage septum, *Helv Odontol Acta* 5:9, 1961.

Baume LJ, Derichsweiler H: Is the condylar growth center responsive to orthodontic therapy? *Oral Surg* 14:347, 1961.

Baume LJ: Häupl L, Stellmach R: Growth and transformation of the TMJ in an orthopedically treated case of Pierre Robin syndrome, *Am J Orthod* 45:90, 1959.

Baumrind S: A reconsideration of the propriety of the "pressure-tension" hypothesis, *Am J Orthod* 55:12, 1969.

Baumrind S, Buck DL: Rate changes in cell replication and protein synthesis in the periodontal ligament incident to tooth movement, *Am J Orthod* 57:109, 1970.

Baumrind S et al: Changes in facial dimensions associated with the use of forces to retract the maxilla, *Am J Orthod* 80:17-30, 1981.

Baumrind S et al: Mandibular plane changes during maxillary retraction, Part 1, *Am J Orthod* 74:32-40, 1978.

Baumrind S et al: Quantitative analysis of the orthodontic and orthopedic effects of maxillary retraction, *Am J Orthod Dentofac Orthop* 84:384-398, 1983.

Bay R, Rakosi T: Fernröntgenologische Untersuchungen von zwei ethnischen Gruppen mit Distalbiss, *Fortschr Kieferorthop* 32:161, 1971.

Becker JJ: Permanent magnet, *Scient Am* 233:92-100, 1970.

Benninghoff A: Architektur der Kiefer und ihre Weichteilbedeckung, *Paradentium* 6:48, 1934.

Benninghoff A: Funktionalle Anpassung, *Handbuch d. Naturften Fische,* 1933.

Bimler HP: Die Elastichen Gebissformer, *Zahnartzl Welt* 19:499-503, 1949.

Bimler HP: Indikation der Gebissformer, *Fortschr Kieferorthop* 25:121, 1964.

Bimler HP: Stomatopedics in theory and practice, *Int J Orthod* 2:5, 1965.

Bishara SE, Ziaja RR: Functional appliances: a review, *Am J Orthod Dentofac Orthop* 95:250, 1989.

Björk A: *The face in profile,* 1947, Lund.

Björk A: Facial development and tooth eruption, *Am J Orthod* 62:339, 1972.

Björk A: Facial growth in man studied with the aid of metallic implants, *Acta Odontol Scand* 13:94, 1955.

Björk A: Prediction of mandibular growth rotation, *Am J Orthod* 55:585, 1969.

Björk A: The principle of the Andresen method of orthodontic treatment. A discussion based on cephalometric x-ray analysis of treated cases, *Am J Orthod* 37:437, 1951.

Björk A: Sutural growth of the upper face studied by the metallic implant method, *Acta Odontol Scand* 24:109, 1966.

Björk A: Variation in the growth pattern of the human mandible: longitudinal radiographic study by the implant method, *J Dent Res* 42:400-411, 1963.

Björk A, Helm S: Prediction of the age of maximum pubertal growth in body height, *Angle Orthod* 37:134-143, 1967.

Björk A, Skieller V: Normal and abnormal growth of the mandible. A synthesis of longitudinal and cephalometric implant studies over a period of 25 years, *Eur J Orthod* 5:1, 1983.

Blackwood HO: Clinical management with the Jasper Jumper, *J Clin Orthodont* 25:755-760, 1991.

Blechman AM: Magnetic force systems in orthodontics. Clinical results of a pilot study, *Am J Orthod* 87:201-210, 1985.

Blechman AM, Smiley M: Magnetic forces in orthodontics, *Am J Orthod* 74:435-443, 1978.

Bluestone CD: The role of tonsils and adenoids in the obstruction of respiration. In McNamara JA, Jr., editor: *Nasorespiratory function and craniofacial growth,* Monograph 9, Craniofacial Growth Series, Ann Arbor, Mich, 1979, Center of Human Growth and Development, University of Michigan.

Blume DG: A study of occlusal equilibration as it relates to orthodontics, *Am J Orthod* 44:575, 1958.

Bolmgran GA, Moshiri F: Bionator treatment in Class II div. 1, *Angle Orthod* 56:255, 1986.

Boman VR: Research studies on the temporomandibular joint, *Angle Orthod* 22:154, 1952.

Bondemark L: Orthodontic magnets: a study of force and field pattern, biocompatibility and clinical effects, *Swed Dent J Supp* 99:1-198, 1994.

Bondemark L, Kurol J, Wennberg A: Biocompatibility of new, clinically used, and recycled orthodontic samarium-cobalt magnets, *Am J Orthod Dentfac Orthop* 105:568-574, 1994.

Bookstein FL: Comment on "Issues related to the prediction of craniofacial growth," *Am J Orthod* 79:442, 1981.

Bookstein FL: The inappropriateness of scientific methods in orthodontics. In Hunter WS, Carlson FS, editors: *Essays in honor of Robert Moyers,* Monograph 24, Craniofacial Growth Series, Ann Arbor, Mich, 1991, Center for Human Growth and Development, University of Michigan.

Bourauel C et al: Das funktionskieferorthopädische Magnetsystem (FMS) nach Vardimon. Teil l. Dreidimensionale Analyse des Kraftsystems anziehender Magnete, *Fortschr Kieferorthop* 56:274-282, 1995.

Brauer JS: Holt TV: Tongue thrust classification, *Angle Orthod* 35:106, 1965.

Breads PR: The Herbst appliance, *Quintessence Dent Tech* 8:249-253, 1984.

Breitner C: Bone changes resulting from experimental orthodontic treatment, *Am J Orthod Oral Surg* 26:521, 1940.

Breitner C: Experimentelle Veränderung der mesiodistalen Beziehungen der oberen and unteren Zahnreihen, *Z Stomatol* 28:134, 1930.

Bringham G et al: Antigenic differences among condylar, epiphyseal, and nasal septal cartilage. In McNamara JA, Jr., editor: *The biology of occlusal development,* Monograph 7, Craniofacial Growth Series, Ann Arbor, Mich, 1977, Center of Human Growth and Development, University of Michigan.

Broadbent BH, Broadbent BH, Jr., Golden W: *Bolton standards of dentofacial development and growth,* St Louis, 1975, Mosby.

Broadbent JM: Crossroads: acceptance or rejection of functional jaw orthopedics, *Am J Orthod Dentofac Orthop* 92:75, 1987.

Brodie AG: On the growth pattern of the human head from the third month to the eighthh year of life, *Am J Anat* 68:209, 1941.

Brodie AG: Some recent observations of the growth of the face and their implications to the orthodontist, *Am J Orthod Oral Surg* 26:741, 1940.

Burstone CJ: Lip posture and its significance in treatment planning, *Am J Orthod* 53:262, 1967.

Bushey R: Personal communication, July 1996.

Carels C, Van der Linden FPGM: Concepts on functional appliances mode of action, *Am J Orthod Dentofac Orthop* 92:162-168, 1987.

Case C: Open-bite malocclusion, *Dent Rev,* July 1894.

Cash RG: Case report: adult nonextraction treatment with a Jasper Jumper, *J Clin Orthod* 25:43-47, 1991.

Cederquist KR, Virolainen K: Craniofacial growth in the squirrel monkey (*Saimiri sciureus*), *Am J Orthod* 69:592, 1976.

Celestin LA: *La thérapeutic Bionator de Wilhelm Balters,* Paris, 1967, Librairie Meloine Sa.

Cerny R: The biological effects of implanted magnetic fields. Part II, mammalian tissues, *Aust J Orthod* 6:114-117, 1980a.

Cerny R: The reaction of dental tissues to magnetic fields, *Aust J Dent* 25:264-268, 1980b.

Champagne M: Herbst appliance therapy related to the mandibular plane angle, *Function Orthod* 6:17-21, 1989.

Chang HW, Cheng K, Cheng M: Effect of activator treatment on Class II div. 1 malocclusion, *J Clin Orthod* 23:560, 1989.

Charlier JP, Petrovic A: *Lack of independent growth potential of rat mandibular condylar cartilage, as revealed in organ culture,* Philadelphia, 1967a, Tissue Culture Association.

Charlier JP, Petrovic A: Recherches sur la mandibule de rat en culture d'organes: le cartilage condylien a-t-il un potentiel de croissance indépendant? *Orthod Fr* 38:165, 1967b.

Charlier JP, Petrovic A, Herrmann J: Déterminisme de la croissance mandibulaire: effets de l'hyperpropulsion et de l'hormone somatotrope sur la croissance condylienne de jeunes rates, *Orthod Fr* 39:567, 1968.

Charlier JP, Petrovic A, Hermann-Stutzmann J: Effects of mandibular hyperpropulsion on the prechondroblastic zone of young rat condyle, *Am J Orthod* 55:71, 1969a.

Charlier JP, Petrovic A, Linck G: La fronde mentonnière et son action sur la croissance mandibulaire. Recherches expérimentales chez le rat, *Orthod Fr* 40:99, 1969b.

Chateau M: Traitement de la retrognatie mandibulaire par l'hyperpropulsion systématique, *Orthod Fr* 36:637, 1955.

Chin GY: New magnetic alloys, *Science* 2108:888-894, 1980.

Clark WJ: *Aspects of twin block functional therapy in orthodontics and dentofacial orthopedics,* doctoral thesis, Dundee, Scotland, 1994, University of Dundee.

Clark WJ: *Magnetic twin block appliances.* Poster clinic presented at the European orthodontics Society meeting, 1990.

Clark WJ: *The twin block technique: applications in dentofacial orthopedics,* London, 1995, Mosby-Wolfe.

Clark WJ: The twin bock technique—a functional orthopedic appliance system, *Am J Orthod Dentofac Orthop* 93:1-18, 1988.

Clark WJ: The twin block traction technique, *Eur J Orthod* 4:129-138, 1982.

Clark WJ, Stirrups DR: A coomaprison of the failure rate of the modified arrowhead clasp and the delta clasp for the retention of the Clark twin bock appliance, *Br J Orthod,* 1995.

Cleall JF: Deglutition: a study of form and function, *Am J Orthod* 51:560, 1965.

Cleall JF; Growth of the palate and maxillary dental arch, *J Dent Res* 53:226, 1974.

Courtney M, Harkness M, Herbison P: Maxillary cranial base changes during treatment with functional appliances, *Am J Orthod Dentofac Orthop* 109:616, 1996.

Craig CE: The skeletal pattern characteristics of Class I and Class II, division, 1, malocclusion in norma lateralis, *Angle Orthod* 21:44, 1951.

Darendeliler MA, Joho JP: Class II bimaxillary protrusion treated with magnetic forces, *J Clinic Orthod* 26:361-368, 1992.

Darendeliler MA, Joho JP: Magnetic activator device II (MAD II) for correction of Class II Division I malocclusions, 103:223-239, 1993.

Dausch-Neuman U: Biometgesicht und Kieferheilkunde, *Fortschr Keiferorthop* 32:353, 1971.

Davies PL: Electromyographic study of superficial neck muscles in mandibular function, *J Dent Res* 58:537, 1979.

Decrue A, Wieslander L: Veränderunger der Fossa articularis nach Vorverlagerung der Mandibula mittels Herbstapparatur, *Zahnärztl Prax* 10:360-365, 1990.

Delaire J: La croissance des os de la voûte du crâne. Principes généraux (introduction à l'étude de la croissance des maxillaires), *Rev Stomatol Chir Maxillofac* 62:518, 1961.

Delaire J: The potential role of facial muscles in monitoring maxillary growth and morphogenesis. In Carlson DS, McNamara JA, Jr., editors: *Muscle adaptation in the craniofacial region,* Monograph 8, Craniofacial Growth Series, Ann Arbor, Mich, 1978, Center of Human Growth and Development, University of Michigan.

Delaire J, Chateau JP: Comment le septum nasal influence-t-il la croissance premaxillaire et maillaire? Déduction en chirurgie des fentes labiomaxillaires, *Rev Stomatol* 78:241, 1977.

Delaire J et al: Quelques résultats des tractions extra-orales à appui fronto-mentonnier dans le traitement orthopédique des malformations maxillo-mandibulaires de Class III et des séquelles osseuses des fentes labio-maxillaires, *Rev Stomatol Chir Maxillofac* 73:633, 1972.

Demisch A: Effects of activator therapy on the craniofacial skeleton in Class II, Division 1, malocclusion, *Eur Orthod Soc Rep Cong,* p. 295, 1972.

Demisch A: Langzeitbeobchtungen über die Stabilität der Okklusion nach Distalbisstherapie mit dem Berner Aktivator, *Schweiz Monatsschr Zahneilkd* 90:867, 1980.

Demner LM: Nassibulin GG: Kiefergelenkumbau bei der Behandlung sagittaler Bissanomalien, *Stomatol DDR* 27:693, 1977.

DeVincenzo JP: Changes in mandibular length before, during and after successful orthopedics correction, *Am J Orthod Dentofac Orthop* 99:241, 1991.

De Vincenzo JP, Huffer R, Winn M: A study in human subjects using a new device designed to mimic the protrusive functional appliances used previously in monkeys, *Am J Orthod Dentofac Orthop* 91:213-224, 1987.

De Vincenzo JP, Winn MW: Orthodontics and orthopedics effect resulting from the use of functional appliances, *Am J Orthod Dentofac Orthop* 96:181, 1989.

Dickson GC et al: Symposium on functional therapy, *Dent Prac* 15:255, 1965.

Downs WB: The role of cephalometrics in orthodontic case analysis and diagnosis, *Am J Orthod* 38:162, 1952.

Drage KJ: Overjet relapse following functional appliance therapy, *Br J Orthod* 17:205, 1990.

Droschl H: The effect of heavy orthopedic forces on the maxilla in the growing *Saimiri sciureus* (squirrel monkey), *Am J Orthod* 63:449, 1973.

Easton JW, Carlson DS: Adaptation of the lateral pterygoid and superficial masseter muscles to mandibular protrusion in the rat, *Am J Orthod Dentofac Orthop* 97:149-158, 1990.

Eckhardt L, Kanitz G, Harzer W: Veranderungen bei Klasse II Behandlung mit dem offenen Aktivator nach Klammt, *Fortschr Kieferorthop* 56:339, 1995.

Egermark I et al: A longitudinal study on malocclusion in relation to signs and symptoms of craniomandibular disorders in children and adolescents, *Eur J Orthod* 12:339-407, 1990.

Egermark I, Thilander B: Craniomandibular disorders with special reference to orthodontic treatment: an evaluation from childhood to adulthood, *Am J Orthod Dentofac Orthop* 101(1):28-34, 1992.

Egermark-Eriksson I, Carlsson GE, Ingervall B: Function and dysfunction of the masticatory system in individuals with dual bite, *Eur J Orthod* 1:107-117, 1979.

Eirew H: Dynamic functional appliances, *Trans BR Soc Stud Orthod* 19:287, 1969.

Elgoyen JC et al: Craniofacial adaptation to protrusive function in young rhesus monkeys, *Am J Orthod* 62:469-480, 1972.

Enlow D: *Handbook of facial growth,* ed 2, Phildelphia, 1982, Saunders.

Eschler J: *Die funktionelle Orthopädie des Kausystems,* Munich, 1952, Leonhard Hanser.

Eschler J: Die muskuläre Wirkungsweise des Andresen-Häuplschen Apparates, *Oesteer Z Stomatol* 49:79, 1952.

Falk F: Vergleichende Untersuchungen über die Entwicklung der apical Basis nach kieferorthopädischer Behandlung mit der aktiven Platten und dem Funktionsregler, *Fortschr Kieferorthop* 30:225, 1969.

Falk F, Fränkel R: Clinical relevance of step-by-step mandibular advancement in the treatment of mandibular retrusion using the Fränkel appliance, *Am J Orthod Dentofac Orthop* 96:333-341, 1989.

Fox J: *Natural history of the human teeth,* London, 1803, Cox.

Fränkel R: The applicability of the occipital reference base in cephalometrics, *Am J Orthod* 77:379, 1980a.

Fränkel R: A functional approach to orofacial orthopaedics, *Br J Orthod* 7:41, 1980b.

Fränkel R: The functional matrix and its practical importance in orthodontics, *Eur Orthod Soc Rep Cong* 18:207, 1969a.

Fränkel R: *Funktionskieferorthopädie und der Mundvorhof als apparative Basis,* Berlin, 1967, V.E.B. Verlag Volk & Gesundheit.

Fränkel R: The guidance of eruption without extraction, *Eur Orthod Soc Rep Cong* 47:3031971.

Fränkel R: Lip seal training in the treatment of the skeletal open bite, *Eur J Orthod* 2:219, 1980c.

Fränkel R: Maxillary retrusion in Class III and treatment with the function corrector III, *Eur Orthod Soc Rep Cong* 46:249, 1970.

Fränkel R: The practical meaning of the functional matrix in orthodontics, *Eur Orthod Soc Rep Cong* 45:207, 1969b.

Fränkel R: *Technik und Handhabung der Funktionsregler,* Berlin, 1973, V.E.B. Verlag Volk & Gesundheit.

Fränkel R: The theoretical concept underlying treatment with function correctors, *Eur Orthod Soc Rep Cong* 42:233, 1966.

Fränkel R: The treatment of Class II Division I malocclusions with functional correctors, *Am J Orthod* 57:265-275, 1969c.

Fränkel R, Fränkel C: A functional approach to treatment of skeletal open bite, *Am J Orthod* 84:54, 1983.

Fränkel R, Fränkel C: *Orofacial orthopedics with the function regulator,* Munich, 1989, S. Karger.

Fraser ED: *A pilot study on the evaluation of short-term effects of Jasper Jumper therapy,* master's thesis, Loma Linda, Calif, 1992, Loma Linda University.

Frass K: Die Kieferorthopädie in der Zahntechnik, *Verlag Neuer Merkur GmbH* 311-325, 1992.

Freunthaller P: Cephalometric observations in Class II, Division 1, malocclusions treated with the activator, *Angle Orthod* 37:18, 1967.

Frislid G, Rakosi T: Analysen und Ergebnisse nach Headgearbehandlung, *Fortschr Kieferorthop* 37:184, 1976.

Ganz C: *Moyers growth seminar,* Ann Arbor, Mich, February 1996, University of Michigan.

Gasson N: *Les rotations de croissance des deux maxillaires: études céphalométrique sui matériel avec implants et confrontation avec les données expérimentales,* doctoral thesis, Strasbourg, France, 1977a, Université Louis-Pasteur.

Gasson N: Utilisation des implants métalliques dans l'étude céphalométrique de la croissance: l'application à l'analyse des rotations de la face, *Orthod Fr* 48:289, 1977b.

Gasson N, Lavergne J: Maxillary rotation during human growth: variations and correlations with mandibular rotation, *Acta Odontol Scand* 35:13, 1977b.

Gasson N, Lavergne J: Maxillary rotation: its relation to the cranial bse and the mandibular corpus. An implant study, *Acta Odontol Scand* 35:89, 1977a.

Gasson N, Petrovic A: Mécanismes et régulation de la croissance antéro-postérieure du maxillair supérieur. Recherches expérimentales chez le jeune rat, sur le rôle de l'hormone somatotroe et du cartilage de la cloison nasale, *Orthod Fr* 43:271, 1972.

Gasson N, Stutzmann JJ: Petrovic A: Les mécanismes régulateurs de l'ajustement occlusal intervieeent: ils dans le contrôle de la croissance du cartilage condylien? Expériences d'administration d'hormone somatotrope et de résection du cartilage septal chez le jeune rat, *Orthod Fr* 46:77, 1975.

Geering-Gaerny M, Rakosi T: Initialsymptome von Kiefergelenkstörungen bei Kindern im Alter von 8-14 Jahren, *Schweiz Monatsschr Zahnheilkd* 81:691, 1971.

Gianelly AA: Force-induced changes in the vascularity in the periodontal ligament, *Am J Orthod* 55:5, 1969.

Gianelly AA et al: Mandibular growth, condylar position and the Frankel appliance, *Angle Orthod* 53:131, 1983.

Gianelly AA: One-phase versus two-phase treatment, *Am J Orthod Dentofac Orthop* 108:556, 1995.

Gibbs CH, Mahan PE: Brehnan K: Occlusal forces during chewing: influence on biting strength and food consistency, *J Prosthet Dent* 46:561-567, 1981.

Gibbs CH et al: Comparison of typical chewing patterns in normal children and adults, *J Am Dent Assoc* 105:33042, 1982.

Graber LW: The alterability of mandibular growth. In McNamara JA, Jr., editor: *Determinants of mandibular form and growth,* Monograph 4, Craniofacial Growth Series, Ann Arbor, Mich, 1975, Center of Human Growth and Development, University of Michigan.

Graber LW: *The variability of treatment response in 50 treated Frankel appliance cases,* Boston, May 1983a, American Association of Orthodontists.

Graber TM: A critical review of clinical cephalometric radiography, *Am J Orthod* 40:1, 1954.

Graber TM: Evolution of the concepts underlying craniofacial growth. In McNamara JA, Jr., et al, editors: *Clinical alteration of the growing face,* Monograph 13, Craniofacial Growth Series, Ann Arbor, Mich, 1983b, Center for Human Growth and Development, University of Michigan.

Graber TM: *Experimental and clinical studies of the effect of the Frankel FR appliance in primates and humans,* Boston, May 1983c, American Association of Orthodontists.

Graber TM: Extra-oral force—facts and fallacies, *Am J Orthod* 41(1):490-505, 1955.

Graber TM: Extrinsic factors influencing craniofacial growth. In McNamara JA, Jr., editor: *Determinants of mandibular form and growth,* Monograph 4, Craniofacial Growth Series, Ann Arbor, Mich, 1975, Center for Human Growth and Development, University of Michigan.

Graber TM: Functional appliances: an overview. In Graber TM, Swain BF, editdors: *Orthodontics: current principles and techniques,* St Louis, 1985, Mosby.

Graber TM: *Orthodontics: principles and practice,* ed 3, Philadelphia, 1972, Saunders.

Graber TM: *A study of the congenital cleft palate deformity,* doctoral dissertation, Chicago, 1950, Northwestern University Medical School.

Graber TM: Temporomandibular joint disturbances in the periodontium, *Int J Periodont Restor Dent* 6:8, 1984.

Graber TM: The "three M's": muscles, malformation, and malocclusion, *Am J Orthod* 49:418, 1963.

Graber TM, Chung DBB, Aoba JM: Dentofacial orthopedics versus orthodontics, *J Am Dent Assoc* 75:1145, 1967.

Graber TM, Neumann N: *Removable orthodontic appliances,* ed 2, Philadelphia, 1984, Saunders.

Grude R: Myo-functional therapy. A review of various cases some years after their treatment by the Norwegian system had been completed, *Nor Tannlaegeforen Tid* 62:1, 1952.

Gwynne-Evans E: An analysis of the orofacial structures with special reference to muscle behavior and dental alignment, *Am J Orthod* 40:715, 1954.

Hägg U: Change in mandibular growth direction by means of a Herbst appliance? A case report, *Am J Orthod Dentofac Orthop* 102:456-463, 1992.

Hägg U, Pancherz H: Dentofacial orthopedics in relation to chronological age, growth period, and skeletal development. An analysis of 72 male patients with Class II division 1 malocclusion treated with the Herbst appliance, *Eur J Orthod* 10:169-176, 1988.

Hägg U, Taranger J: Dental development assessed by tooth counts and its correlation to somatic development during puberty, *Eur J Orthod* 6:55-64, 1984.

Hägg U, Taranger J: Skeletal stages of the hand and wrist as indicators of the pubertal growth spurt, *Acta Odont Scand* 38:187-200, 1980.

Hamilton DG: *The expansion-activator system,* Boston, May 1983, American Association of Orthodontists.

Hansen K, Ieamnuseiuk P, Pancherz H: Long-term effects of the Herbst appliance on the dental arches and arch relationships: a biometric study, *Br J Orthod* 22:123-134, 1995.

Hansen K, Pancherz H: Long-term effects of Herbst treatment in relation to normal growth development: a cephalometric study, *Eur J Orthod* 14:285-295, 1992.

Hansen K, Pancherz H, Hägg U: Long-term effects of the Herbst appliance in relation to the treatment growth period. A cephalometric study, *Eur J Orthod* 13:471-481, 1991.

Hansen K, Pancherz H, Petersson A: Long-term effects of the Herbst appliance on the carniomandibular system with special reference to the TMJ, *Eur J Orthod* 12:244-253, 1990.

Harvold EP: *The activator in interceptive orthodontics,* St Louis, 1974, Mosby.

Harvold EP: Primate experiments on oral sensation and morphogenesis, *Trans Eur Orthod Soc,* pp. 431-434, 1973.

Harvold EP: The role of function in the etiology and treatment of malocclusion, *Am J Orthod* 54:883, 1968.

Harvold EP: Vargervik K: Morphogenetic response to activator treatment, *Am J Orthod* 60:478, 1971.

Hasund A: The use of activator in a system employing fixed appliances, *Eur Orthod Soc Rep Cong* 41:329, 1969.

Häupl K: *Gewebsumbau und Zahnveränderung in der Funktionskieferorthopädie,* Leipzig, 1938, Johann Ambrosius Barth.

Hauser E: Functional orthodontic treatment with the activator, *Eur Orthod Soc Trans,* p. 427, 1973.

Hauser E: Variationskombinationen im Aufbau des Gesichtsschädels, *Fortschr Kieferorthop* 32:425, 1971.

Held AJ, Spirgi M, Cimasoni G: AN orthopedically treated adult case of Class II malocclusion, *Am J Orthod* 49:761-765, 1963.

Henry H: An experimental study of external force application to the maxillary complex. In McNamara JA, Jr., editor: *Factors affecting the growth of the midface,* Monograph 6, Craniofacial Growth Series, Ann Arbor Mich, 1976, Center for Human Growth and Development, University of Michigan.

Herbst E: *Atlas und Grundis der Zahnärztlichen Orthopadie,* Munich, 1910, JF Lehmann Verlag.

Herbst E; Dreissigjährige Erfahrungen mit dem Retentionsscharnier, *Zahnärztl Rundschau* 43:1515, 1934.

Herren P: The activator's mode of action, *Am J Orthod* 45:512, 1959.

Herren P: Die Wirkungsweise des Aktivators, *Schweiz Monatsschr Zahnheilkd* 63:829, 1953.

Heusner A, Petrovic A: Appareil de culture d'organes en milieu liquide continuellement oxygéné, *Med Electron Biol* 2:381, 1964.

Hickham JH: Activators for the fixed appliance orthodontist, *J Clin Orthod* 14:529, 1980.

Hickham JH: *Combined extraoral force and activator systems,* continuing education course, Chicago, June 1982, Kenilworth Research Foundation, University of Chicago.

Hiniker JJ, Ramfjord SP: Anterior displacement of the mandible in adult rhesus monkeys, *J Dent Res* 43(suppl):811, 1964.

Hiniker JJ, Ramfjord SP: Anterior displacement of the mandible in adult rhesus monkeys, *J Prosthet Dent* 16:503, 1966.

Hirschfelder U, Fleischer-Peters A: Funktionelle Behandlung des tiefen Bisses, *Fortschr Kieferorthop* 53:313, 1992.

Hirschfelder U, Fleischer-Peters A: Kritische Bewertung funktionskieferorthopadischer Klasse II Anomalien, *Fortschr Kieferorthop* 54:273, 1993.

Hirzel HC, Grewe JM: Activators: a practical approach, *Am J Orthod* 6:557, 1974.

Hockenjos C et al: Fernröntgenologischer und klinischer Befund bei erschwerter Nasenatmung, *Fortschr Kieferorthop* 35:391, 1974.

Holdaway RA: Soft-tissue cephalometric analysis and its use in orthodontic treatment, *Am J Orthod* 84:1, 1983.

Holdaway RA: *The "VTO,"* Houston, 1976, University of Texas.

Hopkin GB: Neonatal and adult tongue dimensions, *Angle Orthod* 37:132, 1967.

Hotz R: Application and appliance manipulation of functional forces, *Am J Orthod* 58:459, 1970a.

Hotz R: Guidance of eruption versus serial extraction, *Am J Orthod* 58:1, 1970b.

Hotz R: *Orthodontia in everyday practice,* ed 1, Bern, 1961, Hans Huber AG.

Hotz R: *Orthodontics in daily practice: possibilities and limitations in the area of children's dentistry,* ed 5, Baltimore, 1980, Williams and Wilkins.

Houston WJB: The current status of facial growth prediction: a review, *Br J Orthod* 6:11, 1979.

How RP: The acrylic splint Herbst: problem solving, *J Clin Orthod* 18:497-501, 1984.

How RP: The bonded Herbst appliance, *Am J Orthod* 16:663-667, 1982.

How RP: Lower premolar extraction/removable plastic Herbst treatment for mandibular retrognathia, *Am J Orthod Dentofac Orthop* 92:275-285, 1987.

How RP: Updating the bonded Herbst appliance, *J Clin Orthod* 17:122-124, 1983.

Humphreys E: An improved method for determining calcium 45 in biological materials, *Int J Appl Rad Isot* 16:345, 1965.

Ingreval B, Bitsanis E: Function of masticatory muscles during initial phase of activator treatment, *Eur J Orthod* 8:172, 1986.

Isaacson RJ et al: Effect of rotational jaw growth on the occlusion and profile, *Am J Orthod* 72:276, 1977.

Jacobsson SO: Cephalometric evaluation of treatment effect on Class II, Division 1, malocclusions, *Am J Orthod* 53:446, 1967.

Jacobsson SO, Paulin G: The influence of activator treatment on skeletal growth in Angle Class II div. 1 cases, *Eur J Orthod* 12:174, 1990.

Jann GR, Jann HW: Orofacial muscle imbalance, *J Am Dent Assoc* 65:767, 1962.

Janson I: Cephalometric study of the efficiency of the Bionator, *Eur Orthod Soc Rep Cong* 54:283, 1978a.

Janson I: Skeletal and dentoalveolar changes in patients treated with a Bionator during prepubertal and pubertal growth. In McNamara JA, Jr., Ribbens KA, How RP, editors: *Clinical alteration of the growing face,* Monograph 14, Craniofacial Growth Series, Ann Arbor, Mich, 1983, Center for Human Growth and Development, University of Michigan.

Janson I: *Skelettale und dentoalveolare Anderungen durch die Bionatorebehndlung in der vorpubertaren und pubertären Wachstumszeit,* Berlin, 1982, Quintessenz Verlag.

Janson I: Skelettale und dentoalveolare Anderungen durch die Bionatorbehandlung in der vorpubertaren Wachstumzeit, *Fortschr Kieferorthop* 39:62, 1978b.

Janson I, Hasund A: Indikation und Grenzen der Funktionskieferorthopädie in der taglichen Praxis. In *Deutscher Zahnärztekalender Ketterl,* Munich, 1979, Carl Hanser Verlag.

Janzen E, Bluher J: The cephalometric, anatomic, and histologic changes in *Macaca mulatta* after application of a continuous acting reaction force on the mandible, *Am J Orthod* 51:823, 1965.

Jarabak JR, Fizzel JA: *Light-wire edgewise appliance,* St Louis, 1972, Mosby.

Jasper JJ: *The Jasper Jumper—a fixed functional appliance,* Sheboygan, Wisc, 1987, American Orthondontics.

Joho JP: Changes in form and size of the mandible in the orthopaedically treated *Macaca irus* (an experimental study), *Eur Orthod Soc Rep Cong* 44:161, 1968.

Joho JP, Derendeliler MA: Correction of Class II/I malocclusions with the help of a magnetic field. In Hosl E, Baldauf A, editors: *Mechanical & biological basic in orthodontic therapy,* Heidelberg, Germany, 1991, Huthig.

Johnston LE, Jr.: The functional matrix hypothesis: reflections in a jaundiced eye. In McNamara JA, Jr., editor: *Factors affecting the growth of the midface,* Monograph 6, Craniofacial Growth Series, Ann Arbor Mich, 1976, Center for Human Growth and Development, University of Michigan.

Johnston LE, Jr.: Personal communication, 1983.

Jonas I: Die Auswirkungen des Übungseffektes auf die Genauigkeit Röntgenkephalometrischer Durchzeichnungen in der Kieferorthopädie, *Radiologe* 16:427, 1976.

Jonas I: Histomorphologische Untersuchungen über das destruktive und restitutive Verhalten des Ligamentum parodontale unter kieferorthopädischen Zahnbewegungen, *Fortschr Keiferorthop* 39:398, 1978.

Jonas I: Die Reaktionsweise des Parodonts auf Kraftapplikation, *Fortschr Kieferorthop* 41:228, 1980.

Jonas I, Debrunner M, Rakosi T: Wirkungsweise abnehmbarer Behandlungsmittel, *Fortschr Kieferorthop* 37:277, 1976.

Jonas I, Mann W, Münker G: Relationship between tubal function, craniofacial morphology and disorders of deglutition, *Arch Otorhinolaryngol* 218:151, 1978.

Jonas I, Mann W, Schlenter W: Hals-Nasen-Ohren-ärztliche Befunde beimm offenen Biss, *Fortschr Kieferorthop* 43:127, 1982.

Jonas I, Schlenter W, Mann W: The effect of the perforated vestibular screen on nasal respiration, *Eur J Orthod* 5:59, 1983.

Kawata T et al: A new orthodontic force system of magnetic brackets, *Am J Orthod Dentofac Orthop* 92:241-248, 1987.

Kingler E: *Étude de l'ostéoclasie alvéolaire par contrainte,* doctoral thesis, Paris, 1971, Faculté de Médecine de Paris.

Kingsley NW: *Oral deformities,* New York, 1880, D. Appleton & Son.

van der Klaauw CJ: Cerebral skull and facial skull, *Arch Neerl Zool* 7:16, 1946.

Klammt G: Der offene Aktivator, *Stomatol DDR* 5:332, 1955.

Kloehn SJ: Analysis and treatment in mixed dentitions, a new approach, *Am J Orthod* 39:161-186, 1953.

Komposch G: *Reaktionsfähigkeit temporomandibulären Strukturen auf kieferorthopädische Massnahem. Eine Tierexperimentelle Studie,* doctoral thesis, Brisgau, Germany, 1978, Albert-Ludwigs-Universität zu Freiburg.

Komposch G, Hockenjos C: Die Reaktionsfähigkeit des temporomandibulären Knorpels, *Fortschr Kieferorthop* 38:121, 1979.

Korkhaus G: Die Auswertung des Fernröntgenbildes in der Kieferorthopädie, *Dtsch Zahn Mund Kieferheilkd* 3:714, 1936.

Kortsch WE: The tongue and its implications in Class II malocclusions, *J Wisc Dent Soc* 41:261, 1965.

Koski K: Analysis of profile roentgenograms by means of a new "circle" method, *Dent Rec* 73:704, 1953.

Koski K: Cranial growth centers: facts or fallacies? *Am J Orthod* 54:566, 1968.

Kraus F: *Prevence a náprava vyojových nad orofacialní soustavy,* Prague, 1856, Verlag SZN.

Kreiborg S et al: Craniofacial growth in a case of congenital muscular dystrophy. A roentgenographic and electromyographic investigation, *Am Orthod* 74:207, 1978.

Krogman WM, Sassouni V: *Syllabus in roentgenographic cephalometry,* Philadelphia, 1957, Center of Research in Child Growth.

Kuhn TS: *The structure of scientific revolutions,* Chicago, 1962, University of Chicago.

Kühn U, Rakosi T: Palatographische Untersuchungen der Beziehungen zwischen Zungenlage und Dysgnathien an 30 Patienten der Angle Klasse II, 1, *Fortschr Kieferorthop* 36:474, 1975.

Kühn U, Rakosi T: Palatographische Untersuchungen über den Einfluss kieferorthopädisher Apparate auf die Zungenlage, *Fortschr Kieferorthop* 38:36, 1977.

Kühne K, Jonas I, Rakosi T: Weichteilmorphologie bei der Progenie, *Fortschr Kieferorthop* 36:474, 1975.

Kuster R, Ingervall B, Bürgin W: Laboratory and intra-oral tests of the degradation of elastic chains, *Eur J Orthod* 8:202-208, 1986.

Kvam E: A study of the cell-free zone following experimental tooth movement in the rat, *Eur Orthod Soc Rep Cong* 45:419, 1970.

Kvinnsland S: Partial resection of the cartilaginous nasal septum in rats: its influence on growth, *Angle Orthod* 44:135, 1974.

Kydd WL, Neff CW: Frequency of deglutition of tongue thrusters compared to sample population of normal swallowers, *J Dent Res* 43:363-369, 1964.

Lagerstrom LO et al: Dental and skeletal contributions to occlusal correction in patients treated with the high-pull headgear-activator combination, *Am J Orthod Dentofac Orthop* 97:495, 1990.

Langford NM: The Herbst appliance, *J Clin Orthod* 15:558-661, 1981.

Langford NM: Updating fabrications of the Herbst appliance, *J Clin Orthod* 16:173-174, 1982.

Latham RA: Maxillary development and growth: the septopremaxillary ligament, *J Anat* 107:471, 1970.

Lavergne J: Morphogenetic classification of malocclusion as a basis for growth prediction and treatment planning, *Br J Orthod* 9:132, 1982.

Lavergne J, Gasson N: Analysis and classification of the rotational growth pattern without implants, *Br J Orthod* 9:51, 1982.

Lavergne J, Gasson N: Direction and intensity of mandibular rotation in the sagittal adjustment during growth of the jaws, *Scand J Dent Res* 85:193, 1977b.

Lavergne J, Gasson N: Maxillary rotation during human growth, *Acta Odontol Scand* 35:13, 1977.

Lavergne J, Gasson N: A metal implant study of mandibular rotation, *Angle Orthod* 46:144, 1976.

Lavergne J, Gasson N: Operational definitions of mandibular morphogenetic and positional rotations, *Scand J Dent Res* 85:185, 1977.

Lavergne J, Petrovic A: Discontinuities in occlusal relationship and the regulation of facial growth. A cybernetic view, *Eur J Orthod* 5:269, 1983.

Lavergne J, Petrovic A: Pathogenesis and treatment conceptulization of dentofacial malrelations as related to the pattern of occlusal relationship. In Dixon AD, Sarnat BG, editors: *Second international conference on clinical factors and mechanisms influencing bone growth, 1985.*

Lear CSC, Flanagan JB, Moorrees CFA: The frequency of deglutition in man, *Arch Oral Biol* 10:83-99, 1965.

Lemoine C: *Remaniements des maxillaire consécutifs aux transplantations dentaires chez le rat,* doctoral thesis, 1970.

Lemoine C, Charlier JP, Petrovic A: Réaction condylienne à la déviation mandibulaire provoquée chez le rat. Nouvelles donées sur le rôle des facteurs mécaniques dans le croissance mandibulaire, *Orthod Fr* 39:147, 1968.

Lemoine C, Petrovic A: Le marquage à la tetracycline dans les expériences de transplantation dentaires et d'orthodontie chez le rat blanc, *Rev Fr Odontostomatol* 9:1191, 1969.

Lemoine C, Petrovic A, Stutzmann JJ: Inflammatory process of the rat maxilla after molar autotransplantation, *J Dent Res* 49:1175, 1970.

Lewis A, Roche Af, Wagner B: Growth of the mandible during pubescence, *Angle Orthod* 52:325-342, 1982.

Lieb L, Schlagbauer P: Möglichkeiten einer Beeinflussung des Gesichtsschädels am Rhesusaffen, *Fortschr Keiferorthop* 33:113, 1972.

von Limbourg J: The regulations of the embryonic development and the skull, *Acta Morphol Neerl Scand* 7:101, 1968.

von Limbourg J: The role of genetic and local environmental factors in the control of postnatal craniofacial morphogenesis, *Acta Morphol Neerl Scand* 10:37-47, 1972.

Linder-Aronson S: Adenoids—their efforts on mode of breathing and nasal airflow and their relationship to characteristics of the facial skeleton and the dentition, *Acta Otolaryngol* 265(suppl.):1, 1970.

Linder-Aronson S: Effects of adenoidectomy on the dentition and facial skeleton over a period of five years, *Trans Third Int Orthod Cong* pp. 85-100, 1975.

Linder-Aronson S: Respiratory function in relation to facial morphology and the dentition, *Br J Orthod* 6:1, 1979.

Linder-Aronson S, Bäckström A: A comparison between mouth and nose breathers with respect to occulusion and facial dimensions, *Odont Rev* 11:343, 1960.

Linder-Aronson S, Woodside DG, Lundstrom A: Mandibular growth direction following adenoidectomy, *Am J Orthod* 89:273, 1986.

Linge L: Klinische tierexperimentelle Untersuchungen (Korreferat zum Vortrag Petrovic), *Fortschr Keiferorthop* 38:253, 1977.

Livieratos FA, Johnston LE: A comparison of one-stage and two-stage non-extraction alternatives in matched Class II samples, *Am J Orthod Dentofac Orthop* 108:118, 1995.

Logan WR: The clinical management of the Frankel appliance. The FR 1, *Trans Br Soc Stud Orthod* 21:205, 1971.

Logan WR: The vestibular appliance, *Trans Br Soc Stud Orthod* 19:287, 1969.

Lowe AA et al: The effect of the tongue retaining device on awake genioglossus muscle activity in patients with obstructive sleep apnea, *Am J Orthod Dentofac Orthop* 110(1):28-35, 1996.

Luder HU: Effects of activator treatment—evidence for the occurrence of two different types of reaction, *Eur J Orthod* 3:205, 1981.

Lundström A: *Malocclusion of the teeth regarded as a problem in connection with the apical base,* Stockholm, 1923.

Lundström A, Woodside DG: Longitudinal changes in facial type in cases with vertical and horizontal mandibular growth direction, *Eur J Orthod* 5:259, 1983.

Macapanpan LC, Weinmann JP, Brodie AG: Early tissue changes following tooth movement in rats, *Angle Orthod* 24:79, 1954.

Mamandras AH, Allen LP: Mandibular response to orthodontic treatment with the Bionator appliance, *Am J Orthod Dentofac Orthop* 97:113-120, 1990.

Mandelbrot BB: *The fractal geometry of nature,* San Francisco, 1982, W.H. Freeman.

Manns A, Miralles R, Guerrero F: The changes in electrical activity of the postural muscles of the mandible upon varying the vertical posture, *J Prosthet Dent* 45:438-445, 1981.

Margolis HI: Personal communications, July 1976, August 1983.

Markostamou K: *Contribution à l'étude des réactions de l'os alvéolaire au cours du déplacement orthodontique expérimental,* doctoral thesis, Paris, 1974, Faculté de Médecine de Paris.

Markostamou K, Baron R: Étude quantitative de l'ostéoclasie sur la paroi alvéolaire au cours de l'orthodontie expérimentale chez le rat, *Orthod Fr* 44:245, 1973.

Marschner JF, Harris JE: Mandibular growth and Class Ii treatment, *Angle Orthod* 36:89, 1966.

Martin JR: The stability of the anterior teeth after treatment, *Am J Orthod* 48:788, 1948.

Martin R, Sauer K: *Lehrbuch der Anthropologie,* ed 6, Stuttgart, 1957, Gustav Fischer Verlag.

Mason RM, Proffit WR: Myofunctional therapy: background and recommendations, *J Speech Hear Disord* 39:115, 1974.

May TW et al: Skeletal and dental changes using a Jasper Jumper appliance, *J Dent Res(IADR Suppl.),* 1992.

McCallin SG: Retraction of maxillary teeth with removable appliances using intermaxillary or extra-oral traction, *Dent Rec* 74:36, 1954.

McDougall PD, McNamara JA, Jr., Dierkes JM: Arch width development in Class II patients treated with the Frankel appliance, *Am J Orthod* 82:10, 1982.

McEwan DC: Some illusory phenomena of importance in orthodontics, *Am J Orthod* 44:46, 1959.

McNamara JA, Jr.: Components of Class II malocclusion in children 8-10 years of age, *Angle Orthod* 51:269, 1981.

McNamara JA, Jr.: Experimentelle Untersuchungen des Unterkieferwachstums, *Inf Orthod Kieferorthop* 3:219-243, 1976.

McNamara JA, Jr.: Fabrication of the acrylic splint Herbst appliance, *Am J Orthod Dentofac Orthop* 94:10-18, 1988.

McNamara JA, Jr.: Functional determinants of craniofacial size and shape, *Eur J Orthod* 2:131-159, 1980.

McNamara JA, Jr.: JCO interviews: Dr. James McNamara on the Frankel appliance, *J Clin Orthod* 14:320, 1980.

McNamara JA, Jr.: Neuromuscular and skeletal adaptations to altered function in the orofacial region, *Am J Orthod* 64:578-606, 1973.

McNamara JA, Jr.: *Neuromuscular and skeletal adaptions to altered orfacial functin,* Monograph 1, Craniofacial Growth Series, Ann Arbor, Mich, 1972, Center for Human Growth and Development, University of Michigan.

McNamara JA, Jr.: On the Fränkel appliance Part 1—Biological basis and appliance design, *J Clin Orthod* 16:320-337, 1982a.

McNamara JA, Jr.: On the Fränkel appliance Part 2—Clinical management, *J Clin Orthod* 16:391-406, 1982b.

McNamara JA, Jr.: On the possibilities of stimulating mandibular growth. In Graber TM, editor: *Orthodontics: state of the art, essence of the science,* St Louis, 1986, Mosby.

McNamara JA, Jr., Bookstein FL, Shaughnessy TG: Skeletal and dental relationships following functional regulator therapy on Class II patients, *Am J Orthod* 88:91, 1985.

McNamara JA, Jr., Bryan FA: Long-term mandibular adaptations to protrusive function: an experimental study in *Macaca mulatta, Am J Orthod Dentofac Orthop* 92:98-108, 1987.

McNamara JA, Jr., Carlson DS: Quantitative analysis of temporomandibular joint adaptations to protrusive function, *Am J Orthod* 76:593, 1979.

McNamara JA, Jr., Connelly TG, McBride MC: Histological studies of temporomandibular joint adaptations. In McNamara JA, Jr., editor: *Control mechanisms in craniofacial growth,* Monograph 3, Craniofacial Growth Series, Ann Arbor, Mich, 1975, Center for Human Growth and Development, University of Michigan.

McNamara JA, Jr., How RP: Clinical management of the acrylic splint Herbst appliance, *Am J Orthod Dentofac Orthop* 94:142-149, 1988.

McNamara JA, Jr., How RP, Dischinger TG: A comparison of the Herbst and Fränkel treatment in Class II malocclusion, *Am J Orthod Dentofac Orthop* 98:134-144, 1990.

McNamara JA, Jr., Huge SA: The Fränkel appliance, *Am J Orthod* 80:478, 1981.

McNamara JA, Jr., Riolo MI, Enlow DH: Growth of the maxillary complex in the rhesus monkey *(Macaca mulatta), Am J Phys Antrhopol* 44:15, 1976.

Meach CL: A cephalometric comparison of bony profile changes in Class II, Division 1 patients treated with extraoral force and functional jaw orthopaedics, *Am J Orthod* 52:353, 1966.

Melson B, Melsen F, Moss ML: Postural development of the nasal septum studied on human autopsy material. In Carlson DS, editor: *Craniofacial biology,* Monograph 10, Craniofacial Growth Series, Ann Arbor, Mich, 1981, Center for Human Growth and Development, University of Michigan.

Merrifield L, Cross J: *The Kloehn headgear effect,* audiovisual series, Chicago, 1961, American Association of Orthodontists.

Milhorn HT: *The application of control theory to physiological systems,* Philadelphia, 1966, Saunders.

Mills CM, Holman RG, Graber TM: Heavy intermittent cervical traction in Class II treatment. A longitudinal cephalometric assessment, *Am J Orthod* 74:361, 1978.

Mills JRE: Clinical control of craniofacial growth: a skeptic view point. In McNamara JA, Jr., editor: *Clinical alteration of the growing face,* Monograph 14, Craniofacial Growth Series, Ann Arbor, Mich, 1983, Center for Human Growth and Development, University of Michigan.

Mills JRE: The effect of functional appliances on skeletal pattern, *Br J Orthod* 18:267-275, 1991.

Mills JRE: The effect of orthodontic treatment on the skeletal pattern, *Br J Orthod* 5:133, 1978.

Mills JRE: The long-term results of the proclination of lower incisors, *Br Dent J* 120:355, 1966.

Mills JRE, Vig KWL: An approach to appliance therapy. II. *Br J Orthod* 2:29, 1975.

Milne JM, Cleall JF: Cinefluorographic study of functional adaptation of the oropharyngeal structures, *Angle Orthod* 40:267, 1970.

Moffett BC: A research perspective on craniofacial morphogenesis, *Acta Morphol Neerl Scand* 10:91, 1972.

Moiroud A: Essai d'utilisation d'une transformation géométrique dans la prévision de la croissance faciale, *Orthod Fr* 52:725, 1981.

Moore RN, Igel KA, Boice PA: Vertical and horizontal components of functional appliance therapy, *Am J Orthod Dentofac Orthop* 96:433-443, 1989.

Moss JP: Cephalometric changes during functional appliance therapy, *Eur Orthod Soc Trans* 38:327, 1962.

Moss ML: The dialectics of craniofacial growth research: Is it time for a new synthesis? In McNamara JA, Jr., Carlson DS, Ribbens KA, editors: *The effect of surgical intervention on craniofacial growth,* Monograph 12, Craniofacial Growth Series, Ann Arbor, Mich, 1982, Center for Human Growth and Development, University of Michigan.

Moss ML: In *First cephalometric workshop,* Cleveland, July 1957, Bolton Brush Foundation.

Moss ML: Functional analysis of human mandibular growth, *J Prosthet Dent* 10:1149, 1960.

Moss ML: The functional matrix. In Kraus BS, Reidel RA, editors: *Vistas in orthodontics,* Philadelphia, 1962, Lea & Febiger.

Moss ML: The pathogenesis of artificial cranial deformation, *Am J Phys Anthropol* 16:269, 1958.

Moss ML: The role of nasal septal cartilage in mid-face. In McNamara JA, Jr., editor: *Factors affecting the growth of the mid-face,* Monograph 6, Craniofacial Growth Series, Ann Arbor, Mich, 1976, Center for Human Growth and Development, University of Michigan.

Moss ML et al: The passive role of nasal septal cartilage in mid-facial growth, *Plast Reconstr Surg* 41:536, 1968.

Moss ML et al: A three dimensional study of treatment with magnetic and non-magnetic twin blocks, *Eur J Orthod* 15:342, 1993.

Moss ML, Salentijn L: The capsular matrix, *Am J Orthod* 56:474, 1969.

Moss ML, Salentijn L: The logarithmic growth of the human mandible, *Acta Anat* 77:341, 1970.

Moss ML, Salentijn L: The primary role of functional matrices in facial growth, *Am J Orthod* 55:566, 1969.

Moss ML et al: Craniofacial growth in space and time. In McNamara JA, Jr., et al, editors: *Craniofacial biology,* Monograph 10, Craniofacial Growth Series, Ann Arbor, Mich, 1981, Center for Human Growth and Development, University of Michigan.

Moyers RE: *Handbook of orthodontics,* ed 3, Chicago, 1973, Year Book Medical.

Moyers RE: The infantile swallow, *Eur Orthod Soc Trans* 40:180, 1964.

Moyers RE: Skeletal contributions to occlusal development. In McNamara JA, Jr., editor: *The biology of occlusal development,* Monograph 7, Craniofacial Growth Series, Ann Arbor, Mich, 1977, Center for Human Growth and Development, University of Michigan.

Moyers RE et al: Experimental production of Class III in rhesus monkeys, *Eur Orthod Soc Rep Cong* 46:61, 1970.

Nelson C, Harkness M, Herbison P: Mandibular changes during functional appliance treatment, *Am J Orthod Dentofac Orthop* 104:153, 1993.

Neumann B: Funktionskieferorthopädie. Rückblick und Ausblick, *Fortschr Kieferorthop* 36:73, 1975.

Noro T, Tanne K, Sakuda M: Orthodontic forces exerted by activators with varying construction bite heights, *Am J Orthod Dentofac Orthop* 105:169, 1990.

O'Bryn BL et al: An evaluation of mandibular asymmetry in adults with unilateral posterior crossbite, *Am J Orthod Dentofac Ortoph* 107:394, 1995.

Oppenheim A: *Die Krise in der Orthodontie,* Berlin, 1933, Urban & Schwarzenberg.

Oppenheim A: Die Krisis in der Orthodontie, *Z Stomatol,* 1933.

Oppenheim A: Tissue changes, particulary of the bone, incident to tooth movement, *Eur Orthod Soc Trans,* pp. 303-359, 1911.

Organ G: An experimental model to study the effects of the functional regulator in the Macaca monkey, diploma thesis, Toronto, 1979, University of Toronto.

O'Ryan F et al: The relation between nasorespiratory function and dentofacial morphology: a review, *Am J Orthod* 82:403, 1982.

Oudet C: *Régulations de la longeur anatomique du muscle ptérygoïdien latéral de jeune rat au cours de la croissance. Variations du nombre de sarcomères en série consécutives à des perutrbations de la posture de la mandibule,* Mémoire de DERBH, Strasbourg, France, 1979a, Université Louis Pasteur.

Oudet C: *Rythmes ncythéméral et saisonnier de la vitesse de croissance du squelette et de la susceptibilité du cartilage condylien de la mandibule àl'égard des dispositifs orthopédiques,* doctoral thesis, Strasbourg, France, 1979b, Université Louis Pasteur.

Oudet C, Petrovic A: Circannual growth variations of the mandibular condylar cartilage in the young rat, *J Interdiscipl Cycle Res* 8:338, 1977a.

Oudet C, Petrovic A: Daytime and seasons are sources of variations for cartilage and bone growth rate. In Dixon AD, Sarnat BG, editors: Factors and mechanisms influencing bone growth, *Prog Clin Biol Res* 101:659, 1982.

Oudet C, Petrovic A: Effects of a postural hyperpropulsor in the growth of the mandibular condylar cartilage of the young rat during circadian cycle. In Lassmann G, Seitelberger F, editors: *Rhythmische Funktionen in Biologischen Systemen. Ihre Bedeutung fauur Theorie und Klinik,* vol 2, Vienna, 1977b, Facultas-Verlag.

Oudet C, Petrovic A: Effets de l'hyperpropulseur postural sur la croissance du cartilage condylien de la mandibule de jeune rat au cours du cycle circadien, *J Physiol (paris)* 71:34, 1975.

Oudet C, Petrovic A: Effets d'un rétropulseur actif sur la vitesse de croissance du cartilage condylien de jeune rat au cours du nycthémère et de l'année, *Orthod Fr* 47:15, 1976.

Oudet C, Petrovic A: Growth rhythms of the cartilage of the mandibular condyle. Effects of orthopedic appliances, *Int J Chronobiol* 5:545, 1978a.

Oudet C, Petrovic A: Regulation of the anatomical length of the lateral pterygoid muscle in the growing rat. In Guba F, Marechal G, Takacs O, editors: Mechanisms of muscle adaptation to functional requirements, *Adv Physiol Sci* 24:403, 1981a.

Oudet C, Petrovic A: Seasonal variations of the growth rate of the condylar cartilage of the mandible in the young rat. In Halber F et al, editors: *Proceedings, twelfth international conference, International Society for Chronobiology,* Milan, 1981b, Il Ponte.

Oudet C, Petrovic A: Tages- und Jahresperiodische Schwankungen der Reakton des Kondylenknorpels bei der kieferorthopädischen Behandlung, *Fortschr Kieferorthop* 42:1, 1981c.

Oudet C, Petrovic A: Variations in the number of sarcomeres in series and in the lateral pterygoid muscle as a function of the longitudinal deviation of the mandibular position produced by the postural hyperpropulsor. In Carlson D, McNamara JA, Jr., editors: *Muscle adaptation in the craniofacial region,* Monograph 8, Craniofacial Growth Series, Ann Arbor, Mich, 1978b, Center for Human Growth and Development, University of Michigan.

Oudet C, Petrovic A, Garcia P: An experimental orthopedic treatment of the rat mandible with a functional appliance alters the fiber- and myosin-types in masticatory muscles, *Reprod Nutr Dev* 28:795-803, 1988.

Oudet C, Petrovic A, Stutzmann JJ: Time-dependent effects of a "functional"-type orthopedic appliance on rat mandible growth, *Chronobiol Int,* 1985.

Pancherz H: Activity of the temporal and masseter muscles in Class II, Division 1 malocclusions, *Am J Orthod* 77:679-688, 1980.

Pancherz H: The effect of continuous bite-jumping on the dentofacial complex: a follow-up study after Herbst appliance treatment of Class II malocclusion, *Eur J Orthod* 3:49-60, 1981.

Pancherz H: Früh- oder Spätbehandlung mit der Herbst-Apparatur— Stabilität oder Rezidiv, *Inf Orthod Kieferorthop* 26:437-445, 1994.

Pancherz H: The Herbst appliance—its biologic effects and clinical use, *Am J Orthod* 87:1-20, 1985.

Pancherz H: Long-term effects of activator treatment, *Odontol Rev* 27(suppl. 35), 1976.

Pancherz H: The mechanism of Class II correction and Herbst appliance treatment: a cephalometric investigation, *Am J Orthod* 87:1-20, 1982a.

Pancherz H: The nature of Class II relapse after Herbst appliance treatment: a cephalometric long-term investigation, *Am J Orthod Dentofac Orthop* 100:220-233, 1991.

Pancherz H: Treatment of Class II malocclusion by jumping the bite with the Herbst appliance: a cephalometric investigation, *Am J Orthod* 76:432-442, 1979.

Pancherz H: Vertical dentofacial changes during Herbst appliance treatment, *Swed Dent J Suppl* 15:189-196, 1982b.

Pancherz H, Anehus-Pancherz M: The effect of continuous bite jumping with the Herbst appliance on the masticatory system: a functional analysis of treated Class II malocclusions, *Eur J Orthod* 4:37-44, 1982.

Pancherz H, Anehus-Pancherz M: Facial profile changes during and after Herbst appliance treatment, *Eur J Orthod* 16:275-286, 1994.

Pancherz H, Anehus-Pancherz M: The head-gear effect of the Herbst appliance, *Am J Orthod Dentofac Orthop* 103:510-520, 1993.

Pancherz H, Anehus-Pancherz M: Muscle activity in Class II, Division 1 malocclusions treated by bite jumping with the Herbst appliance, *Am J Orthod* 78:321-329, 1980.

Pancherz H, Fackel U: The skeletofacial growth pattern pre- and post-dentofacial orthopaedics. A long-term study of Class Ii malocclusions treated with the Herbst appliance, *Eur J Orthod* 12:209-218, 1990.

Pancherz H, Hägg U: Dentofacial orthopedics in relation to somatic maturation. An analysis of 70 consecutive cases treated with the Herbst appliance, *Am J Orthod* 88:273-287, 1985.

Pancherz H, Hansen K: Mandibular anchorage in Herbst treatment, *Eur J Orthod* 10:149-164, 1988.

Pancherz H, Hansen K: Occlusal changes during and after Herbst treatment: a cephalometric investigation, *Eur J Orthod* 8:215-228, 1986.

Pancherz H, Littmann C: Morphologie and Lage des Unterkiefers bei der Herbst-Behandlung. Eine kephalometrische Analyse der Veränderungen bis zum Wachstumsabschluss, *Inf Orthod Kieferorthop* 21:493-513, 1989.

Pancherz H, Littmann C: Somatische Reife und morphologische Veränderungen des Unterkiefers bei der Herbst-Behandlung, *Inf Orthod Kieferorthop* 20:455-470, 1988.

Pancherz H et al: Class II correction in Herbst and Bass therapy, *Eur J Orthod* 11:17-30, 1989.

Pancherz H, Stickel A: Lageveränderungen des Condylus Mandibulae bei der Herbst-Behandlung, *Inf Orthod Kieferorthop* 21:515-557, 1989.

Pangrazio-Kulbersch V, Berger JL: Treatment of identical twins with Fränkel and Herbst appliances: a comparision of results, *Am J Orthod Dentofac Orthop* 103:131-137, 1993.

Paulsen HU: A laminagraphic study of condylar changes with mandibular advancement, *Am J Orthod Dentofac Orthop,* August 1996 (in press).

Paulsen HU et al: CT-scanning and radiographic analysis of temporomandibular joints and cephalometric analysis in a case of Herbst treatment in late puberty, *Eur J Orthod* 17:165-175, 1995.

Pauwels F: Eine Theorie über den Einfluss mechanischer Reize auf Differenzierung des Stützgewebes, *Z Anat Entwicklung-Gesch* 121:478, 1960.

Persson M: Structure and growth of facial sutures: histologic microangiographic and arthrographic studies in rats and histologic study in man, *Odontol Rev* 24(suppl. 26):1, 1973.

Peterson TM, Rugh JD, McIver JE: Mandibular rest position in subjects with high and low mandibular plane angles, *Am J Orthod* 83:318-320, 1983.

Petrovic AG: L'ajustement occlusal: son rôle dans les processus physiologiques de contrôle de la croissance du cartilage condylien, *Orthod Fr* 48:23, 1977.

Petrovic AG: Auxologic categorization and chronologic specification for the choice of appropriate orthodontic treatment, *Am J Orthod Dentofac Orthop* 105;192-205, 1994.

Petrovic AG: Control of postnatal growth of secondary cartilages of the mandible by mechanisms regulating occlusion. Cybernetic model, *Trans Eur Orthod Soc* 50:69, 1974.

Petrovic AG: An experimental and cybernetic approach to the mechanism of action of functional appliances on the manbidular grwoth. In McNamara JA, Jr., edidtor: *Malocclusion and the periodontium,* Monograph 15, Craniofacial Growth Series, Ann Arbor, Mich, 1984a, Center for Human Growth and Development, University of Michigan.

Petrovic AG: Mechanisms and regulation of mandibular condylar growth, *Acta Morphol Neerl Scand* 10:25, 1972.

Petrovic AG: Point de vue d'un chercheur sur le rat comme modèle expérimental en orthodontie, *Rev Orthop Dentofac* 19:101-113, 1985.

Petrovic AG: Postnatal growth of bone: a perspective of current trends, new approaches, and innovations. In Dixon AD, Sarnat BG, editors: Factors and mechanisms influencing bone growth, *Prog Clin Biol Res* 101:297, 1982.

Petrovic AG: Recherches sur les mécanismes histophysiologiques de la croissance osseuse cranio-faciale, *Ann Biol* 9:303, 1970.

Petrovic AG: Types d'explication dans les sciences biomédicales et en médecine. In Barreau H, editor: *Séminaire sur les fondements des sciences. L'explication dans les sciences de la vie,* Paris, 1983, Editions du CNRS.

Petrovic AG: Zweckmässigkeit, Bedeutung, und Gültigkeit der experimentellen Forschung auf dem Gebiet der Kieferorthopädie und Orthodontie, *Fortschr Kieferorthop* 45:165, 1984b.

Petrovic AG, Charlier JP: La synchondrose sphéno-occipitale de jeune rat en culture d'organes: mise en évidence d'un potentiel de croissance indépendant, *C R Acad Sci (series D)* 265:1511, 1967.

Petrovic AG, Charlier JP, Herrmann J: Les mécanismes de croissance du crâne. Recherches sur le cartilage de la cloison nasale et sur les sutures craniennes et faciales de jeunes rats en culture d'organes, *Bull Assoc Anat* 143:1376, 1969.

Petrovic AG, Gasson N: Aspects biologiques de la rotation de croissance postérieure ou antérieure de la mandibule, *Bull Orthod Soc Yugoslav* 8:33, 1975.

Petrovic AG, Gasson N, Oudet C: Wirkung der übertriebenen posturalen Vorschubstellung des Unterkiefers auf das Kondylenwachstum der normalen under der mit Wachstumshormon behandelten Ratte, *Fortschr Kieferorthop* 36:86, 1975a.

Petrovic AG, Gasson N, Schlienger A: Dissymétrie mandibulaire consécutive à la perturbation occlusale unilatérale provoquée expérimientalement chez le rat. Conception cybernétique des systèmes de contrôle de la croissance des cartilages condylien et angulaire, *Orthod Fr* 45:409, 1974a.

Petrovic AG, Heusner A: Oxygénation d'un fragment d'organe *in vitro:* principe de la culture organotypique en suspension en phase liquide, *C R Acad Sci (series D)* 253:3066, 1961.

Petrovic AG, Lavergne J, Stutzmann JJ: Diagnostic et traitement en orthopédie dento-faciale: principles et diagramme de décision, *Orthod Fr* 58:517-542, 1987.

Petrovic AG, Lavergne J, Stutzmann JJ: Tissue-level growth and responsiveness potential, growth rotation, and treatment decision. In Vig PS, Ribbens KA, editors: *Science and clinical judgment in orthodontics,* Monograph 19, Craniofacial Growth Series, Ann Arbor, Mich, 1986, Center for Human Growth and Development, University of Michigan.

Petrovic AG, Oudet C, Gasson N: Effets des appareils de propulsion et de rétropulsion mandibulaires sur le nombre de sarcomères en série du muscle ptérygoïdien externe et sur la croissance du cartilage condylien de jeune rat, *Orthod Fr* 44:191, 1973.

Petrovic AG, Oudet C, Gasson N: Unterkieferpropulsion durch eine im Oberkiefer fixierte Vorbissführung mit seitlicher Biss-sperre von unterschiedlicher Höhe. Auswirkungen bei Ratten während der Wachsteumsperiode und bei erwachsenen Tieren, *Fortschr Kieferorthop* 43:329, 1982a.

Petrovic AG, Oudet C, Shaye R: Unterkieferpropulsion durch eine im Oberkiefer fixierte Vorbissführung mit seitlicher Biss-sperre von unterschiedlicher Höhe hinsichtlich der täglichen Dauer der Behandlung, *Fortschr Kieferorthop* 43:243, 1982b.

Petrovic AG, Oudet C, Stutzmann JJ: Behandlungsergebnisse in Bezug zur Dauer der über triebenen posturalen Vorschubstellung des Unterkiefers, *Fortschr Kieferorthop* 37:40, 1976.

Petrovic AG, Oudet C, Stutzmann JJ: Temporal organization of rat and human skeletal cells: circadian frequency and quantizement of cell generation time. In Edminds L, editor: *Cell cycle clocks,* New York, 1984, Marcel Dekker.

Petrovic AG, Shambaugh GE, Jr.: Promotion of bone calcification by sodium flouride, *Arch Otolaryngol* 83:162, 1966.

Petrovic AG, Shambaugh GE, Jr.: Studies on sodium flouride effects (a) on human sclerotic bone; (b) on prevention of experimental osteoporosis in rats; (c) synergistic action with phosphates, *Acta Otolaryngol* 65:120, 1968.

Petrovic AG, Stutzmann JJ: Auxologic categorizationa s a prognosticative basis for the choice of appropriate orthodontic treatment. From cognitive to accomplishment, *Acta Med Rom* 32:250-263, 1994.

Petrovic AG, Stutzmann JJ: The concept of the mandibular tissue-level growth potential and the responsiveness to a functional appliance. In Graber TM, editor: *Orthodontics: state of the art, essence of the science,* St Louis, 1986, Mosby.

Petrovic AG, Stutzmann JJ: Contrôle de la croissance post-natale du squelette facial. Données expérimentales et modèle cybernétique, *Acta Odontostomatol* 128:811, 1979a.

Petrovic AG, Stutzmann JJ: A cybernetic view of facial growth mechanisms. In Kehrer B et al, editors: *Long-term treatment in cleft lip and palate,* Bern, 1981, Hans Huber.

Petrovic AG, Stutzmann JJ: Effects on the rat mandible of a chincup-type appliance and of partial or complete immobilization, *Proc Finn Dent Soc* 87:85-91, 1991.

Petrovic AG, Stutzmann JJ: Experimentelle Untersuchung der kieferorthopädischen Beeinflussbarkeit des Geisichtswachstums, *Fortschr Kieferorthop* 41:212, 1980a.

Petrovic AG, Stutzmann JJ: Further investigations into the functioning of the "comparator" of the servosystem (respective positions of the upper and lower dental arches) in the control of the condylar cartilage growth rate and of the lengthening of the jaw. In McNamara JA, Jr., editor: *The biology of occlusal development,* Monograph 6, Craniofacial Growth Series, Ann Arbor, Mich, 1977, Center for Human Growth and Development, University of Michigan.

Petrovic AG, Stutzmann JJ: Hormone somatotrope: modalités d'action des diverses variétés de cartilage, *Pathol Biol* 28:43, 1980b.

Petrovic AG, Stutzmann JJ: Hormone somatotrope: modalités d'acrion sur la croissance des diverses variétés de cartilage, *Sem Hop* 56:1307, 1980c.

Petrovic AG, Stutzmann JJ: Le muscle ptérygoïdien externe et las croisssance du condyle mandibulaire. Recherches expérimentales chez le jeune rat, *Orthod Fr* 43:271-285, 1972.

Petrovic AG, Stutzmann JJ: New ways in orthodontic diagnosis and decision making: physiologic basis, *J Japan Orthod Soc* [special issue] 51:3-25, 1992.

Petrovic AG, Stutzmann JJ: Potencial de crecimiento del nivel tisular mandibular, rotacion de crecimiento y respuesta a aparatos funcionales, *Orthodoncia* 48(96): 26-34, 1984.

Petrovic AG, Stutzmann JJ: Die Progenie, experimentelle Untersuchungen über Pathogenese und Therapie, *Fortschr Kieferorthop* 40:372, 1979b.

Petrovic AG, Stutzmann JJ: Reaktionsfähigkeit des tierischen und menschlichen Kondylenknorpels auf Zell- und Molekularebene im Lichte einer kybernetischen Auffassung des fazialen Wachstums, *Fortschr Kieferorthop* 49:405-425, 1988b.

Petrovic AG, Stutzmann JJ: *Récentes acquisitions biologiques sur la morphogenèse de la mandibule. Le menton,* Paris, 1988a, Masson.

Petrovic AG, Stutzmann JJ: Teoría cibernética del cercimiento craneo-facial, post-natal y mecanismos de acción de los aparatos ortopédicos y orthodónticos, *Rev Assoc Argent Ortoped Func Maxil* 15:7, 1982.

Petrovic AG, Stutzmann JJ: Tierexperimentelle untersuchungen über das Geischts-Schädelwachstum und seine Beeinflussung. Eine biologische Erklärung der sogenannten Wachstumsrotation des Unterkiefers, *Fortschr Kieferorthop* 40:1, 1979c.

Petrovic AG, Stutzmann JJ: Timing aspects of orthodontic treatment, *Bull Orthod Soc Yugoslav* 26(1-2):25-36, 1993.

Petrovic AG, Stutzmann-Herrmann JJ: *Action of rat growth hormone on young rat mandibular condylar cartilage in tissue and organ culture,* Detroit, 1969, American society of Cellular Biologists.

Petrovic AG, Stutzmann JJ, Gasson N: The final length of the mandible: is it genetically predetermined? In Carlson DS, editor: *Craniofacial biology,* Monograph 10, Craniofacial Growth Series, Ann Arbor, Mich, 1981, Center of Human Growth and Development, University of Michigan.

Petrovic AG, Stutzmann JJ, Lavergne J: Biologische Grundlage für die unterschiedliche interindividuelle Gewebereaktion auf eine Kieferorthopädische Behandlung mit dem Bionator. In Harzer W, editor: *Kieferorthopädischer Gewebeumbau,* Berlin, 1991a, Quintessenz Verlag.

Petrovic AG, Stutzmann JJ, Lavergne J: Mechanisms of craniofacial growth and modus operandi of functional appliances: a cell-level and cybernetic approach to orthodontic decision making. In Monograph 23, Craniofacial Growth Series, Ann Arbor, Mich, 1990, Center for Human Growth and Development, University of Michigan.

Petrovic AG, Stutzmann JJ, Lavergne J: Nuevo enfoque del diagnostico y toma de decisiones biologica y cefalométricamente. In Aguila FJ, editor: *Manual de cefalometrica,* Barcelona, 1993, Editorial Aguiram.

Petrovic AG et al: Is it possible to modulate the growth of the human mandible with a functional appliance? *Bull Orthod Yugoslav* 11(1):15-20, 1988.

Petrovic AG, Stutzmann JJ, Oudet C: Condylectomy and mandibular grwoth in young rats. A quantitative study, *Proc Finn Dent Soc* 77:139, 1981b.

Petrovic AG, Stutzmann JJ, Oudet C: Control processes in the postnatal growth of the condylar cartilage of the mandible. In McNamara JA, Jr., editor: *Determinants of mandibular form and growth,* Monograph 4, Craniofacial Growth Series, Ann Arbor, Mich, 1975, Center of Human Growth and Development, University of Michigan.

Petrovic AG, Stutzmann JJ, Oudet C: La culture organotypique en milieu liquide avec renouvellement continu de l'apport gazeux. Un nouveau moyen d'étude des variations de la formation et de la résorption de l'os humain normal ou pathologique, *ITBM* 3:594, 1982e.

Petrovic AG, Stutzmann JJ, Oudet C: Defects in mandibular growth resulting from condylectomy and resection of the pterygoid and masseter muscles. In McNamara JA, Jr., Carlson DS, Ribbens KA, editors: *The effect of surgical interenetion on craniofacial growth,* Monograph 12, Craniofacial Growth Series, Ann Arbor, Mich, 1982c, Center for Human Growth and Development, University of Michigan.

Petrovic AG, Stutzmann JJ, Oudet C: Effets de l'hormone somatotrope sur la croissance du cartilage condylien mandibulaire et de la synchondrose sphéno-occipitale de jeunes rats, en culture organotypique, *C R Acad Scie (series D)* 276:3053, 1973.

Petrovic AG, Stutzmann JJ, Oudet C: Experimentelle Untersuchungen zur Wirkung intraoraler Gummizüge auf den Unter- und Oberkiefer bei wachsenden und ausgewachsenen Ratten, *Fortschr Kieferorthop* 42:209, 1981c.

Petrovic AG, Stutzmann JJ, Oudet C: Orthopedic appliances modulate the bone formation in the mandible as a whole, *Swed Dent J* 15(suppl.):197, 1982d.

Petrovic AG, Stutzmann JJ, Oudet C: Seasonal variations in the direction of growth of the mandibular condyle. In Vidrio A, editor: Biological rhythms in structure and function, *Prog Clin Biol Res* 59C: 195, 1981d.

Petrovic AG, Stutzmann JJ, Oudet C: Turnover of human alveolar bone removed either in the day or in the night, *J Interdiscipl Cycle Res* 12:161, 1981e.

Petrovic AG et al: Kontrollfaktoren des Kodylenwachstums: Wachstumshormon, musculi pterygoidei laterales, und Vor- und Rückschubgerte des Unterkiefers, *Fortschr Keiferorthop* 35:347, 1974b.

Petrovic AG et al: Does the Fränkel appliance produce forward movements of mandibular premolars? *Eur J Orthod* 4:173, 1982f.

Pfeiffer JP, Grobety D: The Class II malocclusion: differential diagnosis and clinical application of activators, extraoral traction, and fixed appliances, *Am J Orthod* 68:499, 1975.

Pfeiffer JP, Grobety D: Removable appliances and extraoral force. In Graber TM, Neumann B, editors: *Removable orthodontic appliances*, ed 2, Philadelphia, 1984, Saunders.

Pfeiffer JP, Grobety D: Simultaneous use of cervical appliance and activator: an orthodontic approach to fixed appliance therapy, *Am J Orthod* 61:353, 1972.

Plaice CH: A note on the determination of serum beta-glucuronidase activity, *J Clin Pathol* 14:661, 1961.

Popper KR: *Conjectures and refutations. The growth of scientific knowledge,* London, 1963, Routledge & Kegan Paul.

Posen AL: The application of quantitative perioral assessment to orthodontic case analysis and treatment planning, *Angle Orthod* 46(2):118, 1976.

Posen AL: The influence of maximum perioral and tongue force on the incisor teeth, *Angle Orthod* 42:285, 1972.

Posselt U: Studies in the mobility of the human mandible, *Acta Odontol Scand* 10(suppl. 10):90-118, 1952.

Poulton DL: The influence of extraoral traction, *Am J Orthod* 53:1-18, 1967.

Powell RN: Tooth contact during sleep: association with other events, *J Dent Res* 44:959-967, 1965.

Prahl B: *Sutural growth. Investigations on the growth mechanism of the coronal suture and its relation to cranial growth in the rat,* doctoral thesis, 1968, University of Nijmegan.

Proffit WR: *Contemporary orthodontics,* ed 2, St Louis, 1993, Mosby.

Proffit WR: Equilibrium theory revisited: factors influencing position of the teeth, *Angle Orthod* 48:175, 1978.

Proffit WR, Field HW: Occlusal force in normal- and long-face children, *J Dent Res* 62:571-574, 1982.

Rakosi T: Ätiologie und diagnostische Beurteilung des offenen Bisses, *Fortschr Kieferorthop* 43:68, 1982a.

Rakosi T: *An atlas and manual of cephalometric radiography,* Philadelphia, 1982b, Lea & Febiger.

Rakosi T: *Atlas und Anleitung zur praktischen Fernröntgenanalyse,* Munich, 1979, C. Hasner Verlag.

Rakosi T: Bedeutung des Säuglings- und Kleinkindalters für die Entstehung von Bissanomalien, *Zahnaertzl Prax* 23:12, 1972a.

Rakosi T: Bedeutung der Wachstumsachse des Unterkiefers für die Therapieplanung, *Fortschr Kieferorthop* 33:31, 1972b.

Rakosi T: Die Bewertung des Zeitfaktors bei der Progeniebehandlung, *Fortschr Kieferorthop* 27:66, 1966a.

Rakosi T: *Cephalometric radiography,* London, 1982c, Wolfe Medical.

Rakosi T: Einführung in die Problematik der Befunderhebung in der Kieferorthopädie, *Fortschr Kieferorthop* 38:115, 1977.

Rakosi T: Extraktion im Milchgebiss, *Fortschr Kieferorthop* 29:16, 1968a.

Rakosi T: Funktionelle Kiefergelensstörungen bei Kindern, *Fortschr Kieferorthop* 32:37, 1971a.

Rakosi T: Grenzen und Möglichkeiten der kieferorthopädischen Spätbehandlung, *Fortschr Kieferorthop* 41:590, 1980.

Rakosi T: Heredität, Weichteilmorphologie, und Bewegungsablauf, *Fortschr Kieferorthop* 30:46, 1969.

Rakosi T: Indikation der Extraktion in der kieferorthopädie, *Zahnaertzl Prax* 21:145, 1970a.

Rakosi T: Kieferorthopädische Apparate mit apparativer Basis im Mundvorhof, *Zahntechnik* 29:125, 1971b.

Rakosi T: Metrische Untersuchung der Lippen-Lagen bei verschiedenen Gebissanomalien, *Fortschr Kieferorthop* 27:470, 1966b.

Rakosi T: Möglichkeiten und Grenzen der kierferorthopädischen Prävention im Milchgebiss, *Dtsch Zahnaertzel Z* 21:848, 1966c.

Rakosi T: The principles of functional appliances. In McNamara JA, Jr., Ribbens KA, Howe RP, editors: *Clinical alteration of the growing face,* Monograph 14, Craniofacial Growth Series, Ann Arbor, Mich, 1983, Center for Human Growth and Development, University of Michigan.

Rakosi T: Das Problem der Zunge in der Kieferorthopädie, *Fortschr Kieferorthop* 36:220, 1975a.

Rakosi T: Progenie im Fernrontgenbild, *Fortschr Kieferorthop* 39:486, 1978.

Rakosi T: Röntgenzephalometrische Untersuchungen über die Änderung der Zungenlage bei kieferorthopädischer Therapie, *Fortschr Kieferorthop* 27:234, 1966d.

Rakosi T: Die Ruhelage am Fernröntgenseiten (FRS)-Bild und ihre Bedeutung für die Kieferorthopädie, *Fortschr Kieferorthop* 22:409, 1961.

Rakosi T: The scope of mechanotherapy and functional treatment in the mixed dentition, *Trans Eur Orthod Soc,* p. 209, 1975b.

Rakosi T: The scope of orthodontic treatment in adults maintained by oral surgery. Indications, *Eur Orthod Soc Rep Cong,* p. 333, 1971c.

Rakosi T: The significance of roentgenographic cephalometrics in the diagnosis and treatment of Class III malocclusions, *Eur Orthod Soc Rep Cong,* p. 155, 1970c.

Rakosi T: Therapie der Klasse-II-Dysgnathien: Möglichkeiten und Grenzen, *Oesterr Z Stomatol* 75:171, 1978.

Rakosi T: Therapie des offenen Bisses, *Fortschr Kieferorthop* 43:171, 1982d.

Rakosi T: Über die Lippenmorphologie und Lippenfunktion, *Zahnaerztl Welt* 77:671, 1968b.

Rakosi T: Über die Möglichkeiten der Progenie-Behandlung, *Schweiz Monatsschr Zahnheilkd* 80:1021, 1970b.

Rakosi T: Über die Problematik der Diagnostik und Behandlung des tiefen Bisses, *Fortschr Kieferorthop* 34:94, 1973.

Rakosi T: Über die Schädelbasis-bezüglichen Rotationen des Unterkiefers, *Fortschr Kieferorthop* 33:177, 1972c.

Rakosi T: Variationen des Schluckaktes, *Fortschr Kieferorthop* 31:81, 1970d.

Rakosi T: Die Wirkungsweise und Konstruktionselemente des Funktionsreglers, *Zahnaertzl Prax* 23:285, 1970e.

Rakosi T, Bäuerle H: Retrospektive Beurteilung der Wachstumsprognose nach Holdaway, *Fortschr Kieferorthop* 39:133, 1978.

Rakosi T, Jonas, I, Burgert R: Simplified postioner construction, *J Clin Orthod* 15:206, 1981.

Rakosi T, Jonas, I, Burgert R: Vereinfachte Anfertigung von Gaumennaht-Sprengungsplatten, *Fortschr Kieferorthop* 44:71, 1983.

Rakosi T, Jonas, I, Graber TM: *Orthodontics—Diagnosis Color Atlas of Dental Medicine,* 1993, Thieme.

Rakosi T et al: Vereinfachte Anfertigung eines Positioners, *Fortschr Kieferorthop* 44:71, 1981.

Rakosi T, Rahn BA: Metallimplantate und Knochenwachstum, *Fortschr Kieferorthop* 39:196, 1978.

Rakosi T, Schilli W: Class II anomalies: a coordinated approach to skeletal, dental, and soft tissue problems, *Oral Surg* 39:860, 1981.

Rakosi T, Schmidt H, Debrunner M: Kriterien für die Beurteilung des Behandlungszieles, *Fortschr Kieferorthop* 37:405, 1976.

Rakosi T, Witt E: Grundelemente der festsitzenden Apparaturen, *Zahnaertzl Prax* 22:19, 1971.

Ramel U: *Symptome sogenannter Kiefergelenksbeschwerden dei einer Gruppe Schweizer Rekruten,* thesis, Bern, 1976, University of Bern.

Randow K et al: The effect of an occlusal interference on the masticatory system, *Odontol Rev* 27:245, 1975.

Rebholz K, Rakosi T: Extraorale Kräfte und die Wirbelsäule, *Fortschr Kieferorthop* 38:324, 1977.

Reitan K: Biomechanical principles and reactions. In Graber TM, Swain BF, editdors: *Orthodontics: current principles and techniques,* St Louis, 1985, Mosby.

Reitan K: Continuous bodily tooth movement and its histological significance, *Acta Odontol Scand* 7:115, 1947.

Reitan K: Effects of force magnitude and direction of tooth movement on different alveolar bone types, *Angle Orthod* 34:244, 1964.

Reitan K: Initial tissue behavior during apical root resorption, *Angle Orthod* 44:68, 1974.

Reitan K: The initial tissue reaction of orthodontic tooth movement, *Acta Odontol Scan* 9(suppl. 6):240, 1951.

Reitan K: Tissue behavior during orthodontic tooth movement, *Am J Orthod* 46:881, 1960.

Remmelink HJ, Tan BG: Cephalometric changes during headgear-reactivator treatment, *Eur J Orthod* 13:466-470, 1991.

Richardson MP: A classificaiton of open bite, *Eur J Orthod* 3:289, 1981.

Richardson MP: Measurement of dental base relationship, *Eur J Orthod* 4:151, 1982.

Richardson MP: Spontaneous changes in incisor relationship following extraction of lower first permanent molars, *Br J Orthod* 6:85, 1979.

Ricketts RM: The influence of orthodontic treatment on facial growth and development, *Angle Orthod* 30;103, 1960.

Ricketts RM: Respiratory obstruction syndrome, *Am J Orthod* 54:495, 1968.

Ricketts RM: Respiratory obstructions and their relation to the tongue posture, *Cleft Palate Bull* 8:4, 1958.

Ricketts RM: A study of changes in temporomandibular relations associated with the treatment of Class II malocclusion (Angle), *Am J Orthod* 38:918, 1952.

Rider EA: Removable Herbst appliance for treatment of obstructive sleep apnea, *J Clin Orthod* 22:256-257, 1988.

Riedel RA: Diagnosis and treatment planning in orthodontics, *Dent Clin North Am* 12:175, 1969.

Riolo ML et al: *An atlas of craniofacial growth,* Monograph 2, Craniofacial Growth Series, Ann Arbor, Mich, 1974, Center for Human Growth and Development, University of Michigan.

Rix RE: Some observations upon the environment of the incisors, *Dent Res* 73:427-441, 1953.

Robin P: Observation sur un novel appareil de redressement, *Rev Stomatol* 9:423, 1902.

Robinson AL: Powerful new magnet material found, *Science* 223:920-922, 1984.

Ronning O: *Alterations in craniofacial morphogenesis induced by parenterally administered papain. An experimental study on the rat,* doctoral dissertation, 1971, University of Turku.

Rose JM et al: Mandibular skeletal and dental asymmetry in Class II subdivision malocclusions, *Am J Orthod Dentofac Orthop* 105:489, 1994.

Rosenblum RE: Class II malocclusion: mandibular retrusion or maxillary protrusion? *Angle Orthod* 65:49, 1995.

Roux W: *Gesammelte Abhandlungen über Entwicklungsmechanik der Organismen,* Leipzig, 1895, W. Englemann.

Rugh JD, Drago CJ: Vertical dimension: a study of clinical rest position and jaw muscle activity, *J Prosthet Dent* 45:670-675, 1981.

Rygh P: Elimination of hyalinized periodontal tissues associated with orhtodontic tooth movement, *Acta Odontol Scand* 31:109, 1973.

Rygh P: Orthodontic root resorption occurring during orthodontic treatment, *Angle Orthod* 47:1, 1977.

Sander FG: The effects of functional appliances and Class II elastics on masticatory patterns. In McNamara JA, Jr., et all, editors: *Clinical alteration of the growing face,* Monograph 14, Craniofacial Growth Series, Ann Arbor, Mich, 1983, Center for Human Growth and Development, University of Michigan.

Sander FG: Neue Elemente für Vorschubdoppelplatten, *Quintessenz* 39:871-883, 1988b.

Sander FG: Die Vorschubdoppelplatten, Ein hervorragender Behandlungsbehelf, *Dent Labor* 36:75-758, 1988a.

Sander FG: *Zur Frage der Biomechanik des Aktivators: Entwicklung und Erprobung neuer Untersuchungsmethoden,* Wiesbaden, 1980, Westdeutscher Verlag, GmbH.

Sander FG, Schmuth GPF: Der Einfluss Verscheidener Bissperren auf die Muskelaktivität bei Aktivatorträgern, *Fortschr Kieferorthop* 40:107-11, 1979.

Sandler PJ: An attractive solution to uneruupted teeth, *Am J Orthod Dentofac Orthop* 100:489-493, 1991.

Sandstedt C: Einige Beitrage zur Theorie der Zahnregulierung, *Nord Tan Tidskr* 5:236, 1904.

Sandstedt C: Einige Beitrage zur Theorie der Zahnregulierung, *Nord Tan Tidskr* 6:1, 1905.

Sarnäs K-V et al: Hemifacial microsomia treated with the Herbst appliance, *Am J Orthod* 82:68-74, 1982.

Sassouni V: A classification of skeletal facial types, *Am J Orthod* 55:109, 1969.

Schiavoni R: A method used to anchor the Herbst appliance, *J Craniomand Prac* 6:245-251, 1988.

Schiavoni R, Grenga V, Macri V: Treatment of Class II high angle malocclusions with the Herbst appliance: a cephalometric investigation, *Am J Orthod Dentofac Orthop* 102:393-409, 1992.

Schlienger A: *Effets des perturbations unilatérales du niveau du plan d'occlusion sur la vitesse et la direction de croissance du condyle et sur l'allongement de la mandibule. Etude expérimentale chez le jeune rat,* doctoral thesis, Strasbourg, France, 1978, Université Louis-Pasteur.

Schmuth GPF: *Kieferorthopädie,* Bonn, 1995, Quintessenz Verlag.

Schmuth GPF: *Kieferorthopädie Grundzüge und Probleme,* Stuttgart, Germany, 1983, Georg Thieme Verlag.

Schmuth GPF: Milestones in the development and practical application of functional appliances, *Am J Orthod* 84:48, 1983.

Schmuth GPF: Das Verhalten der Zunge bei verchieden Funktionsabläufen, *Fortschr Kieferorthop* 28:271, 1967.

Schneider E, Schmidt H, Rakosi T: Die Korrelation zwischen dem Zungepressen und dem Aufbau des Geischtsschädels, *Fortschr Kieferorthop* 36:379, 1975.

Schwartz AM: Erfahrungen mit dem Herbstschen Scharnier zur Behandlung des Distalbisses, *Zahnärztl Rundschau* 43:47-54, 91-100, 1934.

Schwartz AM: *Lehrgang der Gebissregelung. Band II. Die Behandlung,* Vienna, 1956, Urban and Scwarzenberg.

Schwartz AM: *Die Röntgendiagnostik,* Vienna, 1958, Urban & Schwarzenberg.

Schwartz AM: Tissue changes incidental to orthodontic tooth movement, *Int J Orthodont* 18:331-352, 1932.

Schwartz AM: Wirkungsweise des Aktivators, *Fortschr Kieferorthop* 13:117, 1952.

Schwartz AM, Gratzinger M: *Removable orthodontic appliances,* Philadelphia, 1966, Saunders.

Scott J: Cartilage of the nasal system, *Br Dent J* 95:37, 1953.

Scott J: *Dento-facial development and growth,* Oxford, 1967, Pergamon Press.

Scott J: Growth at facial sutures, *Am J Orthod* 42:381, 1956.

Scott J: The growth of the human face, *Proc R Soc Med* 47:91, 1954.

Scott J: The growth of the nasal cavities, *Acta Otolaryngol* 50:215, 1959.

Sectakof PA: The effects of functional appliances on functional activities of jaw muscles in Macaca fascicularis, master's thesis, Toronto, 1992, University of Toronto.

Sessle BJ et al: Effect of functional appliances on jaw muscle activity, *Am J Orthod Dentofac Orthop* 3:222-230, 1990.

Shapera N: A post-retention study: a radiographic evaluation of the long-term changes in the ANS-subnasale area after orthodontic movement, diploma thesis, toronto, 1974, University of Toronto.

Shaye R: CO interviews: Dr. Robert Shaye on functional appliances, *J Clin Orthod* 17:330, 1983.

Shaye R, Schwaninger B, Hoffmann D: Activator construction simplified, *J Clin Orthod* 13:773, 1979.

Sheppard IM, Markus N: Total time of tooth contacts during mastication, *J Prosthet Dent* 12:460-463, 1962.

Sidhu MS, Kharabanda OP, Sidhu SS: Cephalometric analysis of changes produced by a modifed Herbst appliance in the treatment of Class II Division 1 malocclusion, *Br J Orthod* 22:1-12, 1995.

Simon PW: *Grundzüge einer systematischen Diagnostick,* Berlin, 1922, H. Meuser.

Simon PW: *System einer biologisch-mechanischen Therapie der Gesichtsanomalien,* Berlin, 1933, Herman Meusser.

Solow B, Greve E: The effect of adenoidectomy on head posture and nasal respiratory resistance. In McNamara JA, Jr., editor: *Nasorespiratory function and craniofacial growth,* Monograph 9, Craniofacial Growth Series, Ann Arbor, Mich, 1979, Center for Human Growth and Development, University of Michigan.

Spengeman WM: Personal communication, 1967.

Stein G, Weinmann J: Die physiologische Wanderung der Zahne, *Z Stomatol* 23:733, 1925.

Steiner CC: Cephalometrics for you and me, *Am J Orthod* 39(10:729-755, 1953.

Stockfisch H: The kinetor. In Graber TM, Neumann B, editors: *Removable orthodontic appliances,* Philadephia, 1977, Saunders.

Stockfisch H: *The principles and practice of dentofacial orthopaedics,* London, 1995, Quintessence.

Stöckli PW, Dietrich UC: Experimental and clinical findings following functional forward displacement of the mandible, *Trans Eur Orthod Soc,* p. 435, 1973.

Stöckli P, Teuscher UM: *The activator-headgear combination in skeletal Class II treatment.* Mershon memorial lecture, presented at the annual meeting of the American Association of Orthodontists, Atlanta, 1982.

Stöckli P, Teuscher UM: Combined activator-headgear orthopedics. In Graber TM, Swain BF, editors: *Orthodonticss: current principles and techniques,* St Louis, 1985, Mosby.

Stöckli P, Teuscher UM: *Rationale for activator-headgear use.* Chilean Orthodontic Congress, Santiago, September 1994.

Stöckli P, Willert HG: Tissue reactions in the temporomandibular joint resulting from anterior displacement of the mandible in the monkey, *Am J Orthod* 60:142-155, 1971.

Storey AT: Maturation of the orofacial musculature. In Moyers RE, editor: *Handbook of orthodontics,* Chicago, 1988, Year Book.

Storey E: Bone changes associated with tooth movement. A histological study of the effect of force for varying duration in the rabbit, guinea pig, and rat, *Aust J Dent* 59:209, 1955.

Straub W: Malfunction of the tongue, *Am J Orthod* 48:486, 1962.

Stutzmann JJ: *Particularités de la croissance postnatale des cartilages secondaires du squelette facial. Recherches in vivo et en culture organotypique chez le jeune rat, sur les processus du commande et de régulation,* doctoral thesis, Strasbourg, France, 1976, Université Louis-Pasteur.

Stutzmann JJ, Petrovic AG: Auxologic categorization, turnover of the alveolar bone and orthodontic or functional treatment, *Acta Med Rom* 32:264-278, 1994.

Stutzmann JJ, Petrovic A: Bone cell histogenesis: the skeletoblast as a stem-cell for preosteoblasts and for secondary-type prechondroblasts. In Dixon AD, Sarnat BG, editors: *Mechanisms influencing bone growth progress in clinical and biological research,* vol 101, 1982, A. Liss.

Stutzmann JJ, Petrovic A: Effets de la résection du muscle ptérygoïdien externe sur la croissance du cartilage condylien du jeune rat, *Bull Assoc Anat* 58:1107, 1974a.

Stutzmann JJ, Petrovic A: Einfluss von Testosteron auf die Wachstumsgeschwindigkeit des Kondylenknorpels der jungen Ratte. Rolles des "Vergleicher" des Servosystems welches die Verlängerung des Unterkiefers kontrollert, *Fortschr Kieferorthop* 39:345, 1978a.

Stutzmann JJ, Petrovic A: Experimental analysis of general and local extrinsic mechanisms controlling upper jaw growth. In McNamara JA, Jr., editor: *Factors affecting the growth of the midface,* monograph 6, Craniofacial Growth Series, Ann Arbor, Mich, 1976, Center for Human Growth and Development, University of Michigan.

Stutzmann JJ, Petrovic A: Human alveolar bone turn-over rate. A quantitative study of spontaneous and therapeutically induced variations. In McNamara JA, Jr., editor: *Malocclusions and the periodontium,* Monograph 15, Craniofacial Growth Series, Ann Arbor, Mich, 1984, Center for Human Growth and Development, University of Michigan.

Stutzmann JJ, Petrovic A: Intrinsic regulation of the condylar cartilage growth rate, *Eur J Orthod* 1:41, 1979a.

Stutzmann JJ, Petrovic A: Le muscle ptérygoïdien externe, un relais du l'action de la langue sur la croissance du condyle mandibulaire. Données expérimentales, *Orthod Fr* 45:385, 1974b.

Stutzmann JJ, Petrovic A: Nature et aptitudes évolutives des cellules du compartiment mitotique des cartilages secondaires de la mandibule et du maxillaire de jeune rat. Expériences en culture cytotypique et d'homotransplantation, *Bull Asso Anat* 59:467, 1975a.

Stutzmann JJ, Petrovic A: Particularités de croissance de la suture palatine sagittale de jeune rat, *Bull Assoc Anat* 148:552, 1970.

Stutzmann JJ, Petrovic A: Persistence in organ culture of a growth rate circadian rhythm, *Chronobiologia* 5:183, 1978b.

Stutzmann JJ, Petrovic A: Le pic de croissance pubertaire du cartilage condylien chez le mâle: mise en évidence d'une interaction positive entre les effets d'un hyperpropulseur postural et de la testostérone, *Orthod Fr* 48:12, 1977.

Stutzmann JJ, Petrovic A: Régulation intrinséque de la croissance du cartilage condylien de la mandibule: inhibition de la prolifération préchondroblastique par les chondroblasts, *CR Acad Sci (series D)* 281:175, 1975b.

Stutzmann JJ, Petrovic A: Tierexperimentelle Untersuchungen über das Gesichts-Schadelwachstum und seine Beeinflussung. Eine biologische Erklarung der sogenannte Wachstumsrotation des Unterkiefers, *Fortschr Kieferorthop* 40:1, 1979b.

Stutzmann JJ, Petrovic A: Tierexperimentelle Untersuchungen über Zusammenhänge Zwischen Zunge, Musculus pterygoideus lateralis, mandibulärem Kondylenknorpel, und Gaumennaht, *Fortschr Kieferorthop* 59:523, 1975c.

Stutzmann JJ, Petrovic A: Die Umbaugeschwindigkeit des Alveolarknochens beim Erwachsenen vor und nach orthodontischer Behandlung, *Fortschr Kieferorthop* 42:386, 1981.

Stutzmann JJ, Petrovic A: Young rat spheno-occipital synchrondrosis: a circadian rhythm of the growth rate and susceptibility to STH and its mediators, *Chronbiologia* 5:183, 1979c.

Stutzmann JJ, Petrovic A, George D: Effets du rétropulsseur actif sur la croissance de la mandibule du jeune rat. Rôle du muscle ptérygoïdien externe et du frein élastique méniscotemporal sur la vitesse et la direction de la croissance condylienne, *Orthod Fr* 47:1, 1976.

Stutzmann JJ, Petrovic A, George D: Life cycle length, number of cell generations, mitotic index, and modal chromosome number as estimated in tissue culture of normal and sarcomatous bone cells. In Donath A, Courvoisier B, editors: *Third symposium CEMO, Bone and tumors,* Geneva, 1980a, Editions Médecine & Hygiene.

Stutzmann JJ, Petrovic A, Graber TM: Effects of the Fränkel lateral vestibular shields on the widening of the upper jaw: an experimental investigation in the rate, *Stomatol DDR* 33:753, 1983.

Stutzmann JJ, Petrovic A, Malan A: Seasonal variations of the human alveolar bone turnover. A quantitative evaluation in organ culture, *J Interdiscipl Cycle Res* 12:177, 1981.

Stutzmann JJ, Petrovic A, Oudet C: Effets de la thyroxine sur la croissance du cartilage condylien de jeune rat, *J Physiol (Paris)* 71:347a, 1975.

Stutzmann JJ, Petrovic A, Shaye R: Analyse en culture organotypique de la vitesse de formation-résorption de l'os alvéolaire humain prélevé avant et pendant un traitement comprenant le déplacement des dents: nouvelle voie d'approche en recherche orthodontique, *Orthod Fr* 50:399, 1979.

Stutzmann JJ, Petrovic A, Shaye R: Analyse der Resorptionsbildungsgeschwindigkeit des menschlichen Alveolarknochens in organotypischer Kultur, entnommen vor und während der Durchführung einer Zahnbewegung. Ein neuer Anblick in der orthodontischen Forschung, *Fortschr Kieferorthop* 41:236, 1980b.

Stutzmann JJ, Petrovic A, Shaye R: Extrinsic origin of bone resorbing cells in orthodontic tooth movement, *J Dent Res* 59:440, 1980c.

Stutzmann JJ, Petrovic A, Shaye R: Relationship between mandibular growth rotation and alveolar bone turnover rate, *J Dent Res* 59:448, 1980d.

Subtelny JD: The significance of adenoid tissue in orthodontia, *Angle Orthod* 24:59, 1954.

Subtelny JD, Daniel S: Examination of current philosophies associated with swallowing behavior, *Am J Orthod* 51:161, 1965.

Subtelny JD, Sakuda M: Open-bite: diagnosis and treatment, *Am J Orthod* 50:337, 1964.

Symons NB: Studies on the growth and form of the mandible, *Dent Rec* 71:41, 1951.

Tanner JM: *Fetus into man,* Cambridge, Mass, 1978, Harvard University Press.

Taranger J, Hägg U: The timing and duration of adolescent growth, *Acta Odont Scand* 38:57-67, 1980.

Tennebaum M, Gabriel R: Orthodontic treatment with removable plates and extraoral forces, *Trans Eur Orthod Soc,* p. 199, 1973.

Tuescher U: Edgewise therapy with cervical and intermaxillary traction—influence on the bony chin, *Angle Orthod* 53:212, 1983.

Tuescher U: *Quantitative resultate einer wachstumsbezogenen Behandlungsmethode des Distalbisses bei jugendlichen Patiente. Habilitationsschrift zur Erlangung der venia legendi der Medizinsischen Fakultät der Universität Zürich,* Zürich, 1986, University of Zürich.

Thilander B, Filipsson R: Muscle activity related to activator and intermaxillary traction in Angle Class II, Division 1, malocclusions. An electromyographic study of the temporal, masseter, and suprahyoid muscle, *Acta Odontol Scand* 24:142, 1966.

Thom R: *Stabilité structurelle et morphogénèse,* Reading, Mass, 1972, W.A. Benjamin Advanced Book Program.

Thompson JR: The rest position of the mandible and its significance of dental science, *J Am Dent Assoc* 33:151, 1946.

Todd J, Mark L: Issues related to the prediction of craniofacial growth, *Am J Orthod* 79:63, 1981a.

Todd J, Mark L: A reply to Dr. Bookstein, *Am J Orthod* 79:449, 1981b.

Todd J et al: The perception of human growth, *Sci Am* 242:106, 1980.

Tsutsui H et al: Studies on the SmCo magnet as a dental material, *J Dent Res* 58:1597-1606, 1979.

Tulley WJ: Adverse muscle forces—their diagnostic significance, *Am J Orthod* 42:801, 1956.

Tulley WJ: A critical appraisal of tongue-thrusting, *Am J Orthod* 55:640, 1969.

Tulley WJ: The scope and limitation of treatment with the activator, *Am J Orthod* 61:562, 1972.

Vaes G, Jacques P: Studies on bone enzymes. The assay of acid hydrolases and other enzymes in bone tissues, *Biochem J* 97:380, 1965.

Valant JR: Case report: increasing maxillary arch length with a modified Herbst appliance, *J Clin Orthod* 23:810-814, 1989.

Valant JR, Sinclair PM: Treatment effects of the Herbst appliance, *Am J Orthod Dentofac Orthop* 95:138-147, 1989.

Van Beek H: Overjet correction by a combined head-gear and activator, *Eur J Orthod* 4:279-290, 1982.

Van der Linden FPGM: *Gesichtswachstum un faziale Orthopädie,* 1984, Quintessenz.

Van Sickels JE et al: Electromyographic relaxed mandibular position in long-faced subjects, *J Prosthet Dent* 54:578-581, 1985.

Vardimon AD, Mueller HJ: In-vivo and in-vitro corrosion of permanent magnets in orthodontic therapy, *J Dent Res* 64:185, 1985.

Vardimon AD et al: 3-D force and moment analysis of repulsive magnetic appliances to correct dentofacial vertical excess, *J Dent Res* 73:67-74, 1994.

Vardimon AD et al: Rare earth magnets and impaction, *Am J Orthod Dentofac Orthop* 100:494-512, 1991.

Vardimon AD et al: Functional orthopedic magnetic appliance (FOMA) II—modus operandi, *Am J Orthod Dentofac Orthop* 95:371-387, 1989.

Vardimon AD et al: Functional orthopedic magnetic appliance (FOMA) III—modus operandi, *Am J Orthod Dentofac Orthop* 97:135-148, 1990.

Vardimon AD et al: Magnetic versus mechanical expansion with different force thresholds and points of force application, *Am J Orthod Dentofac Orthop* 92:455-466, 1987.

Vardimon AD et al: Functional orthopedic magnetic appliance (FOMA) II—modus operandi, *Am J Orthod Dentofac Orthop* 95:371-387, 1989.

Vargervik K, Harvold EP: Response to activator treatment in Class II malocclusion, *Am J Orthod* 88:242-251, 1985.

Vig PS et al: Quantitative evaluation of nasal airflow in relation to facial morphology, *Am J Orthod* 77:258, 1980.

Voudouris JC: Glenoid fossa and condylar remodeling following progressive mandibular protrusion in the juvenile Macaca fascicularis, master's thesis, Toronto, 1988, University of Toronto.

Wachsman C: Treatment of irregularities of the teeth and jaws by mens of activators, *Am J Orthod* 35:61, 1949.

Watson W: A computerized appraisal of high-pull headgear, *Am J Orthod* 62:561-579, 1972.

Watt DD, Williams CH: The effects of the physical consistency of food on the growth and development of the mandible and the maxilla of the rat, *Am J Orthod* 37:895, 1951.

Weilan FJ, Bantleon H-P: Treatment of Class II malocclusions with the Jasper Jumper appliance—a preliminary report, *Am J Orthod Dentofac Orthop* 108:341, 1995.

Weinmann JP, Sicher H: *Bone and bones: fundamentals of bone biology,* St Louis, 1955, Mosby.

Wexler MR, Sarnat BG: Rabbit snout growth: effect of injury to the septovomeral region, *Arch Otolarnygol* 74:305, 1961.

Whitney EF, Sinclair PM: An evaluation of combination second molar extraction and functional appliance therapy, *Am J Orthod Dentofac Orthop* 91:188, 1987.

Wieslander L: The effect of force on cranio-facial development, *Am J Orhtod* 65:531, 1974.

Wieslander L: Intensive treatment of severe Class II malocclusions with a headgear-Herbst appliance in the early mixed dentition, *Am J Orthod* 86:1-13, 1984.

Wieslander L: Long-term effects of treatment with the headgear-Herbst appliance in the early mixed dentition. Stability or relapse? *Am J Orhtod Dentofac Orthop* 104:319, 1994.

Wilson GH: The anatomy and physiology of the temporomandibular joint, *J Nat Dent Assoc* 7:414, 1920.

Winders RV: Forces exerted on the dentition by perioral and lingual musculature during swallowing, *Angle Orthod* 28:226, 1958.

Windmiller EC: The acrylic-splint Herbst appliance: a cephalometric evaluation, *Am J Orthod Dentofac Orthop* 104:73-84, 1993.

Witt E: Grundprinzipien der Aktivator- und Bionatortherapie, *Zahnaertzl Prax* 22:1, 1971.

Witt E: Investigations into orthodontic forces of different appliances, *Eur Orthod Soc Rep Cong* p. 391, 1966.

Witt E, Gehrle ME: *Leitfaden der Kieferorthopädischen Technik,* Berlin, 1988, Quintessenz Verlag.

Witt E, Komposch G: Intermaxilläre Kraftwirkung bimaxillarer Geräte, *Fortschr Keiferorthop* 32:345-352, 1971.

Witt E, Meyer U: Indications for a working action of bimaxillary appliances, *Eur Orthod Soc Rep Cong* p. 321, 1972.

Wolff J: *Das Gesetz der Transformation der Knochen,* Berlin, 1892, Hirschwold.

Woodside DG: The activator. In Salzmann JA, editor: *Orthodontics in daily practice,* Philadelphia, 1974, Lippincott.

Woodside DG: *Distance, velocity and relative growth rate standards for mandibular growth,* thesis, Toronto, 1969.

Woodside DG: The Harvold-Woodside activator. In Graber TM, Neumann B, editors: *Removable orthodontic appliances,* Philadelphia, 1984, Saunders.

Woodside DG: Some effects of activator treatment on the mandible and the midface, *Trans Eur Orthod Soc* p. 443, 1973.

Woodside DG: Studies in functional appliance therapy. In Graber TM, editor: *Physiologic principles of functional appliances,* St Louis, 1985, Mosby.

Woodside DG et al: Primate experiments in malocclusion and bone induction, *Am J Orthod* 83:460, 1983.

Woodside DG, Linder-Aronson S: The channelization of upper and lower anterior face heights compared to population standards in boys between ages 6-20 years, *Eur J Orthod* 1:25, 1979.

Woodside DG et al: Mandibular and maxillary growth after changed mode of breathing, *Am J Orthod Denteofac Orthop* 100(1):1-18, 1991.

Woodside DG, Metaxas A, Altuna G: The influence of functional appliance therapy on glenoid fossa remodeling, *Am J Orthod Dentofac Orthop* 92:181-198, 1987.

Woodside DG, Metaxas A, Altuna G: Some effects of activator treatment on the growth rate of the mandible and the position of the midface, *Trans Third Inter Orthodont Cong* 443, 1973.

Woodside DG et al: Some effects of activator treatment on the growth rate of the mandible and the position of the midface, *Trans Third Inter Orthod Cong* pp. 459-480, 1975.

Yamin C: Effects of functional appliances on the temporomandibular joint and masticatory muscles in Macaca fascicularis, master's thesis, Toronto, 1991, University of Toronto.

Zeemann EC: Catastrophe theory, *Sci Am* 234:65, 1976.

Zreik T: Fixed-removable Herbst appliance, *J Clin Orthod* 28:246-298, 1994.

# Index